Polysaccharide-based Nano-Biocarrier in Drug Delivery

Polysaccharide-based Nano-Biocarrier in Drug Delivery

Edited by
Tapan Kumar Giri and Bijaya Ghosh

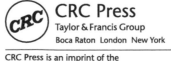

CRC Press
Taylor & Francis Group
Boca Raton London New York

CRC Press is an imprint of the
Taylor & Francis Group, an **informa** business

CRC Press
Taylor & Francis Group
6000 Broken Sound Parkway NW, Suite 300
Boca Raton, FL 33487-2742

First issued in paperback 2020

ISBN 13: 978-0-367-57101-6 (pbk)
ISBN 13: 978-1-138-48111-4 (hbk)

**Visit the Taylor & Francis Web site at
http://www.taylorandfrancis.com**

**and the CRC Press Web site at
http://www.crcpress.com**

Contents

Preface

With the growing awareness of drug-induced diseases in the last few decades, the trend of pharmaceutical research had shifted to drug targeting. The research community seems to be fascinated with idea of delivering drugs at an optimal rate to their exact site of action. Once considered wishful thinking, nanotechnology has made this a reality. Many drug-loaded nanostructures have already demonstrated their superiority over their conventional counterparts. Inspired by this success, work is ongoing to develop nanosized dosage forms for almost all the important drugs that have significant delivery problems.

However, materials employed in the fabrication of nanostructures determine their properties.

Being pharmaceutical ingredients, these materials have to meet stringent regulatory standards of safety. Cost is also an important factor that determines the feasibility of mass production and marketing. So stress is given to usage of easily available natural substances such as nanomaterials.

Bio-based natural polysaccharides are excellent candidate materials for these purposes. As nanocarriers, polysaccharides have greater stability in the blood as they can bypass the reticuloendothelial system. Further, the existence of several functional groups in their structure make them modifiable chemically and biochemically. The presence of hydrophilic moieties in their structure, such as carboxyl, hydroxyl, and amino groups, improves the bioavailability of the drugs by increasing their bioadhesion with the cells and tissues. Due to their natural origin and ease of availability, they have been widely employed in the design of nanocarriers loaded with antimicrobial drugs. Finally, as the most abundant material found in nature, they are much cheaper than other nanomaterials. Hence a nanodosage form developed in the laboratory has high potential for being upgraded to a marketed product.

All these factors have influenced us in our review of the recent advances in polysaccharide-based nano-biocarriers in drug delivery application and we have compiled them in this book

This book is organized to provide the most relevant and realistic information on polysaccharide-based nanocarriers for different types of drug delivery. The current state-of-the-art research has been accumulated in 17 chapters.

To make this book reader friendly and useful, we have provided some in-depth literature. The chapters discuss the fundamental ideas as well as the development and application of these systems for the delivery of small molecules, proteins, peptides, oligonucleotides, and genes. We hope that this book will meet the demands of a reference book for concerned professionals and researchers who intend to conceptualize and develop nano delivery systems for drugs using polysaccharides as nanomaterials.

Preparation of this book would not have been possible without the valuable contributions from various experts in the field. We would like to thank the authors who took time from their busy schedules and responded to our request. We deeply appreciate their timely contributions. We are thankful to the management of the NSHM Knowledge Campus, Kolkata-Group of Institutions and our colleagues for their continued support. We are grateful to our family members for their continuous moral support and inspiration during the preparation of this book. We are thankful to CRC Press for extending this opportunity to us and their expert assistance. Constructive comments and suggestions from readers in improving the quality of this book are welcome.

Tapan Kumar Giri
Bijaya Ghosh

About the Editors

Tapan Kumar Giri was educated at Jadavpur University, Kolkata, India, where he received pharmacy degrees in B.Pharm, M.Pharm and a Ph.D. He has held academic posts in various pharmacy institutes of North India and is currently working as an Assistant Professor in Pharmaceutics at NSHM Knowledge Campus, Kolkata-Group of Institutions, Kolkata, India. His main research interests are formulation development and drug delivery. He has mentored over 20 Master's students. He has published around 60 research papers, 7 book chapters and 2 pharmacy books. He has served as a guest editor for the *Current Chemical Biology Journal*, Bentham Science. He has received the prestigious highly cited article award from Elsevier as well as the teacher of the year 2017 award from Maulana Abul Kalam Azad University of Technology, West Bengal, India.

Bijaya Ghosh has been teaching for the last 30 years and has taught pharmacy to undergraduates and graduate students in some of the premier institutions of North and South India. Currently she is working as a Professor in Pharmaceutics at NSHM Knowledge Campus, Kolkata-Group of Institutions, Kolkata, India. She received her B.Pharm, M.Pharm and Ph.D. degrees from Jadavpur University in the years 1983, 1986 and 1994, respectively. She has authored 2 pharmacy text books and has published some 40 research papers in national and international journals. Her research interests involve various streams of novel drug delivery like sustaining drug release, passive and iontophoretic drug delivery and nanobiotechnology. Ever interested in experimenting with new concepts, currently she is working on the reverse iontophoretic extraction of small molecules for therapeutic drug monitoring.

Contributors

Kiran S. Avadhani
Biocon Research Limited
Bengaluru, India

Hemant Ramchandra Badwaik
Department of Pharmaceutical Chemistry
Rungta College of Pharmaceutical Sciences
    and Research
Bhilai, India

Subham Banerjee
Department of Pharmaceutics
National Institute of Pharmaceutical Education
    and Research (NIPER)-Guwahati
Assam, India

María E. Berrio
Department of Chemistry
Universidad del Valle
Cali, Colombia

Yamini S. Bobde
Department of Pharmacy
Birla Institute of Technology and
    Science-Pilani
Hyderabad, India

Debanjana Chakraborty
Department of Chemistry
Indian Institute of Chemical Biology
Kolkata, India

Debarupa Dutta Chakraborty
Department of Pharmaceutical Chemistry
Himalayan Pharmacy Institute
Majhitar, India

Prithviraj Chakraborty
Department of Pharmaceutics
Himalayan Pharmacy Institute
Majhitar, India

Tania Chakraborty
NSHM Knowledge Campus
Kolkata-Group of Institutions
Kolkata, India

Indranil Chanda
Department of Examination
Assam Science and Technology University
Guwahati, India

Urmi Chaurasia
Department of Pharmaceutical Science
S. Bhagwan Singh PG Institute of Biomedical
    Sciences and Research
Dehradun, India

Moumita Das
School of Pharmaceutical Technology
Adamas University
Barasat, India

Vaswati Rita Das
Department of Pharmaceutics
Bharat Technology
Howrah, India

Sandipan Dasgupta
NSHM Knowledge Campus
Kolkata-Group of Institutions
Kolkata, India

Arnab De
Department of Pharmaceutical Technology
Jadavpur University
Kolkata, India

Prasanta Dey
School of Pharmacy
Sungkyunkwan University
Suwon, Republic of Korea

Dibyendu Dutta
NSHM Knowledge Campus
Kolkata-Group of Institutions
Kolkata, India

Angelica García-Quintero
Department of Chemistry
Universidad del Valle
Cali, Colombia

Animesh Ghosh
Department of Pharmaceutical Sciences
    and Technology
Birla Institute of Technology Mesra
Ranchi, India

Balaram Ghosh
Department of Pharmacy
Birla Institute of Technology and
    Science-Pilani
Hyderabad, India

Lakshmi Kanta Ghosh
Department of Pharmaceutical Technology
Jadavpur University
Kolkata, India

Miltu Kumar Ghosh
NSHM Knowledge Campus
Kolkata-Group of Institutions
Kolkata, India

Srijita Halder
NSHM Knowledge Campus
Kolkata-Group of Institutions
Kolkata, India

Shah Hiral
Arihant School of Pharmacy & BRI
Gandhinagar, India

Chethan Gejjalagere Honnappa
Biocon Research Limited
Bangalore, India

Shah Jigar
Institute of Pharmacy
Nirma University
Ahmedabad, India

Narayanan Kasinathan
Biocon Research Limited
Bengaluru, India

Hyung Sik Kim
School of Pharmacy
Sungkyunkwan University
Suwon, Republic of Korea

Leena Kumari
Department of Pharmaceutical Technology
Jadavpur University
Kolkata, India

Amit Kundu
School of Pharmacy
Sungkyunkwan University
Suwon, Republic of Korea

Tulio A. Lerma
Mindtech Research Group
Mindtech-RG, Mindtech S. A. S.
Cali, Colombia

Amit Maity
School of Pharmacy
Seacom Skills University
Bolpur, India

Arindam Maity
School of Pharmaceutical Technology
Adamas University
Barasat, India

Anroop B. Nair
College of Clinical Pharmacy
King Faisal University
Al-Ahsa, Saudi Arabia

Kartik Nakhate
Department of Pharmacology
Rungta College of Pharmaceutical Sciences
    and Research
Bhilai, India

Manuel Palencia
Department of Chemistry
Universidad del Valle
Cali, Colombia

Falguni Patra
NSHM Knowledge Campus
Kolkata-Group of Institutions
Kolkata, India

Anupam Roy
Laboratory of Food Chemistry and Technology
Department of Chemical Engineering
Birla Institute of Technology
Ranchi, India

Souvik Roy
NSHM Knowledge Campus
Kolkata-Group of Institutions
Kolkata, India

Sreyajit Saha
Laboratory of Food Chemistry and Technology
Department of Chemical Engineering
Birla Institute of Technology
Ranchi, India

Kalyani Sakure
Department of Pharmaceutics
Rungta College of Pharmaceutical Sciences
    and Research
Bhilai, India

Nilanjan Sarkar
NSHM Knowledge Campus
Kolkata-Group of Institutions
Kolkata, India

Pradipta Sarkar
Department of Pharmaceutical
    Technology
Jadavpur University
Kolkata, India

Pallavi Krishna Shetty
Apotex Research Private Limited
Bommasandra Industrial Area
Bangalore, India

Patel Snehal
Institute of Pharmacy
Nirma University
Ahmedabad, India

Chavda Vishal
Institute of Pharmacy
Nirma University
Ahmedabad, India

1 Oral Delivery of Proteins and Polypeptides through Polysaccharide Nanocarriers

Hemant Ramchandra Badwaik, Kartik Nakhate,
Leena Kumari, and Kalyani Sakure

CONTENTS

1.1 INTRODUCTION

Due to advancements in the field of biotechnology, a plethora of therapeutic proteins and peptides are now being produced on a commercial basis (Renukuntla et al. 2013). More than 90% of approved therapeutic proteins and peptides are parenteral formulations since this method of administration circumvents hurdles related to degradation by physical and enzymatic means in the gastrointestinal tract (Lalatsa 2013). In contrast, the oral delivery of therapeutic molecules provides numerous benefits including self-administration, patient acceptability, and compliance. However, breakthroughs in the advancement of an attractive protein delivery vehicle have been hindered by numerous aspects such as toxicities related to absorption-enhancing agents, differences in bioavailability among individual patients, and the high cost of production. Implementation of a suitable delivery vehicle that can safeguard peptide drugs from the degradation caused by enzymatic activities and also sustain and control the release rate, is required for the extended retention and therapeutic response of peptide drugs in the human body (Hamman et al. 2005). Numerous approaches have so far been investigated to meet these criteria. Of these, polysaccharide-based nanocarriers seem to offer a promising novel approach for oral delivery of protein and peptide drugs. Polysaccharides are biocompatible, biodegradable, non-toxic, and ubiquitous in nature and can be easily derivatized by chemical and biochemical means. This chapter highlights the intestinal mucosal barriers which prevent peptide and protein absorption and the novel polysaccharide-based nanotechnologies for overcoming the hurdles in absorption of peptide drugs.

1.2 THERAPEUTIC IMPORTANCE OF PROTEINS AND PEPTIDES FOR THE TREATMENT OF DISEASES

Recently, the pharmaceutical sector based on peptides has been very optimistic. In 1970, just one peptide was entered into the clinical phase but the number has now reached to about 20 peptides per year (Lax 2010). In 2017, about 688 peptidergic agents were undergoing clinical trials and more than 100 drugs based on peptides are available commercially. The global peptide therapeutics market in 2016 was worth US$21.12 billion, which is expected to grow with a compound annual growth rate (CAGR) of between 9.0% and 9.5% from 2017 to 2023. The world market has been dominated by North America, and Asia Pacific is anticipated to grow at the highest CAGR over the forecast period. Some illnesses treated with peptides are presented in the following sections.

1.2.1 INFECTIONS

Worldwide, infectious diseases have been accountable for 16% of total deaths every year (Center for Strategic and International Studies, n.d.). Moreover, resistance to antimicrobial drugs developed by microorganisms has prompted researchers to investigate new treatment strategies (Mahlapuu et al. 2016). The antimicrobial peptides (AMP) are cationic peptides with a small number of amino acids (12–50) synthesized by cells like epithelial cells, neutrophils, monocytes, macrophages, and keratinocytes. The peptides are either constitutively present or induced during infection, to kill or to hamper the multiplication of Gram +ve and Gram –ve bacteria, yeasts, parasites, fungi, viruses, and even cancerous cells (Zhang and Gallo 2016). The biological function of antimicrobial peptides is demonstrated in Figure 1.1. The cationic properties of AMP permit their insertion into phospholipid membranes and anionic walls that trigger bacterial cell death. They can also induce the immune cells to release cytokines, angiogenesis, and chemotaxis, which aids in the healing of wounds (Hancock 2001; Izadpanah and Gallo 2005).

Among several types of AMPs, the defensins and the cathelicidins are the most important classes. Defensins are categorized into constitutive α-defensins and inducible β-defensins (Guaní-Guerra et al. 2010). While α-defensins are expressed in the neutrophils, in some types of macrophages, in intestinal Paneth cells, and in the female genital tract, β-defensins are found in the skin epithelial cells, the genitourinary tract, the respiratory tract, and granulocytes (Bals 2000; Reddy et al. 2004). They promote the secretion of tumor necrosis factors, chemokines, histamine, and prostaglandins, and also the activation of T cells and other immune cells that exhibit an antimicrobial effect (Izadpanah and Gallo 2005; Gallo et al. 2002). The cathelicidin, LL-37, is produced mainly in T cells, B cells, neutrophils, monocytes, myeloid cells, and mast cells (Izadpanah and Gallo 2005; Steinstraesser et al. 2011). It is also present in bone marrow, plasma, enterocytes of the colon, epithelial cells of the respiratory (including the nose and lungs) and urinary tracts, and the keratinocytes. They exhibit antimicrobial activity by virtue of the effects like chemotaxis,

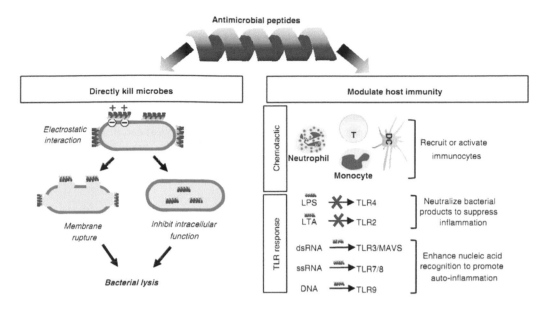

FIGURE 1.1 Biological function of antimicrobial peptides. AMPs bind to bacterial membranes through electrostatic interactions either to disrupt the membrane or to enter the bacterium to inhibit intracellular function. Some AMPs also modulate host immunity by recruiting/activating immunocytes or by influencing Toll-like receptor (TLR) recognition of microbial products and nucleic acids released upon tissue damage. DC, dendritic cell; LPS, lipopolysaccharide; LTA, lipoteichoic acid; MAVS, mitochondrial antiviral signaling protein. (Reprinted from *Curr Biol* 26, Zhang, L. and Gallo, R.L. Antimicrobial peptides, R14–R19, Copyright 2016, with permission from Elsevier.)

angiogenesis, apoptosis, interleukins release, pro-inflammatory cytokines inhibition, antiendotoxic action, and histamine release (Steinstraesser et al. 2011). Analogues of several AMPs are currently undergoing preclinical and clinical trials in order to test their effectiveness with diseases like acne infections, oral and systemic candidiasis, type 1 diabetes mellitus, diabetic foot ulcers, peritoneal infections, pneumonia, meningitis, gingivitis, Crohn's disease, *gastric H. pylori* infections, and ulcers (Reddy et al. 2004; Greber and Dawgul 2017).

1.2.2 Cancer

Cancer represents about 21% of the global peptide market, followed by metabolic disorders, gastrointestinal problems, and respiratory diseases (Uhlig et al. 2014). Due to the hazardous effects of chemotherapy, efforts are being made to develop highly specific drugs with fewer propensities to induce adverse effects, which mainly include monoclonal antibodies, peptidergic hormones, and peptide vaccine (Thundimadathil 2012; Shin et al. 2014; Marqus et al. 2017). Peptides are found to be more effective than antibodies due to their smaller size, which permits superior penetration into the tumor with excellent biocompatibility. They are also easy to synthesize and modify and can act as a carrier for cytotoxic drugs and radionuclides (Thundimadathil 2012). Some cancerous cells express the receptors for specific endogenous peptides, therefore, to target cytotoxic drugs to a specific cell, they can be can be conjugated to a peptide. For example, prostate and breast cancer cells express receptors for the peptide bombesin, which can be attached to doxorubicin (Lin et al. 2016). Similarly, peptides can be used to carry radioactive elements into the target cancerous cell. After binding to a cell, peptides can release anticancer drugs, or emit radiation based on its complexation, to destroy the cancerous cell. This strategy is used to destroy neuroendocrine tumors as most of them over-express somatostatin receptors. Therefore, somatostatin-analog peptides bound to radioactive substances are used as an anticancer approach (Kaspar and Reichert 2013). Hormone-based therapy has also been used for the treatment of cancers. For example, depot formulations of luteinizing hormone-releasing hormone (LHRH) ago-nists (leuprolide, buserelin, nafarelin, gonadorelin, and goserelin) and antagonists (abarelix, ganirelix, degarelix, and cetrorelix) have been employed for prostate and ovarian cancer (Thundimadathil 2012). Tumor cells express tumor-associated antigens, which are recognized by the T cells. Therefore, anti-cancer immunity can be induced by injecting peptides derived from tumor cell antigens as a vaccine (Tagliamonte et al. 2014). Some peptides can be given therapeutically to suppress the tumor growth. Buforin II, a peptide obtained from the *Bufo bufo gargarizans* stomach with antimicrobial properties, has the ability to induce the extrinsic apoptotic pathway in human cervical carcinoma, leukemia, and lung cancer cells by interacting with plasma membrane gangliosides (Cho et al. 2009).

1.2.3 CARDIOVASCULAR DISEASES

According to a World Health Organization (WHO) report (2017a), cardiovascular diseases are the foremost cause of death globally and about 17.7 million deaths occurred due to cardiovascular diseases in 2015, which is about 31% of the total deaths worldwide. Bioactive peptides as neu-traceuticals have attracted a large amount of attention as several of them can act as antioxidant, antithrombotic, antihypertensive, and antihyperlipidemic agents (Marcone et al. 2017). Although synthetic angiotensin-converting enzyme (ACE) inhibitors have long been used as antihyperten-sives, some food peptides with ACE inhibitory activity are considered as effective antihypertensive agents. Casokinins and lactokinins obtained from caseins and whey proteins in milk, respectively, are potent ACE inhibitor peptides. They are effective in hypertensive patients, but do not alter blood pressure in normotensive people. Further, they are devoid of the side effects of ACE inhibitors (for example captopril), which includes, dry cough, angioedema, and skin rashes (Erdmann et al. 2008). Milk peptides can also produce the antihypertensive effect through inhibition of endothelin-1 release by the endothelial cells. Moreover, by inhibiting release of endothelin-1 and by augment-ing activity of bradykinin and endothelium-derived nitric oxide, milk peptides produce an antihy-pertensive effect (Maes et al. 2004; Korhonen and Pihlanto 2006). Natural peptides found in soy proteins, fish, and eggs also have antioxidant properties. The antioxidant activities are associated with protection against peroxidation of lipids, synthesis of the intracellular antioxidants, free radical scavenging, and quenching of singlet oxygen (Kitts and Weiler 2003). By virtue of these activities, peptides can be used for the management of atherosclerosis. Bioactive peptides also possess anti-thrombotic properties by initiating enzymatic hydrolysis. Casoplatelin isolated from bovine casein inhibits the aggregation of platelets to produce an antithrombotic effect (Phelan and Kerins 2011). KRDS derived from human lactoferrin also prevents platelets aggregation. Antihyperlipidemic activities have been observed in soy, whey, and fish protein (Lammi et al. 2015). This effect might be attributed to the induction of LDL receptors expression and bile synthesis, and reduction in lipids absorption (Erdmann et al. 2008). The glycinin-derived peptides, LPYPR and IAVPGEVA exhibit hypocholesterolemic effects. These peptides act by inhibiting 3-hydroxy-3-methylglutaryl CoA (HMG-CoA) reductase, which is a rate-limiting enzyme in the biosynthesis of cholesterol and the key target for statins (Lammi et al. 2015). Peptide IIAEK (lactostatin) obtained from bovine milk β-lactoglobulin produced strong cholesterol-lowering effects (Marcone et al. 2017). The peptides obtained from the globin hydrolysis produce antihyperlipidemic effects by attenuating fat absorp-tion through the intestine and promoting lipolysis akin to soy protein (Erdmann et al. 2008). The atrial natriuretic peptides like α-NP and β-NP are secreted by the wall of the atria in response to an acute increase in stretching forces on the ventricular walls during hypertension. These peptides promote excretion of Na+ through the kidneys and the dilation of arteries and veins to reduce blood pressure. The effect is further aided due to their inhibitory effect on the sympathetic nervous system and renin-angiotensin-aldosterone pathway (Daniels and Maisel 2007). Such agents may be ideal to treat heart failure and hypertension. Based on this, the recombinant human β-NP nesiritide was developed and approved by the USFDA in 2002 for the treatment of patients with acutely decom-pensate heart failure (Richards et al. 2004).

1.2.4 ENDOCRINE DISORDERS

Therapeutic benefits of peptidergic agents have been reported in several endocrine disorders. Nowadays, diabetes has become one of the major public health problems. According to a WHO report (2017b), the number of diabetes patients has increased from 108 million in 1980 to 422 million in 2014, and about 1.6 million deaths occurred due to diabetes in 2015. In recent times, peptide-based therapeutic strategies for type 2 diabetes have been widely explored, which includes glucagon-like peptide (GLP)-1 analogues (semaglutide, liraglutide, and exenatide) and dipeptidyl peptidase (DPP-IV) inhibitors (gemigliptin, sitagliptin, and vildagliptin). These agents improve diabetes by promoting glucose-induced insulin secretion and suppressing glucagon secretion and appetite, without causing hypoglycemia, the most common adverse effect of insulin and oral hypoglycemic drugs (Hemmingsen et al. 2017). Obesity has become an important risk factor for the pathological conditions, like type 2 diabetes, stroke, cardiovascular diseases, and cancers (Troke et al. 2014). Neuropeptides are important regulators of feeding and energy homeostasis, and strategies targeting hypothalamic neuropeptides may be fruitful for the management of obesity. For example, antagonists of potent orexigenic agents like neuropeptide Y (Nakhate et al. 2009) and positive modulators of the anorexic neuropeptide CART (Nakhate et al. 2011) may be effective antiobesity agents. Similarly, peripherally secreted peptides like PYY-36 (released by intestinal L-type cells) caused anorexia, prolonged gastric emptying, and inhibited ghrelin secretion (Valderas et al. 2010). Intestinal entero-endocrine cells also release satiety-triggering peptides like cholecystokinin and GLP-1. Moreover, appetite-suppressing peptides secreted by the pancreatic endocrine cells, including pancreatic poly-peptide, amylin, and glucagon, can also be targeted for the development of antiobesity medications (Guyenet and Schwartz 2012). Osteoporosis is the most commonly evident metabolic disease of the bones with the highest propensity for causing osteoporotic fractures in women aged 50 and above. Calcitonin obtained from salmon is found to be 20–40 times more potent than human calcitonin, and is therapeutically used in the treatment of osteoporosis. It acts by promoting calcium deposition in the bones by activating osteoblasts. Similarly, parathormone (PTH) analogs also produce beneficial effects in patients of osteoporosis by enhancing osteoblast activity. In Europe, while two derivatives of PTH (teriparatide and PTH 1-84) have been approved, only teriparatide has been approved by the USFDA (Daroszewska 2012; Luhmann et al. 2012).

1.2.5 IMMUNOMODULATION

The peptidergic antiviral agent seems to look promising in the treatment of viral infections. Enfuvirtide (or T20), synthetic peptide obtained from the gp41 (HIV-1 protein), blocks the fusion of the virus with cells and, consequently, its replication. It is an approved antiretroviral drug in the USA and Europe (Wang et al. 2009). T1249 (second-generation inhibitor) is a potent variant of peptide T20 (first-generation inhibitor) with more stability and increased activity against T20 resistant virus variants. Third-generation inhibitors, T2635 and sifuvirtide, showed a further increase in thermal stability, plasma half-life, and potent antiviral activity against resistant virus variants as compared to previous peptide generations (Berkhout et al. 2012). P9, a short peptide derived from mouse β-defensin-4, exhibited a broad spectrum of antiviral activity against numerous respiratory viruses like H1N1, H3N2, H5N1, H7N7, H7N9, MERS-CoV, SARS-CoV, and influenza A. The antiviral effect of P9 is attributed to prevention of the acidification of endosomes, which blocks the fusion of viruses in the membrane and consequentially prevents the release of viral RNA (Zhao et al. 2016). Multiple sclerosis, a chronic inflammatory condition triggered by a T cell-mediated autoimmune attack against a myelin sheath of neurons, results in neurological deficits like sensory disturbances, paralysis, blindness, and dysfunction of the bowel and bladder (Kolb-Mäurer et al. 2015). Glatiramer acetate, which is a mixture prepared from some synthetic peptides comprising the four amino acids alanine, lysine, tyrosine, and glutamate, mimics the fundamental proteins of the myelin sheath (Farina et al. 2005). The peptides promote the formation of suppressor T cells that consequently suppress the pathogenic T cells; thus, contributing to the beneficial actions of the glatiramer acetate (Van Kaer 2011).

1.3 HURDLES IN ORAL PROTEINS/PEPTIDES DELIVERY

The major glitches in the optimal utilization of therapeutic proteins and peptides, such as vaccines, antigens, and hormones by the oral route, are their large molecular size, poor permeation, destruction of the gastrointestinal tract, and extensive first pass metabolism in liver. These hurdles can be overcome by adopting techniques such as mucoadhesive polymers, enzyme inhibitors, permeation enhancers, and chemical transformation of protein structures (Muheem et al. 2016).

1.3.1 THE PHYSICAL BARRIER OF THE MUCOSAL LAYER

The intestinal mucosa, consisting of mucus gel and the underlying epithelia, acts as the most important physical barrier for the absorption of macromolecules (Figure 1.2) (Bourganis et al. 2017). Mucus is a non-Newtonian and thixotropic jelly-like substance. It serves as the major defensive layer against the influx of foreign entities, while concurrently allowing the selective flux of nutrients, immune cells, and antibodies (Lai et al. 2009b). This is attributed to a dense network of mucin, which causes the entrapment of the foreign molecules by two mechanisms, viz., steric obstruction due to limited mesh-spacing among the mucin fibers and adhesive interactions due to the adhesive hydrophobic or electrostatic interactions (Olmsted et al. 2001).

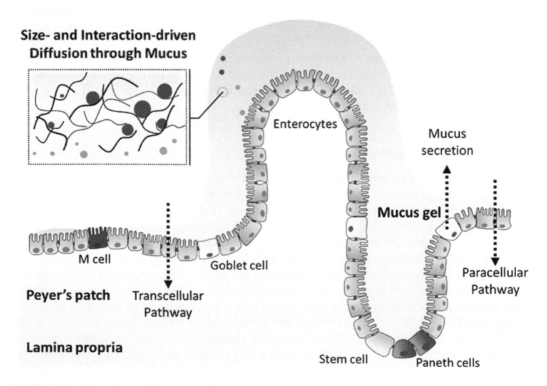

FIGURE 1.2 The physical barrier of the mucosa, comprised by the mucus gel layer and the underlying epithelia. Macromolecules have to diffuse through mucus according to their size or surface properties and follow a certain absorption pathway across the epithelial layer. (Reprinted from *Eur J Pharm Biopharm*, 111, Bourganis, V., Karamanidou, T., Kammona, O., and Kiparissides, C. Polyelectrolyte complexes as prospective carriers for the oral delivery of protein therapeutics, 44–60, Copyright 2017, with permission from Elsevier.)

Permeability through this absorption-limiting barrier depends on particle size (the larger the particle diameter, the lower the particle mobility) and the pH-sensitive charge on the particle surface (Cone 2005). Positively charged molecules are immobilized in the mucus layer because of their electrostatic adhesive interactions with negatively charged mucins and are rapidly eliminated through the normal mucus clearance mechanisms. Thus, macromolecules administered via oral route must penetrate through the dense mucin mesh to be absorbed into the circulatory system (Bansil and Tumer 2006). After mucus, the underlying intestinal epithelium acts as a major barrier for the macromolecules as it has the ability to selectively prevent the entry of molecules identified as potentially harmful. It consists of a single layer of tightly bound columnar epithelial cells (Boegh et al. 2013). The lymphatic tissue called Peyer's patches are covered with specialized epithelial M cells that transport antigens present in the intestinal lumen to the immune system cells to trigger an immune response. The M cells play a pivotal role in drug absorption, as they are slightly covered with mucus and have a high capacity to execute transcytosis. Passive transport through the epithelial membrane occurs by transcellular or paracellular mechanisms. Moreover, transportation of macromolecules is also possible by carrier- and receptor-mediated uptake and transcytosis, as well as lymphatic and vesicular transport by M cells. Small hydrophilic entities (MW < 500 Da) are preferentially transported by the paracellular route, however charged entities or molecules with a higher weight follow alternative routes (Elsayed 2012). Most of the therapeutic macromolecules, due to their hydrophilic nature, cannot cross the lipoidal cell membrane, thus precluding the possibility of absorption via transcellular pathway. Such agents follow the paracellular mechanism, especially molecular diffusion, through the aqueous channels. Moreover, the epithelial passage of therapeutic agents depends on molecular weight and leads to heavier molecules only achieving partial absorption. In addition, the negatively charged membrane significantly immobilized positively charged molecules (Lewis and Richard 2015).

1.3.2 THE ENZYMATIC BARRIER

The digestion of dietary proteins into smaller subunits takes place in the gastrointestinal tract (GIT). Therefore, inherent susceptibility of proteins and peptides to proteolytic degradation poses a major challenge to their oral delivery (Langguth et al. 1997). Proteolytic enzymes like endopeptidases, exopeptidases (carboxypeptidases and aminopeptidases), prolinases, prolidases, etc. are widely distributed (Zhou 1994). They cause the breakdown of proteins into smaller amino acid fragments by hydrolyzing peptide bonds, with wide substrate specificity. The proteolytic process in the stomach is initiated by certain aspartic proteases (i.e. pepsins) that remain active at pH 2–3. Moreover, gastric lipase hydrolyzes triglycerides are present in lipid formulations. When partially degraded proteins from the stomach reach the duodenum, they are mixed with proteases secreted by the pancreas like trypsin, α-chymotrypsin, serin endopeptidases, elastase, exopeptidases and carboxypeptidase A and B, and enterocyte-associated enzymes. The majority of the internal bonds in most of the proteins and peptides are cleaved by endopeptidases (Lee and Yamamoto 1990). This results in the formation of free amino acids and 2–6 residue containing small peptides. In the brush border epithelium, the small peptides are further cleaved by carboxypeptidases and aminopeptidases to form free amino acids. These enzymes act on the terminal ends of peptides to cleave the individual amino acids (Gruber et al. 1987). The enzymes like pancreatic lipase and nucleases also participate in the digestive activities. While the pancreatic lipases hydrolyze triglycerides into fatty acids and monoglycerides, the nucleases cause hydrolysis of phosphodiester linkages in the nucleic acids. Even after endocytosis, the macromolecular agents face the harsh environment triggered by lysosomal and cytosolic enzymes like nucleases and peptidases. While nucleases pose a barrier to the transfection of cells by the therapeutic nucleic acids, the lysosomal peptidases cause the breakdown of peptides to their constituent amino acids. Bourganis et al. (2017) explains the fate of proteins after their administration by oral route as shown in Figure 1.3.

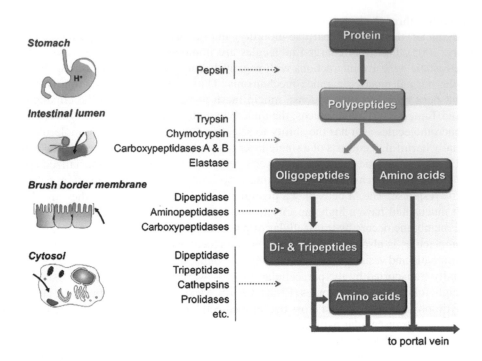

FIGURE 1.3 The fate of orally administered proteins after several stages of proteolysis along the GIT. (Reprinted from *Eur J Pharm Biopharm* 111, Bourganis, V., Karamanidou, T., Kammona, O., and Kiparissides, C. Polyelectrolyte complexes as prospective carriers for the oral delivery of protein therapeutics, 44–60, Copyright 2017, with permission from Elsevier.)

1.3.3 THE CHEMICAL BARRIER

Variations in pH is observed along the length of the GIT. The pH ranges from 6.5 to 6.9 in the oral cavity, which is reduced in the stomach (pH 1–3). This harsh acidic environment is responsible for protein denaturation, pepsin activation, and inhibition of bacterial growth (Bernkop-Schnürch 2009). The pH is subsequently neutralized (6.0–6.5) as approaching the first segment of small intestine (i.e. duodenum), and ultimately reaches between 7 and 8 in the colon and rectum. Most of the proteins show a charge density that is dependent on pH. Moreover, the proteins are ampholytic with side chains that carry both a positive and a negative charge. Therefore, the conformational integrity and stability of the proteins is significantly modulated by the pH of the surrounding medium and the interactions between amino acid residues with an opposite charge. Conformational changes in the proteins result in their unfolding and denaturation, and consequently leads to an increase in the propensity of degradation by hydrolysis and enzymes (Mahato 2003). Thus, the stability of the macromolecules in a wide range of pH is essential for their increased efficacy after oral administration.

1.3.4 THE UNSTIRRED AQUEOUS LAYER

In the intestinal lumen, the bulk of the fluid is combined with glycocalyx and mucus to form a stagnant aqueous layer adjacent to the epithelial brush border membrane. The aqueous nature of the boundary layer can significantly hinder hydrophobic molecule diffusion (Hamman 2005). However, this layer has almost no effect on the absorption of most therapeutically used macromolecules, which possess a hydrophilic character enabling free diffusion through aqueous media (Thompson and Ibie 2011).

1.4 TRANSPORT MECHANISMS IN THE GI TRACT

In GIT, four mechanisms (i.e. transcellular, paracellular, carrier-, and receptor-mediated transport mechanisms) are involved in the crossing of therapeutic agents through the cell membrane in the GIT (Yun et al. 2013) as shown in Figure 1.4. A detailed understanding of biomolecules along with their distinctive transport mechanisms is necessary in designing delivery systems for oral peptidergic drugs.

1.4.1 TRANSCELLULAR TRANSPORT

Transcellular transport refers to the movement of substances through a cell, both the apical membrane and basolateral membrane. In the basolateral membrane, the protein lipid ratio is very low, and hence it is comparatively thinner with higher permeable as compared to the apical membrane. Transcellular transport of molecules depend on lipophilicity, charge, surface hydrophobicity, hydrogen bond potential, size, or the presence of a ligand on the surface of a particle (Mahato 2003). Enterocytes comprise the majority of the absorptive cells of the intestinal lining and a very small proportion (about 1%) of M cells that are located in the epithelium of the Peyer's patches (Van de Graaff 1986). Peyer's patches, small masses of lymphatic tissue in the mucosal lining of the ileum, are covered by a specialized follicle associated epithelial layer that contains M cells. Since M cells in the Peyer's patches are highly specialized for antigens, they can transport peptides from the intestinal lumen to the immune system cells to initiate an immune response. Therefore, due to their high endocytosis ability, M cells may be a potential portal for the oral delivery of large molecules like proteins and peptides, including nanoparticles (Dobrynin and Rubinstein 2005). Nevertheless, this mechanism is restricted to the absorption of lipophilic drugs with a relatively low molecular weight.

1.4.2 PARACELLULAR TRANSPORT

Paracellular transport represents the movement of substances through the spaces in between epithelial cells. The paracellular transport of molecules is not dependent on the lipophilicity and hydrogen bonding capacity. Therefore, tight junctions are the main rate-limiting barrier for permeation of ions and larger molecules for paracellular transport. The biophysical properties of junctions are shared with ion channels, which include ion concentration dependent permeability, size and charge

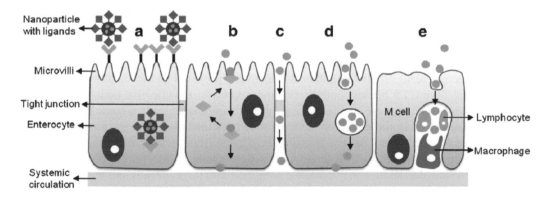

FIGURE 1.4 Schematic representation of transport mechanisms: (a) receptor-mediated transport; (b) carrier-mediated transport; (c) paracellular transport; (d) transcellular transport; and (e) M cell mediated transport i.e. phagocytosis by M cells. (Reprinted from *Adv Drug Deliv Rev* 65, Yun, Y., Cho, Y.W., and Park, K. Nanoparticles for oral delivery: targeted nanoparticles with peptic ligands for oral protein delivery, 822–32, Copyright 2013, with permission from Elsevier.)

selectivity, competition among permeant molecules, anomalous mole-fraction effects, and pH-sensitivity (Aungst 2000). Tight junctions between epithelial cells permit ions but exclude macromolecules (Tiwari et al. 2012). The paracellular space dimensions lie between 10 and 50 Å with an average size of 7–9 Å for the jejunum, 3–4 Å for the ileum, and 8–9 Å for the colon (Gupta et al. 2009). Therefore, substances with more than 15 Å (~3.5 kDa) of a molecular radius are unable to penetrate through this route. Moreover, since tight junctions comprise only around 0.01% of the total absorptive surface of the intestine (Pereira De Sousa et al. 2015), the paracellular transport of proteins across mucosal epithelia is highly restricted. The paracellular mechanism complements transportation through transcellular process by defining the selectivity and degree of reverse leak for solutes and ions, making a significant contribution to overall tissue-specific transport. Moreover, transcellular absorption showed a significant reduction in the colon, while such gradient does not exist for paracellular transport (Gruber et al. 1987).

1.4.3 CARRIER- AND RECEPTOR-MEDIATED TRANSPORT

Carriers transport small hydrophilic molecules across the cell and release them from the basal enterocytes surface into circulation (Lai et al. 2009a). Active absorption of specific molecules by carriers is an energy dependent process. Target molecules are recognized by carriers through membrane receptors, and transport them across the epithelial membranes, against the direction of the concentration gradient and usually in trace quantities. Small dipeptides, tripeptides, amino acids, and monosaccharides are transported via transcellular mechanisms though carrier-mediated transport processes. In receptor-mediated transport, proteins act as a ligand for specific surface-attached receptors or as a surface-attached receptor for specific ligands. This strategy can be used to increase the oral bioavailability of therapeutic proteins by modification such as receptor-specific ligands (therapeutic peptides or proteins). This transportation involves membrane invagination to form a vesicle and initiates the endocytosis process, which comprises pinocytosis, phagocytosis, potocytosis, and receptor-mediated endocytosis (Lai et al. 2009b). During the process, ligands bind to a specific cell-surface receptor forming a cluster with the receptor that is subsequently internalized through coated vesicles into endosomal acidic compartments.

1.5 FORMULATION STRATEGIES FOR EFFECTIVE ORAL PROTEINS AND PEPTIDES DELIVERY

As discussed earlier in this chapter, due to various hurdles (absorption, enzymatic degradation, and low bioavailability) several strategies were adopted by researchers to enable the significant delivery of proteins and peptides by oral route. Such strategies include, use of enzyme inhibitors, absorption enhancers and use of mucoadhesive polymers, cell permitting peptides, and novel nanocarrier systems. Muheem et al. (2016) and Renukuntla et al. (2013) prepared an excellent review explaining these strategies. Figure 1.5 broadly outlines the approaches for the effective understanding of the different strategies. Out of these strategies the polymeric nanocarrier system has attracted the most attention of researchers in the field. Polymeric nanocarriers tend to protect the encapsulated drug from the external environment, thereby isolating the peptide from various enzymes, including peptidases, and promote their uptake by enterocyte cells. Subsequent to absorption, polymeric nanocarriers undergo a slow degradation in accordance with their kinetic properties and the characteristics of the polymer, thereby allowing a controlled and sustained release of proteins and peptide drugs (Delie and Balanco-Príeto 2005).

Among the polymeric nanocarrier strategies investigated for attaining effective oral delivery of proteins and peptides, those implementing polysaccharide excipients are generally more encouraging since they are widely diverse, biocompatible, and possess peculiar features.

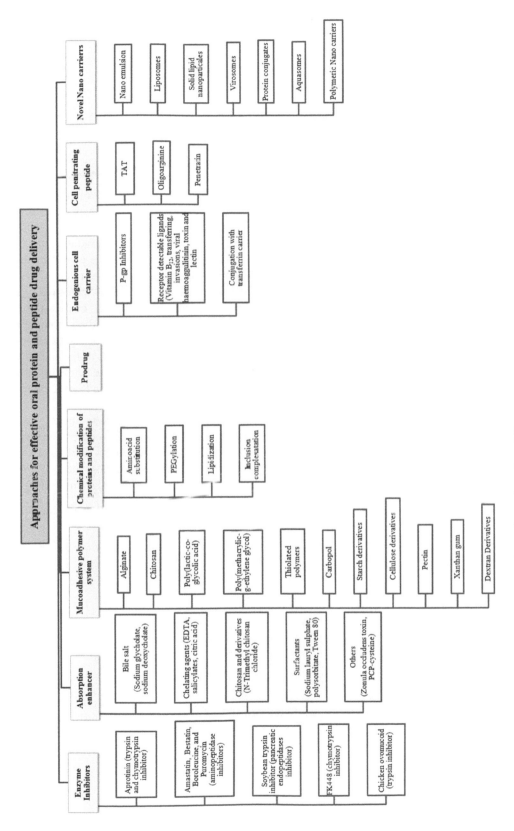

FIGURE 1.5 Formulation strategies for effective oral proteins and peptices delivery.

In this chapter, we shall emphasize the different polysaccharide-based nanocarriers used for the oral delivery of proteins and polypeptides.

1.6 POLYSACCHARIDE NANOCARRIERS FOR ORAL PROTEIN AND POLYPEPTIDE DELIVERY

Various polysaccharides have been successfully utilized by researchers for successful protein and peptide delivery through nanocarriers systems (Figure 1.6).

1.6.1 ALGINATE NANOCARRIER

Alginates (ALs) are one of the most widely investigated natural polysaccharides for peroral protein and peptide delivery (George and Abraham 2006; Gombotz and Wee 2012). Alginates are naturally occurring anionic polysaccharides comprising two distinct monosaccharide units, (1–4)-linked β-D-mannuronic acid and α-L-guluronic acid. AL possesses outstanding biodegradable, biocompatible, and mucoadhesive characteristics, and finds significant applications in the pharmaceutical field including the formulation of novel drug delivery vehicles and other controlled release devices (Dong et al. 2006). Alginate-based micro and nanoformulations can be prepared with ease by the induction of ionotropic gelation with calcium ions. The gel forming ability of AL enables the formation of a pre-gel comprising of minute agglomerates of gel fragments, which then promote the incorporation of an aqueous solution of polycations to form a coating of polyelectrolyte complex (De and Robinson 2003). Recently, chitosan has been utilized for combining AL to form nanoparticles. Alginate and chitosan have the ability to crosslink with each other via an electrostatic force to form nanoparticles with the potential to enhance permeability and bioadhesion (Sarmento et al. 2007b; Yin et al. 2009; Sarmento et al. 2007c; Zhang et al. 2011).

Numerous investigations have reported on the oral administration of insulin by alginate nanocarriers. In an interesting piece of research by Sarmento et al. (2007b), insulin-encapsulated alginate/chitosan nanocarriers were prepared for oral administration in diabetic rats. Orally delivered alginate/chitosan nanoparticles diminished glucose levels of basal serum by greater than 40% with an administration of 50 and 100 IU/kg doses, thereby maintaining the hypoglycemic effect for

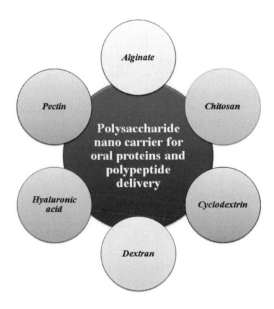

FIGURE 1.6   Polysaccharide nanocarrier for oral proteins and polypeptide delivery.

a prolonged duration (~ 18 hours) (Sarmento et al. 2007b). The same authors published another work in which insulin-loaded alginate nanoparticles were prepared by ionotropic pregelation of calcium chloride with dilute aqueous AL solution, followed by the formation of a polyelectrolyte complex with the aid of chitosan. The loading capacity of insulin into the core of alginate nanoparticles, and also the entrapment efficiency, mostly depends upon the mass ratio of alginate:chitosan. The formulation of alginate/chitosan nanoparticles protects the insulin from the extremely acidic pH of the stomach upon oral administration. Approximately, 50% retention of insulin was observed in the gastric fluid of the stomach for up to 24 hours whereas, with prolonged release up to 75% was noticed in the intestinal environment (Sarmento et al. 2007c).

In another work, Li et al. (2007) successfully formulated bovine serum albumin-loaded quater-nized chitosan (QCS)/alginate (AL) nanoparticles (QCS/AL). The encapsulation of bovine serum albumin (BSA) was influenced by average molecular weight (M_w) and degree of substitution (DS) of QCS, and also on BSA concentration. High M_w QCS promotes BSA release in an acidic medium, whereas, high DS decelerate BSA release in both 0.1M hydrochloric acid (HCl) and 0.1M phosphate buffer saline (PBS) (Li et al. 2007). A recent report is available on the formulation of nanoemul-sions coated with alginate/chitosan for oral administration of insulin (Li et al. 2013). This study was aimed at reducing the size of minute droplets of multiple emulsion by the homogenization technique. It also aimed to coat the nanoemulsion surface with alginate/chitosan via an electrostatic crosslinking technique, in order to stabilize the nanoemulsion in the GIT. The *in vivo* bioavailability study of alginate/chitosan-coated nanoemulsion was carried out in normal as well as diabetic rats, following administration by oral route (Li et al. 2013).

Another work was published by Masalova et al. (2013) in which they formulated and evalu-ated alginate and chitosan gel nanoparticles in the presence of stabilizers (PEG 1500, PEG 6000, TWEEN 80) for efficient oral administration of BSA.

Alginate-based nanocarriers also find promising application in food technology. A novel approach based on alginate-chitosan-pluronic composite nanoparticles can be used for encapsulat-ing nisin, a natural polycyclic antibacterial peptide used as food preservative. *In vitro* drug release testing of nanocarriers performed for two weeks exhibited an initial burst pattern release of nisin, and then a more sustained release from the formulation (Bernela et al. 2014).

1.6.2 Chitosan Nanocarriers

Chitosan, a cationic polysaccharide, is an attractive polymer with significant applications in oral protein and peptide delivery (Zhang et al. 2010; Jing et al. 2017). The controlled delivery systems based on chitosan have already been explored widely for the transport of numerous drugs and bioactives (Giri et al. 2012). Among various drug delivery applications, chitosan nanocarriers have been found to be quite promising in the improvement of the transmucosal delivery of proteins and peptides across diverse mucosal membranes (Saikia et al. 2015; Makhlof et al. 2011).

There are various chitosan-based nanocarriers that have exhibited attractive outcomes in the oral delivery of proteins, these include CS-coated nanocapsules (Prego et al. 2005; Prego et al. 2006), CS-coated liposomes (Werle and Takeuchi 2009; Thongborisute et al. 2006; Carvalho et al. 2009), CS-coated lipid nanoparticles (Garcia-Fuentes et al. 2005; Fonte et al. 2011), CS-coated gold nanoparticles (Bhumkar et al. 2007), self-assembled nanocarriers made with hydrophobically mod-ified CS (Rekha and Sharma 2009), CS nanocarriers formed by interpolymer complexation (Lin et al. 2007; Sarmento et al. 2007a; Sarmento et al. 2007b; Sonaje et al. 2009; Sonaje et al. 2010a; Sonaje et al. 2010b), and nanoparticles based on ionically crosslinked CS (Pan et al. 2002; Alonso-Sande et al. 2006).

Among numerous proteins and peptides encapsulated by chitosan nanocarriers, insulin is one of the proteins that has been most widely investigated by researchers in the pharmaceutical field. In a research work by Pan et al. (2002), insulin encapsulated bioadhesive chitosan nanocarriers were formulated by an ionic gelation method with the aid of tripolyphosphate anions. The absorption of insulin by the intestines was greatly enhanced in case of CS-NPs as compared to the aqueous CS solution *in vivo*. Administering 21 IU/kg of insulin in the form of CS-NPs, prolonged the hypoglycemic effect beyond 15 hours and up to 14.9% average bioavailability in comparison to the subcutaneous preparation of insulin solution (Pan et al. 2002).

In spite of being the most widely explored polymer for oral insulin delivery, researchers are nowadays mainly focusing on CS derivatized biopolymers for delivering various proteins and peptide drugs by oral route (Bernkop-Schnürch 2000; Chen et al. 2003). The shift to the derivatized form might be attributable to the necessity of nanoparticles to remain intact in the acidic pH of the stomach and also to combat against them being degraded by proteolytic enzymes. However, at a low pH condition, the solubility of CS increases, which in turn retards the transportation of proteins to the intestines (Chaudhury and Das 2011). To overcome this difficulty, CS derivatives with improved physicochemical properties have been developed, which prevents the degradation of proteins in the GI tract and also imparts a sustained release of proteins (Agnihotri et al. 2004). CS possesses free hydroxyl and amino groups that facilitates modification or substitution with varying chemical moieties for the formation of CS derivatives with suitable characteristics for the oral delivery of drugs (Aranaz et al. 2010).

In another interesting work by Bayat et al. (2008), an insulin-loaded nanoparticulate system was synthesized by implementing chitosan (CS), triethylchitosan (TEC), and dimethylethylchitosan (DMEC, a novel quaternized derivative of chitosan) for delivery to the colon. *Ex vivo* studies have shown the remarkable transport of insulin via colon absorption in rat models for nanocarriers formulated with quaternized derivatives as compared to those formulated with native chitosan. Moreover, *in vivo* investigations in rat models have revealed significant insulin absorption via the colon by implementing these nanocarriers in comparison with free insulin administered to diabetic rats (Bayat et al. 2008).

For oral delivery of nanocarriers, the other peptide that has gained an increasing amount of interest with researchers is calcitonin. In a study by Garcia-Fuentes et al. (2005), preparation and characterization of poly(ethylene glycol) (PEG)-coated and chitosan (CS)-coated lipid nanoparticles for the effective oral administration of salmon calcitonin (sCT) was reported. Subsequent to oral delivery of the sCT-loaded CS-coated nanoparticles, they interacted favorably with the intestinal mucosal layer, and subsequently allowed for site-specific delivery of sCT for a longer duration, This then lead to a prolonged pharmacological effect as compared to PEG-coated nanoparticulate formulations (Garcia-Fuentes et al. 2005).

Yet, in another case, Prego et al. (2006) formulated and investigated salmon calcitonin encapsulated chitosan-PEG nanocapsules and PEG-coated nanoemulsions as a control by the method of solvent displacement, resulting in the size ranging 160–250 nm. It was noted that the existence of PEG, in either native form or grafted to chitosan, stabilizes the nanocapsules in the gastrointestinal fluids. The *in vivo* investigation exhibited the potential of chitosan-PEG nanocapsules to intensify and sustain the intestinal absorption of salmon calcitonin for a prolonged duration. Therefore, it was noted that by regulating the degree of pegylation of chitosan, highly stable and less cytotoxic nanocapsules were obtained with absorption enhancing properties (Prego et al. 2006).

Chitosan decorated nanocarriers are also known to encapsulate elcatonin, a derivative form of calcitonin. In a research work by Kawashima et al. (2000), a novel mucoadhesive chitosan coated poly-DL-lactide/glycolide copolymer (PLGA) nanospheres was developed for oral elcatonin delivery. It was observed that the chitosan-coated nanospheres remarkably minimized the calcium level of blood in comparison with uncoated nanospheres and elcatonin solution, and sustained the effect for a period of 48 hours in fasted Wistar rats (Kawashima et al. 2000).

Similarly, CS-coated liposomes were also designed and evaluated for their promising application in oral calcitonin delivery. In this instance, an improved enteral absorption of calcitonin, in rats, was achieved based on their mucoadhesive properties (Werle and Takeuchi 2009).

A novel silk peptide is also known to be encapsulated within the stimuli-responsive nanocarrier system for oral delivery. For instance, Hu et al. (2002) explored the release behavior of an *in vitro* silk peptide (SP) from the core of chitosan (CS)-poly(acrylic acid) (PAA) complex nanoparticulate formulations. The peptide release from nanoparticles was sensitive to alteration in the pH of the medium and was sustained for up to 10 days. Owing to their pH-responsive ability, CS-PAA nanoparticles are known to be suitable vehicles for peptide delivery in the GIT (Hu et al. 2002).

So far, numerous investigations have provided remarkable evidence for the effectiveness of CS nanocarriers for oral transportation of protein and peptides. However, for significant advancement in preclinical development of chitosan-based nanoparticulate formulations, it is essential to comprehend the various driving mechanisms governing the drug release from CS-based nanocarriers. During the past few decades, several interesting works have unveiled insights related to these issues. On the basis of preliminary experiments with animal models, it is highly believed that protein and peptide drugs could be successfully delivered via oral route by employing CS nanoparticles exerting the desired pharmacological response. However, more progress and validation of the implementation of these nanoparticles is to be carried out in large animal models.

1.6.3 Cyclodextrin Nanocarrier

Cyclodextrins (CDs) are cyclic oligosaccharides comprising of a glucopyranose unit which has a hydrophobic central core and hydrophilic exterior surface. The native form of CDs comprises of 6, 7, or 8 glucopyranose units and are designated as alpha, beta, and gamma CDs, respectively. Numerous derivatives of CDs are available and possess excellent pharmaceutical applications, but quite few of them, mostly those bearing the methyl (M), hydroxypropyl (HP), and sulfobutylether (SBE) groups, are utilized on a commercial scale as novel pharmaceutical excipients (van de Manakker et al. 2009; Zhou and Ritter 2010). The versatile functional properties of CDs have enabled them to be employed in various oral drug delivery applications, including protein and peptide delivery (Sajeesh and Sharma 2006; Trapani et al. 2010). CDs are mainly implemented as complexing agents in drug transportation vehicles for enhancing the aqueous solubility of protein drugs and also to increase their stability and bioavailability. Moreover, CDs are also used for minimizing gastrointestinal irritation, masking the unpleasant taste or smell, and also for preventing drug interactions. The CDs incorporated in the nanocarriers are meant to provide modification to the carriers for improving encapsulation capacity for poorly soluble drugs (Salústio et al. 2011).

A novel hydroxypropyl-β-cyclodextrin-insulin (HPβCD-I) complex loaded in a polymethacrylic acid-chitosan-polyether (polyethylene glycol-polypropylene glycol copolymer) (PMCP) nanocarriers has been developed for oral delivery. CDs elevate the solubilization capacity of insulin while PMCP decreases degradation by proteolytic enzymes and increases the duration of nanoparticle retention (Sajeesh and Sharma 2006).

In another work, chitosan/cyclodextrin nanoparticles have also shown to be a promising vehicle for the oral transportation of heparin and insulin. For instance, Krauland and Alonso (2007) generated nanoparticulate formulations consisting of chitosan (CS) and carboxymethyl-β-cyclodextrin (CM-β-CD) or a physical mixture of CM-β-CD/tripolyphosphate (TPP) via the ionotropic gelation technique and to characterize their association potential for the delivery of insulin and heparin. The release of the macromolecules was governed by the type of molecule and its interaction with the matrix of the nanoparticles: insulin was released rapidly (84%–97% insulin was released within 15 minutes) while the release of heparin was retarded owing to its high association with the nanoparticles for a prolonged period of time (8.3%–9.1% heparin was released within 8 hours) (Krauland and Alonso 2007).

In other research, Trapani et al. (2010) designed and investigated novel nanocarriers comprising of chitosan (CS), or CS/cyclodextrin (CDs), and characterized their ability for orally delivering the peptide glutathione (GSH). The *ex vivo* studies carried out in the intestinal model of a frog demonstrated that in the case of CS as well as CS/CDs nanocarriers possessed the ability to enhance permeation across the intestinal epithelial region. Hence, it was suggested that the inclusion of this small peptide within the cavity of CDs prevents its degradation by endopeptidases

(Trapani et al. 2010). Since cyclodextrins (CDs) enhances the absorption by modifying the fluidity of the mucosal membrane and also shielding the insulin against degradation and thermal denaturation, an approach was initiated to entrap insulin complexed with β-cyclodextrin into the trimethylchitosan and alginate hydrogel nanoparticles. Permeability studies have been performed across caco-2 and the observations have revealed that approximately 8.41% ± 0.39% of the drug was permeated in 240 minutes (Mansourpour et al. 2015).

1.6.4 DEXTRAN NANOCARRIER

Dextran is another biodegradable, biocompatible, highly branched polyanionic polysaccharide possessing the potential to form nanocarrier delivery vehicles for oral transportation of peptide drug molecules (Van Tomme and Hennink 2007; Chen et al. 2009). It comprises of 1→6 and 1→4 glycosidic linkage bearing 2.3 sulfate moieties per glucosyl residue and its synthesis is carried out by a plethora of bacterial strains such as *Gluconobacter oxydans*, *Leuconostoc mesenteroides*, and *Streptococcus mutans* (Heinze et al. 2006). Numerous polymer chains grafted with dextran sulfate possess the ability to undergo hydrophilic to hydrophobic transition by altering temperature. Recently, numerous dextran-grafted copolymers have been outlined for their application in the fabrication of nanocarriers, including dextran-g-poly(N-isopropylacrylamide) (Patrizi et al. 2009), dextran-poly(N-isopropylacrylamide) (Otsuka et al. 2012), and dextran- PMAA-PNIPAM-iron oxide (Feng et al. 2012) segments. The application of dextran is not only restricted to the formation of nanocarriers but is also utilized as a coating material for various nanocarriers (Yu et al. 2012).

Chen et al. (2003) prepared an antiangiogenesis peptide-loaded nanoparticle delivery vehicle via a simple coacervation process by implementing two polysaccharides chitosan (CS) and dextran sulfate (DS) carrying opposite charges. The weight ratio of two polysaccharides determines the surface charge, particle size, encapsulation efficiency, and drug release behavior of the prepared nanoparticles. The maximum entrapment efficiency obtained by the antiangiogenesis peptide was 75% with a 0.59:1 CS:DS weight ratio showing prolonged and sustained peptide release for over 6 days (Chen et al. 2003).

In another work, an aqueous nanocarrier system was synthesized by implementing the differentially charged polymers DS and polyethylenimine (PEI) where zinc acted as a stabilizer for oral insulin delivery. *In vivo* analysis in steptozotocin-induced diabetic rats demonstrated a hypoglycemic response for a longer duration (Tiyaboonchai et al. 2003). Similarly, an insulin incorporated nanoparticle delivery vehicle was formulated by complex formation between dextran sulfate and chitosan in aqueous media. The study revealed that DS/chitosan nanoparticles are responsive to changes in pH and the release of insulin is governed by a dissociation mechanism (Sarmento et al. 2006).

Vitamins are also utilized for the coating of dextran nanoparticles. For example, Chalasani et al. (2007) revealed the potential of vitamin B_{12} coated dextran nanoparticles using varying levels of crosslinking as an efficient insulin carrier in animal models for the treatment of diabetes. The polydisperse NPs were produced exhibiting large-sized particles, high entrapment of insulin, and rapid release due to their low crosslinking levels. They depicted extensive (70%–75%) reductions in blood glucose level and extended (54 hours) the antidiabetic response showing biphasic behavior in the case of streptozocin induced diabetic rats. In addition, the nanoparticles also showed an identical potency of orally administered insulin in congenital diabetic mice with a 60% decline in blood sugar level at 20 hours (Chalasani et al. 2007). Bovine serum albumin (BSA) and rhodamine 6G (R6G) were also employed for encapsulation within chitosan (CS)-dextran sulfate (DS) nanoparticles. In case of both R6G and BSA, high entrapment efficiency (98%) was achieved when the charge ratio of the two oppositely charged polysaccharides was > 1.12. The mechanism of release of both BSA and R6G from the nanocarriers was governed by the ion-exchange mechanism and the release was sustained for up to 7 days (Chen et al. 2007).

1.6.5 Hyaluronic Acid Nanocarrier

In recent years, hyaluronic acid (HA) has garnered enormous interest from researchers designing nanocarriers for peptide delivery (Leach and Schmidt 2005; Oh et al. 2010). It is a natural acidic polysaccharide, generally comprising of a N-acetylglucosamine and D-glucuronic acid disaccharide unit. It possesses the unique characteristics of being non-adhesive, non-toxic, non-immunogenic, and biodegradable, and is best suited for the fabrication of varying controlled release formulations (Kogan et al. 2007). HA bears a negative charge in a neutral pH environment that enables it to be uniformly coated on the exterior surface of positively charged nanocarriers. It is known to be related to various cellular processes, such as angiogenesis and the regulation of inflammatory pathways (Pardue et al. 2008; Petrey and Carol 2014). However, HA due to its short duration of half-life lessens its suitability for long-term applications in the clinical field. For the purpose of prolonging the retention of HA in systemic circulation, various modifications of carboxyl and hydroxyl moieties are employed by the esterification process (Della Valle and Romeo 1989), dialdehyde crosslinking (Shu et al. 2002), and carbodiimide reaction (Kuo et al. 1991). HA bears a negative charge which can be utilized for safeguarding the positive charge of polycationic nanoparticulate formulations. The modification of HA enables it to become responsive to several stimuli including changes in pH, enzyme, and redox potential and thus, renders it a suitable polymer for developing nanoscale peptide-delivery vehicles.

HA-based nanoparticles have successfully encapsulated insulin for oral administration. For instance, Han et al. (2012) have developed and evaluated novel insulin-incorporated HA nanocarriers with the technique of reverse emulsion freeze drying. The pH-sensitive HA nanoparticles protected insulin against the harsh acidic pH of the stomach and did not disrupt the junction integrity of epithelial cells, thereby indicating long-term safety for chronic treatment. Permeability studies via rat small intestine revealed that HA nanoparticles significantly elevated the transport of insulin through the ileum and duodenum. Subsequent to administration of insulin-loaded HA nanocarriers by oral route, diabetic rats treated with oral insulin also exhibited a stronger hypoglycemic response than with insulin solution (Han et al. 2012). Hence, these HA-based nanocarriers could be an attractive polysaccharide for the oral delivery of proteins and peptides.

1.6.6 Pectin Nanocarrier

Pectin is another attractive polysaccharide obtained from natural sources and is one of the major constituents of the cell wall of plants (Xiao and Anderson 2013). Chemically, pectin comprises of poly-α-1–4-galacturonic acid, bearing different degrees of methylated carboxylic acid groups. Pectins, having a low degree of methylation, possess the ability to form gel in the environment of multivalent ions, while pectins, having a higher degree of methylation, also lead to the formation of gel in acidic environment by adding various sugars, such as glucose or sucrose. The most crucial factor which governs the pectin solubility and its unique ability to form gel and film is the degree of esterification of its glacaturonic acid residues. From a traditional point of view, pectin finds widespread application in the food industry (Luzio and Cameron 2013; Ström et al. 2014).

Owing to their excellent stability in acidic environment even at extreme temperatures, pectin becomes one of the ideal candidates to be utilized in various drug delivery systems (DDS). Pectin possesses the distinctive capability of forming gel in the presence of divalent cations. Several studies have noted that pectin is resistant to various GI enzymes such as proteases and amylase and it is usually degraded by microbial flora present in the colon (Sadeghi 2011; Mishra et al. 2012). Recently intensive interest by researchers has been shown for developing pectin formulations for sustained and controlled drug delivery. Among them various pectin-based vehicles (microspheres, films, hydrogels, and nanoparticles) have been developed for delivering several drugs and proteins (Liu et al. 2007; Sriamornsak 2011).

Various pectin-based nanoformulations for oral protein and peptide delivery have been reviewed. In a study by Cheng and Lim (2004), the effect of the molecular mass of pectin and formulation pH was investigated on insulin encapsulated calcium pectinate nanoparticles. These nanoparticles were formulated by ionotropic gelation with calcium ions for efficient insulin delivery to the colon. The investigators concluded that insulin release from nanoparticulate formulations was influenced by the magnitude of nanoparticle dilution and pH of dissolution media (Cheng and Lim 2004).

In another interesting investigation by Thirawong et al. (2008), self-assembled pectin-liposome nanocomplexes (PLNs) were synthesized by blending together positively charged liposomes and pectin solution, for enhancing the absorption of calcitonin (eCT) by the intestines. The eCT-incorporated PLNs displayed a strong pharmacological effect in comparison to the eCT-encapsulated liposomes and eCT solution, and prolonged decrease in plasma level of calcium was noticed in rats. The response was attributable to the pectin's potential to stick to the mucus membrane and extend the retention time in the intestine (Thirawong et al. 2008).

1.7   FUTURE PERSPECTIVES AND CONCLUSION

Owing to their unique properties, polysaccharide-based delivery systems have recently emerged as one of the most widely investigated natural polymers in the nanomedicine domain. On the basis of the recent advancements in biotechnology, numerous nanoparticulate drug delivery vehicles have been formulated for the oral transportation of protein drugs. However, synthetic polymers employed in protein delivery possess several drawbacks which cannot be ignored. The major concern related to these synthetic polymers is their low biodegradability and biocompatibility. The introduction of several biodegradable polymers, including lactide/glycolide copolymers, polyanhydrides and poly(ortho esters) could partially solve these issues, but some problems may still arise, such as possible toxicity after degradation, non-uniformity in degradation, and drug release.

Polysaccharides are the natural polymers that have proven to be an attractive substitute for the synthetic polymers in designing nanoparticulate delivery systems for oral protein and peptide delivery. They are quite safe, non-toxic, stable, hydrophilic, and of a biodegradable and biocompatible nature. They are also amenable to various chemical modifications and provide greater flexibility in designing drug delivery. After oral administration, the protein drugs must enter blood circulation by traversing the intestinal barricade layer including mucus membrane, tight epithelial junctions, and proteolytic enzymes present in the intestines. The overall aim of polysaccharide-based nanocarrier systems is to improve the protein bioavailability *in vivo* and also to improve the residence time. Nevertheless, several unsolved issues must be addressed in the near future, such as the mechanism of interaction of the nanoparticles with various cells, tissues, and organs of human body, the influence of nanoparticles on the human metabolic system, and further enhancement of the poor bioavailability for oral delivery of proteins.

REFERENCES

Agnihotri, S.A., Mallikarjuna, N.N., and Aminabhavi, T.M. 2004. Recent advances on chitosan-based micro- and nanoparticles in drug delivery. *J Controlled Release* 100: 5–28.

Alonso-Sande, M., Cuña, M., Remuñán-López, C., Teijeiro-Osorio, D., Alonso-Lebrero, J.L., and Alonso, M.J. 2006. Formation of new glucomannan-chitosan nanoparticles and study of their ability to associate and deliver proteins. *Macromolecules* 39: 4152–8.

Aranaz, I., Harris, R., and Heras, A. 2010. Chitosan amphiphilic derivatives. Chemistry and applications. *Curr Org Chem* 14: 308–30.

Aungst, B.J. 2000. Intestinal permeation enhancers. *J Pharm Sci* 89: 429–42.

Bals, R. 2000. Epithelial antimicrobial peptides in host defense against infection. *Respir Res.* 1: 141–50.

Bansil, R. and Turner, B.S. 2006. Mucin structure, aggregation, physiological functions and biomedical applications. *Curr Opin Colloid Interface Sci* 11: 164–70.

Bayat, A., Dorkoosh, F.A., Dehpour, A.R. et al. 2008. Nanoparticles of quaternized chitosan derivatives as a carrier for colon delivery of insulin: *ex vivo* and *in vivo* studies. *Int J Pharm* 356: 259–66.

Berkhout, B., Eggink, D., and Sanders, R.W. 2012. Is there a future for antiviral fusion inhibitors? *Curr Opin Virol* 2 (1): 50–9.

Bernela, M., Kaur, P., Chopra, M., and Thakur R. 2014. Synthesis, characterization of nisin loaded alginate-chitosan-pluronic composite nanoparticles and evaluation against microbes. *LWT-Food Sci Tech* 59: 1093–9.

Bernkop-Schnürch, A. 2000. Chitosan and its derivatives: Potential excipients for peroral peptide delivery systems. *Int J Pharm* 194: 1–3.

Bernkop-Schnürch, A. 2009. *Oral Delivery of Macromolecular Drugs. Barriers, Strategies and Future Trends*. New York: Springer.

Bhumkar, D.R., Joshi, H.M., Sastry, M., and Pokharkar, V.B. 2007. Chitosan reduced gold nanoparticles as novel carriers for transmucosal delivery of insulin. *Pharm Res* 24: 1415–26.

Boegh, M., Foged, C., Müllertz, A., and Nielsen, H.M. 2013. Mucosal drug delivery: Barriers, in vitro models and formulation strategies. *J Drug Del Sci Technol* 23: 383–91.

Bourganis, V., Karamanidou, T., Kammona, O. and Kiparissides, C. 2017. Polyelectrolyte complexes as prospective carriers for the oral delivery of protein therapeutics. *Eur J Pharm Biopharm* 111: 44–60.

Carvalho, E.L., Grenha, A., Remuñán-López, C., Alonso, M.J. and Seijo, B. 2009. Mucosal delivery of liposome–chitosan nanoparticle complexes. *Methods Enzymol* 465: 289–12.

Center for Straetgic and International Studies. (n.d.) https://www.csis.org/.

Chalasani, K.B., Russell-Jones, G.J., Jain, A.K., Diwan, P.V., and Jain, S.K. 2007. Effective oral delivery of insulin in animal models using vitamin B12-coated dextran nanoparticles. *J Controlled Release* 122: 141–50.

Chaudhury, A. and Das, S. 2011. Recent advancement of chitosan-based nanoparticles for oral controlled delivery of insulin and other therapeutic agents. *Aaps Pharmscitech*: 1210–20.

Chen, F.M., Ma, Z.W., Dong, G.Y., and Wu, Z.F. 2009. Composite glycidyl methacrylated dextran (Dex-GMA)/gelatin nanoparticles for localized protein delivery. *Acta Pharmacol Sin* 30: 485–93.

Chen, Y., Mohanraj, V.J., Parkin, J.E. 2003. Chitosan-dextran sulfate nanoparticles for delivery of an anti-angiogenesis peptide. *Letters in Peptide Science*. 10 (5–6): 621–9.

Chen, Y., Mohanraj, V.J., Wang, F. and Benson, H.A. 2007. Designing chitosan-dextran sulfate nanoparticles using charge ratios. *AAPS Pharm Sci Tech* 8: 131–9.

Cheng, K. and Lim, L.Y. 2004. Insulin-loaded calcium pectinate nanoparticles: Effects of pectin molecular weight and formulation pH. *Drug Dev Ind Pharm* 30: 359–67.

Cho, J.H., Sung, B.H. and Kim, S.C. 2009. Buforins: Histone H2A-derived antimicrobial peptides from toad stomach. *Biochim Biophys Acta* 1788: 1564–9.

Cone, R.A. 2005. Mucus. In J. Mestecky, M.E. Lamm, W. Strober, J. Bienenstock, J.R. McGhee, and L. Mayer (Eds.), *Mucosal Immunology*, 49–72. Burlington, MA: Elsevier Academic Press.

Daniels, L.B. and Maisel, A.S. 2007. Natriuretic peptides. *J Am Coll Cardiol* 50: 2357–68.

Daroszewska, A. 2012. Prevention and treatment of osteoporosis in women: An update. *Obstet Gynaecol Reprod Med* 22: 162–9.

De, S. and Robinson, D. 2003. Polymer relationships during preparation of chitosan-alginate and poly-l-lysine–alginate nanospheres. *J Controlled Release* 89: 101–12.

Delie, F. and Balanco-Príeto, M.J. 2005. Polymeric particulates to improve oral bioavailability of Peptide drugs. *Molecules* 10: 65–80.

Della Valle, F. and Romeo, A. 1989. Esters of hyaluronic acid. United States patent US 4,851,521.

Dobrynin, A.V. and Rubinstein, M. 2005. Theory of polyelectrolytes in solutions and at surfaces. *Prog Polym Sci* 30: 1049–118.

Dong, Z., Wang, Q., and Du, Y. 2006. Alginate/gelatin blend films and their properties for drug controlled release. *J Membrane Sci* 280: 37–44.

Elsayed, A. 2012. Oral delivery of insulin: Novel Approaches. In *Recent Adv Nov Drug Carr Syst*. InTech, pp. 281–314.

Erdmann, K., Cheung, B.W.Y., and Schröder, H. 2008. The possible roles of food-derived bioactive peptides in reducing the risk of cardiovascular disease. *J Nutri Biochem* 19: 643–54.

Farina, C., Weber, M.S., Meinl, E., Wekerle, H., and Hohlfeld, R. 2005. Glatiramer acetate in multiple sclerosis: Update on potential mechanisms of action. *Lancet Neurol* 4: 567–75.

Feng, W., Lv, W., Qi, J., Zhang, G., Zhang, F. and Fan, X. 2012. Quadruple responsive nanocomposite based on Dextran-PMAA-PNIPAM, iron oxide nanoparticles, and gold nanorods. *Macromol Rapid Commun* 33: 133–9.

Fonte, P., Nogueira, T., Gehm, C., Ferreira, D., and Sarmento, B. 2011. Chitosan-coated solid lipid nanoparticles enhance the oral absorption of insulin. *Drug Deliv Transl Res* 1: 299–308.

Gallo, R.L., Murakami, M., Ohtake, T., and Zaiou M. 2002. Biology and clinical relevance of naturally occurring antimicrobial peptides. *J Allergy Clin Immunol* 110: 823–31.

Garcia-Fuentes, M., Torres, D., and Alonso, M.J. 2005. New surface-modified lipid nanoparticles as delivery vehicles for salmon calcitonin. *Int J Pharm* 296: 122–32.

George, M. and Abraham, T.E. 2006. Polyionic hydrocolloids for the intestinal delivery of protein drugs: Alginate and chitosan-a review. *J Controlled Release* 114: 1–4.

Giri, T.K., Thakur, A., Alexander, A., Ajazuddin., Badwaik, H., and Tripathi, D.K. 2012. Modified chitosan hydrogels as drug delivery and tissue engineering systems: Present status and applications. *Acta Pharm Sin B* 2: 439–49.

Gombotz, W.R. and Wee, S.F. 2012. Protein release from alginate matrices. *Adv Drug Deliv Rev* 64: 194–205.

Greber, K.E. and Dawgul, M. 2017. Antimicrobial peptides under clinical trials. *Curr Top Med Chem* 17: 620–8.

Gruber, P., Longer, M.A. and Robinson, J.R. 1987. Some biological issues in oral, controlled drug delivery. *Adv Drug Deliv Rev* 1: 1–18.

Guaní-Guerra, Santos-Mendoza, T., Lugo-Reyes, S.O., and Teŕan, L.M. 2010. Antimicrobial peptides: General overview and clinical implications in human health and disease. *Clin Immunol* 135: 1–11.

Gupta, H., Bhandari, D., and Sharma, A. 2009. Recent trends in oral drug delivery: A review. *Recent Pat Drug Deliv Formul* 3: 162–73.

Guyenet, S.J. and Schwartz, M.W. 2012. Regulation of food intake, energy balance, and body fat mass: Implications for the pathogenesis and treatment of obesity. *J Clin Endocrinol Metab* 97 (3): 745–55.

Hamman, J.H., Enslin, G.M., and Kotzé, A.F. 2005. Oral delivery of peptide drugs: Barriers and developments. *BioDrugs* 19: 165–77.

Han, L., Zhao, Y., Yin, L. et al. 2012. Insulin-loaded pH-sensitive hyaluronic nanoparticles enhance transcellular delivery. *AAPS Pharm Sci Tech* 13: 836–45.

Hancock, R.E.W. 2001. Cationic peptides: Effectors in innate immunity and novel antimicrobials. *Lancet Infect Dis* 1: 156–64.

Heinze, T., Liebert, T., Heublein, B., and Hornig, S. 2006. Functional polymers based on dextran. In *Polysaccharides Ii*, D. Klemm (Ed.), 199–291. Berlin Heidelberg: Springer.

Hemmingsen, B., Sonne, D.P., Metzendorf, M.I., and Richter, B. 2017. Dipeptidyl-peptidase (DPP)-4 inhibitors and glucagon-like peptide (GLP)-1 analogues for prevention or delay of type 2 diabetes mellitus and its associated complications in people at increased risk for the development of type 2 diabetes mellitus. *Cochrane Database Syst Rev* 5: CD012204.

Hu, Y., Jiang, X., Ding, Y., Ge, H., Yuan, Y., and Yang, C. 2002. Synthesis and characterization of chitosan–poly (acrylic acid) nanoparticles. *Biomaterials* 23: 3193–201.

Izadpanah, A. and Gallo, R.L. 2005. Antimicrobial peptides. *J Am Acad Dermatol* 52: 381–90.

Jing, Z.W., Ma, Z.W., Li, C. et al. 2017. Chitosan cross-linked with poly (ethylene glycol) dialdehyde via reductive amination as effective controlled release carriers for oral protein drug delivery. *Bioorganic Med Chem Lett* 27: 1003–6.

Kaspar, A.A. and Reichert, J.M. 2013. Future directions for peptide therapeutics development. *Drug Discov Today* 18 (17–18): 807–17.

Kawashima, Y., Yamamoto, H., Takeuchi, H., and Kuno, Y. 2000. Mucoadhesive DL-lactide/glycolide copolymer nanospheres coated with chitosan to improve oral delivery of elcatonin. *Pharm Dev Technol* 5: 77–85.

Kitts, D.D. and Weiler, K. 2003. Bioactive proteins and peptides from food sources. Applications of bioprocesses used in isolation and recovery. *Curr Pharm Design* 9: 1309–23.

Kogan, G., Šoltés, L., Stern, R., and Gemeiner, P. 2007. Hyaluronic acid: A natural biopolymer with a broad range of biomedical and industrial applications. *Biotechnol Lett* 29: 17–25.

Kolb-Mäurer, A., Goebeler, M., and Mäurer, M. 2015. Cutaneous adverse events associated with interferon- β treatment of multiple sclerosis. *Int J Mol Sci* 16: 14951–60.

Korhonen, H. and Pihlanto, A. 2006. Bioactive peptides: Production and functionality. *Int Dairy J* 16: 945–60.

Krauland, A.H. and Alonso, M.J. 2007. Chitosan/cyclodextrin nanoparticles as macromolecular drug delivery system. *Int J Pharm* 340: 134–42.

Kuo, J.W., Swann, D.A. and Prestwich, G.D. 1991. Chemical modification of hyaluronic acid by carbodiimides. Bioconjugate Chem 2: 232–41.

Lai, S.K., Wang, Y.Y., Wirtz, D. and Hanes, J. 2009a. Micro- and macrorheology of mucus. *Adv Drug Deliv Rev* 61: 86–100.

Lai, S.K., Wang, Y.Y., Cone, R., Wirtz, D., and Hanes, J. 2009b. Altering mucus rheology to "solidify" human mucus at the nanoscale. *PLoS ONE* 4: 1–6.

Lalatsa, A. 2013. Peptide, proteins and antibodies. In *Fundamentals of Pharmaceutical Nanoscience*. I.F. Uchegbu, A.G. Schatzlein, W.P Cheng, and A. Lalatsa (Eds.), 511–42. New York: Springer Science + Business Media.

Lammi, C., Zanoni, C., Arnoldi, A., and Vistoli, G. 2015. Two peptides from soy β-conglycinin induce a hypocholesterolemic effect in hepg2 cells by a statin-like mechanism: Comparative in vitro and in silico modeling studies. *J Agric Food Chem* 63: 7945–51.

Langguth, P., Bohner, V., Heizmann, J. et al. 1997. The challenge of proteolytic enzymes in intestinal peptide delivery. *J Control Release* 46: 39–57.

Lax, R. 2010. The future of peptide development in the pharmaceutical industry. *Phar Manufacturing* 1: 10–5.

Leach, J.B. and Schmidt, C.E. 2005. Characterization of protein release from photocrosslinkable hyaluronic acid-polyethylene glycol hydrogel tissue engineering scaffolds. *Biomaterials* 26: 125–35.

Lee, V.H.L. and Yamamoto, A. 1990. Penetration and enzymatic barriers to peptide and protein absorption. *Adv Drug Deliv Rev* 4: 171–207.

Lewis, A.L. and Richard, J. 2015. Challenges in the delivery of peptide drugs: An industry perspective. *Ther Delivery* 6: 149–63.

Li, T., Shi, X.W., Du, Y.M., and Tang, Y.F. 2007. Quaternized chitosan/alginate nanoparticles for protein delivery. *J Biomed Mater Res A* 83 (2): 383–90.

Li, X., Qi, J., Xie, Y. et al. 2013. Nanoemulsions coated with alginate/chitosan as oral insulin delivery systems: Preparation, characterization, and hypoglycemic effect in rats. *Int J Nanomedicine* 8: 23–32.

Lin, W., Xie, X., Deng, J. et al. 2016. Cell-penetrating peptide doxorubicin conjugate loaded NGR-modified nanobubbles for ultrasound triggered drug delivery. *J Drug Target* 24 (2): 134–46.

Lin, Y.H., Mi, F.L., Chen, C.T. et al. 2007. Preparation and characterization of nanoparticles shelled with chitosan for oral insulin delivery. *Biomacromolecules* 8 (1): 146–52.

Liu, L., Fishman, M.L., and Hicks, K.B. 2007. Pectin in controlled drug delivery-a review. *Cellulose* 14 (1): 15–24.

Luhmann, T., Germershaus, O., Groll, J., and Meinel, L. 2012. Bone targeting for the treatment of osteoporosis. *J Control Release* 161 (2): 198–213.

Luzio, G.A. and Cameron, R.G. 2013. Determination of degree of methylation of food pectins by chromatography. *J Sci Food Agric* 93 (10): 2463–9.

Maes, W., Camp, J.A., Vermeirssen, V. et al. 2004. Influence of the lactokinin Ala-Leu-Pro-Met-His-Ile-Arg (ALPMHIR) on the release of endothelin-1 by endothelial cells. *Regul Pept* 118 (1–2): 105–9.

Mahato, R.I., Narang, A.S., Thoma, L., and Miller, D.D. 2003. Emerging trends in oral delivery of peptide and protein drugs. *Crit Rev Ther Drug Carr Syst* 20: 153–214.

Mahlapuu, M., Håkansson, J., Ringstad, L., and Björn, C. 2016. Antimicrobial peptides: An emerging category of therapeutic agents. *Front Cell Infect Microbiol* 6: 194.

Makhlof, A., Tozuka, Y., and Takeuchi, H. 2011. Design and evaluation of novel pH-sensitive chitosan nanoparticles for oral insulin delivery. *Eur J Pharm Sci* 42 (5): 445–51.

Mansourpour, M., Mahjub, R., Amini, M. et al. 2015. Development of acid-resistant alginate/trimethyl chitosan nanoparticles containing cationic β-cyclodextrin polymers for insulin oral delivery. *AAPS Pharm Sci Tech* 16 (4): 952–62.

Marcone, S., Belton, O., and Fitzgerald, D.J. 2017. Milk-derived bioactive peptides and their health promoting effects: A potential role in atherosclerosis. *Br J Clin Pharmacol* 83 (1): 152–162.

Marqus, S., Pirogova, E., and Piva, T.J. 2017. Evaluation of the use of therapeutic peptides for cancer treatment. *J Biomed Sci* 24: 21.

Masalova, O., Kulikouskaya, V., Shutava, T., and Agabekov, V. 2013. Alginate and Chitosan gel nanoparticles for efficient protein entrapment. *Physics Procedia* 40: 69–75.

Mishra, R.K., Banthia, A.K., and Majeed, A.B. 2012. Pectin based formulations for biomedical applications: A review. *Asian J Pharm Clin Res* 5 (4): 1–7.

Muheem, A., Shakeel, F., Jahangir, M.A. et al. 2016. A review on the strategies for oral delivery of proteins and peptides and their clinical perspectives. *Soudi Pharm J* 24: 413–28.

Nakhate, K.T., Dandekar, M.P., Kokare, D.M., and Subhedar, N.K. 2009. Involvement of neuropeptide Y Y(1) receptors in the acute, chronic and withdrawal effects of nicotine on feeding and body weight in rats. *Eur J Pharmacol* 609 (1–3): 78–87.

Nakhate, K.T., Kokare, D.M., Singru, P.S., and Subhedar, N.K. 2011. Central regulation of feeding behavior during social isolation of rat: Evidence for the role of endogenous CART system. *Int J Obes* 35 (6): 773–84.

Oh, E.J., Park, K., Kim, K.S et al 2010. Target specific and long-acting delivery of protein, peptide, and nucleotide therapeutics using hyaluronic acid derivatives. *J Control Release* 141 (1): 2–12.

Olmsted, S.S., Padgett, J.L., Yudin, A.I., Whaley, K.J., Moench, T.R., and Cone, R.A. 2001. Diffusion of macromolecules and virus-like particles in human cervical mucus, *Biophys J* 81: 1930–7.

Otsuka, I., Travelet, C., Halila, S. et al. 2012. Thermoresponsive self-assemblies of cyclic and branched oligosaccharide-block-poly (N-isopropylacrylamide) diblock copolymers into nanoparticles. *Biomacromolecules* 13 (5): 1458–65.

Pan, Y., Li, Y.J., Zhao, H.Y. et al. 2002. Bioadhesive polysaccharide in protein delivery system: Chitosan nanoparticles improve the intestinal absorption of insulin in vivo. *Int J Pharm* 249 (1): 139–47.

Pardue, E.L., Ibrahim, S., and Ramamurthi, A. 2008. Role of hyaluronan in angiogenesis and its utility to angiogenic tissue engineering. *Organogenesis* 4 (4): 203–14.

Patrizi, M.L., Piantanida, G., Coluzza, C., and Masci, G. 2009. ATRP synthesis and association properties of temperature responsive dextran copolymers grafted with poly (N-isopropylacrylamide). *Eur Polym J* 45 (10): 2779–87.

Pereira De Sousa, I., Steiner, C., Schmutzler, M. et al. 2015. Mucus permeating carriers: Formulation and characterization of highly densely charged nanoparticles. *Eur J Pharm Biopharm* 97: 273–9.

Petrey, A.C. and Carol A. 2014. Hyaluronan, a crucial regulator of inflammation. *Front Immunol* 5: 101.

Phelan, M. and Kerins, D. 2011. The potential role of milk-derived peptides in cardiovascular disease. *Food Funct* 2: 153–67.

Prego, C., Garcia, M., Torres, D., and Alonso, M.J. 2005. Transmucosal macromolecular drug delivery. *J Control Release* 101 (1): 151–62.

Prego, C., Torres, D., Fernandez-Megia, E., Novoa-Carballal, R., Quiñoá, E., and Alonso, M.J. 2006. Chitosan-PEG nanocapsules as new carriers for oral peptide delivery: Effect of chitosan pegylation degree. *J Control Release* 111 (3): 299–308.

Reddy, K.V.R., Yedery, R.D., and Aranha, C. 2004. Antimicrobial peptides: Premises and promises. *Int J Antimicrob Ag* 24: 536–47.

Rekha, M.R. and Sharma, C.P. 2009. Synthesis and evaluation of lauryl succinyl chitosan particles towards oral insulin delivery and absorption. *J Control Release* 135 (2): 144–51.

Renukuntla, J., Vadlapudi, A.D., Patel, A., Boddu, S.H.S., and Mitra, A.K. 2013. Approaches for enhancing oral bioavailability of peptides and proteins. *Int J Pharm* 447: 75–93.

Richards, A.M., Lainchbury, J.G., Troughton, R.W. et al. 2004. Clinical applications of B-type natriuretic peptides. *Trends Endocrinol Metab* 15 (4): 170–4.

Sadeghi, M. 2011. Pectin-based biodegradable hydrogels with potential biomedical applications as drug delivery systems. *J Biomater Nanobiotechnol* 2 (01): 36.

Saikia, C., Gogoi, P., and Maji, T.K. 2015. Chitosan: A promising biopolymer in drug delivery applications. *J Mol Genet Med S* 4: 006.

Sajeesh, S. and Sharma, C.P. 2006. Cyclodextrin–insulin complex encapsulated polymethacrylic acid based nanoparticles for oral insulin delivery. *Int J Pharm* 325 (1): 147–54.

Salústio, P.J., Pontes, P., Conduto, C. et al. 2011. Advanced technologies for oral controlled release: Cyclodextrins for oral controlled release. *AAPS Pharm Sci Tech* 12 (4): 1276–92.

Sarmento, B., Ferreira, D., Veiga, F., and Ribeiro, A. 2006. Characterization of insulin-loaded alginate nanoparticles produced by ionotropic pre-gelation through DSC and FTIR studies. *Carbohydr Polym* 66 (1): 1–7.

Sarmento, B., Ribeiro, A., Veiga, F., Ferreira, D.C., and Neufeld, R. 2007a. Oral bioavailability of insulin contained in polysaccharidenanoparticles. *Biomacromolecules* 8 (10): 3054–60.

Sarmento, B., Ribeiro, A., Veiga, F., Sampaio, P., Neufeld, R., and Ferreira, D. 2007b. Alginate/chitosan nanoparticles are effective for oral insulin delivery. *Pharm Res* 24 (12): 2198–206.

Sarmento, B., Ribeiro, A.J., Veiga, F., Ferreira, D.C., and Neufeld, RJ. 2007c. Insulin-loaded nanoparticles are prepared by alginate ionotropic pre-gelation followed by chitosan polyelectrolyte complexation. *J Nanosci Nanotechnol* 7 (8): 2833–41.

Shin, M.C., Zhang, J., Min, K.A. et al. 2014. Cell-penetrating peptides: Achievements and challenges in application for cancer treatment. *J Biomed Mater Res A* 102 (2): 575–87.

Shu, X.Z., Liu, Y., Luo, Y., Roberts, M.C., and Prestwich, G.D. 2002. Disulfide cross-linked hyaluronan hydrogels. *Biomacromolecules* 3 (6): 1304–11.

Sonaje, K., Chen, Y.J., Chen, H.L. et al. 2010a. Enteric-coated capsules filled with freeze-dried chitosan/poly (γ-glutamic acid) nanoparticles for oral insulin delivery. *Biomaterials* 31 (12): 3384–94.

Sonaje, K., Lin, K.J., Wey, S.P. et al. 2010b. Biodistribution, pharmacodynamics and pharmacokinetics of insulin analogues in a rat model: Oral delivery using pH-responsive nanoparticles vs. subcutaneous injection. *Biomaterials* 31 (26): 6849–58.

Sonaje, K., Lin, Y.H., Juang, J.H., Wey, S.P., Chen, C.T., and Sung, H.W. 2009. *In vivo* evaluation of safety and efficacy of self-assembled nanoparticles for oral insulin delivery. *Biomaterials* 30 (12): 2329–39.

Sriamornsak, P. 2011. Application of pectin in oral drug delivery. *Expert Opin Drug Deliv* 8 (8): 1009–23.

Steinstraesser, L. Kraneburg, U. Jacobsen, F., and Al-Benna, S. 2011. Host defense peptides and their antimicrobial-immunomodulatory duality. *Immunobiol* 216 (3): 322–33.

Ström, A., Schuster, E., and Goh, S.M. 2014. Rheological characterization of acid pectin samples in the absence and presence of monovalent ions. *Carbohydr Polym* 113: 336–43.

Tagliamonte, M., Petrizzo, A., Tornesello, M.L., Buonaguro, F.M., and Buonaguro, L. 2014. Antigen-specific vaccines for cancer treatment. *Hum Vaccin Immunother* 10 (11): 3332–46

Thirawong, N., Thongborisute, J., Takeuchi, H., and Sriamornsak, P. 2008. Improved intestinal absorption of calcitonin by mucoadhesive delivery of novel pectin–liposome nanocomplexes. *J Control Release* 125 (3): 236–45.

Thompson, C. and Ibie, C. 2011. The oral delivery of proteins using interpolymer polyelectrolyte complexes. *Ther Deliv* 2: 1611–31.

Thongborisute, J., Takeuchi, H., Yamamoto, H., and Kawashima, Y. 2006. Visualization of the penetrative and mucoadhesive properties of chitosan and chitosan-coated liposomes through the rat intestine. *J Liposome Research* 16 (2): 127–41.

Thundimadathil, J. 2012. Cancer treatment using peptides: Current therapies and future prospects. *J Amino Acids* 2012: 1–13.

Tiwari, G., R. Tiwari, B., Sriwastawa, L. et al. 2012. Drug delivery systems: An updated review. *Int J Pharm Investig* 2012: 2–11.

Tiyaboonchai, W., Woiszwillo, J., Sims, R.C., and Middaugh, C.R. 2003. Insulin containing polyethylenimine–dextran sulfate nanoparticles. *Int J Pharm* 255 (1): 139–51.

Trapani, A., Lopedota, A., Franco, M. et al. 2010. A comparative study of chitosan and chitosan/cyclodextrin nanoparticles as potential carriers for the oral delivery of small peptides. *Eur J Pharm Biopharm* 75 (1): 26–32.

Troke, R.C., Tan, T.M., and Bloom, S.R. 2014. The future role of gut hormones in the treatment of obesity. *Ther Adv Chronic Dis* 5 (1): 4–14.

Uhlig, T., Kyprianou, T., Martinelli, F.G. et al. 2014. The emergence of peptides in the pharmaceutical business: From exploration to exploitation. *EuPA Open Proteom* 4: 1–12.

Valderas, J.P., Irribarra, V., Boza, C. et al. 2010. Medical and surgical treatments for obesity have opposite effects on peptide YY and appetite: A prospective study controlled for weight loss. *J Clin Endocrinol Metab* 95 (3): 1069–75.

Van de Graaff, K.M. 1986. Anatomy and physiology of the gastrointestinal tract. *Pediatr Infect Dis* 5. S11–S16.

Van de Manakker, F., Vermonden, T., Van Nostrum, C.F., and Hennink, W.E. 2009. Cyclodextrin-based polymeric materials: Synthesis, properties, and pharmaceutical/biomedical applications. *Biomacromolecules* 10 (12): 3157–75.

Van Kaer, L. 2011. Glatiramer acetate for treatment of MS: Regulatory B cells join the cast of players. *Exp Neurol* 227 (1): 19–23.

Van Tomme, S.R. and Hennink, W.E. 2007. Biodegradable dextran hydrogels for protein delivery applications. *Expert Rev Med Devices* 4 (2): 147–64.

Wang, R., Yang, L.M., Wang, Y.H. et al. 2009. Sifuvirtide, a potent HIV fusion inhibitor peptide. *Biochem Biophys Res Commun* 382 (3): 540–4.

Werle, M. and Takeuchi, H. 2009. Chitosan–aprotinin coated liposomes for oral peptide delivery: Development, characterisation and *in vivo* evaluation. *Int J Pharm* 370 (1): 26–32.

WHO Report. 2017a. Cardiovascular diseases. Fact sheet.

WHO Report. 2017b. Diabetes. Fact sheet.

Xiao, C. and Anderson, C.T. 2013. Roles of pectin in biomass yield and processing for biofuels. *Front Plant Sci* 4: 67.

Yin, L., Ding, J., He, C., Cui, L., Tang, C., and Yin, C. 2009. Drug permeability and mucoadhesion properties of thiolated trimethyl chitosan nanoparticles in oral insulin delivery. *Biomaterials* 30 (29): 5691–700.

Yu, M., Huang, S., Yu, K.J., and Clyne, A.M. 2012. Dextran and polymer polyethylene glycol (PEG) coating reduce both 5 and 30 nm iron oxide nanoparticle cytotoxicity in 2D and 3D cell culture. *Int J Mol Sci* 13 (5): 5554–70.

Yun, Y., Cho, Y.W., and Park, K. 2013. Nanoparticles for oral delivery: Targeted nanoparticles with peptic ligands for oral protein delivery. *Adv Drug Deliv Rev* 65: 822–32.

Zhang, H.L., Wu, S.H., Tao, Y., Zang, L.Q., and Su, Z.Q. 2010. Preparation and characterization of water-soluble chitosan nanoparticles as protein delivery system. *J Nanomater* 2010: 1–5.

Zhang, L. and Gallo, R.L. 2016. Antimicrobial peptides. *Curr Biol* 26: R14–R19.

Zhang, Y., Wei, W., Lv, P., Wang, L., and Ma, G. 2011. Preparation and evaluation of alginate-chitosan micro-spheres for oral delivery of insulin. *Eur J Pharm Biopharm* 77 (1): 11–9.

Zhao, H., Zhou, J., Zhang, K. et al. 2016. A novel peptide with potent and broad-spectrum antiviral activities against multiple respiratory viruses. *Sci Rep* 6: 22008.

Zhou, J. and Ritter, H. 2010. Cyclodextrin functionalized polymers as drug delivery systems. *Polym Chem* 1 (10): 1552–9.

Zhou, X.H. 1994. Overcoming enzymatic and absorption barriers to non-parenterally administered protein and peptide drugs. *J Control Release* 29: 239–52.

2 Oral Absorption of Polysaccharide Nanoparticles Loaded with Drug Molecule across the GIT

Tapan Kumar Giri

CONTENTS

2.1 INTRODUCTION

Oral administration of the drug represents the most frequent and suitable drug delivery route. However, the oral route is not always feasible due to various problems including lack of drug absorbability, gastrointestinal drug instability, and short residence time in the gastrointestinal tract. These problems can be overcome by using colloidal drug delivery systems (Kreuter 1983; Kreuter 1990). Nanoparticles are drug-loaded colloidal polymeric carriers with a high stability and so are not quickly digested in the gastrointestinal tract (Giri et al. 2016a; Giri et al. 2017). They are taken up from the intestine in particulate form and reach the blood, lymph nodes, spleen, and liver. Oral administrations of nanoparticles are taken up in the gastrointestinal tract via intercellular, intracellular, paracellular, M cells, and Peyer's patches (Kreuter 1991). Uptake of a nanoparticle is dependent on size; a smaller particle is taken up more easily in comparison to larger particle. Moreover, the incorporation of drugs into nanoparticles augments the oral bioavailability of various drugs. The impact of nanoparticles delivered orally on drug pharmacokinetics and pharmacodynamics can be extensively different from that observed with a conventional dosage form (Figure 2.1). Recently, polysaccharide-based nanoparticles have gained much attention for the oral delivery of drugs. Polysaccharides are natural polymers exhibiting good biocompatibility and biodegradability (Giri et al. 2015; Giri et al. 2016b). Nanoparticles prepared from natural polysaccharides have the prospective to maintain drug stability and augment the duration of the drugs therapeutic effect when administered through oral routes (Florence 1997). Moreover, polysaccharide can be simply modified and is non-toxic, stable, safe, with gel forming properties which all signify its suitability for oral drug delivery (Sinha and Kumria 2001).

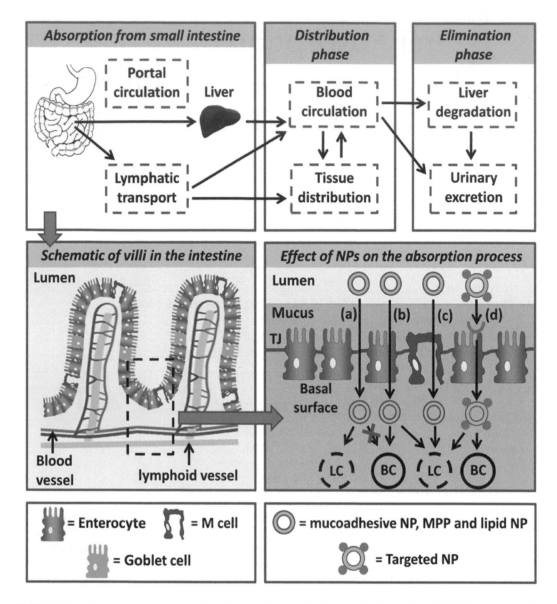

FIGURE 2.1 Mechanisms of absorption, distribution, metabolism, and elimination (ADME) of nanoparticle formulations following oral administration. (Reprinted from *Adv Drug Deliv Rev*, 106, Griffin, B.T., Guo, J., Presas, E., Donovan, M.D., Alonso, M.J., and O'Driscoll, C.M. Pharmacokinetic, pharmacodynamic and biodistribution following oral administration of nanocarriers containing peptide and protein drugs, 367–80, Copyright 2016, with permission from Elsevier.)

2.2 PHYSICOCHEMICAL PROPERTIES OF ORALLY ADMINISTERED NANOPARTICLES ON A PHARMACOKINETIC PROFILE

Size, surface charge, bioadhesiveness, lipophilicity, and functional modification of nanoparticles affect the pharmacokinetic profile. Nanoparticle size influences the uptake by enterocytes and M cells (Gaumet et al. 2009; Verma et al. 2012). Different size ranges (300, 600, and 1000 nm) of carboxylated chitosan-grafted poly(methyl methacrylate) nanoparticles were studied to investigate size-dependent absorption mechanisms (He et al. 2012). It was observed that smaller particles were transported to a larger extent in comparison to the larger nanoparticles. The biodistribution and elimination of nanoparticles is also dependent on size. It was observed that <6 nm size nanoparticles are typically filtered, but >8 nm size is not proficient for glomerular filtration (Longmire et al. 2008). Nanoparticle charges promote aggregation in the gut's luminal fluids and influence uptake. After absorption cationic nanoparticles interact with plasma proteins resulting in aggregation. Moreover, larger charged nanoparticles undergo improved clearance by the reticuloendothelial system prior to target tissues uptake (Guo et al. 2010). Pegylation of the nanoparticle surface changes the surface polarity and promotes mucus penetration (Xu et al. 2015). Moreover, pegylated nanoparticles protect against gastrointestinal lumen aggregation and diminished enzymatic degradation (Prego et al. 2006; Jevsevar et al. 2010; Pawar et al. 2014). After absorption, pegylated nanoparticles are retained in the blood for a prolonged time and decreased clearance of the nanoparticles (Veronese and Pasut 2005).

2.3 UPTAKE OF NANOPARTICLES FROM THE GASTROINTESTINAL TRACT

The intestinal epithelium which covers the surfaces of the gastrointestinal tract is a proficient barrier for allowing absorption of fluids, electrolytes, and nutrients (Walker and Owen 1990; Watson et al. 2009). The intestinal epithelial cell layer consists of secretory cells (Paneth cells and goblet cells) and absorptive cells (enterocytes) (Balcerzak et al. 1970; Cheng and Leblond 1974). Enterocytes are specialized cells consisting of organized microvilli on their apical surfaces responsible for transporting nutrients (Figure 2.2) (Hellmich and Evers 2006). Fatty acids are absorbed through enterocytes via passive diffusion, and monosaccharides and amino acids are absorbed through active transport by the specific receptors located on enterocytes (Wright et al. 2006). The intestinal epithelium also consists of M cells residing in the Peyer's patches which can take up antigens and microorganisms and deliver them to immune system (Cornes 1965).

The strength of the intestinal epithelium can be attributed to the existence of tight junctions. Tight junctions consist of transmembrane proteins including occludins, claudins, and junctional adhesion molecules along with numerous intracellular plaque proteins and different regulatory

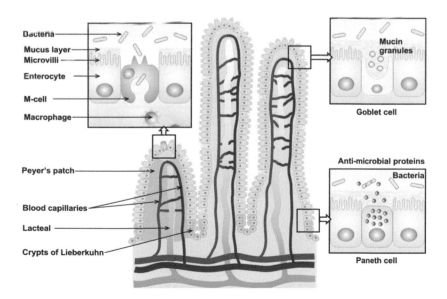

FIGURE 2.2 Schematic illustrations of the structure of the intestinal epithelium and its barrier function against exogenous pathogens; the cell types shown are enterocytes, goblet cells, Paneth cells and the M cells in Peyer's patches. (Reprinted from *Biomaterials*, 32, Chen, M.C., Sonaje, K., Chen, K.J., Sung, H.W. A review of the prospects for polymeric nanoparticle platforms in oral insulin delivery, 9826–38, Copyright 2011, with permission from Elsevier.)

proteins (Figure 2.3) (Ward et al. 2000; Laukoetter et al. 2006). Claudins form the seal between adjacent cells, plaque proteins give structural support, and regulatory proteins regulate signal transductions (Ma and Anderson 2006).

The polymeric nanoparticles protect the drug from degradative enzymes present in the gastrointestinal tract and low pH of the stomach and have the ability to improve their transmucosal transport (des Rieux et al. 2006; Plapied et al. 2011; Florence 2012). However, intestinal mucosa is the major barrier to the uptake of the nanoparticle. For uptake, the nanoparticles must stick to and cross this viscoelastic layer that is perpetually secreted and cleared. Mucoadhesive nanoparticles with a positive charge have been developed to increase the interaction with the mucus and extend the mucosal retention of the nanoparticles. However, developed nanoparticles are attached in loosely adherent mucus layer and cleared rapidly (Ensign et al. 2012). Therefore, nanoparticles should be designed in such a way that penetrates the mucus and releases the drugs and/or nanoparticles containing drugs closer to the epithelium. Lai et al. developed pegylated muco-inert nanoparticles by attaching dense, low-molecular-weight polyethylene glycol that penetrated the mucus (Lai et al. 2009). Moreover, nanoparticles of smaller sizes are rapidly taken up in comparison to larger particles (des Rieux et al. 2006). Specific cells in the gastrointestinal tract such as M cells, enterocytes, and goblet cells are involved in the uptake and transcytosis of orally delivered nanoparticles (Figure 2.4). M cells are a particularly attractive target for oral nanoparticulate drug delivery. M cells are located in the gut-associated lymphoid tissue or follicle associated epithelium

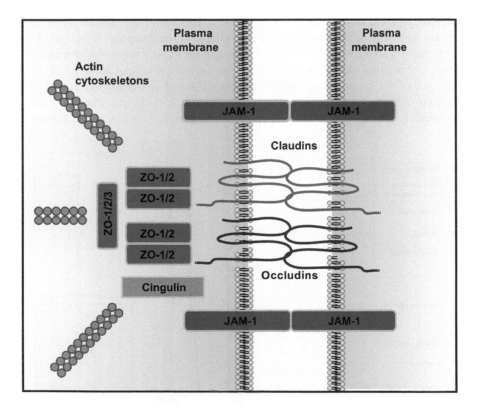

FIGURE 2.3 Schematic illustrations of the tight junctions (TJs) between contiguous epithelial cells. TJs located at the apical domains of epithelial cells consist of a complex of transmembrane [e.g., claudins, occludins and junctional adhesion molecules (JAMs)] and cytoplasmic (e.g., ZO-1, ZO-2, ZO-3, cingulin) proteins. ZO-1 proteins are a linkage molecule between transmembrane proteins and actin cytoskeletons and play an important role in the rearrangement of cell-cell contacts. (Reprinted from *Biomaterials*, 32, Chen, M.C., Sonaje, K., Chen, K.J., Sung, H.W. A review of the prospects for polymeric nanoparticle platforms in oral insulin delivery, 9826–38, Copyright 2011, with permission from Elsevier.)

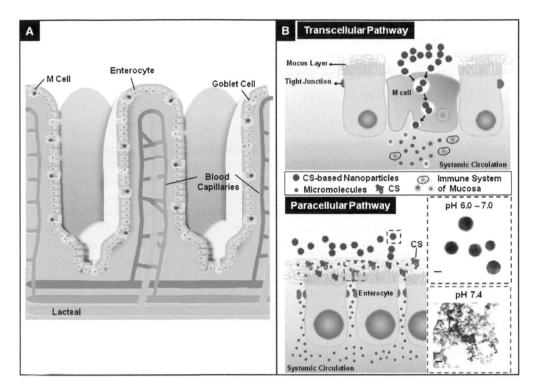

FIGURE 2.4 Schematic illustrations of (A) the structure of the intestinal epithelium comprising enterocytes, goblet cells and M cells in Peyer's patches; (B) the presumed mechanisms of the transcellular and paracellular transport of macromolecules. (Reprinted from *Adv Drug Deliv Rev*, 65, Chen, M.C., Mi, F.L., Liao, Z.X., Hsiao, C.W., Sonaje, K., Chung, M.F., Hsu, L.W., and Sung, H.W. Recent advances in chitosan-based nanoparticles for oral delivery of macromolecules, 865–79, Copyright 2013, with permission from Elsevier.)

of Peyer's patches (Azizi et al. 2010; Brayden et al. 2005; Corr et al. 2005). To induce immune responses, M cells deliver foreign material from the intestinal lumen to the lymphoid tissues. They also transport a wide range of materials including viruses, bacteria, and antigens from the intestinal lumen to the lymphoid tissues (des Rieux et al. 2006).

Enterocytes in the intestine are accountable for transporting nutrients and nanoparticles via passive diffusion or active transport (Johnson et al. 2006). Goblet cells are the second most abundant cells in the intestine that produce barriers against pathogens by secreting mucus (Neutra et al. 1977; Neutra and Leblond 1966).

The paracellular or transcellular route are present in the intestine for the uptake of nanoparticles (Bourdet et al. 2006). Paracellular and transcellular transport of macromolecules can be increased by using chitosan polysaccharide (Lin et al. 2007; Angelova and Hunkeler 2001). Chitosan-based nanoparticles are taken up through transcellular pathways by enterocytes or M cells (Figure 2.1) (Behrens et al.2002). Kadiyala et al. showed that nanoparticle transport is increased 5-fold through the M cell co-culture model in comparison to intestinal caco-2 cell monolayers (Kadiyala et al. 2010). Nanoparticle uptake through intestinal epithelial cells can be improved by increasing the mucoadhesive ability of the nanoparticles (Acosta 2009; Takeuchi et al. 2001; Yin et al. 2009). Various studies have demonstrated the efficiency of the mucoadhesive chitosan-based nanoparticle in augmenting their intestinal transcellular permeability (Magdalena Canali et al. 2012; Borges et al. 2006; Woitiski et al. 2011).

In spite of the hopeful results obtained for nanoparticles with suitable size, surface properties, and mucoadhesiveness, the *in vivo* therapeutic efficacy of the drugs in general remains low (Florence 2005; McNeela et al. 2012; Mrsny 2012; O'Donnell and Williams 2011; Florence 2012). Conjugation of the nanoparticle surface with specific ligands for epithelial receptors might enhance the transepithelial transport of the nanoparticles (Plapied et al. 2011; Devriendt et al. 2012) (Figure 2.5).

2.4 ORAL DELIVERY OF POLYSACCHARIDE NANOPARTICLE-LOADED BIOACTIVE AGENTS

2.4.1 CHITOSAN NANOPARTICLES

Chitosan is a natural polysaccharide obtained from the partial deacetylation of chitin. It is a mucoadhesive polymer widely used to augment cellular permeability and increase the oral bioavailability of administered drugs. It was reported that chitosan binds to cell membranes and reduces cell monolayer transepithelial electrical resistance as well as to augment paracellular permeability (Dodane et al. 1999; Artursson et al. 1994). Moreover, paracellular and transcellular transport of chitosan solutions depends on the chitosan's degree of deacetylation and molecular weight (Schipper et al 1996). Positive charges on the chitosan interact with membrane's tight junction protein resulting in plasma membrane destabilization and an increase in permeability (Fang et al. 2001; Dodane et al. 1999).

Modifications to chitosan have been made to improve permeation and mucoadhesion. Incorporation of thiol groups enhanced mucoadhesion through disulfide bond formation with cysteine residues present in mucin (Bernkop-Schnürch et al. 2004). Moreover, thiolated polymers with reduced glutathione improve permeability by interfering with closing of the tight junctions (Bernkop-Schnürch et al. 2003). Chitosan nanoparticles are an ideal oral delivery vehicle because of their ultrafine size, increased retention in oral mucosa, and longer release times of the drug.

Chitosan nanoparticles enhanced protein drug uptake more efficiently than chitosan solutions (Fernandez-Urrusuno et al. 1999; Pan et al. 2002; Ma et al. 2005). Chitosan nanoparticles loaded with insulin and incubated in caco-2 cells resulted in greater cell binding and uptake in comparison

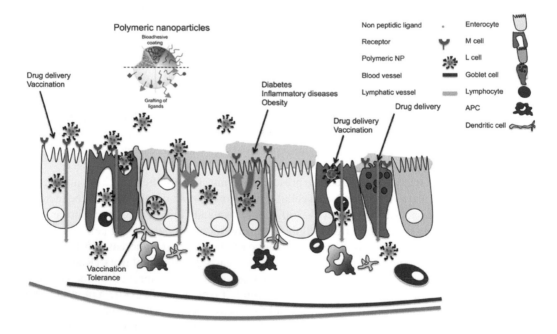

FIGURE 2.5 Schematic representation of polymeric nanoparticle targeting for oral drug delivery as a function of cell type. (Reprinted from *Adv Drug Deliv Rev*, 65, des Rieux, A., Pourcelle, V., Cani, P.D., Marchand-Brynaert, J. and Préat, V. Targeted nanoparticles with novel non-peptidic ligands for oral delivery, 833–44, Copyright 2013, with permission from Elsevier.)

to chitosan solution containing insulin (Ma and Lim 2003). It was observed that after 2 h incubation, chitosan nanoparticles localized inside the cell, however chitosan in solution remained extracellular. Chitosan nanoparticles loaded with cyclosporine A have been developed and orally administered to dogs (El-Shabouri 2002). Chitosan nanoparticles improved the bioavailability of the drug 73% in comparison to the commercial microemulsion product Neoral®. Oral delivery of calcitonin-loaded chitosan-coated lipid nanoparticles to rats reduced the serum calcium level 27% (Prego et al. 2005). This reduction of calcium was considerably greater in comparison to calcitonin solution containing calcitonin or un-coated lipid nanoemulsion containing calcitonin.

Chitosan nanoparticles containing catechins were prepared by the ionic gelation method (Dudhani and Kosaraju 2010). The prepared nanoparticles were in the size range of 110–130 nm. An *in vitro* release study revealed that chitosan nanoparticles have the potential for the sustained release of catechin in the gastrointestinal tract (Dudhani and Kosaraju 2010). Similarly, chitosan nanoparticles were used as carriers for delivery of tea catechins (Hu et al. 2008). Tea polyphenols degradation risk in the gastrointestinal tract was reduced by encapsulating tea polyphenols in chitosan nanoparticles (Sang et al. 2005; Kim and Hong 2010). *In vitro* gastrointestinal absorption of epigallocatechin gallate and green tea catechin can be enhanced by incorporating into chitosan nanoparticles (Dube et al. 2010). The main goal of the development of chitosan nanoparticles for insulin oral delivery is to protect the drug from the harsh acidic environment of the stomach. The pH responsive chitosan nanoparticles were prepared to improve oral insulin delivery (Pan et al. 2002). It was observed that the release of insulin was faster at pH 4.0 whereas slower at pH 5.8 and release of the drug followed the dissociation mechanism. Tokumitsu et al. also observed similar results (Tokumitsu et al. 1999). For successful oral delivery of insulin, self-assembled chitosan nanoparticles were prepared (Mao et al. 2006). It was observed that polyelectrolyte complexation was formed between negatively charged insulin and positively charged chitosan. Furthermore, polyelectrolyte complex was proficient in defending insulin from degradation for 6 h at 50 °C. In addition, nanoparticles could be effectively frozen and dried without compromising the size of the particles and insulin stability. Effects of polyethylene glycol-grafted trimethyl chitosan on insulin uptake were investigated (Mao et al. 2005). Nanocomplexes were synthesized by the self-assembling of the negatively charged insulin and the positively charged chitosan. The nanoparticles released insulin in a pH-dependent manner. Recent advances in using chitosan-based nanoparticles loaded with bioactive agents are represented in Table 2.1.

2.4.2 ALGINATE NANOPARTICLES

Alginate is anionic polysaccharide derived from marine brown algae. It is a natural, biodegradable, and mucoadhesive polymer devoid of toxicity after oral administration (Draget and Tylor 2011; Downs et al. 1992). Alginate has been widely investigated as a nanocarrier in drug delivery devices in which the release rate of the drug can be improved by varying the interaction of the drug and polymer (Nair and Laurencin 2007). Moreover, it is mucoadhesive and used in a controlled drug delivery system to enhance drug bioavailability (Pandey and Ahmad 2011). Alginate nanoparticles can be prepared easily using the ionotropic gelation method with calcium ions (Li et al. 2008; Machado et al. 2012). This technique offers several advantages including being a single step process, not requiring specialized equipment, requiring less toxic reagents, and having a low cost. Sarmento et al. prepared alginate nanoparticles loaded with insulin with an iontotropic gelation method for oral insulin delivery (Sarmento et al. 2007). The prepared nanoparticles showed an entrapment efficiency of 72.8% with a diameter of 750 nm. To improve the oral bioavailability of antifungal drugs, econazole and clotrimazole was encapsulated in alginate-stabilized nanoparticles or polylactide-co-glycolide nanoparticles (Pandey et al. 2005). More than 90% drug entrapment was obtained in alginate nanoparticulate formulation, whereas only about 50% occurred in the case of polylactide-co-glycolide nanoparticulate formulation. An *in vivo* pharmacokinetic and biodistribution study on mice suggested that the drug was released for 5–6 days with each of the nanoparticulate

TABLE 2.1

Examples of Chitosan-Based Nanoparticulate System for Oral Delivery of Bioactive Agent

Bioactive Agent	Research Finding	Reference
Insulin	Hypoglycemic effect lasted for at least 10 h	Sonaje et al. 2009
Exeddin	Bioavailability was 15%	Nguyen et al. 2011
Heparin	Anti-factor Xa activity in plasma was maintained for up to 12 h	Chen et al. 2009
Epigallocatechin gallate	Efficacy of epigallocatechin gallate against rabbit atherosclerosis was considerably enhanced	Hong et al. 2014
Epigallocatechin gallate	Intestinal permeability and absorption of epigallocatechin gallate was improved	Hu et al. 2012
Insulin	Greater hypoglycemic effect for a long period of time	Sonaje et al. 2010
Insulin	Prolong and control the release of insulin	Cui et al. 2006
Quercetin	Nanoparticles exhibited non-toxic behavior in HepG2 liver cells	Aluani et al. 2017
Naringenin	Naringenin nanoparticles have better effectiveness in lowering blood glucose levels in comparison to free drug	Maity et al. 2017
Fucoidan	Release of the drug from nanoparticles increased when pH levels changed from 2.5 to 7.4.	Huang et al. 2014
Sunitinib	Sustained release was obtained with 69% released within 72 h.	John et al. 2016
Tamoxifen citrate	Nanoparticles improved the drug passage across the rat intestinal tissue.	Barbieri et al. 2015
Scutellarin	Bioavailability of drug was increased 2–3 fold	Wang et al. 2017
Enoxaparin	Only 2% drug was released in simulated gastric fluid but 60% in simulated intestinal fluid	Bagre et al. 2013
Tamoxifen	Permeation of drug across the intestinal epithelium was increased	Barbieri et al. 2015
Alendronate sodium	Release of drug was dependent on pH	Miladi et al. 2015

formulations. Moreover, bioavailability of the drug was increased from both nanoparticulate formulations. The drugs were detected in the liver, lungs, and spleen for 6–8 days in the case of nanoparticles while free drugs were cleared by 12 h. Alginate nanoparticles were prepared for the oral delivery of the anti-tubercular drugs rifampicin, ethambutol, isoniazid, and pyrazinamide (Ahmad et al. 2006). The average size of a nanoparticle was 235.5 nm with a polydispersity index of 0.44. The bioavailabilities of all drugs entrapped in the alginate nanoparticles were considerably higher in comparison to free drugs. Nanoparticulate formulation maintains drug levels above the minimum inhibitory concentration for up to 15 days whereas free drugs stayed for only 1 day.

Existing drug delivery systems for the treatment of *H. pylori*-induced disorders have failed due to either inappropriate mucoadhesion or mucopenetration. Novel mucopenetrating alginate-chitosan polyelectrolyte complex nanoparticles were prepared to eradicate *H. pylori*-induced disorders (Arora et al. 2011). The prepared nanoparticles showed low *in vitro* mucoadhesion in comparison to chitosan nanoparticles. However, the prepared nanoparticles exhibited outstanding mucopenetration and localization in the gastric mucosa constantly for over 6 h, which clinically can help in the eradication of *H. pylori*.

2.4.3 DEXTRAN NANOPARTICLES

Dextran is a polysaccharide made of various glucose molecules. The natural dextran structure can be modified by reacting various hydrophobic molecules with its various hydroxyl groups (Lemarchand et al. 2003). It is neutral, biocompatible, water soluble, and biodegradable. Both dextran and its derivatives have prospective application in the novel drug delivery system, and particularly the nanodrug delivery system, for the oral delivery of bioactive agents (Coviello et al. 2007; Aumelas et al. 2007; Chen et al. 2003; Gavory et al. 2011). Dextran is a very useful biomaterial in the nanomedicine field and a lot of researchers are currently working on the preparation of nanosystems.

Nanoparticles were prepared using dextran sulfate and polyethylenimine for oral insulin delivery (Tiyaboonchai et al. 2003). The prepared nanoparticles were spherical in shape with an average particle size of 250 nm and +30 mV zeta potential. The highest encapsulation efficiency was 90%. The rapid release of insulin was observed in an *in vitro* dissolution study. The *in vivo* study in rats exhibited a prolonged hypoglycemic effect. Vitamin B12-conjugated dextran nanoparticles were prepared for the oral delivery of insulin (Chalasani et al. 2007). The prepared nanoparticles exhibited intense blood glucose reductions (70%–75%) and anti-diabetic effects in streptozotocin-induced diabetic rats for about 54 h.

Nanoparticles were prepared using periodate-oxidized dextran to improve nanoformulation stability and a sustained oral delivery of the hydrophobic drug indomethacin (Yuan et al. 2006; Xu et al. 2005). Nanoformulations served as good depots for indomethacin and released the drug up to 14 days.

2.4.4 PECTIN NANOPARTICLES

Pectin is a plant cell wall structural component obtained from natural resources (May 1990). It is extracted from various citrus products including the pomace, apple, and orange under slightly acidic conditions. Pectin is divided into low methoxyl pectin and high methoxyl pectin (Grant et al. 1973). Pectin has been extensively studied in drug delivery. Pectin is a prospective carrier for colon targeted drug delivery due to the degradation of pectin in colonic microorganisms. β-lactoglobulin is the whey protein that binds to hydrophobic ligands, giving it potential for transporting drugs, specifically for colon cancer. Pectin nanoparticles containing β-lactoglobulin were prepared to deliver anticancer platinum complex to the colon (Izadi et al. 2016). Release of the drug in simulated gastrointestinal conditions showed that β-lactoglobulin is stable in acidic conditions but is capable of releasing the drug at pH 7. Citrus pectin nanoparticles coated with Eudragit S100 were prepared for the delivery of 5-fluorouracil to the colon (Subudhi et al. 2015). Galectin-3 receptors are over expressed in colorectal cancer cells and citrus pectin acts as a ligand for these receptors. More than 70% of the drug was released in the colonic region after 24 h. *In vitro* cytotoxicity assay showed 1.5-fold higher cytotoxicity of nanoparticles in comparison to the solution of 5-fluorouracil against HT-29 cancer cells. *In vivo* data showed that eudragit S100 shielded nanoparticles in the harsh environment of the stomach to help the particles reach the colon.

2.5 CONCLUSION

Numerous studies suggest that nanoparticles may be useful in oral drug delivery systems. Nanoparticles based on natural polymers such as polysaccharides have emerged as the preferred choice of material due to their low/non-toxicity and immunogenicity. Additionally, polysaccharide nanoparticles also exhibit greater advantages in biocompatibility, biodegradability, and the ability to adhere to the body's mucosal linings. The uptake of nanoparticles is clearly size-dependent and smaller nanoparticles are taken up to a much greater degree in comparison to larger nanoparticles. Encapsulation of a bioactive agent into nanoparticles was shown to improve the efficacy and bioavailability of a number of drugs compared to a conventional dosage form.

REFERENCES

Acosta, E. 2009. Bioavailability of nanoparticles in nutrient and nutraceutical delivery. *Colloid Interface Sci* 14: 3–15.
Ahmad, Z., Pandey, R., Sharma, S., and Khuller, G.K. 2006. Pharmacokinetic and pharmacodynamic behaviour of antitubercular drugs encapsulated in alginate nanoparticles at two doses. *Int J Antimicrob Agents* 27 (5): 409–16.

Aluani, D., Tzankova, V., Kondeva-Burdina, M., Yordanov, Y., Nikolova, E., Odzhakov, F. et al. 2017. Evaluation of biocompatibility and antioxidant efficiency of chitosan-alginate nanoparticles loaded with quercetin. *Int J Biol Macromol* 103: 771–82.

Angelova, N. and Hunkeler, D. 2001. Effect of preparation conditions on properties and permeability of chito-sansodium hexametaphosphate capsules. *J Biomater Sci Polym Ed* 12: 1317–37.

Arora, S., Gupta, S., Narang, R.K., and Budhiraja, R.D. 2011. Amoxicillin loaded chitosan-alginate poly-electrolyte complex nanoparticles as mucopenetrating delivery system for h. Pylori. *Sci Pharm* 9 (3): 673–94.

Artursson, P., Lindmark, T., Davis, S.S., and Illum, L. 1994. Effect of chitosan on the permeability of mono-layers of intestinal epithelial cells (Caco-2). *Pharm Res* 11: 1358–61.

Aumelas, A., Serrero, A., Durand, A., Dellacherie, E., and Leonard, M. 2007. Nanoparticles of hydrophobi-cally modified dextrans as potential drug carrier systems. *Colloids Surf B Biointerfaces* 59: 74–80.

Azizi, A., Kumar, A., Diaz-Mitoma, F., and Mestecky, J. 2010. Enhancing oral vaccine potency by targeting intestinal M cells. *PLoS Pathog* 6: e1001147.

Bagre, A.P., Jain, K., and Jain, N.K. 2013. Alginate coated chitosan core shell nanoparticles for oral delivery of enoxaparin: In vitro and in vivo assessment. *Int J Pharm* 456: 31–40.

Balcerzak, S.P., Lane, W.C., and Bullard, J.W. 1970. Surface structure of intestinal epithelium. *Gastroenterology* 1970 (58): 49–55.

Barbieri, S., Buttini, F., Rossi, A., Bettini, R., Colombo, P., Ponchel, G. et al. 2015. Ex vivo permeation of tamoxifen and its 4-OH metabolite through rat intestine from lecithin/chitosan nanoparticles. *Int J Pharm* 491: 99–104.

Behrens, I., Pena, A.I.V., Alonso, M.J., and Kissel, T. 2002. Comparative uptake studies of bioadhesive and non-bioadhesive nanoparticles in human intestinal cell lines and rats: The effect of mucus on particle adsorption and transport. *Pharm Res* 19: 1185–93.

Bernkop-Schnürch, A., Guggi, D., and Pinter, Y. 2004. Thiolated chitosans: Development and in vitro evalua-tion of a mucoadhesive, permeation enhancing oral drug delivery system. *J Control Release* 94: 177–86.

Bernkop-Schnürch, A., Kast, C.E., and Guggi, D. 2003. Permeation enhancing polymers in oral delivery of hydrophilic macromolecules: Thiomer/GSH systems. *J Control Release* 93: 95–103.

Borges, O., Cordeiro-da-Silva, A., Romeijn, S.G., Amidi, M., De Sousa, Borchard, G., and Junginger, H.E. 2006. Uptake studies in rat Peyer's patches, cytotoxicity and release studies of alginate coated chitosan nanoparticles formucosal vaccination. *J Control Release* 114: 348–58.

Bourdet, D.L., Pollack, G.M., and Thakker, D.R. 2006. Intestinal absorptive transport of the hydrophilic cat-ion ranitidine: A kinetic modeling approach to elucidate the role of uptake and efflux transporters and paracellular vs. transcellular transport in Caco-2 cells. *Pharm Res* 23: 1178–87.

Brayden, D.J., Jepson, M.A., and Baird, A.W. 2005. Keynote review: Intestinal Peyer's patch M cells and oral vaccine targeting. *Drug Discov Today* 10: 1145–57.

Chalasani, K.B., Russell-Jones, G.J., Jain, A.K., Diwan, P.V. and Jain, S.K. 2007. Effective oral delivery of insulin in animal models using vitamin B_{12}-coated dextran nanoparticles. *J Control Release* 122 (2): 141–50.

Chen, M.C., Wong, H.S., Lin, K.J., Chen, H.L., Wey, S.P., Sonaje, K. et al. 2009. The characteristics, biodis-tribution and bioavailability of a chitosan-based nanoparticulate system for the oral delivery of heparin. *Biomaterials* 30: 6629–37.

Chen, X.G., Lee, C.M., and Park, H.J. 2003. O/W emulsification for the self-aggregation and nanoparticle formation of linoleic acid-modified chitosan in the aqueous system. *J Agric Food Chem* 51: 3135–9.

Cheng, H. and Leblond, C.P. 1974. Origin, differentiation and renewal of the four main epithelial cell types in the mouse small intestine I. Columnar cell. *Am J Anat* 141: 461–79.

Cornes, J.S. 1965. Number, size, and distribution of Peyer's patches in the human small intestine. *Gut* 6: 225–9.

Corr, S.C., Gahan, C.C., and Hill, C. 2008. M-cells: Origin, morphology and role inmucosal immunity and microbial pathogenesis, FEMS Immunol. *Med Microbiol* 52: 2–12.

Coviello, T., Matricardi, P., Marianecci, C., and Alhaique, F. 2007. Polysaccharide hydrogels for modified release formulations. *J Control Release* 119: 5–24.

Cui, F., Shi, K., Zhang, L., Tao, A., and Kawashima, Y. 2006. Biodegradable nanoparticles loaded with insu-lin–phospholipid complex for oral delivery: Preparation, in vitro characterization and in vivo evalua-tion. *J Controlled Release* 114: 242–50.

des Rieux, A., Fievez, V., Garinot, M., Schneider, Y.J., and Préat, V. 2006. Nanoparticles as potential oral delivery systems of proteins and vaccines: A mechanistic approach. *J Control Release* 116: 1–27.

Devriendt, B., De Geest, B.G., Goddeeris, B.M., and Cox, E. 2012. Crossing the barrier: targeting epithelial receptors for enhanced oral vaccine delivery. *J Control Release* 160: 431–9.

Dodane, V., Khan, M.A., and Merwin, J.R. 1999. Effect of chitosan on epithelial permeability and structure. *Int J Pharm* 182: 21–32.

Downs, E.C., Robertson, N.E., Riss, T.L., and Plunkett, M.L. 1992. Calcium alginate beads as a slowrelease system for delivering angiogenic molecules *in vivo* and *in vitro*. *J Cell Physiol* 152: 422–9.

Draget, K.I. and Tylor, C. 2011. Chemical, physical and biological properties of alginates and their biomedical implications. *Food Hydrocoll* 25: 251–6.

Dube, A., Nicolazzo, J.A., and Larson, I. 2010. Chitosan nanoparticles enhance the intestinal absorption of the green tea catechins (þ)-catechin and (-)-epigallocatechin gallate. *Eur J Pharm Sci* 41 (2): 219–25.

Dudhani, A.R. and Kosaraju, S.L. 2010. Bioadhesive chitosan nanoparticles: Preparation and characterization. *Carbohydr Polym* 81(2): 243–51.

El-Shabouri, M.H. 2002. Positively charged nanoparticles for improving the oral bioavailability of cyclosporin-A. *Int J Pharm* 249: 101–8.

Ensign, L.M., Schneider, C., Suk, J.S., Cone, R., and Hanes, J. 2012. Mucus penetrating nanoparticles: Biophysical tool and method of drug and gene delivery. *Adv Mater* 24: 3887–94.

Fang, N., Chan, V., Mao, H.Q., and Leong, K.W. 2001. Interactions of phospholipid bilayer with chitosan: Effect of molecular weight and pH. *Biomacromolecules* 2: 1161–8.

Fernández-Urrusuno, R., Calvo, P., Remuñán-López, C., Vila-Jato, J.L., and Alonso, M.J. 1999. Enhancement of nasal absorption of insulin using chitosan nanoparticles. *Pharm Res* 16: 1576–81.

Florence, A. 1997. The oral absorption of Micro- and Nanoparticulates: Neither exceptional nor Unusual. *Pharm Res* 14: 259–66.

Florence, A.T. 2005. Nanoparticle uptake by the oral route: fulfilling its potential? *Drug Discov Today Technol* 2: 75–81.

Florence, A.T. 2012. "Targeting" nanoparticles: The constraints of physical laws and physical barriers. *J Control Release* 164: 115–24.

Gaumet, M., Gurny, R., and Delie, F. 2009. Localization and quantification of biodegradable particles in an intestinal cell model: The influence of particle size. *Eur J Pharm Sci* 36: 465–73.

Gavory, C., Durand, A., Six, J.L., Nouvel, C., Marie, E., and Leonard, M. 2011. Polysaccharide-covered nanoparticles prepared by nanoprecipitation. *Carbohydr Polym* 84: 133–40.

Giri, T.K., Bhowmick, S., and Maity, S. 2017. Entrapment of capsaicin loaded nanoliposome in pH responsive hydrogel beads for colonic delivery. *J Drug Deliv Sci Technol* 39: 417–22.

Giri, T.K., Giri, A., Barman, T.K., and Maity, S. 2016a. Nanoliposome is a promising carrier of protein and peptide biomolecule for the treatment of cancer. *Anticancer Agents Med Chem* 16: 816–31.

Giri, T.K., Pradhan, M., and Tripathi, D.K. 2016b. Synthesis of graft copolymer of kappa-carrageenan using microwave energy and studies of swelling capacity, flocculation properties, and preliminary acute toxicity. *Turk J Chem* 40: 283–95.

Giri, T.K., Verma, D., and Tripathi, D.K. 2015. Effect of adsorption parameters on biosorption of Pb^{++} ions from aqueous solution by poly (acrylamide)-grafted kappa-carrageenan. *Polym Bull* 72: 1625–46.

Grant, G.T., Morris, E.R., Rees, D.A., Smith, P.J.C., and Thom, D. 1973. Biological interactions between polysaccharides and divalent cations: The Egg-box model. *Febs Lett* 32: 195–98.

Guo, J., Fisher, K.A., Darcy, R., Cryan, J.F., and O'Driscoll, C. 2010. Therapeutic targeting in the silent era: Advances in non-viral siRNA delivery. *Mol BioSyst* 6: 1143–61.

He, C., Yin, L., Tang, C., and Yin, C. 2012. Size-dependent absorption mechanism of polymeric nanoparticles for oral delivery of protein drugs. *Biomaterials* 33: 8569–78.

Hellmich, M.R. and Evers, B.M. 2006. Regulation of gastrointestinal normal cell growth. In: Johnson, L. (Ed.), *Physiology of the Gastrointestinal Tract*, 435–58. 4th ed. Burlington, MA: Academic Press.

Hong, Z., Xu, Y., Yin, J.F., Jin, J., Jiang, Y., and Du, Q. 2014. Improving the effectiveness of (-)-epigallocatechin gallate (EGCG) against rabbit atherosclerosis by EGCG loaded nanoparticles prepared from chitosan and polyaspartic acid. *J Agric Food Chem* 62 (52): 12603–9.

Hu, B., Pan, C., Sun, Y., Hou, Z., Ye, H., and Zeng, X. 2008. Optimization of fabrication parameters to produce chitosan-tripolyphosphate nanoparticles for delivery of tea catechins. *J Agric Food Chem* 56 (16): 7451–8.

Hu, B., Ting, Y.W., Zeng, X.X., and Huang, Q.R. 2012. Cellular uptake and cytotoxicity of chitosan-caseinophosphopeptides nanocomplexes loaded with epigallocatechin gallate. *Carbohydr Polym* 89 (2): 362–70.

Huang, Y.C., Chen, J.K., Lam, U.I., and Chen, S.Y. 2014. Preparing, characterizing and evaluating chitosan/fucoidan nanoparticles as oral delivery carriers. *J Polym Res* 21: 415.

Izadi, Z., Divsalar, A., Saboury, A.A., and Sawyer, L. 2016. β-lactoglobulin-pectin nanoparticle-based oral drug delivery system for potential treatment of colon cancer. *Chem Biol Drug Des* 88 (2): 209–16.

Jevsevar, S., Kunstelj, M., and Porekar, V.G. 2010. PEGylation of therapeutic proteins. *Biotechnol J* 5: 113–28.

John, J., Sangeetha, D., and Gomathi, T. 2016. Sunitinib loaded chitosan nanoparticles formulation and its evaluation. *Int J Biol Macromol* 82: 952–58.

Johnson, L.R., Barret, K.E., Gishan, F.K., Merchant, J.L., Said, H.M., and Wood, J.D. 2006. *Physiology of the gastrointestinal tract*. In: Wright, E.M., Loo, D.D.F., Hirayama, B.A., and Turk, E. (Eds.), *Sugar Absorption*, 1653–65. 4th ed. San Diego: Elsevier Inc.

Kadiyala, I., Loo, Y., Roy, K., Rice, J., and Leong, K.W. 2010. Transport of chitosan–DNA nanoparticles in human intestinal M-cell model versus normal intestinal enterocytes. *Eur J Pharm Sci* 39: 103–9.

Kim, M.R. and Hong, J. 2010. Analysis of chemical interactions of (-)-epigallocatechin- 3-gallate, a major green tea polyphenol, with commonly consumed over-the counter drugs. *Food Sci Biotechnol* 19 (2): 559–64.

Kreuter, J. 1983. Evaluation of nanoparticles as drug-delivery systems. II. Comparison of the body distribution of nanoparticles with the body distribution of microspheres (diameter & gt; 1 μm), liposomes, and emulsions. *Pharm Acta Helv* 58: 217–26.

Kreuter, J. 1990. Large-scale production problems and manufacturing of nanoparticles. In: P. Tyle (Ed.), *Specialized drug delivery systems*, 257–66. New York: Marcel Dekker.

Kreuter, J. 1991. Peroral administration of nanoparticles. *Adv Drug Deliv Rev* 7: 71–86.

Lai, S.K., Wang, Y.Y., and Hanes, J. 2009. Mucus-penetrating nanoparticles for drug and gene delivery to mucosal tissues. *Adv Drug Deliv Rev* 61: 158–71.

Laukoetter, M.G., Bruewer, M., and Nusrat, A. 2006. Regulation of the intestinal epithelial barrier by the apical junctional complex. *Curr Opin Gastroenterol* 22: 85–9.

Lemarchand, C., Couvreur, P., Vauthier, C., Costantini, D., and Gref, R. 2003. Study of emulsion stabilization by graft copolymers using the optical analyzer Turbiscan. *Int J Pharm* 254: 77–82.

Li, X., Kong, X., Shi, S., Zheng, X., Guo, G., Wei, Y., et al. 2008. Preparation of alginate coated chitosan microparticles for vaccine delivery. *BMC Biotechnol* 8: 89–99.

Lin, Y.H., Mi, F.L., Chen, C.T., Chang, W.C., Peng, S.F., Liang, H.F., and Sung, H.W. 2007. Preparation and characterization of nanoparticles shelled with chitosan for oral insulin delivery. *Biomacromolecules* 8: 146–52.

Longmire, M., Choyke, P.L., and Kobayashi, H. 2008. Clearance properties of nano-sized particles and molecules as imaging agents: Considerations and caveats. *Nanomedicine-UK* 3: 703–17.

Ma, T.Y. and Anderson, J.M. 2006. Tight junctions and the intestinal barrier. In: Johnson, L. (Ed.), *Physiology of the Gastrointestinal Tract*. 4th ed., 1559–94 Burlington, MA: Academic Press.

Ma, Z. and Lim, L.Y. 2003. Uptake of chitosan and associated insulin in Caco-2 cell monolayers: A comparison between chitosan molecules and chitosan nanoparticles. *Pharm Res* 20: 1812–9.

Ma, Z., Lim, T.M., and Lim, L.Y. 2005. Pharmacological activity of peroral chitosaninsulin nanoparticles in diabetic rats. *Int J Pharm* 293: 271–80.

Machado, A.H., Lundberg, D., Ribeiro, A.J., Veiga, F.J., Lindman, B., Miguel, M.G., et al. 2012. Preparation of calcium alginate nanoparticles using waterinoil (W/O) nanoemulsions. *Langmuir* 28: 4131–41.

Magdalena Canali, M., Pedrotti, L., Balsinde, J., Ibarra, C., and Correa, S.G. 2012. Chitosan enhances transcellular permeability in human and rat intestine epithelium. *Eur J Pharm Biopharm* 80: 418–25.

Maity, S., Mukhopadhyay, P., Kundu, P.P., and Chakraborti, A.S. 2017. Alginate coated chitosan core-shell nanoparticles for efficient oral delivery of naringenin in diabetic animals—An in vitro and in vivo approach. *Carbohydr Polym* 170: 124–32.

Mao, S., Bakowsky, U., Jintapattanakit, A., and Kissel, T. 2006. Self-assembled polyelectrolyte nanocomplexes between chitosan derivatives and insulin. *J Pharm Sci* 95: 1035–48.

Mao, S., Germershaus, O., Fischer, D., Linn, T., Schnepf, R., and Kissel, T. 2005. Uptake and transport of PEG-graft-trimethyl-chitosan copolymer–insulin nanocomplexes by epithelial cells. *Pharm Res* 22: 2058–68.

May, C.D. 1990. Industrial pectins, sources, production and applications. *Carbohy Polym* 12: 91–107.

McNeela, E.A. and Lavelle, E.C. 2012. Mucosal vaccines. In: Kozlowski, P.A. (Ed.), *Recent Advances in Microparticle and Nanoparticle Delivery Vehicles for Mucosal Vaccination Mucosal Vaccines*. Berlin Heidelberg: Springer, pp. 75–99.

Miladi, K., Sfar, S., Fessi, H., and Elaissari, A. 2015. Enhancement of alendronate encapsulation in chitosan nanoparticles. *J Drug Deliv Sci Technol* 30: 391–96.

Mrsny, R.J. 2012. Oral drug delivery research in Europe. *J Control Release* 161: 247–53.

Nair, L.S. and Laurencin, C.T. 2007. Biodegradable polymers as biomaterial. *Prog Polym Sci* 6: 762–98.

Neutra, M., Grand, R., and Trier, J. 1977. Glycoprotein synthesis, transport, and secretion by epithelial cells of human rectal mucosa: Normal and cystic fibrosis. *Lab Invest* 36: 535–46.

Neutra, M. and Leblond, C. 1966. Synthesis of the carbohydrate of mucus in the Golgi complex as shown by electron microscope radioautography of goblet cells from rats injected with glucose-H3. *J Cell Biol* 30: 119–36.

Nguyen, H.N., Wey, S.P., Juang, J.H., Sonaje, K., Ho, Y.C., Chuang, E.Y. et al. 2011. The glucose-lowering potential of exendin-4 orally delivered via a pH-sensitive nanoparticle vehicle and effects on subsequent insulin secretion in vivo. *Biomaterials* 32: 2673–82.

O'Donnell, K.P. and Williams, R.O. 2011. Nanoparticulate systems for oral drug delivery to the colon. *Int J Nanotechnol* 8: 4–20.

Pan, Y., Li, Y.J., Zhao, H.Y., Zheng, J.M., Xu, H., Wei, G. et al. 2002. Bioadhesive polysaccharide in protein delivery system: Chitosan nanoparticles improve the intestinal absorption of insulin in vivo. *Int J Pharm* 249: 139–47.

Pandey, R. and Ahmad, Z. 2011. Nanomedicine and experimental tuberculosis: Facts, flaws, and future. *Nanomedicine* 7: 259–72.

Pandey, R., Ahmad, Z., Sharma, S., and Khuller, G.K. 2005. Nano-encapsulation of azole antifungals: Potential applications to improve oral drug delivery. *Int J Pharm* 301: 268–76.

Pawar, V.K., Meher, J.G., Singh, Y., Chaurasia, M., Surendar Reddy, B., and Chourasia, M.K. 2014. Targeting of gastrointestinal tract for amended delivery of protein/peptide therapeutics: Strategies and industrial perspectives. *J Control Release* 196: 168–83.

Plapied, L., Duhem, N., des Rieux, A., and Préat, V. 2011. Fate of polymeric nanocarriers for oral drug delivery. *Curr Opin Colloid Interface Sci* 16: 228–37.

Prego, C., Garcia, M., Torres, D., and Alonso, M.J. 2005. Transmucosal macromolecular drug delivery. *J Control Release* 101: 151–62.

Prego, C., Torres, D., Fernandez-Megia, E., Novoa-Carballal, R., Quinoa, E., and Alonso, M.J. 2006. Chitosan-PEG nanocapsules as new carriers for oral peptide delivery-effect of chitosan pegylation degree. *J Control Release* 111: 299–308.

Sang, S.M., Lee, M.J., Hou, Z., Ho, C.T., and Yang, C.S. 2005. Stability of tea polyphenol (-)-epigallocatechin-3-gallate and formation of dimers and epimers under common experimental conditions. *J Agric Food Chem* 53 (24): 9478–84.

Sarmento, B., Ribeiro, A., Veiga, F., Sampaio, P., Neufeld, R., and Ferreira, D. 2007. Alginate/chitosan nanoparticles are effective for oral insulin delivery. *Pharm Res* 24: 2198–206.

Schipper, N.G., Vårum, K.M. and Artursson, P. 1996. Chitosans as absorption enhancers for poorly absorbable drugs. 1: Influence of molecular weight and degree of acetylation on drug transport across human intestinal epithelial (Caco-2) cells. *Pharm Res* 13: 1686–92.

Sinha, V.R. and Kumria, R. 2001. Polysaccharides in colon-specific drug delivery. *Int J Pharm* 224: 19–38.

Sonaje, K., Lin, K.J., Wey, S.P., Lin, C.K., Yeh, T.H. et al. 2010. Biodistribution, pharmacodynamics and pharmacokinetics of insulin analogues in a rat model: Oral delivery using pH-responsive nanoparticles vs. subcutaneous injection. *Biomaterials* 31: 6849–58.

Sonaje, K., Lin, Y.H., Juang, J.H., Wey, S.P., Chen, C.T., and Sung, H.W. 2009. In vivo evaluation of safety and efficacy of self-assembled nanoparticles for oral insulin delivery. *Biomaterials* 30: 2329–39.

Subudhi, M.B., Jain, A., Jain, A., Hurkat, P., Shilpi, S., Gulbake, A., and Jain, S.K. 2015. Eudragit S100 coated citrus pectin nanoparticles for colon targeting of 5-fluorouracil. *Materials* 8 (3): 832–49.

Takeuchi, H., Yamamoto, H., and Kawashima, Y. 2001. Mucoadhesive nanoparticulate systems for peptide drug delivery. *Adv Drug Deliv Rev* 47: 39–54.

Tiyaboonchai, W., Woiszwillo, J., Sims, R.C., and Middaugh, C.R. 2003. Insulin containing polyethylenimine-dextran sulfate nanoparticles. *Int J Pharm* 255 (1–2): 139–51.

Tokumitsu, H., Ichikawa, H., and Fukumori, Y. 1999. Chitosan–gadopentetic acid complex nanoparticles for gadolinium neutron-capture therapy of cancer: Preparation by novel emulsion-droplet coalescence technique and characterization. *Pharm Res* 16: 1830–5.

Verma, M.S., Liu, S.Y., Chen, Y.Y., Meerasa, A., and Gu, F.X. 2012. Size-tunable nanoparticles composed of dextran-b-poly(D,L-lactide) for drug delivery applications. *Nano Res* 5: 49–61.

Veronese, F.M. and Pasut, G. 2005. PEGylation, successful approach to drug delivery. *Drug Discov Today* 10: 1451–1458.

Walker, R.I. and Owen, R.L. 1990. Intestinal barriers to bacteria and their toxins. *Annu Rev Med* 41: 393–400.

Wang, J., Tan, J., Luo, J., Huang, P., Zhou, W., Chen, L. et al. 2017. Enhancement of scutellarin oral delivery efficacy by vitamin B12-modified amphiphilic chitosan derivatives to treat type II diabetes induced-retinopathy. *J Nanobiotechnol* 15: 18.

Ward, P.D., Tippin, T.K., and Thakker, D.R. 2000. Enhancing paracellular permeability by modulating epithe-
    lial tight junctions. *Pharm Sci Technolo Today* 3: 346–58.
Watson, A.J., Duckworth, C.A., Guan, Y., and Montrose, M.H. 2009. Mechanisms of epithelial cell shedding
    in the mammalian intestine and maintenance of barrier function. *Ann N Y Acad Sci* 1165: 135–42.
Woitiski, C.B., Sarmento, B., Carvalho, R.A., Neufeld, R.J., and Veiga, F. 2011. Facilitated nanoscale delivery
    of insulin across intestinal membrane models. *Int J Pharm* 412: 123–31.
Wright, E.M., Loo, D.D.F., Hirayama, B.A., and Turk, E. 2006. Sugar Absorption. In: Johnson, L (Ed.),
    Physiology of the Gastrointestinal Tract. 4th ed., 1653–65. Burlington, MA: Academic Press.
Xu, Q., Ensign, L.M., Boylan, N.J., Schon, A., Gong, X., Yang, J.C., et al. 2015. Impact of surface polyethylene
    glycol (PEG) density on biodegradable nanoparticle transport in mucus ex vivo and distribution in vivo.
    ACS Nano 9: 9217–27.
Xu, Q.G., Yuan, X.B., and Chang, J. 2005. Self-aggregates of cholic acid hydrazide-dextran conjugates as drug
    carriers. *J Appl Polym Sci* 95: 487–93.
Yin, L., Ding, J., He, C., Cui, L., Tang, C., and Yin, C. 2009. Drug permeability and mucoadhesion properties
    of thiolated trimethyl chitosan nanoparticles in oral insulin delivery. *Biomaterials* 30: 5691–700.
Yuan, X.B., Li, H., Zhu, X.X., and Woo, H.G. 2006. Self-aggregated nanoparticles composed of periodate-
    oxidized dextran and cholic acid: Preparation, stabilization and in-vitro drug release. *J Chem Technol
    Biotechnol* 81: 746–54.

3 Cellulose-Based Nanocomposites for Pharmaceutical and Biomedical Applications

Manuel Palencia, María E. Berrio,
Angelica García-Quintero, and Tulio A. Lerma

CONTENTS

3.1   INTRODUCTION

It has been reported that changes in the properties of particles can be observed when particle size is less than what is termed "the critical size". For example, catalytic activity (5 nm), paramagnetism and other electromagnetic phenomena (<100 nm), refractive index changes (50 nm), or modifying hardness and plasticity (<100 nm). Additionally, as dimensions reach nanometer level, interactions at phase interfaces become largely improved, and this is important to enhance the materials properties. In this context, the surface area/volume ratio of reinforcement materials employed in the preparation of nanocomposites is crucial to the understanding of their structure-property relationship. Also, it has been reported that the addition of particles to the continuous phase can improve the properties of the material and increase the range of applications (Peigney et al. 2000; Gangopadhyay and Amitabha 2000; Gall et al. 2002).

A nanocomposite can be defined as a solid multiphase structure, where at least one of its phases has dimensions on the nanometer scale (i.e., <100 nm in at least one dimension) (Ray and Okamoto 2003; Pandey et al. 2005; Park et al. 2003; Koo 2006). However, this concept is under discussion because though nanometer scale can be easily defined for systems with defined shapes (particulates, rods, wires, etc.), in many researches, greater dimensions have been used to define the nanometric nature of particles. Recently, an interest in the study of nanocomposite materials has increased due to the excellent mechanical and thermal properties they show in comparison with those observed in their respective source materials when considered individually (Müller et al. 2017). In general, the study of nanocomposites is an interdisciplinary area, including physics, chemistry, biology, materials science, and engineering. Thus, bringing together knowledge from scientists with different backgrounds is a fundamental aspect in the development and application of new nanocomposite materials.

Presently, different types of cellulose at the nanometric scale (i.e., nanocrystals and cellulose nanofibers) have been used as precursors for obtaining nanocomposites. The use of nanocellulose as a filling material has attracted the attention of researchers because it presents a series of advantages, such as, biodegradability, low density, large specific surface area, high relative abundance, easy processability and a wide reactive surface allowing for easy modification. However, the nanocellulose has a high hydrophilicity and there are also a number of important disadvantages that must be mentioned and analyzed with careful consideration because these could affect some applications. For example, the incompatibility of phase between nanocellulose and most polymer matrices has been described, the above is related with phase segregation during the composite preparation, in consequence, a previous stage of compatibilization should be analyzed for many formulations. But also, as a result of the high hydrophilicity, the capture of humidity from the environment by the nanocellulose can be an undesired effect (Ray and Okamoto 2003; Pandey et al. 2005; Park et al. 2003; Moon et al. 2011). In order to account for some of these weaknesses, various nanocellulose types, routes of attainment, and modification strategies have been developed (see Figure 3.1). These aspects will be described in the sections below. Below, a general description of nanocellulose is developed to ease the understanding of its use in the making of nanocomposites and demonstrate the applicability of these materials for pharmaceutical and biomedical applications.

3.2 NANOCELLULOSE TYPES AND PREPARATION METHODS

Cellulose is a homopolysaccharide consisting of a linear chain of several hundred to many thousands of $\beta(1\rightarrow4)$-linked D-glucose units, this biopolymer is the main structural unit of plant cells, as well as fungi, algae, and other living organisms. Its degree of polymerization depends on its origin; it has been estimated that wood cellulose has about 10,000 units of glucopyranose whereas cotton cellulose has ~15,000 (Habibi 2014). Cellulose has the particularity that each monomer unit has three hydroxyl groups (OH), which play an important role in the formation of fibrillar and semicrystalline assemblies, and can also act as reaction sites for chemical modifications (Dufresne 2017). On the other hand, when transverse or longitudinal dissociation of the fibers is generated in the fibrillar-type cellulose assemblies, either by mechanical, chemical or enzymatic processes, new cellulosic structures in nanometric scale are produced and these are known under the term "nanocellulose". These nanostructures can be classified into three categories which are *cellulose nanocrystals* (these nanocrystals exhibit high specific strength, modulus, high surface area, and unique liquid crystal properties), *cellulose nanofibers* (a lightweight material, with a high elastic modulus, which exhibits thermal expansion similar to glass and presents high barrier properties for gases such as oxygen) and *bacterial nanocellulose* (which is clearly defined in function of origin; unlike plant cellulose, this type of nanocellulose is produced in a pure form, without lignin, hemicellulose, pectin or any other compound usually present in plants) (Klemm et al. 2011).

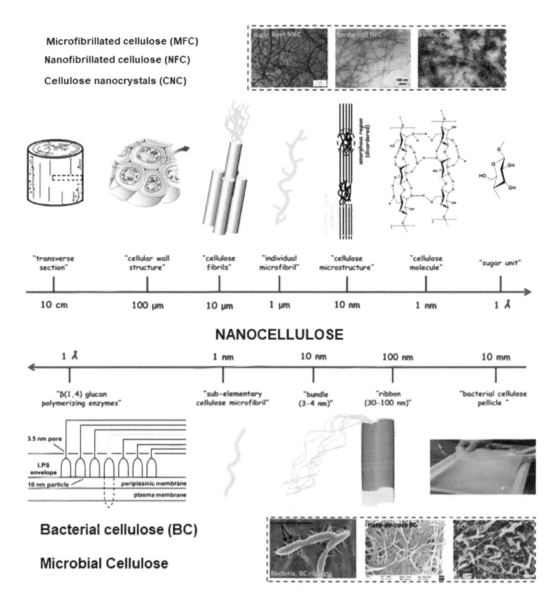

FIGURE 3.1 Hierarchical structure of cellulose; top image (from large unit to small unit): cellulose nanocrystals (CNC), micro/nanofibrillated cellulose (MFC and NFC); bottom image (from tiny unit to small unit): bacterial cellulose (BC). Transmission electron micrographs of sugar beet MFC, hardwood MFC, ramie CNC; and scanning electron micrographs of BC ribbons, nata-de-coco BC, BC pellicle. (Reprinted from *Eur Polym J* 59, Lin, N. and Dufresne, A. Nanocellulose in biomedicine: Current status and future prospect, 302–25, Copyright 2014, with permission from Elsevier.)

A schematic representation of the chemical structure and intra-, inter-molecular hydrogen bonds in crystalline cellulose is shown in Figure 3.2.

The synthesis of cellulose nanocrystals is carried out by acid hydrolysis and the subsequent depolymerization of the cellulose chains. During this process, nanocrystals are formed from hydrolytic rupture and the elimination of biomolecules such as polysaccharides which are attached to the surface of the coarse fibers; when the rupture and elimination of amorphous cellulose regions are produced, the acid can be accessed more easily and generate crystalline sections of smaller cellulose. The process requires control of the degree of depolymerization of the glucose chains in order

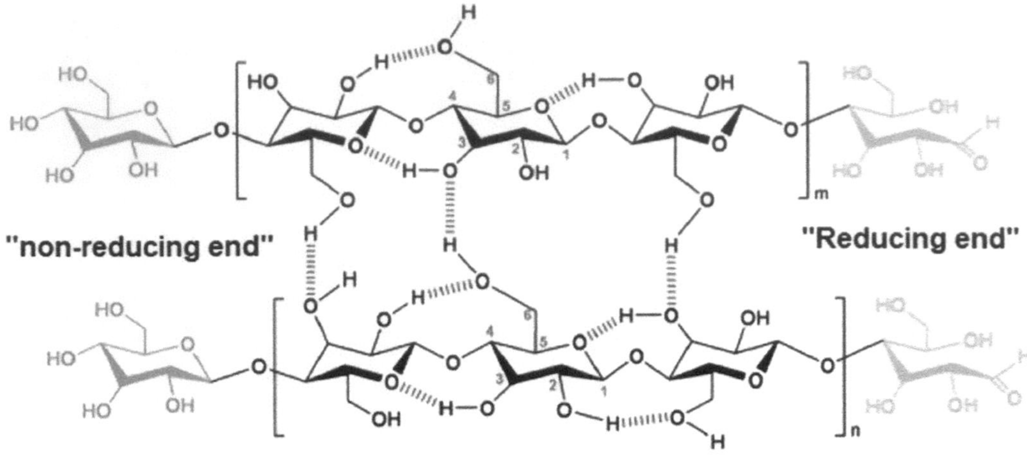

FIGURE 3.2 Schematic representation of the chemical structure and intra-, inter-molecular hydrogen bonds in crystalline cellulose. (Reprinted from *Eur Polym J* 59, Lin, N. and Dufresne, A. Nanocellulose in biomedicine: Current status and future prospect, 302–25, Copyright 2014, with permission from Elsevier.)

to achieve the desired size and can be stopped by diluting the acid mixture. Finally, the nanocrystals are purified by centrifugation and filtration processes (Ferreira et al. 2017). The dimensions, morphology, and yield of the nanocrystals will depend on the source of cellulose and its degree of crystallinity, thus, a higher yield is expected if the degree of crystallinity is higher (Trache et al. 2017). Transmission of electron micrographs from a dilute suspension of nanocellulose are shown in the Figure 3.3.

On the other hand, cellulose nanofibers, in combination with chemical or enzymatic pretreatments, can be easily obtained through a mechanical process. During this process, cellulose fibers are disintegrated into sub-fibers having micrometric lengths and nanometric thicknesses; like cellulose nanocrystals, the dimensions of the nanofibers will depend on the nature of the origin cellulose. Among others, the general methods for the mechanical treatment of cellulose are high-pressure homogenization, microfluidization, and microgrinding (Moon et al. 2011). In order to increase the yield in the production of cellulose nanofibers, several strategies have been proposed to decrease the defibrillation energy to reduce the of rigidity of the fibers (e.g., enzymatic pretreatment, vapor explosion, alkaline, and acid treatment, among others) (Wei et al. 2014).

Cellulose is not only a structural component of plants, it is also synthesized and excreted as cellulose nanofibers by various microorganisms such as *Gluconacetobacter xylinus* (which has the ability to produce a layer of bacterial nanocellulose with a thicknesses of less than 100 nm in the liquid-air interface) (Jozala et al. 2016). Bacterial nanocellulose has the advantage of having a finer structure, greater water absorption capacity, and higher crystallinity when compared with nanocellulose obtained by chemical and physical methods, in addition, its purification process is simple and fast. However, the lack of development in biotechnological processes has limited production yields up to 40% (Ciolacu and Darie 2016). Some general applications of cellulose and their composites are summarized in Table 3.1.

3.3   NANOCELLULOSE MODIFICATION

The high hydrophilicity of nanocellulose produces a high dispersion capacity in water and polar solvents such as dimethyl sulfoxide or dimethylformamide. However, in non-polar solvents, nanocellulose tends to form aggregates which produces drawbacks in the synthesis of non-polar nanocomposites. Aggregates of nanocellulose are a result of a lack of stability in organic solutions

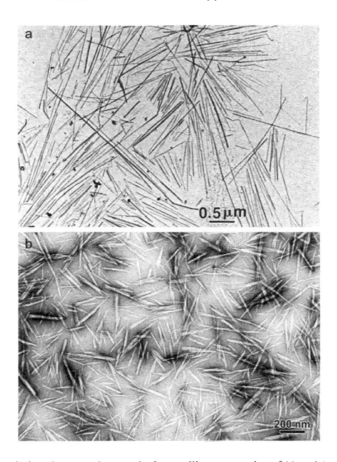

FIGURE 3.3 Transmission electron micrographs from a dilute suspension of (a) tunicin, and (b) ramie nanocrystals. (Reprinted from *Mater Today* 16, Dufrene, A. Nanocellulose: A new ageless biomaterial, 220–27, Copyright 2013, with permission from Elsevier.)

TABLE 3.1
Some of Applications of Nanocellulose and Its Composites

Application	Description
Emulsion stabilizer	Cellulose nanocrystal has been used as a surfactant for food, drugs and cosmetic applications.
Substrate for catalyst	Deposition of substances on the surface of the cellulose nanocrystal has been used as heterogeneous catalyst.
Template for materials	Because nanocellulose exhibits nematic behavior at low concentrations and less viscosity than other forms of cellulose has been proposed as template for different materials.
Wastewater treatment	Since nanocellulose is non-toxic and has high surface area can be used as an adsorbent, in addition, it can be functionalized with organic substances to enhance this adsorption characteristics.
Super capacitor	Bacterial cellulose and nanofiber-supported in polyaniline nanocomposites have been synthesized in situ.

Source: (Ferraz et al. 2012; Jozala et al. 2016; Dufresne 2017).

or through the incompatibility of phases with hydrophobic matrices (Pandey et al. 2013). However, hydroxyl groups on the surface of nanocellulose offer the possibility to carry out superficial chemical modifications with the aim to incorporate non-polar chains on the surface and improve the compatibility between phases of different natures (Oksman et al. 2016).

A schematic summary of the main methods of surface modification via the use of functional polymers is shown in the Figure 3.4. Between different functional polymers and products resulting from the surface modification of cellulose nanocomposites are: acetylated cellulose nanocomposite, TEMPO oxidative cellulose nanocomposite, silylated cellulose nanocomposite, poly(ethylene glycol) grafted onto cellulose nanocomposite, poly(ethylene oxide) grafted onto cellulose nanocomposite, aliphatic polymers grafted onto cellulose nanocomposite, poly(lactic acid) grafted onto cellulose nanocomposite, poly(methyl methacrylate) grafted from cellulose nanocomposite, poly(N,N-dimethylaminoethyl methacrylate) grafted from cellulose nanocomposite, polystyrene grafted from cellulose nanocomposite,

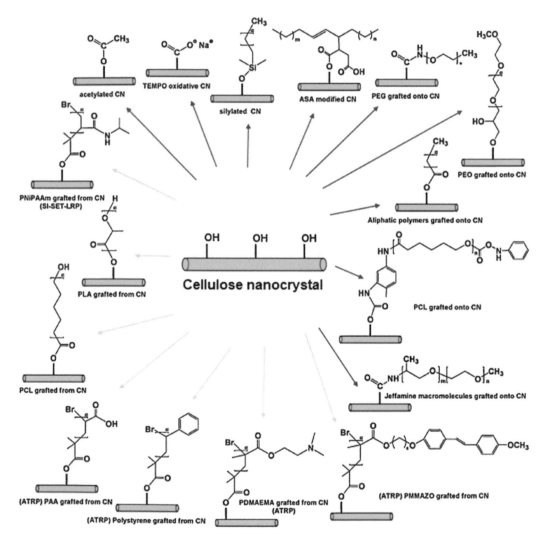

FIGURE 3.4 Surface covalent chemical modifications of cellulose nanocrystals by the use of functional polymers: poly(ethylene glycol) (PEG), poly(ethylene oxide) (PEO), poly(lactic acid) (PLA), poly(acrylic acid) (PAA), poly(N-isopropylacrylamide) (PNiPAAm), poly(N,N-dimethylaminoethyl methacrylate) (PDMAEMA). (Reprinted from *Mater Today* 16, Dufrene, A. Nanocellulose: A new ageless biomaterial, 220–27, Copyright 2013, with permission from Elsevier.)

poly(lactic acid) grafted from cellulose nanocomposite, poly(N-isopropylacrylamide) grafted from cellulose nanocomposite and acetylated cellulose nanocomposite.

Modifications of the nanocellulose can be classified as covalent or non-covalent modification according to the type of bond formed. The non-covalent modifications are produced through hydrophilic affinity through molecular coating (e.g., by the use of non-ionic surfactants), electrostatic attractions (e.g., by the use of ionic surfactants), hydrogen bonds (e.g., by the surface modification of polymer phase) or van der Walls forces (e.g., by the insertion of hydrophilic segments in the structure of the substrate) (Moon et al. 2011). Various investigations have reported the use of surfactants of mono- and di-esters of phosphoric acid with non-polar tails, which coat the cellulose nanoparticles and allow their dispersion in organic solvents (Kim et al. 2009). Clearly, the hydrophilic-lipophilic balance of the surfactants is an important factor in the selection of a surfactant. On the other hand, covalent modifications are usually produced from sulfonation reactions (e.g., using sulfuric acid), TEMPO-mediated oxidation (e.g., cellulose oxidation with sodium hypochlorite and catalytic amounts of sodium bromide and 2,2,6,6-tetramethylpiperidine-1-oxyl radical), esterification (e.g., using citric acid or acetic acid), etherification (e.g., using triphenylchloromethane), silylation (e.g., using trichloromethylsilane), urethanization (e.g., using methyl isocyanate), among others (Peng et al. 2011). General details about modification strategies are given below.

Sulfonation can be performed during the depolymerization process via hydrolysis with sulfuric acid which occurs with the formation of sulfate esters on the surface of the nanocellulose. Therefore, sulfuric acid carries out two functions: acid hydrolysis and the incorporation of sulfonic groups. However, the cellulose surface becomes strongly hydrophilic but adsorption is seen to be favored on cationic substrates (Ruiz-Palomero et al. 2016). The TEMPO-mediated oxidation is used for the conversion of hydroxymethyl groups into carboxylic form, which has the advantage of being highly selective with primary hydroxyl groups and easy to implement. By this procedure, cellulose becomes strongly hydrophilic but not only the adsorption is seen to be favored on cationic substrates, they can also be mediated by pH (Lin and Dufresne 2013). The hydroxyl groups on nanocellulose can be esterificated by acetylation reactions. Essentially, hydroxyl and carboxylic acid groups react to form esters and, in consequence, the reaction yield is affected by the presence of water in the reactor (Ashori et al. 2014). Etherification is widely used as a chemical pretreatment to favor defibrillation in the attainment of cellulose nanofibers; usually a base such as sodium hydroxide and an acid such as monochloroacetic acid are used, however, this has the limitation that it generates mainly nanofibers with a greater hydrophilicity (Habibi 2014). The use of alkyl chlorosilanes of variable length, due to the high reactivity of chlorosilane groups toward hydroxyl groups, allows the modification of nanocellulose and causes the consequent increase in its hydrophobicity and dispersibility in low polarity solvents. However, it is important to control the degree of silylation since it can bring about disintegration of the nanostructure (Khalil 2014). Reactions of urethanization are also used for the superficial modification of nanocellulose by means of the reaction of the hydroxyl groups with the isocyanate groups of the modifying agent, in order to increase the material hydrophobicity (Natterodt et al. 2017). This procedure is seen to be similar to the urethanization of other surfaces based on glucose units (Benitez et al. 2017; Arbelaez et al. 2017). Additionally, amidation reactions, polymer anchoring, and click chemistry processes are also used with the aim of generating surface modifications and increasing the compatibility of phases in the process of the synthesis of the nanocomposites (Boujemaoui et al. 2017; Habibi 2014).

3.4 SYNTHESIS OF CELLULOSE NANOCOMPOSITES

As previously mentioned, one of the main challenges during the synthesis of cellulose-based nanocomposites is related to the adequate homogeneous dispersion of nanoparticles within the polymer matrix. A correct dispersion is needed in order to avoid the aggregation of the nanoparticles because this could produce the loss of its nanometric scale, and in consequence, the effect on nanocomposite properties is limited (Oksman et al. 2016).

Cellulose-based nanocomposites can usually be obtained using four techniques: casting-evaporation (Flauzino et al. 2016), electrospinning (Mariano and Dufresne 2017), melt compounding (Kargarzadeh et al. 2017), and impregnation (Peng et al. 2011).

3.4.1 Casting-Evaporation

Casting-evaporation is one of the most widely used techniques for the production of cellulose-based nanocomposites. This technique is based on the dispersion of the nanocellulose particles in water, or a suitable organic solvent, followed by mixing it with the polymer matrix and then lyophilization or slow evaporation of the solvent. Change by:

The evaporation stage can be a delayed process which should allow the interaction and progressive reorganization of the nanoparticles within the matrix (Flauzino et al. 2016). One of the limitations of this technique is the compatibility between the nanocellulose, the solvent, and the polymeric matrix. It is clear that water is the most suitable solvent because of the highly hydrophilic nature of nanocellulose. However, in experiments where the use of water as a solvent is not possible, surface modification of nanocellulose appears as a practical alternative for the compatibilization of the phases (Peng et al. 2011). Different morphological features can be obtained depending on a specific procedure; for example, films can be obtained by casting, whereas spherical shape particles can be obtained by emulsion systems (see Figure 3.5).

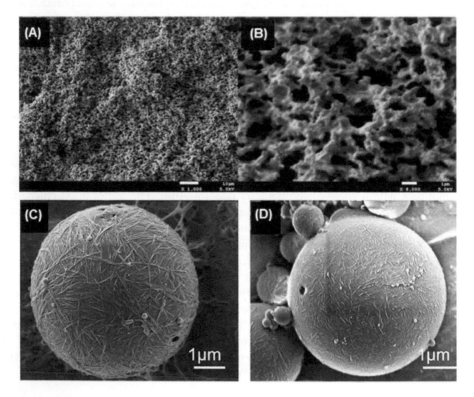

FIGURE 3.5 SEM images of poly(aniline)-cellulose nanocomposite structure at (A) 10 μm and (B) 1 μm by Casting-evaporation; and SEM images of polymerized styrene/water emulsions stabilized by (C) bacterial cellulose nanocrystals (CNF) and (D) cotton cellulose nanocrystals. (Reprinted from *Polymer* 132, Kargarzadeh, H., Mariano, M., Huang, J., Lin, N., Ahmad, I., Dufresne, A., and Thomas, S. Recent developments on nanocellulose reinforced polymer nanocomposites: A review, 368–97, Copyright 2017, with permission from Elsevier.)

3.4.2 ELECTROSPINNING

This is a method of fiber production which uses an electric force to draw charged threads from polymer solutions or molten polymers; the fiber diameters obtained are in the order of some 100 nanometers. Thus, electrospinning emerges as a simple and efficient method for the production of cellulose-based nanocomposite fibers. Fibers are gained by dispersing nanocellulose into a suitable solvent followed by the addition of the polymer solution. Later, the solution is rotated using a high electric field in order to apply a high electric force that exceeds the forces of the surface tension of the polymer solution, and to generate a thin stream of solution from the capillary to the collector plate. Finally, by evaporation of the solvent, fibers are deposited on a suitable substrate (Mariano and Dufresne 2017).

3.4.3 MECHANICAL MELT MIXING

This method is based on the incorporation of nanocellulose into the polymeric matrix of thermo-plastic polymers via the use of mechanical mixing at high temperatures, extrusion of the mixture, and finally the molding of the material. A typical instrument for mechanical melt mixing is the torque rheometer, which is a batch mixer used originally to measure the torque required to rotate its blades at a fixed rotor speed during the mixing process. It is necessary to carry out a pretreatment for the modification of the surface functional groups in order to avoid agglomeration and evaluate adequately the working temperatures because these can affect the properties of nanocellulose (Ferrer et al. 2017; Kargarzadeh et al. 2017).

3.4.4 IMPREGNATION

This technique consists of generating a nanocellulose network, which is subsequently impregnated with a low viscosity and cured resin. For this, the generation of the thin cellulose film is commonly carried out by the membrane filtration of a nanocellulose solution or by applying pressure to a medium without solvent. Subsequently, the thermosetting resin is impregnated at a low pressure, to finally perform the curing process and the generation of the nanocomposite. Several studies have shown layer assembly can be easily made with this method, and further that alternating layers of polymer and nanocellulose have been obtained (Ferrer et al. 2017; Peng et al. 2011).

3.5 CHARACTERIZATION OF CELLULOSE-BASED NANOCOMPOSITES

Cellulose-based nanocomposites can be characterized by various techniques, where the choice of technique will depend mainly on the researcher's criteria, their interest in a specific characteristic of the material, or the application that the researcher wants to give it. Next, the most popular techniques for the characterization of nanocomposites are cataloged and briefly described.

3.5.1 MORPHOLOGICAL CHARACTERIZATION

Morphological characterization begins with a visual examination of the material. Mainly it is directed toward the identification of heterogeneity on the surface of the material obtained. For example, if the thin nanocomposite cellulose films have opacity, this suggests the presence of aggregates at a micrometric scale. Macroscopically, the digital image analysis technique can be used to explore the surface anisotropy when changes in the visual appearance are detected (Palencia et al. 2016). On the other hand, microscopically, techniques such as scanning electron microscopy (SEM), atomic force microscopy (AFM), and electron transmission microscopy (TEM) can be used to obtain information about the homogeneity of the material, identification of pores, degree of dispersion, identification of aggregates and possible orientations of the nanomaterial within the polymeric matrix (Karimi 2017).

3.5.2 MECHANICAL CHARACTERIZATION

Mechanical characterizations are classified according to changes in temperature. Those where the temperature remains constant throughout the experiment are denominated as mechanical characterizations to constant temperature; in this case, generally a universal testing machine is used to study both the tensile and compressive strength of materials. Also, mechanical characterizations can be performed by considering the effects of temperature; for this dynamic mechanical thermal analyzers (DMTA) are used. In general, mechanical tests are carried out in order to determine parameters such as Young modulus elastic limit, tensile modulus, and proportionality limit, among others, in order to evaluate the effect of the incorporation of the nanocellulose into the material (Dufresne 2017). Other techniques such as indentation hardness tests by AFM microscopy can be used in the determination of mechanical parameters for small volumes of nanocomposites (Díez-Pascual et al. 2015).

3.5.3 THERMAL CHARACTERIZATION

Thermogravimetric analysis (TGA) and differential scanning calorimetry (DSC) are widely used for the analysis of both precursor materials and nanocomposite materials. The DSC analysis allows for glass transition temperatures, T_g, to be obtained which is a determining factor in the mechanical behavior of materials and can be altered by the interactions between the polymeric matrix and the nanocellulose particles. On the other hand, TGA analysis is commonly used for determining the thermal stability of the materials and can show decomposition temperature, water contents of the nanocomposites and thermal degradation sequence of the components (Sheltami et al. 2017).

3.5.4 BARRIER PROPERTIES

The measurement of the barrier properties of cellulose nanocomposites is essential in evaluating their potential uses and limitations. These properties are influenced by parameters of process during production stage and by working temperatures during its use. Thus, for example, at high temperatures, a greater permeation of liquids or vapors can produce plasticization and cause the mechanical properties of the material to become degraded. In particular, the importance of barrier properties for cellulose-based nanocomposites, lies in the fact that by interacting mainly with water, water absorption can be generated due to the high hydrophilicity of the nanocellulose, this leads to changes in the properties of the nanocomposites, and enables microbial colonization to be enhanced (Moon et al. 2011). The implementation of this type of test is simple and can be carried out through permeation studies when porous layers have been made or by analogous experiments through determination of water absorption capacity. Some studies have examined the water absorption capacity through the use of dry samples of nanocomposites, which were subsequently immersed in deionized water for specific periods of time and removed from the aqueous medium to be gravimetrically characterized (Slavutsky and Bertuzzi 2014; Palencia et al. 2017).

It is important to highlight that other techniques can be used to achieve these objectives, such as electrochemical impedance spectroscopy, Raman microscopy, protein adsorption tests, nuclear magnetic resonance in solid-state, microbial colonization susceptibility, enzymatic degradations, and contact angle, among others (Cheremisinoff 1996; Palencia 2017).

3.6 PHARMACEUTICAL AND BIOMEDICAL APPLICATIONS

Pharmaceutical and biomedical applications of cellulose-based nanocomposites are very wide and have been described in terms of their biocompatibility and hemocompatibility. Usually, biocompatibility studies are based on cell models (human dermal fibroblasts, human monocytic cell line, and human osteoblastic cell line), indirect cytotoxicity tests and cell culture on nanocellulose films. Though biocompatibility of cellulose has been evidenced in several studies using different methodologies, cellulose is not readily degraded by the human body due to it lacking in cellulolytic enzymes. Therefore, it is clear that some grade of incompatibility should exist (i.e., cellulose may be considered as non-biodegradable *in vivo* or as a slowly degradable material) (Dugan et al. 2013; Lin and Dufresne 2014; Miyamoto et al. 1989). In consequence, it is important to carry out a careful review of the methodological approach used before fully accepting the conclusions on biocompatibility, since, unlike other types of biocompatible materials such as polylactic acid or chitosan, assimilation by the human body is not complete. For example, some studies on cellulose nanocomposites with hydrogel properties were only based on experiments of cell cultivation, where the growth, propagation, and activity of cells were analyzed in order to evaluate the conditions of material biocompatibility (Lin and Dufresne 2014; Miyamoto et al. 1989). In another study, *in vivo* biocompatibility of bacterial nanocellulose membranes were studied through the histological analysis of long-term subcutaneous implants in mice. It was concluded that implants based on bacterial nanocellulose caused a mild and benign inflammatory reaction which did not elicit a foreign body reaction. However, no differences were observed between the control group and implanted animals (Lin and Dufresne 2014; Märtson et al. 1999). Recently, from *in vitro* experiments, it was concluded that oxidized cellulose became more vulnerable to hydrolysis and therefore potentially more degradable by the human body (Li et al. 2009; Luo et al. 2013). This result suggests that through oxidation, the biodegradability of nanocellulose can be enhanced and, through this method, nanocellulose degradability *in vitro* can be improved in water, phosphate buffered saline, and simulated body fluid by periodate oxidation (which is a classical method used to determine the structure of complex carbohydrates).

In contrast to potential incompatibility arguments, depending on the type of cellulose used in the fabrication of the nanocomposite, different results related to toxicity should be taken into consideration. For example, for cellulose nanocrystalline, toxicological experiments such as acute lethal tests, multitrophic assay, animal experiments with fathead minnows and Zebrafish, reproduction tests, *in vitro* rainbow trout hepatocyte assay, respiratory toxicity of aerosolized cellulose nanocrystalline on the human airways with a co-culture of human monocyte-derived macrophages, dendritic cells, and a bronchial epithelial cell line, (pro-)inflammatory cytokines, *in vitro* gene mutations, *in vitro* and *in vivo* chromosomal tests, skin irritation and sensitization tests, and cytotoxicity evaluations with different cell lines, concluded that there was a low toxicity potential, low environmental risk, and low cytotoxicity (O'Connor and Schwartz 1993; Baumann et al. 2009; Knight et al. 2009; Pan et al. 2010; Jackson et al. 2011). But also, for cellulose nanofibers, from cytotoxicity evaluations with human monocytes and mouse macrophages, kinetic luminescent bacteria tests for acute environmental toxicity, *in vitro* genotoxicity with enzyme comet assay, neurotoxicity and systemic effects with a nematode models, *in vitro* pharyngeal aspiration studies for pulmonary immunotoxicity and genotoxicity with mice, cytotoxicity evaluations with 3T3 fibroblast cells (including the test of cell membrane, cell mitochondrial activity and DNA proliferation), cytotoxicity evaluations with bovine fibroblasts cells, and effects of gene expression *in vitro*, concluded that there was no evidence of inflammatory effects or cytotoxicity, no DNA and chromosome damage, low cytotoxicity at low concentrations of nanocellulose, and no evidence of cytotoxicity for pure cellulose nanofibers. Finally, for bacterial nanocellulose, from cytotoxicity evaluations with osteoblast cells and L929 fibroblast and with human umbilical vein endothelial cells, animal experiments with C57/Bl6 male mice, and *in vivo* intraperitoneal injection studies with BALB/c male mice concluded that there was no evidence of toxicity *in vitro* and *in vivo*, and non-immunogenicity (Lin and Dufresne 2014).

On the other hand, hemocompatibility is another important property associated with biocompatibility; a hemocompatible material can potentially be used for blood-contacting biomaterials such as artificial blood vessels, blood bags, and pumps, as well as for the making of artificial organs (e.g., artificial hearts) (Lin and Dufresne 2014; Palencia et al. 2016). Recently, studies have reported that by the oral incorporation of cellulose nanofibers it is possible to promote the regulation of blood metabolic variables such as postprandial blood glucose, plasma insulin, glucose-dependent insulinotropic polypeptide, and triglyceride concentrations (Ferraz et al. 2012; Lin and Dufresne 2014; Pértile et al. 2012).

For biomedical applications, some authors use the term "biocellulose" to refer to nanocellulose. Biocelluose is a term that can appear redundant if the chemical definition of cellulose is used. However, it can be useful to the reader to be familiar with the term in order to look for further information. Some examples of biomedical applications are: tissue bioscaffolds for cellular culture, drug excipient, and drug delivery; immobilization and recognition of enzyme/protein; substitutes/medical biomaterials, blood vessel replacement, soft tissue-ligament, meniscus, and cartilage replacements; skin tissue repair and wound healing; advanced nanomaterials for tissue repair, regeneration, and healing; bone tissue regeneration and healing; and antimicrobial nanomaterials (mainly involving silver particles and their derivatives), among others (Feese et al. 2011; Ferraz et al. 2012; Hagiwara et al. 2010; Jackson et al. 2011; Kim et al. 2013; Klemm et al. 2001; Klemm et al. 2006; Kolakovic et al. 2013; Kowalska-Ludwicka et al. 2013; Liebert et al. 2011; Mahmoud et al. 2010; Mathew et al. 2012; Varjonen et al. 2011; Villanova et al. 2011; Wei et al. 2011).

On the other hand, for drug release, different types of nanocellulose-polymer systems have been studied. For example, composites of cellulose nanocrystals and chitosan, alginate and cyclodextrine have been evaluated for drug release in different dosage forms (e.g., microspheres, hydrogel microparticulate, and supramolecular hydrogel) and drug release mechanisms (e.g., diffusional transport, Fickian diffusion, and diffusion-swelling). Also, cellulose nanofibers and bacterial cellulose hydrogels have been studied for drug release (Lin and Dufresne 2014).

It is clear that through the incorporation of cellulose nanocrystals, hydrogels of superabsorbent nanocomposites can be easily obtained, for example, poly(acrylamide-co-acrylate)-cellulose nanocrystal, which has been widely studied in the development of biological tissues due to its null toxicity, its high resistance to deformation, and high cell proliferation (Wu and Zhou 2012).

In particular, the polymeric matrix of poly(acrylamide-co-acrylate) is a polymer with a high hydrophilic nature similar to the cellulose nanocrystal; as the above suggests the function of nanocellulose is not related to hydrophobicity but rather to the effect of nanostructuration on the mechanical properties of hydrogels (e.g., the incorporation of cellulose nanocrystals into the polymer matrix increases the density of effective crosslinking of the hydrogel and therefore decreases the gelation time). Clearly, nanocellulose could be replaced by another nanostructure, however, hemocompatibility, an innocuous nature, and cellular compatibility are warranted with the use of nanocellulose (Wu and Zhou 2012, Quinn et al. 2014).

Another example are composites of cellulose nanocrystals and poly(3-hydroxybutyrate-co-3-hydroxyvalerate) where the hydrophobic properties of the compound are further modulated by the varied contents of the nanomaterial easing the use of the nanocomposite and hydrophobic drug release systems (some hydrophobic drugs are anticancer drugs such as paclitaxel, docetaxel, and etoposide, etc.) (Quinn et al. 2014). For hydrophilic drugs, such as doxorubicin hydrochloride (DOX) and tetracycline, poly(acrylamide-co-acrylate)-cellulose nanocrystal could be used. Some applications of nanocellulose composites are shown in Table 3.2.

TABLE 3.2

Some of Applications of Nanocellulose Composites

Nanocomposite	Application	Description
Cellulose nanocrystal + Ag nanoparticles	Antimicrobial biomaterials	Cellulose nanocrystal functionalized with aldehydes in order to reduce cations of silver and obtain a composite with antimicrobial properties.
Cellulose nanocrystal + flourophore surface	Florescence biomarker	Fluorophores on the nanocellulose surface generates a potential biomarkers used for the quantification of a variety of nanoparticles within the cell.
Bacterial cellulose nanofiber + polyvinyl alcohol	Tissue engineering	Production of polymeric material with broad range of mechanical properties. Nanocomposites have the similar properties than soft tissue as cardiovascular and connective tissues.
Bacteria cellulose networks + hydroxyapatite	biomedical materials	Nanocomposites were produced by introducing the mineral phase into the bacteria culture medium during the formation of cellulose fibrils. The studies suggest the biocompatibility of the materials and the bioactivity of hydroxyapatite.
Cellulose nanofibers functionalized + methylene diphenyl diisocyanate	Medical implants	Nanocomposites were prepared by compression molding and stacking of nanocellulose fiber between polyurethane films. The developed composites were utilized to fabricate various versatile medical implants, because their mechanic and biocompatibility properties.
Nanocrystal + chitin fibers	Medical sutures	Bacterial cellulose nanocrystals and chitin fibers show considerable enzymatic degradation, suggesting a good biodegradability, low cytotoxicity and ability to promote the cell proliferation for the development of medical sutures.
Cellulose nanocrystals + cetyltrimethylammoniu bromide	Drug delivery	Zeta potential was increased in a concentration dependent manner, the surface bound with significant quantities of the hydrophobic anticancer drugs such as docetaxel, paclitaxel, and etoposide was achieved. But also, water soluble antibiotics such as tetracycline and doxorubicin.

Source: (Peng et al. 2011; Moon et al. 2011; Ferraz et al. 2012; Sheltami et al. 2017; and Dufresne 2017).

3.7 STUDY OF CYTOCOMPATIBILITY *IN VITRO* OF SCAFFOLDS BASED ON CHITOSAN, POLYVINYL ALCOHOL, METHYLCELLULOSE, AND NANOCELLULOSE NANOCOMPOSITES USING L929 FIBROBLAST CELLS-K

Kanimozhi et al. evaluated the cytocompatibility of a nanocomposite scaffold made of chitosan, polyvinyl alcohol, methylcellulose, and nanocellulose obtained from *Hibiscus cannabinus*; the method of obtaining the nanocellulose consisted of the extraction of fibers from the leaves of the plant, which were then scrutinized, dried, and hydrolyzed in acid media using a solution of 70% H_2SO_4, then the nanocellulose was washed, neutralized, and dialyzed with distilled water at a constant pH (Kanimozhi et al. 2017). Material used for the synthesis of the nanocomposite was obtained from a mixture of chitosan in a solution of acetic acid, polyvinylalcohol, and methylcellulose in purified water; later, the nanocellulose nanoparticles were mixed with the solution in order to obtain the composite, finally, the solvent was evaporated under a vacuum; the scaffold was obtained using NaCl particles and the composite mixture. For characterization studies, the researchers employed ATR-FTIR, X-ray diffraction, scanning electron microscopy, Raman spectroscopy, atomic force microscopy, and transmission electron microscopy. They found an increase in the chemical interactions between the nanocellulose and the polymer scaffold, a low aggregation, and uniform distribution of the nanocellulose having a cubical shape. The authors evaluated the degree of swelling of the materials finding that nanocellulose produces an increase in degradation and swelling, but also it facilitates the cell growth. The bioassay employed included an antibacterial activity tested against *Staphylococcus aureus* and *Escherichia coli*, which were made using a disk diffusion method. Results showed an increase in the antibacterial activity of the scaffold as the concentration of nanocellulose nanoparticles were increased. The biocompatibility and cytotoxicity were evaluated through cell cultures and an MTT assay, which is a colorimetric assay for assessing cell metabolic activity. The results showed evidence that L929 cells had a performance equivalent to those observed for the collagen scaffolds with respect to cell migration and proliferation rate on the scaffold; the cell adhesion was evaluated by culturing cells in a thin scaffold and the surface morphology was evaluated by scanning electron microscopy evidencing a non-porous cell surface. In addition, fluorescence images showed that L929 could attach and grow well on the material demonstrating a potential biocompatibility. The results of the investigation indicated that this nanocomposite is a material with potential biomedical applications oriented to cell adhesion and skin tissue engineering.

3.8   *IN VITRO* DELIVERY OF AMPICILLIN BY NANOCOMPOSITES BASED ON CELLULOSE

Ampicillin is an antibiotic used to prevent and treat a number of bacterial infections because it is able to penetrate Gram positive and some Gram negative bacteria. This drug is used in medical treatments such as the infections of respiratory and urinary tracts, meningitis, salmonellosis, and endocarditis, among others. Nanostructured materials have been studied for the release of sodium ampicillin, these systems have been made from poly(caprolactone) and titanium dioxide by the sol-gel method using multicomponent solutions containing titanium butoxide, poly(caprolactone), water, and chloroform (Tang et al. 2015; Deepa and Pothan 2016; Poonguzhali et al. 2017).

However, other materials have been used in conjunction with nanocellulose to develop controlled release systems, for example, alginate. In particular, alginate is an anionic polysaccharide distributed widely in the cell walls of brown algae with the potential for a broad range of applications as a biomaterial, especially as a supporting material or delivery system for tissue engineering. The greatest advantage of using alginate for controlled release formulations is its biodegradability, good mechanical strength, and non-toxicity properties; recently, it has been proposed that the use of alginate in combination with nanocellulose is the most efficient controlled release system for drugs such as ampicillin. It is expected that for this specific application, any type of nanocellulose can be used; however, a comparison of differences resulting of nanocellulose type has not been performed (Jeon and Bouhadir 2009; Chaa et al. 2012; Hakkarainen et al. 2016; Poonguzhali et al. 2017).

Poonguzhali et al. describe the isolation of nanocellulose from *Hibiscus sabdariffa* fibers using acid hydrolysis, to ensure the correct diffusion of the acid molecules into the fibers and the adequate cleavage of glycosidic bonds. Afterward, the *H. sabdariffa* fiber is cut into small pieces (~2 cm) in order to sterilize it using NaOH (2%) in water and an autoclave (15 lbs and at a temperature of 120°C for a period of 1 h). Then, the sterilized fibers are washed with water several times, then dried and bleached with a mixture of sodium hydroxide, acetic acid, and sodium hypochlorite in 1:3 ratios for 1 h. Washing with water is required to remove the bleaching agent. Finally, the bleached cellulose fibers are hydrolyzed with oxalic acid for 5 h in an autoclave under a pressure of 20 lb. The fibers are then neutralized and the suspension is diluted with water and kept in a magnetic stirrer for 8 h. The pH of the suspension is around 6.7. The nanocellulose is then obtained from the suspension by drying it at room temperature (Poonguzhali et al. 2017).

On the another hand, alginate nanocellulose nanocomposite films can be prepared by a casting method. For this, alginate is dissolved in deionized water at room temperature and continuously stirred using a homogenizer for 2 h. The pure alginate film is prepared using the above solution. To the alginate solution, nanocellulose (0.5%) is added and stirred for 2 h. The solutions are then cast on Teflon-coated plates and the film forms over a 48 h period. The dried films are then removed from the plates and placed inside an oven in order to evaporate residual solvents completely (~2 days). Preparation of the corresponding drug-loaded alginate and alginate nanocellulose nanocomposite films should be similarly performed to evidence the difference and effect of nanocellulose on release. Finally, 1% of ampicillin is dissolved in 50 mL of the above prepared alginate and alginate nanocellulose materials. The mixture is thoroughly stirred and left overnight to remove air bubbles before being cast onto Teflon plates at room temperature (Tang et al. 2015; Deepa and Pothan 2016; Poonguzhali et al. 2017).

The main results obtained by Poonguzhali et al. are shown below. Images of SEM of alginate nanocellulose film can be seen in Figure 3.6. Nanocellulose can be identified as the small white spots dispersed throughout the film, whereas the alginate does not contain any spots and shows a smooth surface.

For drug-loaded films, a multiphase morphology was evidenced and the surface roughness of the film was enhanced by loading the ampicillin. Moreover, there is a more uniform surface roughness for an alginate nanocellulose film with ampicillin when it is compared with an alginate nanocellulose film. But also, an alginate nanocellulose film had higher swelling when compared with alginate due to ampicillin having a higher solubility than that of nanocellulose and, as a consequence, voids are easily created. The end effect is a higher swelling on the alginate film with ampicillin.

In relation to the mechanical properties of this type of material, it was seen that the tensile strength of the drug-loaded alginate film increased slightly when compared to the alginate nanocellulose film. The above can be explained as a result of the higher incorporation of ampicillin with alginate. But, the addition of nanocellulose as well as ampicillin decreased the elongation at break

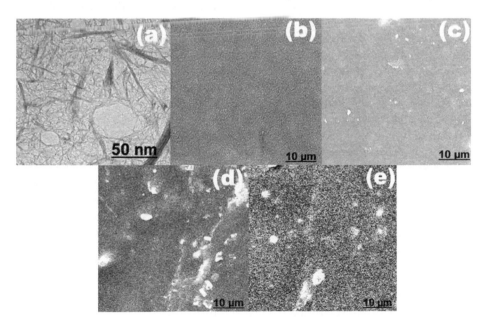

FIGURE 3.6 Micrograph of nanocellulose: (a) SEM image of alginate, (b) alginate nanocellulose film, (c) alginate nanocellulose film + ampicillin and (d), alginate film + ampicillin. (Reprinted from *Polymer* 132, Kargarzadeh, H., Mariano, M., Huang, J., Lin, N., Ahmad, I., Dufresne, A., and Thomas, S. Recent developments on nanocellulose reinforced polymer nanocomposites: A review, 368–97, Copyright 2017, with permission from Elsevier.)

and increased the tensile strength for different films. These results show that nanocellulose and ampicillin have a positive impact on the mechanical stability of the drug-loaded film. In addition, results showed an effect of nanocellulose on the release of ampicillin; thus, the release profile for ampicillin from an alginate film with nanocellulose was higher than that of the film without nano-cellulose. Finally, the presence of nanocellulose in the scaffold leaves free space for the ampicillin causing a faster release of the drug. The release of ampicillin from alginate can easily be explained by diffusion through the film and by an erosion mechanism (in the case of polymer nanocomposites, the ideal case is that the drug is uniformly distributed/dissolved in the polymer matrix, and then drug release occurs via diffusion or erosion of the matrix. If the diffusion of the drug is faster than the matrix degradation, the drug release mechanism occurs mainly by diffusion; but, in the opposite case, the release is defined by a mechanism of erosion). Since it is hydrophilic, it is expected that ampicillin molecules will significantly penetrate the voids of the alginate nanocellulose scaffold (Tang et al. 2015; Deepa and Pothan 2016; Poonguzhali et al. 2017). This suggests that the alginate nanocellulose film with ampicillin can be used as a suitable material for the application of *in vitro* drug release.

3.9 NANOCRYSTALLINE CELLULOSE FOR CONTROLLED RELEASE OF HYDROPHOBIC ANTICANCER DRUGS (DOCETAXEL, PACLITAXEL, AND ETOPOSIDE)

Chemotherapy is a strategy for cancer treatment that uses one or more anticancer drugs or chemo-therapeutic agents as part of a standardized chemotherapy regimen. The use of drugs constitutes a systemic therapy for cancer through the introduction of chemical substances into the blood stream which are then, therefore, in principle, capable of being transported to cancer at any anatomic location in the body. However, though traditional chemotherapeutic agents are cytotoxic by means of interfering with cell division (mitosis), cancer cells vary widely in their susceptibility to these agents. It is widely recognized that the efficacy of chemotherapy depends on the type of cancer and the stage; to determine the correct dosage of chemotherapy can be difficult, and it is clear that if the dose is too low then it will be ineffective against the tumor, whereas, if the dose is excessive then the toxicity and side effects will be intolerable to the patient. Therefore, finding new systems or strategies for drug controlled release is a continuous area of research (O'Connor and Schwartz 1993; Baumann et al. 2009; Knight et al. 2009).

Cellulose and derivatives of cellulose such as ethyl cellulose, methyl cellulose, or carboxy-methyl cellulose have a long history of use in the pharmaceutical industry in numerous forms including oral, topical, and injectable formulations. Thus, for example, cellulose has excellent compaction properties when blended with other pharmaceutical excipients. The form of cellulose used in tablets is usually the microcrystalline cellulose but despite wide use in drug-loaded tablets, there is still strong research into the use of microcrystalline cellulose and other types of cellulose in the development of advanced pelleting systems whereby the rate of tablet disintegration and drug release may be easily controlled (O'Connor and Schwartz 1993; Baumann et al. 2009; Knight et al. 2009; Pan et al. 2010; Jackson et al. 2011).

On the other hand, as a result of its large surface area, stiffness, strength, small size, and phase behavior, nanocellulose is actively being investigated as a material for use in the pack-aging, pharmaceutical, and biomedical industries. The high surface charge of nanocrystalline nanocellulose and the well-established biocompatibility of cellulosic materials suggest signifi-cant potential pharmaceutical applications of nanocellulose. Thus, it is clear that nanocrystalline cellulose offers several potential advantages as a drug delivery excipient: (i) the large surface area and negative charge of nanocrystalline cellulose suggests that large amounts of drugs can be bound to its surface; (ii) biocompatibility of cellulose suggests that nanocrystalline cellulose can be used for purposes like those tested for other biocompatible polymers; (iii) the numerous surface hydroxyl groups on nanocrystalline cellulose provide a site for surface modification of the material with a wide range of chemical functional groups by a variety of methods; and (iv) nanocrystalline cellulose is a low-cost material, and a readily abundant material from a renewable and sustainable resource, in consequence, its use provides a substantial environmental advantage compared with other nanomaterials (Vinatier et al. 2009; Abdalla et al. 2008; Podczeck et al. 2008; Kranz et al. 2009; Jackson et al. 2011).

The use of nanocrystalline cellulose for the controlled release of drugs as docetaxel, paclitaxel, and etoposide performed by Jackson et al. (2011) is an excellent example of studies performed the pharmaceutical field. The main aspects related with the methodology and results obtained by Jackson's research team are described below. First, and maybe foremost, is the nanocrystalline cellulose preparation. A general procedure, for commercial products, starts with commercial softwood which has been fully bleached and milled to pass through a 0.5-mm mill in order to ensure particle size uniformity and an increased surface area. The milled pulp must be hydrolyzed using acids, for example, sulfuric acid at 45°C, and stirred at high speed for 25 min. The cellulose suspension is then diluted with cold, deionized distilled water and allowed to settle overnight. The clear top layer is decanted and the remaining "white cloudy layer" is washed with deionized water and centrifuged three times to remove practically all soluble cellulose materials. The resulting thick, white suspension is dialyzed against slow running deionized water for several days (1–4 days) using dialysis tubing with a molecular weight cutoff of 12–14 kDa. The suspension from the dialysis tubes is dispersed by subjecting it to ultrasound treatment for 10 min at 60% power (Hamad 2006; Podczeck et al. 2008; Pan et al. 2010; Jackson et al. 2011).

For the Jackson et al. study, it is important to note that the nanocrystalline cellulose did not flocculate in water; in consequence, the nanocrystalline cellulose-drug complexes prepared in water could not be effectively separated by microcentrifugation. In this case, the nanocrystalline cellulose-drug suspensions must be transferred to dialysis bags with a molecular weight cutoff of 10 kDa and dialyzed against deionized water overnight in the dark at 4°C. Thus, the concentration of the unbound drug in the dialysate can be easily determined by UV-Vis spectroscopy, allowing for the calculation of the amount of drug bound to the nanocrystalline cellulose by mass balance.

In order to solubilize the hydrophobic drugs, paclitaxel, docetaxel, and etoposide, the surface of the nanocrystalline cellulose is first modified with cetyl trimethylammonium bromide or CTAB. CTAB is a quaternary ammonium surfactant used, in this case, to produce micellar solubilization of drugs and a correct association with the nanocellulose. The nanocellulose/CTAB is incubated with stock solutions of the drugs with increasing concentrations. Because these drugs are characterized by a low solubility in water, they were solubilized in a minimal amount of either DMSO or a solution of diblock copolymer in 10 mM NaCl as previously described. To form the pellets, the system drug/nanocellulose/CTAB suspensions is incubated at 25°C with tumbling at 8 rpm for 30 min and finally centrifuged at 18000 × g for 10 min.

For nanocellulose, the XRPD pattern is characterized by two high intensity peaks, indicating the high degree of crystallinity in the material that can be obtained by the previously described methodology. But also, the SEM images of these fibers are an important tool in demonstrating the nanoscopic dimensions of this material in a deionized water suspension. Some studies have shown that hydrophilic drugs can be bound directly to the surface of nanocellulose at relatively high weight ratios. The two hydrophilic drugs studied (doxorubicin hydrochloride or tetracycline hydrochloride) probably are bound by an ionic interaction with the negatively charged surface of nanocellulose since doxorubicin hydrochloride or tetracycline hydrochloride is a cationic species slightly positively charged and tetracycline hydrochloride is zwitterionic. It was observed that an amount less doxorubicin hydrochloride bound to nanocellulose when dispersed in PBS in comparison with the deionized water. This can be attributed to interference with doxorubicin hydrochloride binding because of the presence of large amounts of counterions in the PBS (Jackson et al. 2011).

The work performed by Jackson et al. demonstrates that nanocrystalline cellulose can be surface-modified to deliver hydrophobic drugs. Thus, by coating the negatively charged nanocellulose with a cationic surfactant it is possible to create a hydrophobic domain on the surface of the nanocellulose. A clear interaction between CTAB and nanocellulose is identified by flocculation phenomena when high CTAB concentrations are used (Jackson et al. 2011).

3.10 COMMERCIAL PRODUCTS BASED ON NANOCELLULOSE COMPOSITES

Nanocellulose is seen to be a potential component for application in many industries such as the packaging industry, the information and communication industry, the automotive industry, the building industry, and in particular industries relying on formulations (chemical, pharmaceutical, cosmetics, food, among others). At the present, nanocellulose is produced on an industrial scale for commercial application and its production is considered a sector of great growth and huge commercial projections. In biomedicine, applications of nanocellulose for composites includes tissue engineering and cellular culture, drug delivery, medical implants and substitute materials, wound healing dressings, and antimicrobial materials. A summary of commercial products and patents is shown in Table 3.3 and 3.4. Other drug carrier systems based on nanocellulose are already available on the market such as microsphere or bead (e.g., propranolol hydrochloride, theophylline, indomethacin, ibuprofen, metoprolol tartrate, and itraconazole), suspensions (e.g., paclitaxel, procaine hydrochloride, and docetaxel), hydrogel or gel (e.g., bovine serum albumin, collagen, and growth factors), membrane or coating for tablets (e.g., paracetamol, lysozyme, caffeine, indomethacin, itraconazole, beclomethasone dipropionate, lidocaine, and ibuprofen), nanofiber (e.g., Columbia blue and riboflavin) and aerogel (e.g., beclomethasone dipropionate) (Lin and Dufresne 2014).

3.11 CONCLUSIONS

In this chapter we have discussed the acquisition of cellulose nanostructures and the development of nanocomposites based on these, their properties, and their most attractive applications. Nanocellulose is characterized as having at least one of its dimensions in the nanometer scale (this is <100 nm).

TABLE 3.3

Commercial Products Based on Nanocellulose

Product	Description	Manufacturer
Biofill®	It is used as a temporary substitute for human skin (in cases of second and third degree burns) as well as bandages and dental implants. It is manufactured in different sizes and shapes.	BioFill Products Bionext
BASYC®	It is a material used for micronerve surgery and as artificial blood vessel.	
XCell®	It is a product for external application, and has been suggested for use as a blood vessel. Also it is used for the treating venous leg ulcer producing a protective, moist, hypoxic environment.	Xylos Corporation
Gengiflex®	It is used in the therapy of burns, ulcers, treatment of periodontal diseases and dental implants, in surgery and dental treatments.	BioFill Products Bionext
Bioprocess®	It is used in the therapy of burn, skin wounds and ulcers as temporary artificial skin.	BioFill Products Bionext
Surgicel®	It is a product widely used to control capillary, venous and small artery hemorrhage in surgical procedures when conventional methods are impractical. This material is available in bands of different sizes and has bacteriostatic characteristics.	Johnson & Johnson Company

TABLE 3.4

Summary of Patents Based on Nanocellulose

Patent Number	Patent Name	Description
US 7832857 B2	Microbial cellulose contact lens	The contact lens is development employed a copolymer of bacterial cellulose and Hioxifilcon B, a copolymer of 2-hydroxyethyl methacrylate and 2,3-dihydroxypropyl methacrylate. This invention has the advantages of producing contact lenses without the cross-ling step.
WO 2016174104 A1	Modified bacterial nanocellulose and its uses in chip cards and medicine	This invention consists of a nanocellulose composite which acts like a chip technology and material engineering. This material is preferably employed in wound healing, tissue engineering and as a transplant. It can also be used in methods of stimulus conduction, muscle stimulation and/or monitoring heartbeat.
EP 2779996 A1	Drug delivery system for sustained delivery of bioactive agents	The drug delivery system is made from a nanofibrillated cellulose, the bioactive agent and a support composed of a synthetic polymer and natural polymers. The material can be synthesized by different methods described in the patent. The system can be a medical device, combination product, implant, transdermal patch or a formulation for oral, sub-lingual, intraocular, in others.
US 20110039744	Personal cleansing compositions comprised of a bacterial cellulose network and cationic polymer	The material is composed of a bacterial cellulose network and a cationic polymer constituting a liquid matrix. The proportions of the two materials and method of obtaining the product have many forms that are described in the patent, these include a proportion to 0.05%–0.5% of one of the reactive.
US 20160198984 A1	Nanocellulose and nanocellulose composites as substrates for conformal bioelectronics	This invention consists of a system for electronic devices using nanocellulose and its composites made from the covalent or physical interaction between polymers. The material is suitable for thin-film electronic devices and can be employed as biological surface.

The attainment of these nanometric structures can be through chemical production, mechanical production, and through natural processes (enzymatic production of fungi or bacteria). From these three processes the crystals of nanocellulose, cellulose nanofibers, and bacterial cellulose is obtained. These three compounds can then be used to produce nanocomposite materials, which are widely applied in the fields of biomedicine and pharmaceutical through the combination of mechanical properties and bioactivity.

To obtain these nanocomposites, it is necessary to have compatibility between the nanocellulose and the matrix in which it is supported (as is the case of the generation of polymeric nanocomposites). However, one of the first obstacles is the high hydrophilicity given by the -OH groups present in cellulose, which in turn gives it high reactivity. Therefore, this allows superficial modifications that allow the insertion of hydrophobic chains into the structure of the nanocellulose. These modifications can be carried out by means of esterification, etherification, urethanization, and silylation reactions, among others. Other ways to obtain nanocomposites based on cellulose are casting-evaporation, electrospinning, melt compounding, and impregnation. Now, the biomedical and pharmaceutical applications are limited to using cellulose-based nanocomposites as supports or scaffolds for the generation of cell culture medium, since they cannot be completely degraded by the biological processes of the human body. However, its low cytotoxicity and its great biocompatibility gives it a wide range of biomedical applications, in tissue reconstruction, wound healing, enzymatic recognition, drug release, and antimicrobial biomaterials, among others.

REFERENCES

Abdalla, A., Klein, S., and Mader, K. 2008. A new self-emulsifying drug delivery system (SEDDS) for poorly soluble drugs: Characterization, dissolution, in vitro digestion and incorporation into solid pellets. *Eur J Pharm Sci* 35 (5): 457–64.

Arbelaez, N., Lerma, T., and Córdoba A. 2017. Modification of membranes by insertion of short-chain alcohols on reactive porous substrates: Effect of chain length on the surface free energy. *J Sci Technol Appl* 2: 75–83.

Ashori, A., Babaee, M., Jonoobi, M., and Hamzeh, Y. 2014. Solvent-free acetylation of cellulose nanofibers for improving compatibility and dispersion. *Carbohyd Polym* 102: 369–75.

Baumann, M.D., Kang, C.E., Stanwick, J.C. et al. 2009. An injectable drug delivery platform for sustained combination therapy. *J Control Release* 138: 205–13.

Benitez E., Lerma T., and Córdoba A. 2017. Making of porous ionic surfaces by sequential polymerization: polyurethanes + grafting of polyelectrolytes. *J Sci Technol Appl* 2: 44–53.

Boujemaoui, A., Cobo, C., Engström, J. et al. 2017. Polycaprolactone nanocomposites reinforced with cellulose nanocrystals surface-modified via covalent grafting or physisorption: A comparative study. *ACS Appl Mat Interf* 9: 35305–18.

Chaa, R., Heb, Z., and Ni, Y. 2012. Preparation and characterization of thermal/pH-sensitive hydrogel from carboxylated nanocrystalline cellulose. *Carbohyd Polym* 1: 16.

Cheremisinoff, N. 1996. *Polymer Characterization: Laboratory Techniques and Analysis*. New Jersey: Elsevier.

Ciolacu, D.E. and Darie, R.N. 2016. Nanocomposites based on cellulose, hemicelluloses, and lignin. In: Visakh, P.M. and Martínez Morlanes, M.J. (Eds.), *Nanomaterials and Nanocomposites: Zero- to Three-Dimensional Materials and Their Composites*, 391–423. Weinheim: Wiley-VCH Verlag GmbH & Co. KGaA.

Deepa, A.E. and Pothan, A. 2016. Biodegradable nanocomposite films based on sodium alginate and cellulose nanofibrils. *Materials* 9: 50.

Díez-Pascual, A., Gómez, M., Ania, F., and Flores, A. 2015. Nanoindentation in polymer nanocomposites. *Progr Mat Sci* 67: 1–94.

Dufresne, A. 2017. Cellulose nanomaterial reinforced polymer nanocomposites. *Curr Opin Colloid Interf Sci* 29: 1–8.

Dugan, J.M., Gough, J.E., and Eichhorn, S.J. 2013. Bacterial cellulose scaffolds and cellulose nanowhiskers for tissue engineering. *Nanomed* 8: 287–98.

Feese, E., Sadeghifar, H., Gracz, H.S., Argyropoulos, D.S., and Ghiladi, R.A. 2011. Photobactericidal porphyrin-cellulose nanocrystals: synthesis, characterization, and antimicrobial properties. *Biomacromol* 12: 3528–39.

Ferraz, N., Carlsson, D.O., Hong, J. et al. 2012. Hemocompatibility and ion exchange capability of nanocellulose polypyrrole membranes intended for blood purification. *J Soc Interf* 9: 1943–55.

Ferreira, F.V., Pinheiro, I.F., Gouveia, R.F., Thim, G.P., and Lona, L.M.F. 2017. Functionalized cellulose nanocrystals as reinforcement in biodegradable polymer nanocomposites. *Polym Compos* 39:1–10.

Ferrer, A., Pal, L., and Hubbe, M. 2017. Nanocellulose in packaging: Advances in barrier layer technologies. *Ind Crops Products* 95: 574–82.

Fluazino, W., Mariano, M., Vieira, I. et al. 2016. Mechanical properties of natural rubber nanocomposites reinforced with high aspect ratio cellulose nanocrystals isolated from soy hulls. *Carbohyd Polym* 153: 143–52.

Gall, K., Dunn, M.L., Liu, Y., Finch, D., Lake, M., and Munshi, N.A. 2002. Shape memory polymer nanocomposites. *Act Materialia*. 50: 5115–26.

Gangopadhyay, R. and Amitabha, D. 2000. Conducting polymer nanocomposites: a brief overview. *Chem Mater* 12: 608–22.

Habibi, Y. 2014. Key advances in the chemical modification of nanocelluloses. *Chem Soc Rev* 43: 1519–42.

Hagiwara, Y., Putra, A., Kakugo, A., Furukawa, H., and Gong, J.P. 2010. Ligament-like tough double-network hydrogel based on bacterial cellulose. *Cellulose* 17: 93–101.

Hakkarainen, T., Koivuniemi, R., and Kosonen, M. 2016. Nanofibrillar cellulose wound dressing in skin graft donor site treatment. *J Control Release* 244: 292–301.

Hamad W. 2006. On the development and applications of cellulosic nanofibrillar and nanocrystalline materials. *Canad J Chem Eng* 84: 513–9.

Jackson, J.K., Letchford, K., Wasserman, B.Z., Ye, L., Hamad, W.Y., and Burt, H.M. 2011. The use of nanocrystalline cellulose for the binding and controlled release of drugs. *Int J Nanomed* 6: 321–30.

Jeon, O. and Bouhadir, K.H. 2009. Photocrosslinked alginate hydrogels with tunable biodegradation rates and mechanical properties. *Biomater* 30: 2724–34.

Jozala, A., Lencastre-Novaes, L., Lopes, A. et al. 2016. Bacterial nanocellulose production and application: A 10-year overview. *Appl Microbiol Biotechnol* 100: 2063–72.

Kanimozhi, K., Khaleel Basha, S., Sugantha Kumari, V., Kaviyarasu, K., Maaza, M. 2017. In vitro cyto-compatibility of chitosan/PVA/methylcellulose–Nanocellulose nanocomposites scaffolds using L929 fibroblast cells. *Appl Surf Sci* 44, 574–583.

Karimi, S. 2017. Thermoplastic cellulose nanocomposites. In: Kargarzadeh, H., Ahmad, I., Thomas, S., and Dufresne, A. (Eds.), *Handbook of Nanocellulose and Cellulose Nanocomposites*, 175–216. Weinheim: Wiley-VCH Verlag GmbH & Co. KGaA.

Kargarzadeh, H., Mariano, M., Huang, Jin. et al. 2017. Recent developments on nanocellulose reinforced polymer nanocomposites: A review. *Polym* 132: 368–93.

Khalil, A., Davoudpour, Y., Islam, N. et al. 2014. Production and modification of nanofibrillated cellulose using various mechanical processes: A review. *Carbohyd Polym* 99: 649–65.

Kim, J., Montero, G., Habibi, Y. et al. 2009. Dispersion of cellulose crystallites by nonionic surfactants in a hydrophobic polymer matrix. *Polym Eng Sci* 49: 2054–61.

Kim, J., Kim, S.W., Park, S., Lim, KT., Seonwoo, H., Kim Y. et al. 2013. Bacterial cellulose nanofibrillar patch as a wound healing platform of tympanic membrane perforation. *Adv Healthcare Mater* 2: 1525–31.

Klemm, D., Kramer, F., Moritz, S. et al. 2011. Nanocelluloses: A new family of nature-based materials. *Angew Chemie Intern Ed* 50: 5438–66.

Klemm, D., Schumann, D., Kramer, F., Heßler, N., Hornung, M., Schmauder, H.P. et al. 2006. Nanocelluloses as innovative polymers in research and application. *Adv Polym Sci* 205: 49–96.

Klemm, D., Schumann, D., Udhardt, U., and Marsch S. 2001. Bacterial synthesized cellulose–artificial blood vessels for microsurgery. *Prog Polym Sci* 26: 1561–03.

Knight, P.E., Podczeck, F., and Newton, J.M. 2009. The rheological properties of modified microcrystalline cellulose containing high levels of model drugs. *J Pharm Sci* 98: 2160–9.

Kolakovic, R., Peltonen, L., Laukkanen, A., Hellman, M., Laaksonen, P., Linder, M.B. et al. 2013. Evaluation of drug interactions with nanofibrillar cellulose. *Eur J Pharm Biopharm* 85: 1238–44.

Koo, J.H. 2006. *Polymer Nanocomposites: Processing, Characterization, and Applications*. New York: McGraw-Hill Professional.

Kowalska-Ludwicka, K., Cala, J., Grobelski, B., Sygut, D., Jesionek-Kupnicka, D., Kolodziejczyk, M. et al. 2013. Modified bacterial cellulose tubes for regeneration of damaged peripheral nerves. *Arch Med Sci* 9: 527–34.

Kranz, H., Jurgens, K., Pinier, M., and Siepmann, J. 2009. Drug release from MCC- and carrageenan-based pellets: Experiment and theory. *Eur J Pharm Biopharm* 73: 302–9.

Li, J., Wan, Y.Z., Li, L.F., Liang, H., and Wang, J.H. 2009. Preparation and characterization of 2,3-dialdehyde bacterial cellulose for potential biodegradable tissue engineering scaffolds. *Mater Sci Eng C* 29: 1635–42.

Liebert, T., Kostag, M., Wotschadlo, J., and Heinze, T. 2011. Stable cellulose nanospheres for cellular uptake. *Macromol Biosci* 11: 1387–92.

Lin, N. and Dufresne A. 2013. Physical and/or chemical compatibilization of extruded cellulose nanocrystal reinforced polystyrene nanocomposites. *Macromol* 46: 5570–83.

Lin, N. and Dufresne, A. 2014. Nanocellulose in biomedicine: Current status and future prospect. *Eur Polym J* 59: 302–25.

Luo, H., Xiong, G., Hu, D., Ren, K., Yao, F., Zhu, Y. et al. 2013. Characterization of TEMPO-oxidized bacterial cellulose scaffolds for tissue engineering applications. *Mater Chem Phys* 143: 373–79.

Mahmoud, K.A., Menam, J.A., Male, K.B., Hrapovic, S., Kamen, A., and Luong, J.H.T. 2010. Effect of surface charge on the cellular uptake and cytotoxicity of fluorescent labeled cellulose nanocrystals. *ACS Appl Mater Interf* 2: 2924–32.

Mariano, M. and Dufresne, A. 2017. Nanocellulose: common strategies for processing of nanocomposites. In: Agarwal, U., Atalla, R., and Isogai, A. (Eds.), *Nanocelluloses: Their Preparation, Properties, and Applications*, 203–25 The American Chemical Society: ACS Symp Series.

Märtson, M., Viljanto, J., Hurme, T., Laippala, P., and Saukko, P. 1999. Is cellulose sponge degradable or stable as implantation material? An in vivo subcutaneous study in the rat. *Biomat* 20: 1989–95.

Mathew, A.P., Oksman, K., Pierron, D., and Harmad, MF. 2012. Fibrous cellulose nanocomposite scaffolds prepared by partial dissolution for potential use as ligament or tendon substitutes. *Carbohydr Polym* 87: 2291–8.

Miyamoto, T., Takahashi, S., Ito, H., Inagaki, H., and Noishiki, Y. 1989. Tissue biocompatibility of cellulose and its derivatives. *J Biomed Mater Res* 23: 125–33.

Moon, R.J., Martini, A., Nairn, J., Simonsen, J., and Youngblood, J. 2011. Cellulose nanomaterials review: Structure, properties and nanocomposites. *Chem Soc Rev* 40: 3941–94.

Müller, Kerstin., Bugnicourt, Elodie, Latorre, Marcos. et al. 2017. Review on the processing and properties of polymer nanocomposites and nanocoatings and their applications in the packaging, automotive and solar energy fields. *Nanomaterials* 74: 1–47.

Natterodt, J., Sapkota, J., Foster, J., and Weder, C. 2017. Polymer nanocomposites with cellulose nanocrystals featuring adaptive surface groups. *Biomacromol* 18: 517–25.

O'Connor, R.E. and Schwartz, J.B. 1993. Drug release mechanism from a microcrystalline cellulose pellet system. *Pharm Res.* 10: 356–61.

Oksman, K., Aitomaki, Y., Mathew, A.P. et al. 2016. Review of the recent developments in cellulose nanocomposite processing. *Compos: Part A* 83: 2–18.

Palencia M. 2017. Surface free energy of solids by contact angle measurements. *J Sci Technol Appl* 2: 84–93.

Palencia M., Berrio M.E., and Melendrez M. 2016. Nanostructured polymer composites with potential applications into the storage of blood and hemoderivates. *J Sci Technol Appl* 1: 4–14.

Palencia, M., Lerma, T., and Combatt, E. 2017. Hydrogels based in cassava starch with antibacterial activity for controlled release of cysteamine-silver nanostructured agents. *Curr Chem Biol* 11: 28–35.

Palencia, M., Lerma, T., and Palencia, V. 2016. Description of fouling, surface changes and heterogeneity of membranes by color-based digital image analysis. *J Membr Sci* 510: 229–37.

Pan, J., Hamad, W., and Straus, S.K. 2010. Parameters affecting the chiral nematic phase of nanocrystalline cellulose films. *Macromol* 43: 3851–58.

Pandey, J.K., Reddy, K.R., Kumar, A.P., and Singh, R.P. 2005. An overview on the degradability of polymer nanocomposites. *Polym Degrad Stability* 88: 234–50.

Pandey, J., Nakagaito, A., and Takagi, H. 2013. Fabrication and applications of cellulose nanoparticle-based polymer composites. *Polym Eng Sci* 53: 1–8.

Park, S.J., Cho, M.S., Lim, L.T., Choi, H.J., and Jhon, M.S. 2003. Synthesis and dispersion characteristics of multi-walled carbon nanotube composites with poly(methyl methacrylate) prepared by in-situ bulk polymerization. *Macromol Rapid Commun.* 24: 1070–73.

Pértile, R., Moreira, S., Gil da Costa, R., Correia, A., Guardão, L., Gartner, F. et al. 2012. Bacterial cellulose: Long-term biocompatibility studies. *J Biomater Sci Polym Ed* 23: 1339–54.

Peigney, A., Laurent, C.H., Flahaut, E., and Rousset, A. 2000. Carbon nanotubes in novel ceramic matrix nanocomposites. *Ceram Int* 26: 677–83.

Peng, B.L., Dhar, N., Liu, H.L., and Tam, K.C. 2011. Chemistry and applications of nanocrystalline cellulose and its derivatives: A nanotechnology perspective. *The Canad J Chem Eng* 89: 1191–1206.

Podczeck, F., Knight, P.E., and Newton, J.M. 2008. The evaluation of modified microcrystalline cellulose for the preparation of pellets with high drug loading by extrusion/spheronization. *Int J Pharm* 350: 145–54.

Poonguzhali, R., Khaleel, S., and Sugantha V. 2017. Synthesis of alginate/nanocellulose bionanocomposite for in vitro delivery of ampicillin. *International Journal of Drug Delivery* 9, 107–111.

Quinn, D.I., Tangen, C.M., Hussain, M., Lara, P.N., Jr, Goldkorn, A., Moinpour, C.M. et al. 2013. Docetaxel and atrasentan versus docetaxel and placebo for men with advanced castration-resistant prostate cancer: A randomised phase 3 trial. *Lancet Oncol* Aug 14(9):893–900.

Ray, S.S., and Okamoto, M. 2003. Polymer—layered silicate nanocomposites: A review from preparation to processing. *Progr Polym Sci* 28: 1539–41.

Ruiz-Palomero, C., Soriano, M., and Valcárcel, M. 2016. Sulfonated nanocellulose for the efficient dispersive micro solid-phase extraction and determination of silver nanoparticles in food products. *J Chromatograph A* 1428: 352–58.

Sheltami, R., Kargarzadeh, H., Abdullah, I., and Ahmad, I. 2017. Thermal properties of cellulose nanocomposites". In: Kargarzadeh, H., Ahmad, I., Thomas, S., and Dufresne, A. (Eds.), *Handbook of Nanocellulose and Cellulose Nanocomposites*, 523–52. Weinheim: Wiley-VCH Verlag GmbH & Co.

Slavutsky, A. and Bertuzzi, M. 2014. Water barrier properties of starch films reinforced with cellulose nanocrystals obtained from sugarcane bagasse. *Carbohyd Polym* 110: 53–61.

Tang S., Zhao Z., and Chen G. 2015. Fabrication of ampicillin/starch/polymer composite nanofibers with controlled drug release properties by electrospinning. *J Sol Gel Sci Technol* 15: 3887–93.

Trache, D., Hazwan, M., Mohamad, M.K., and Kumar, V. 2017. Recent progress in cellulose nanocrystals: Sources and production. *Nanoscale* 9: 1763–86.

Varjonen, S., Laaksonen, P., Paananen, A., Valo, H., Hähl, H., Laaksonen, T. et al. 2011. Self-assembly of cellulose nanofibrils by genetically engineered fusion proteins. *Soft Matter* 7: 2402–11.

Villanova, J., Ayres, E., Carvalho, SM., Patrício, PS., Pereira, F.V., and Oréfice, RL. 2011. Pharmaceutical acrylic beads obtained by suspension polymerization containing cellulose nanowhiskers as excipient for drug delivery. *Eur J Pharm Sci* 42: 406–15.

Vinatier, C, Gauthier, O, Fatimi, A et al. 2009. An injectable cellulose-based hydrogel for the transfer of autologous nasal chondrocytes in articular cartilage defects. *Biotechnol Bioeng* 102: 1259–67.

Wei, B., Yang, G., and Hong, F. 2011. Preparation and evaluation of a kind of bacterial cellulose dry films with antibacterial properties. *Carbohydr Polym* 84: 533–38.

Wei, Haoran, Rodriguez, Katia, Renneckar, Scott, and Vikesland, Peter. 2014. Environmental science and engineering applications of nanocellulose-based nanocomposites. *Environ Sci Nano* 1: 302–16.

Wu, Qinglin and Zhou, Chengjun. 2012. Recent development in applications of cellulose-nanocrystals for advanced polymer-based nanocomposites by novel fabrication strategies. In: Neralla, S. (Ed.), *Nanocrystals: Synthesis, Characterization and Applications*, 103–20. London: InTech.

4 Recent Advances of Chitosan Nanoparticles as a Carrier for Delivery of Antimicrobial Drugs

Bijaya Ghosh and Tapan Kumar Giri

CONTENTS

4.1 INTRODUCTION

The 20th century saw a significant increase in the life span of humans which in turn led to spectacular social and economic growth worldwide. Control of infectious diseases was a key factor in the accomplishment of this increase (Fausi 2001; Kikuchi 2015). Microbial diseases, once the greatest cause of death and disability, had almost lost their bite after the discovery of penicillin. However, in the past few decades the threat has resurfaced. The occurrence of both emerging and re-emerging infectious diseases has substantially increased. Emerging infections are classed as infections that occur in a population for the first time. Whereas, re-emerging infections are the infections that have occurred before and have re-emerged after a decline in incidents (Morens et al. 2008).

One of the crucial factors in antimicrobial therapy is the condition of the patient. It is desirable that the cause of the disease be ascertained and the causative agent identified before the start of the therapy. The results of the diagnostic tests can only be obtained after 24–72 h. Critically ill patients cannot be left untreated during this period. Hence therapy is usually initiated based on clinical manifestation, using broad spectrum antimicrobial agents.

Once the microorganism in question is identified, the next step is to conduct the antibiotic susceptibility testing. However, the choice of dosage form depends upon the urgency, intensity, and site of infection. After the discovery of penicillin, a further number were added to the repertoire of antimicrobial agents in rapid succession; then came the era of computer aided drug design. Super computers aided by knowledge of protein crystallography could tackle the challenge of decoding the complex structures of important proteins, and some new drugs were designed. In fact, the very first drug designed via computer was the antimicrobial drug norfloxacin (Boyd and Marsh 2006). But the simply structured procaryotes had already outsmarted the sophisticated humans in their own game. To defeat the powerful antimicrobials, the microbes started forming biofilms. Submerged in the matrix of multilayered films, they offered concerted resistance in the form of poor antibiotic penetration, adaptive stress response, and altered metabolic pathways (Stewart 2002). Many antibiotic resistant superbugs were born. The war between man and microbe had tilted in the invader's favor.

Thanks to stringent regulatory control, discovery of new antimicrobial agents has become cost prohibitive. Hence, warfare against microbes was focused on the design of newer dosage forms to optimize the usage of existing drugs. Embedding or encapsulating drugs in nanoscale carriers has become an important strategy in the race for victory in this neck to neck struggle (Salouti and Ahanagari 2014).

It was observed that nano delivery systems carrying an antimicrobial payload can increase the overall efficacy of drugs by virtue of their increased surface-to-volume ratio. They release the drug at a therapeutically optimal rate to inhibit the microbial growth with minimum side effects (Chen et al. 2014). However, the ultrafine delivery vehicles have their own constraints. To be successful in the test of risk benefit ratio, these nano-dosage forms have to be biocompatible, stable, non-immunogenic, and target microbial cells, leaving the host cells unaffected. Accordingly, a variety of nano-dosage forms have been developed and evaluated by a host of researchers using almost every conceivable biomolecule. Among these, polysaccharides by virtue of their biodegradability, hydrophilicity, and ease of structural manipulation occupy a prominent position. This chapter reviews the role of a natural polysaccharide—chitosan and chitosan-based nano-dosage forms—targeted against infectious diseases.

4.2 INFECTIOUS DISEASES – THE PRESENT STATUS

Every lifeform has its own challenges and more often than not these challenges force them to form communities. Bacteria is no exception. They too form communities to avoid the attack of antibiotics. These communities are known as biofilms. A biofilm is a matrix-like structure in which bacteria of the same or different species live in close proximity to one another attached to a surface using a sugary substance which they secrete. Sometimes, they get so closely attached that genetic information can be exchanged between them. The structure gives them added immunity against antibiotics because penetration of antibiotics to these layers is often difficult. The formation of biofilm gifts the bacteria added capability to adjust against environmental stress. The resistant superbugs are assisted by evolutionary selection as well as high human mobility. Methicillin-resistant *Staphylococcus aureus*, fluoroquinolone-resistant *S. aureus* (Kaatz 2005), erythromycin-resistant *S. pneumonia*, vancomycin-resistant *Enterococci* (Kayser 2003) are some dreaded examples. The problem has reached such a proportion that in the year 2000, the World Health Organization had to issue an alert that infectious diseases might become non-curable.

4.3 STRATEGIES ADOPTED BY THE MICROBES TO DEFEAT THE ANTIBIOTICS

Currently available antibiotics usually work via three mechanisms: interfering with cell wall synthesis, protein synthesis, and DNA replication. Unfortunately, some bacteria have developed resistance to antibiotics working on each of these processes. They can break down antibiotics, (β-lactamases and aminoglycosides), modify the essential components for protein synthesis (ribosomes in tetracycline resistance), or generate non-specific resistance to antibiotic action by actively removing them from the system (expression of efflux pumps). When a particular bacterium acquires all these resistance capabilities, a multidrug resistant superbug is born (Wang et al. 2017). At a physical level they can form biofilms to make the antibiotic penetration difficult. At the genetic level, resistance can be transferred and spread between bacteria through three mechanisms: plasmids, transposons, and integrons (Coetzee et al. 2016; Liu et al. 2016). Resistance can be mediated through changes in the protein machinery too, such as the alteration of antibiotic targets, inactivation of enzymes, the emergence and elimination of stress activated proteins, like BamA or KatG (Noinaj et al. 2013; Chakraborty et al. 2013) which work by unknown mechanisms.

4.4 MODE OF ACTION OF NANO DELIVERY SYSTEMS

To exert antimicrobial action nanoparticles need to be in contact with the bacterial cells. At the cell wall level, they interact with microbes by electrostatic attraction, Van Der Waal forces, receptor ligands, and hydrophobic interactions (Li et al. 2015; Armentano et al. 2014; Gao et al. 2014; Luan et al. 2016). These interactions weaken the cell wall and pave the way for the entry of nanoparticles within the cytoplasm. Inside the cell, nanoparticles can interact with cellular components like DNA and lysosomes, and protein synthesis machinery.

This results in oxidative stress, electrolyte imbalance, altered membrane permeability, protein inactivation, and sometimes changes in gene expression (Xu et al. 2016; Yang et al. 2009). Usually the most important mechanisms that cause cell death are related to oxidative stress and metal ion release (Gurunathan et al. 2012 Zacharova et al. 2015).

4.5 NATURAL POLYSACCHARIDES AS NANOCARRIERS

The concept of packaging the existing drugs into nanosized vehicles to enhance their efficacy has to balance with safety, stability as well as economic factors involved in their production. The early stage nano-dosage forms developed for microbial diseases usually used inorganic or artificial poly meric materials. But these systems had the drawback of poor biocompatibility and biodegradability (Kang et al. 2015). Hence, there was a constant search for nanomaterials that had chemically well-defined and stable structure, as well as biocompatible, biodegradable, water soluble, protein repel-lent, non-toxic, non-immunogenic, offering the opportunity for easy surface modification (Kang et al. 2015).

A number of naturally occurring substances were screened to assess their feasibility for develop-ing biodegradable nanosystems. Polymeric nanosystems, especially the polysaccharides, are rated highly within these criteria.

Polysaccharides which are abundantly available from plant and bacterial sources are equipped with these sought after properties. Compared to other biomolecules, proteins or nucleic acids, poly-saccharides enjoy more structural flexibility as the linkage points between sugar units are not con-strained to the same positions (Kang et al. 2015). They can either adsorb the drug on the surface or hide it within their core (Kumari et al. 2014). Chitosan—a polysaccharide obtained from natural sources—was found to have antimicrobial properties and be particularly suitable for the develop-ment of nanovehicles for antimicrobial drugs.

4.6 CHITOSAN—AN ANTIMICROBIAL POLYSACCHARIDE

Chitosan is obtained by the controlled deacetylation of chitin, a nitrogen-containing organic compound widely available in animal shells, marine diatoms, as well as fungal cell walls (Singla and Chawla 2001). Cultivation of the fungus *Aspergillus niger* is also projected to be an alternative source of chitosan (Rabea et al. 2003). The quality of chitosan depends on the degree of deacetylation. Usually a product having greater than 60% deacetylation becomes soluble in dilute acid and is called chitosan. Chitosan was first prepared by a French professor H. Braconnot (Dayong 2012). He treated mushrooms repeatedly with warm alkaline solution to get a white fibroid chitosan which he named fungine. The structure of chitin, from which chitosan is derived, is the same as cellulose with only one difference. Instead of hydroxyl [-OH] group at C-2 position, chitin has an acetamido [-NHCOCH3] group. Chitosan is produced when an acetyl group is removed and a NH2 group is exposed. The change confers on the molecule its antimicrobial potential. As the process used for deacetylation of chitin can remove the acetyl groups only partially, chitosan is regarded as a partial N-deacetylated derivative of chitin (Rafaat and Sahl 2009; Khor 2001).

Though chitosan was discovered in 1811, it did not get much attention until the 1970s. Since the 1970s, researchers have started showing an active interest in chitosan which paved the way for its application in different fields of science, including its use in antimicrobial dosage development. Chitosan itself is effective against a broad spectrum of bacteria, fungi, and viruses. The antimicrobial effect of chitosan is mainly dependent on its molecular weight and degree of deacetylation. In acidic solution the amino groups of chitosan get protonated making it a polyelectrolyte. The positively charged amino groups of chitosan get attracted to the negatively charged mucus conferring the molecule its property of mucoadhesiveness (Rafaat and Sahl 2009).

Biodegradability is a desired parameter for dosage forms intended for systemic application. Hence, degradation of chitosan or chitosanolysis has been investigated by a number of researchers (Ulanski et al. 2000; Rhoades and Roller 2000; Kumar et al. 2005). It was shown that chitosan can be degraded by non-specific enzymes (chitinases, cellulases, hemicellulases, glucanases, etc.) from a variety of sources (Vårum et al. 1997; Rhoades and Roller 2000; Kumar et al. 2005; Rafaat and Sahl 2009). Lysozyme, an enzyme found in tears, saliva, and body fluids can break the β 1,4 glycosidic linkage of chitosan to make it biodegradable.

Fukamizo et al. proposed a classification system for chitosanases according to their capacity to cleave the bonds (Fukamizo et al. 1994). Class I chitosanases split the bond between acetylated D-glucosamine (GlcNAc) and D-glucosamine (GlcN), in class II, only GlcN-GlcN linkage and in class III both GlcN-GlcN and GlcN-GlcNAc linkages (Rafaat and Shal 2009).

The polymer can be degraded by UV radiation too, and it increases its antimicrobial potential (Matsuhasi and Kume 1997). Though chitosan has not been officially proclaimed as GRAS (generally recognized as safe) by the FDA, it has approved its use in medical purpose like wound healing and drug encapsulation. Primex Ingredients ASA—a Norwegian manufacturer of chitosan—has claimed that its purified chitosan product (ChitoClear®) has achieved a GRAS self-affirmed status in the US (Rafaat and Sahl 2009).

4.7   NEED FOR NANOPARTICULATE DRUG DELIVERY IN INFECTIOUS DISEASES

Treatments of infection with anti-infective drugs have been around for decades. However, due to the development of antibiotic resistance, infections may now become lethal. A microbial strain is considered resistant when the microbe does not respond to standard treatments and the infection becomes difficult to treat (WHO 2014).

Microbes can become resistant through diverse mechanisms such as permeability modification of the membrane, DNA alterations, changes of intracellular lifecycle, enzyme activation, and multidrug efflux pump development (Alekshun and Levy 2007). Some of the microbes such as *Chlamydophila pneumonia* or *Mycoplasma pneumonia* not only reside in the cytosol but also in the nucleus, endosome, golgi apparatus, and endoplasmic reticulum (Katz and Waites 2004) (Figure 4.1). Inhibiting the growth of these microbes is a challenging task, since most drugs can't go beyond the extracellular space. In addition, the few drugs that can penetrate the cell membrane to enter the cellular space, get quickly degraded and provide a concentration below the therapeutic/inhibitory concentration

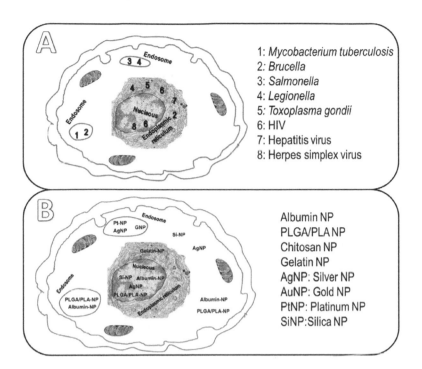

FIGURE 4.1 A. Intracellular localization of different pathogens: 1: *mycobacterium tuberculosis* 2: *brucella*; 3: *salmonella*; 4: *legionella*; 5: *toxoplasma gondii*; 6:HIV; 7: hepatitis C virus 8: herpes simplex virus. B. Intracellular distribution of different kinds of nanoparticles: albumin NP; PLGA/PLA NP; GelatinNP; AgNP: silver NP; AuNP: gold NP; PtNP: platinum NP; SiNP: silica NP. (Reprinted from *J Controlled Release* 224, Zazo, H., Colino, C.I., and Lanao, J.M. Current applications of nanoparticles in infectious diseases, 86–102, Copyright 2016, with permission from Elsevier.)

levels (Briones et al. 2008). Another major difficulty is that the pathogenic microbes present intracellularly can also stay alive and replicate within phagocytic cells. These cells act as a safe-house for microbes, where drugs cannot reach. They protect the microbes from treatment and abet their growth by favoring their replication and the spread of infection (Briones et al. 2008; Mukhopadhyay and Basu 2003).

Development of new drugs is a slower process than in the past (Rai et al. 2013). In addition, developed molecules often fail to perform in the clinical trials owing to their inactivation, degradation or inability to reach the infection site (Chang et al. 2010). Physicochemical limitations of drug molecules such as a short half-life, variable absorption, and low bioavailability are also some major constraints obstructing their clinical acceptability. To conquer these limitations, frequent administrations with high doses have been used for the treatment of infectious diseases. But with high dose comes the burden of toxicity and sometimes severe side effects lead to the discontinuation of therapy (Briones et al. 2008; Lembo and Cavalli 2010). As the loading of drugs in the nanocarriers can solve some of these problems and augment the effectiveness of available drugs (Kingsley et al. 2006), antimicrobial drug delivery research is focused on the development of nanoparticulate drug delivery systems. Nanocarriers allow drugs to be targeted selectively and help them reach the desired target within the cells and release the drugs at therapeutic concentration levels. They protect the drugs from degradation and undesirable interactions prior to reaching the target site. Moreover, they can hold numerous drugs in a single formulation which is exceedingly useful in combating complicated infections like the ones caused by *Helicobacter pylori* or HIV (Destache et al. 2010; Freeling et al. 2014). Figure 4.1 shows some examples of nanoparticles intracellular distribution.

4.8 NANOSYSTEMS CONTAINING CHITOSAN FOR ANTIMICROBIAL DRUG DELIVERY

4.8.1 CHITOSAN-BASED NANOCARRIER SYSTEMS FOR ANTIBACTERIAL DRUG DELIVERY

A sizable section of drug delivery researchers are engaged in developing nanotechnology-based dosage forms to advance the therapeutic effectiveness of existing antibiotics. To treat intracellular infection, antibiotics should be delivered to the exact locations within the host where microbes are present. The use of a nanocarrier to enter the bacteria through endocytic/phagocytic pathways seems to be an attractive move toward the intracellular targeted delivery of antibiotics (Figure 4.2). Characteristics of an "ideal" nanocarrier for intracellular drug delivery are shown in Figure 4.3.

Chitosan nanoparticles use several mechanisms to fight microbes. The antimicrobial action of chitosan can be augmented by preparing nanoparticles. Clinical use of chitosan is limited due to poor solubility in vivo (Friedman et al. 2013). However, in vivo solubility of chitosan can be increased by incorporating chitosan into nanoparticles (Friedman et al. 2013). Encapsulating chitosan into nanoparticles increases its binding to microbial cell walls, surface charge, and surface area-to-volume ratio (Blecher et al. 2011; Friedman et al. 2013).

Chitosan nanoparticles have better effectiveness against *E. coli* and *S. aureus* in comparison to chitosan itself, acetic acid, and even doxycycline (Blecher et al. 2011). Chitosan nanoparticles with a high molecular weight show superior activity against Gram positive bacteria in comparison to Gram negative bacteria. However, chitosan nanoparticles with a low molecular weight have better effectiveness against Gram negative bacteria in comparison to Gram positive bacteria (Huh and Kwon 2011). Chitosan may be more effective on Gram negative bacteria due to the presence of more negative charge on its cell envelope. Amino groups (positively charged) of chitosan also displace the

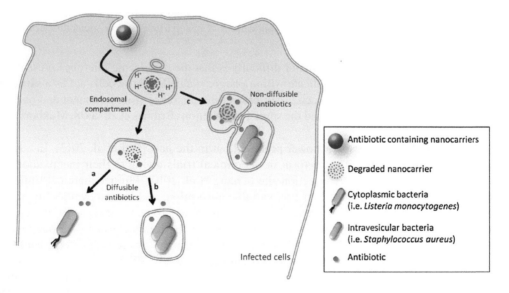

FIGURE 4.2 Intracellular delivery of antibiotics to treat intracellular infections. Following cell internalization through one or several endocytic pathways, nanocarriers should be destabilized and/or degraded by hydrolytic enzymes and/or acidic pH to allow the antibiotic to be released. A diffusible antibiotic will easily escape from endosomes and reach cytoplasmic bacteria (a) or vesicles containing bacteria (b) to exert antimicrobial activity. In some cases, fusion between endosomes (with captured nanocarriers + antibiotic) and vesicles containing bacteria (c) are needed in order to allow non-diffusible antibiotics to exert their antimicrobial activity. (Reprinted from *Int J Antimicrob Agents* 43, Abed, N. and Couvreur, P. Nanocarriers for antibiotics: A promising solution to treat intracellular bacterial infections, 485–96, Copyright 2014, with permission from Elsevier.).

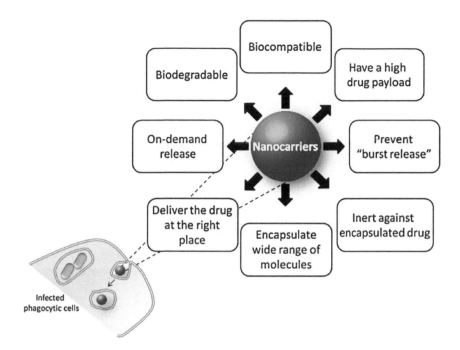

FIGURE 4.3 Characteristics of an "ideal" nanocarrier for intracellular drug delivery. (Reprinted from *Int J Antimicrob Agents* 43, Abed, N., and Couvreur, P. Nanocarriers for antibiotics: A promising solution to treat intracellular bacterial infections, 485–96, Copyright 2014, with permission from Elsevier.)

Mg^{++} and Ca^{++} cations that generally stabilize lipopolysaccharides present in the outer membrane of Gram negative bacteria. Displacement of the Mg^{++} and Ca^{++} cations weakens the cell wall and augments the permeability of the membrane (Friedman et al. 2013; Huang et al. 2011).

Antibacterial activity of chitosan nanoparticles against *Staphylococcus aureus* was much higher in comparison to chitosan solutions (Wazed Ali et al. 2010). Du et al. determined minimal bactericide concentration and minimal inhibitory concentration using chitosan nanoparticles and chitosan solution on *Staphylococcus aureus*, *Salmonella choleraesuis*, and *Escherichia coli* (Du et al. 2009). Minimal bactericide concentration of chitosan nanoparticles was found to be much lower (one-fourth) to that of chitosan solutions. To augment the antibacterial effectiveness Cu^{2+} and Zn^{2+} ions were added to chitosan nanoparticles. Antibacterial activity was augmented by 20–40 times in comparison to simple solutions.

Abelgawad et al. (2014) developed a hybrid nanofiber mat for antimicrobial usage by combining chitosan-based silver nanoparticles with polyvinyl alcohol. Nanofibers with 150 nm average diameter were obtained by electrospinning and crosslinking with glutaraldhyde. The antibacterial efficacy was evaluated for both silver-loaded and control (chitosan/PVA) mats. The results indicated that compared to the control group, the chitosan-PVA hybrid mats containing silver nanoparticles had superior bactericidal activity against the Gram negative bacteria *E. coli*. Synergistic action between silver nanoparticles and chitosan-PVA was suggested as the cause for the potentiating effect (Figure 4.4).

A research group developed triggered-release liposomes stabilized by chitosan-modified gold nanoparticles for selectively delivering a drug to the toxin-releasing bacteria. They used Methicillin-resistant *Staphylococcus aureus* (MRSA) as a model for a toxin-releasing bacterium and vancomycin as the anti-MRSA model drug. The chitosan-gold stabilized liposomes could protect the encapsulated drug during storage and released it completely at the site of infection. The toxins secreted by MRSA got inserted into the liposomal membrane to create pores which acted as the release pathway for drugs (Pornpattanarangkul et al. 2011).

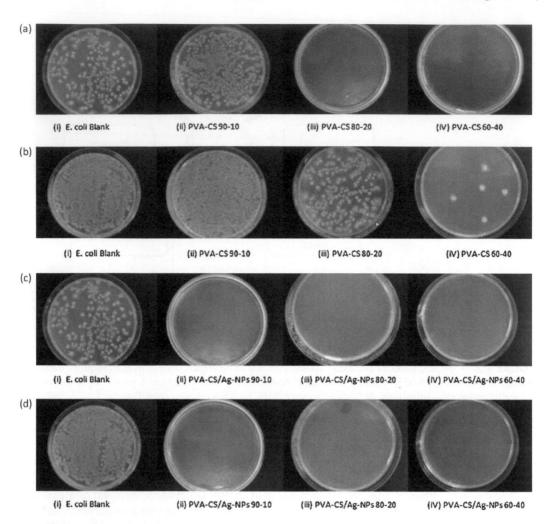

FIGURE 4.4   The antibacterial activity of the e-spun mats against *E. coli*. (a) PVA/CS [9/10, 80/20, and 60/40] weight blending ratios at 7×105 CFU/mL bacteria, (b) PVA/CS [9/10,80/20, and 60/40] weight blending ratios at 7×107 CFU/mL bacteria, (c) PVA/CS-Ag-NPs [9/10, 80/20, and 60/40] weight blending ratios at 7×105 CFU/mL bacteria, and (d)PVA/CS-Ag-NPs [9/10, 80/20, and 60/40] weight blending ratios at 7×107 CFU/mL bacteria. (Reprinted from *Carbohydr Polym* 100, Abdelgawad, A.M., Hudson, S.M., and Rojas, O.J. Antimicrobial wound dressing nanofiber mats from multicomponent (chitosan/silver-NPs/polyvinyl alcohol) systems, 166–78, Copyright 2014, with permission from Elsevier.)

The antibacterial agent levofloxacin was also entrapped into chitosan nanoparticles to treat ocular infections (Ameeduzzafar et al. 2018). The prepared nanoparticles showed a nanometric size range with high encapsulation efficiency. The prepared nanoparticles demonstrated superior antibacterial activity against *S. aureus* and *P. aeruginosa*. Chitosan nanoparticles loaded with ciprofloxacin hydrochloride as an antibacterial agent were prepared via ionotropic gelation method using tripolyphosphate as a crosslinking agent (Sobhani et al. 2017). The antibacterial activity of prepared nanoparticles was evaluated against *S. aureus* and *E. coli*. The minimum inhibitory concentration of chitosan nanoparticles loaded with ciprofloxacin hydrochloride was 50% lower in comparison to the free drug. Chitosan nanoparticles without drugs showed antibacterial activity at higher concentrations.

One of the major problems associated with the treatment of salmonella infection is inadequate penetration into the cell. The penetrability is further reduced when bacteria form biofilms. Flucoidan-coated chitosan nanoparticles were prepared to treat the aforementioned infection

(Elbi et al. 2017). The size range of the fucoidan-coated chitosan nanoparticles were bigger than that of the chitosan nanoparticles (320 vs. 124 nm). Over a period of two weeks, sustained release of ciprofloxacin was observed from both the chitosan nanoparticles and the fucoidan-coated chitosan nanoparticles. Interestingly, in spite of the greater size, the intracellular antibacterial activity of the fucoidan-coated chitosan nanoparticles was two-fold higher than the chitosan nanoparticles and six-fold higher than the drug alone. Vancomycin-loaded chitosan nanoparticles were also prepared to treat MRSA infections (Kalhapure et al. 2017). The prepared nanoparticles were spherical in shape (220.57±5.9 nm) and showed minimum inhibitory concentrations of 7.81 and 62.5 µg/ml against MRSA at pH 6.5 and 7.4 respectively. In vivo antibacterial activity showed that MRSA burden in mice treated with chitosan nanoparticles was reduced by almost eight-fold compared to those treated with pure vancomycin. Various chitosan nanocarrier systems loaded with antibacterial drugs are shown in Table 4.1.

TABLE 4.1
Chitosan Nanocarrier for Delivery of Antibacterial Drug

Drug	Nanocarrier	Research Finding	References
Rifampin	Chitosan/gelatin/lecithin nanoparticles	Nanoparticles release rifampicin at a slow and constant rate	Farnia et al. 2017
Thyme essential oil	Chitosan nanoparticles and nanocapsules	The inhibitory activity against foodborne bacteria was higher for nanoparticles in comparison to nanocapsules	Sotelo-Boyás et al. 2017
Amoxicillin	Genipin-crosslinked fucoidan/chitosan-N-arginine nanogels	Exhibited pH-responsive drug release property	Lin et al. 2017
Thymol	Chitosan silver nanoparticles	Nanoparticles showed efficacy against multiple foodborne pathogens	Manukumar et al. 2017
Vancomycin	N-trimethyl chitosan nanoparticles	Inhibits bacteria and promotes bone repair in vivo in a *Staphylococcus aureus*-induced osteomyelitis rabbit model	Zhang et al. 2017
Ampicillin	Chitosan with super paramagnetic calcium ferrite nanoparticle	Drug was released quickly in acidic medium in comparison to the basic or neutral medium	Bilas et al. 2017
Norfloxacin	Chitosan nanoparticulate in-situ gelling system	The best formulation showed adequate antibacterial activity and was free from ocular irritancy	Upadhayay et al. 2016
Chlorhexidine and silver	Chitosan/poly(ethylene oxide) nanofibrous membrane	Nanofibrous membranes acted as an active antibacterial dressing for the local delivery of antibacterial agents to prevent percutaneous device associated infections	Song et al. 2016
Tigecycline	Lecithin-coated chitosan nanoparticles	Developed nanoparticles effectively cured of *S. aureus* infected wounds	Dhanalakshmi et al. 2016
Amoxicillin	Ureido-conjugated chitosan nanoparticles	Prepared nanoparticles have great potential for effective therapy of *H. pylori* infection	Jing et al. 2016
Tetracycline and lovastatin	Poly(D,L-lactide-co-glycolide acid)-chitosan nanoparticles	Prepared nanoparticles showed good biocompatibility and antibacterial activity	Lee et al. 2016

(*Continued*)

TABLE 4.1 (CONTINUED)

Chitosan Nanocarrier for Delivery of Antibacterial Drug

Drug	Nanocarrier	Research Finding	References
Gentamicin	Chitosan/fucoidan nanoparticles	Nanoparticles effectively deliver gentamicin in the pulmonary region for pneumonia treatment	Huang et al. 2016
Sparfloxacin	Chitosan nanosuspension	Nanosuspension showed higher in vitro and in vivo antimicrobial potential compared to pure drug	Ambhore et al. 2016
Temporin B	Chitosan nanoparticle	Nanocarrier evidenced a sustained antibacterial action against various strains of *Staphylococcus*	Piras et al. 2015
Vancomycin	Chitosan nanoparticle	Nanoparticles showed good bactericidal activity against *S. aureus*	Cerchiara et al. 2015
Daptomycin	Chitosan-coated alginate nanoparticles	The developed nanoparticles effectively delivered daptomycin for treatment of bacterial endophthalmitis	Costa et al. 2015
Isoniazid and rifampicin	Spray dried inhalable chitosan nanoparticles	More effective against the mycobacterium than free drugs	Garg et al. 2016
Daptomycin	Chitosan nanoparticles	Total in vitro release of daptomycin was obtained within 4 h	Silva et al. 2015
Ciprofloxacin	Carboxymethyl chitosan nanoparticles	Nanoparticle showed stronger antibacterial activity against *Escherichia coli* than the free ciprofloxacin	Zhao et al. 2013
Tetracycline	O-carboxymethyl chitosan nanoparticles	Nanoparticles were six-fold more effective in killing intracellular *S. aureus* in comparison to tetracycline alone	Maya et al. 2012
Ceftriaxone sodium	Chitosan nanoparticles	Enhanced the intracellular delivery and antibacterial effect of ceftriaxone sodium in enterocytes and macrophages	Zaki and Hafez 2012

4.8.2 Chitosan-Based Nanocarrier Systems for Antiparacidal Drug Delivery

Parasites are among of the oldest organisms found in nature, occurring all over the world. Their existence has been discovered even in fossil sponges millions of years old (Zapalski and Hubert 2011). A parasitic disease is an infectious disease transmitted or caused by a parasite. Recently, the propensity of these infections have enhanced significantly due to various factors such as the increase in immigration, international tourism, and import of food products. Despite the fast development of science and medicine, parasitic diseases are still an exceptionally serious problem continually contributing to disability and death (Cholewiński et al. 2015).

The antimalarial drug chloroquine was conjugated into chitosan nanoparticles and its efficacy evaluated against liver apoptosis and a reactive oxygen species-mediated caspase activation in the *Plasmodium berghei* infection (Tripathy et al. 2015). Chitosan nanoparticles containing chloroquine improved reactive oxygen species, apoptotic protein level, and mitochondrial membrane potential in comparison to chloroquine. Chitosan nanoparticles containing chloroquine reduced apoptotic cells by 61.56% whereas free chloroquine reduced the same by 25.31%. in *P. berghei* induced liver apoptosis.

Leishmaniasis is a protozoan disease affecting large numbers of people in various regions of the world. Even if numerous drugs have been used to treat disease: limited efficacy, the requirement for prolonged therapy, and resistance development remain the major limitations. Novel chitosan nanoparticles loaded with recombinant leishmania superoxide dismutase were prepared via ionotropic gelation method for treatment of leishmaniasis (Danesh-Bahreini et al. 2011). It was observed that chitosan nanoparticles loaded with recombinant leishmania superoxide dismutase increased the immunogenicity toward cell-mediated immunity that is effective in leishmania eradication.

Lymphatic filariasis is a parasitic infection that also affects large numbers of people, especially those in tropical areas. Eradication of this disease completely can only be possible by the potent vaccine development. Antigen abundant larval transcript and brugia malayi thioredoxin have produced an identifiable level of defense among the numerous filarial antigens, thereby these two antigens are recognized as good vaccine candidates. Malathi et al. tried to enhance the immunoprophylactic activity of these two antigens by entrapping them into chitosan nanoparticles (Malathi et al. 2015). It was observed the immunostimulatory properties of nanoparticles provide an improved level of proliferation for antigens in peripheral blood mononuclear cells from endemic normal personals in comparison to stimulation obtained by antigens alone. Various chitosan nanocarrier systems loaded with antiparasitic drug are shown in Table 4.2.

TABLE 4.2
Chitosan Nanocarriers for Delivery of Antiparasitic Drugs

Drug	Nanocarrier	Research Finding	References
Chloroquine	Chitosan nanoparticle	The nanoparticle is better than free chloroquine in protecting the tissue damage during malarial infection	Tripathy et al. 2014
Amphotericin B	Mannose-anchored thiolated chitosan nanocarrier	Chitosan nanoparticles elicited 90% macrophage viability and 71-fold augmentation in drug uptake in comparison to the free drug	Shahnaz et al. 2017
Amphotericin B	4-sulfated N-acetyl galactosamine anchored chitosan nanoparticles	Highly significant anti-leishmanial activity was observed with nanoparticle in comparison to the free drug	Tripathi et al. 2015
Amphotericin B	Chitosan-chondroitin sulfate nanocarrier	Nanocarriers improved the toxicity profile and lowered LD50 value of the drug considerably in comparison to the free drug	Bose et al. 2016
β-lapachone	Lecithin-chitosan nanoparticles	Nanoparticles reduced inflammatory response without affecting the parasite killing efficacy	Moreno et al. 2015
Amphotericin B	Chitosan and chondroitin sulfate nanoparticles	Nanoparticles significantly reduced the lesion size and the parasite burden in comparison to the free drug	Ribeiro et al. 2014
Amphotericin B	Sodium alginate crosslinked glycol chitosan stearate nanoparticles	Nanoparticles showed more localized distribution toward leishmania infected organs i.e. the spleen and liver while lesser toward kidney	Gupta et al. 2015
Curcumin	Mannosylated chitosan nanoparticles	Nanoparticles showed effective endocytosis within the macrophages of reticuloendothelial system	Chaubey et al. 2014
Rifampicin	Mannose-conjugated chitosan nanoparticles	Accumulation of nanoparticles in macrophage rich organs, particularly in the liver and spleen, were significantly higher in comparison to the free drug	Chaubey and Mishra 2014

4.8.3 Chitosan-Based Nanocarrier Systems for Antifungal Drug Delivery

Unlike bacterial infections, treatment of fungal infections is a challenging job especially in immunocompromised people. Unlike bacteria, fungi is eukaryotic. It contains a membrane-bound nucleus and also mitochondria, endoplasmic reticulum, and a golgi apparatus enclosed within a rigid cell wall, mostly made of the complex polysaccharides—chitin and glucan. Fungi thrive in environments that are wet and slightly acidic in nature. They can grow in both light and dark. Though closely linked with animals, fungi digest their food in a way totally different from animals. They first digest the food and then ingest it later. In spite of a lot of research, the exact molecular architecture of fungal cell walls remains elusive. But it is the most practical medical target for containing an infection because the medicines come in contact with the cell wall first. The fungal cell wall has a unique balance of rigidity and flexibility. Park et al. (2008) prepared a series of low molecular weight (1, 3, 5, and 10 kDa) water-soluble (LMWS) chitosan derivatives to achieve improved penetrability of the fungal membrane. They evaluated their antifungal efficacy against major plant pathogens as well as some fungal species that usually infect immunocompromised people. The strain on which LMWS-chitosan derivatives were tested included *C. albicans* (causative organism of oropharyngeal candidiasis), *T. beigelli* (disseminated infection in immune-compromised patients), the common Baker's yeast, *S. cerevisiae* (causing fungemia or presence of fungus in blood), *A. fumigatus* (saprophytic fungi causing severe lung infection), *A. paraciticus* (produces the carcinogenic compound aflatoxin in plants and cause invasive lung infection), *B. cineria* (a plant pathogen causing serious economic loss), *F.solani* (the reason behind almost 50% of human fungal diseases like corneal infection, osteomyelitis, skin infection, fungemia, and endophthalmitis), *F. oxysporum* (causes wilting of banana plants and oil palms), and *P. verrucosum* (the reason behind a rare type of highly inflammatory cutaneous infection) (Schnadig and Woods 2009; Munoz et al. 2005; Williamson et al. 2007; Zhang et al. 2006; Hafizi et al. 2013; O'Gorman et al. 2015).

It was observed that chitosan derivatives could successfully inhibit the growth of fungus. The derivative with the highest molecular weight (10 kDa) showed maximum antifungal activity. The minimum inhibitory concentration of this derivative was quite low. It could inhibit the growth of all the strains tested at a concentration level less than 0.04 mg/ml which caused no haemolytic effect on the human red blood cells. The lytic effects of chitosan derivates were also assessed by an MTT assay. The cells treated by chitosan derivatives showed distinct morphological changes whereas untreated cells had a normal smooth surface. Lipid membrane-disruption was suggested to be mechanism causing the antifungal effect. The derivatives fared well in terms of safety parameters too. The cell viability assay performed on LMWS-chitosan treated human keratocyte cells (HaCaT cell lines) showed no cytotoxic effect.

4.9 CONCLUSION

The threat of re-emerging microbial diseases and the high costs of drug discovery has caused the scientific community to look for a cure among the existing repertoire of drugs. Focus has shifted to the development of novel dosage forms and newer strategies are being framed to combat diseases caused by microbes using the existing drugs available.

Bacteria are simple prokaryotic lifeforms with highly efficient replication machinery. Apart from genetic code bearing nucleic acids, other components essential for bacterial life are a cell membrane, a ribosome, a few proteins and enzymes and often a sturdy cell wall to keep it protected from the hostile environment. The drugs designed to contain or kill these microbes interfere with the synthesis of these essentially vital components. Unfortunately most of the components of the microbial body are basic in nature and at the molecular level have strong similarities with the host cells that they choose to infect. Hence most of the drugs also have the potential to cause damage to the cellular machineries of the host. More often than not the highly potent antimicrobial agents meant for the microbes, cause significant damage to the host, making the treatment of infectious disease a challenging job. Here's where nanoparticles become useful. Nanoparticles have the advantage of nanometric dimensions and can enjoy high mobility and penetrability through the bio barriers. When custom-made, with optimal size distribution, these drug-loaded vehicles can deliver their payload to the desired site to enhance the therapeutic effect of drugs manifold. With smaller than average microbes also, they can negotiate the cell barriers of the host and interact with the vital machineries of the normal cells and affect their functioning. A sizable fraction of the scientific community is opposed to the use of nanoscale dosage forms because of this possibility.

However with the backdrop of antibiotic resistance and the mutative development of superbugs, nanoscale delivery systems are too powerful a weapon to ignore in the war against the pathogenic microbes. So, research is focused on developing nanosized dosage forms that will have selective toxicity against the pathogens. Chitosan is a rare find gifted with this quality. It has broad spectrum of antimicrobial activity and is equipped with in-built hydroxyl and amino groups that can be attached to drugs with simple chemical reactions. Its antimicrobial properties have already been exploited in wound healing. Presently, researchers are trying to exploit its antimicrobial properties by complexation and molecular weight manipulation. The world is hopeful that that this wonder molecule will form the basis of the proverbial "magic bullet" not only for antimicrobials but also for many other therapeutic molecules. The positive outcomes of numerous chitosan-based nanosystems developed in the laboratory seems to be the reason behind that expectation.

REFERENCES

Abdelgawad, A.M., Hudson, S.M., and Rojas, O.J. 2014. Antimicrobial wound dressing nanofiber mats from multicomponent (chitosan/silver-NPs/polyvinyl alcohol) systems. *Carbohydr Polym* 100: 166–78.

Alekshun, M.N. and Levy, S.B. 2007. Molecular mechanisms of antibacterial multidrug resistance. *Cell* 128: 1037–50.

Ambhore, N.P., Dandagi, P.M., and Gadad, A.P. 2016. Formulation and comparative evaluation of HPMC and water soluble chitosan-based sparfloxacin nanosuspension for ophthalmic delivery. *Drug Deliv Transl Res* 6 (1): 48–56.

Ameeduzzafar., Imam, S.S., Abbas Bukhari, S.N., and Ahmad, J. and Ali, A. 2018. Formulation and optimization of levofloxacin loaded chitosan nanoparticle for ocular delivery: In-vitro characterization, ocular tolerance and antibacterial activity. *Int J Biol Macromol* 108: 650–59.

Armentano, I., Arciola, C.R., Fortunati, E., Ferrari, D., Mattioli, S., Amoroso, C.F. et al. 2014. The interaction of bacteria with engineered nanostructured polymeric materials: A review. *Scientific World J* 2014: 410–23.

Bilas, R., Sriram, K., Maheswari, P.U., and Sheriffa Begum, K.M. 2017. Highly biocompatible chitosan with super paramagnetic calcium ferrite ($CaFe_2O_4$) nanoparticle for the release of ampicillin. *Int J Biol Macromol* 97: 513–25.

Blecher, K., Nasir, A., and Friedman, A. 2011. The growing role of nanotechnology in combating infectious disease. *Virulence* 2: 395–401.

Bose, P.P., Kumar, P., and Dwivedi, M.K. 2016. Hemoglobin guided nanocarrier for specific delivery of amphotericin B to Leishmania infected macrophage. *Acta Trop* 158: 148–59.

Boyd, D.B. and Marsh, M.M. 2006. History of computer in pharmaceutical research and development: A narrative. In: Ekins, S. (Ed.), *Computer Applications in Pharmaceutical Research and Development*, 1–36. Wiley and Sons.

Briones, E., Colino, C.I., and Lanao, J.M. 2008. Delivery systems to increase the selectivity of antibiotics in phagocytic cells. *J Control Release* 125: 210–27.

Cerchiara, T., Abruzzo, A., di Cagno, M., Bigucci, F., Bauer-Brandl, A., Parolin, C. et al. 2015. Chitosan based micro- and nanoparticles for colon-targeted delivery of vancomycin prepared by alternative processing methods. *Eur J Pharm Biopharm* 92: 112–9.

Chakraborty, S., Gruber, T., Barry, C.E., Boshoff, H.I., and Rhee, K.Y. 2013. Para-aminosalicylic acid acts as an alternative substrate of folate metabolism in Mycobacterium tuberculosis. *Science* 339 (6115): 88–91.

Chang, C.H., Lin, Y.H., Yeh, C.L., Chen, Y.C., Chiou, S.F., Hsu, Y.M. et al. 2010. Nanoparticles incorporated in pH-sensitive hydrogels as amoxicillin delivery for eradication of Helicobacter pylori. *Biomacromolecules* 11: 133–42.

Chaubey, P. and Mishra, B. 2014. Mannose-conjugated chitosan nanoparticles loaded with rifampicin for the treatment of visceral leishmaniasis. *Carbohydr Polym* 101: 1101–8.

Chaubey, P., Patel, R.R., and Mishra, B. 2014. Development and optimization of curcumin-loaded mannosylated chitosan nanoparticles using response surface methodology in the treatment of visceral leishmaniasis. *Expert Opin Drug Deliv* 11 (8): 1163–81.

Chen, J., Wang, F., Liu, Q, and Du, J. 2014. Antibacterial polymeric nanostructures forbiomedical applications. *Chem Commun* 50: 14482.

Cholewiński, M., Derda, M., and Hadaś, E. 2015. Parasitic diseases in humans transmitted by vectors. *Ann Parasitol* 61 (3): 137–57.

Coetzee, J., Corcoran, C., Prentice E, Moodley, M., Mendelson, M., and Poirel, L. 2016. Emergence of plasmid-mediated colistin resistance (MCR-1) amongEscherichia coliisolated from South African patients. *S Afr Med J* 106 (5): 449–50.

Costa, J.R., Silva, N.C., Sarmento, B., and Pintado, M. 2015. Potential chitosan-coated alginate nanoparticles for ocular delivery of daptomycin. *Eur J Clin Microbiol Infect Dis* 34 (6): 1255–62.

Danesh-Bahreini, et al. 2011. Nanovaccine for leishmaniasis: preparation of chitosan nanoparticles containing Leishmania superoxide dismutase and evaluation of its immunogenicity in BALB/c mice. *Int J Nanomedicine* 6: 835–42.

Dayong, T. 2012. From chitin to chitosan. In: K.Yao J. Li Y. Fanglian, and Y. Yin (Eds.), *Chitosan Based Hydrogels Functions and Applications*, 1–38. CRC Press.

Destache, C.J., Belgum, T., Goede, M., Shibata, A., and Belshan, M.A. 2010. Antiretroviral release from poly(DL-lactide-co-glycolide) nanoparticles in mice. *J Antimicrob Chemother* 65: 2183–7.

Dhanalakshmi, V., Nimal, T.R., Sabitha, M., Biswas, R., and Jayakumar, R. 2016. Skin and muscle permeating antibacterial nanoparticles for treating Staphylococcus aureus infected wounds. *J Biomed Mater Res B Appl Biomater* 104 (4): 797–807.

Du, W.L., Niu, S.S., Xu, Y.L., Xu, Z.R., and Fan, C.L. 2009. Antibacterial activity of chitosan tripolyphosphate nanoparticles loaded with various metal ions. *Carbohydr Polym* 75: 385–9.

Elbi, S., Nimal, T.R., Rajan, V.K., Baranwal, G., Biswas, R., Jayakumar, R., and Sathianarayanan, S. 2017. Fucoidan coated ciprofloxacin loaded chitosan nanoparticles for the treatment of intracellular and biofilm infections of Salmonella. *Colloids Surf B Biointerfaces* 160: 40–7.

Farnia, P., Velayati, A.A., Mollaei, S., and Ghanavi, J. 2017. Modified rifampin nanoparticles: Increased solubility with slow release Rate. *Int J Mycobacteriol* 6 (2): 171–6.

Fauci, A.S. 2001. Infectious diseases: considerations for the 21st century. *Clininfect Diseases* 32: 675–85.

Freeling, J.P., Koehn, J., Shu, C., Sun, J., and Ho, R.J. 2014. Long-acting three-drug combination anti-HIV nanoparticles enhance drug exposure in primate plasma and cells within lymph nodes and blood. *AIDS* 28: 2625–7.

Friedman, A.J., Phan, J., Schairer, D.O., Champer, J., Qin, M., Pirouz, A. et al. 2013. Antimicrobial and anti-inflammatory activity of chitosan–alginate nanoparticles: A targeted therapy for cutaneous pathogens. *J Investig Dermatol* 133: 1231–9.

Fukamizo, T., Ohkawa, T., Ikeda, Y., and Goto, S. 1994. Specificity of chitosanase from Bacillus pumilus. *Biochim BiophysActa* 1205: 183–8.

Gao, W., Thamphiwatana, S., Angsantikul, P., and Zhang, L. 2014. Nanoparticle approaches against bacterial infections. *Wires Nanomed Nanobi* 6 (6): 532–47.

Garg, T., Rath, G., and Goyal, A.K.2016. Inhalable chitosan nanoparticles as antitubercular drug carriers for an effective treatment of tuberculosis. *Artif Cells Nanomed Biotechnol* 44 (3): 997–1001.

Gupta, P.K., Jaiswal, A.K., Asthana, S., Verma, A., Kumar, V., Shukla, P. et al. 2015. Self assembled ionically sodium alginate cross-linked amphotericin B encapsulated glycol chitosan stearate nanoparticles: Applicability in better chemotherapy and non-toxic delivery in visceral leishmaniasis. *Pharm Res* 32 (5): 1727–40.

Gurunathan, S., Han, J.W., Dayem, A.A., Eppakayala, V., and Kim, J.H. 2012. Oxidative stress-mediated antibacterial activity of graphene oxide and reduced graphene oxide in Pseudomonas aeruginosa. *Int J Nanomedicine* 7:5901–14.

Hafizi, R., Salleh, B. and Latiffah, Z. 2013. Morphological and molecular characterization of Fusarium. solaniand F. oxysporum associated with crown disease of oil palm. *Braz J Microbiol* 44 (3): 959–68.

Huang, L., Dai, T., Xuan, Y., Tegos, G.P., and Hamblin, M.R. 2011. Synergistic combination of chitosan acetate with nanoparticle silver as a topical antimicrobial: Efficacy against bacterial burn infections. *Antimicrob Agents Chemother* 55: 3432–8.

Huang, Y.C., Li, R.Y., Chen, J.Y., and Chen, J.K. 2016. Biphasic release of gentamicin from chitosan/fucoidan nanoparticles for pulmonary delivery. *Carbohydr Polym* 138: 114–22.

Huh, A.J., and Kwon, Y.J. 2011. "Nanoantibiotics": A new paradigm for treating infectious diseases using nanomaterials in the antibiotics resistant era. *J Control Release* 156: 128–45.

Jing, Z.W., Jia, Y.Y., Wan, N., Luo, M., Huan, M.L., and Kang, T.B. et al. 2016. Design and evaluation of novel pH-sensitive ureido-conjugated chitosan/TPP nanoparticles targeted to Helicobacter pylori. *Biomaterials* 84: 276–85.

Kaatz, G.W. 2005. Bacterial efflux pump inhibition. *Curr Opin Investig Drugs* 6: 191–98.

Kalhapure, R.S., Jadhav, M., Rambharose, S., Mocktar, C., Singh, S., Renukuntla, J., and Govender, T. 2017. pH-responsive chitosan nanoparticles from a novel twin-chain anionic amphiphile for controlled and targeted delivery of vancomycin. *Colloids Surf B Biointerfaces* 158: 650–7.

Kang, B.,Opatz, T., Landfester, K., and Wurm, F.R. 2015. Carbohydrate nanocarriers in biomedical applications: functionalization. *Chem Soc Rev* 44: 8301–8325.

Katz, B. and Waites, K. 2004. Emerging intracellular bacterial infections. *Clin Lab Med* 24: 627–49.

Kayser, F.H. 2003. Safety aspects of enterococci from medical point of view. *Int J Food Microbiol* 88: 255–262.

Khor, E. 2001. *Chitin: Fulfilling a Biomaterials Promise*. Elsevier.

Kikuchi, M. 2015. The role of formulation and dosage form in vaccine. *Yakugaku Zasshi* 135 (2): 263–67.

Kingsley, J.D., Dou, H., Morehead, J., Rabinow, B., Gendelman, H.E., and Destache, C.J. 2006. Nanotechnology: A focus on nanoparticles as a drug delivery system. *J Neuro Immune Pharmacol* 1: 340–350.

Kumar, A.B.V., Varadaraj, M.C., Gowda, L.R., and Tharanathan, N. 2005. Characterization of chitooligosaccharides prepared by chitosanolysis with the aid of papain and pronase, and their bactericidal action against Bacillus cereus and Escherichia coli. *Biochem J* 391: 167–175.

Kumari, A., Singla, R., Gulani, A., and Jadav, S.K. 2014. Nanoencapsulation for drug delivery. *J Exp Clin Sci* 13: 265–286.

Lee, B.S., Lee, C.C., Wang, Y.P., Chen, H.J., Lai, C.H., and Hsieh, W.L. et al. 2016. Controlled-release of tetracycline and lovastatin by poly(D,L-lactide-co-glycolide acid)-chitosan nanoparticles enhances periodontal regeneration in dogs. *Int J Nanomedicine* 11: 285–97.

Lembo, D. and Cavalli, R. 2010. Nanoparticulate delivery systems for antiviral drugs. *Antivir Chem Chemother* 21: 53–70.

Li, H., Chen, Q., Zhao, J., and Urmila, K. 2015. Enhancing the antimicrobial activity of natural extraction using the synthetic ultrasmall metal nanoparticles. *Sci Rep* 5: 11033.

Lin, Y.H., Lu, K.Y., Tseng, C.L., Wu, J.Y., Chen, C.H., and Mi, F.L. 2017. Development of genipin-crosslinked fucoidan/chitosan-N-arginine nanogels for preventing Helicobacter infection. *Nanomedicine (Lond)* 12: 1491–510.

Liu, Y.Y., Wang, Y., Walsh, T.R, Yi, L.X., Zhang, R., Spencer, J. et al. 2016. Emergence of plasmid-mediated colistin resistance mechanism MCR-1 in animals and human beings in China: A microbiological and molecular biological study. *Lancet Infect Dis* 16: 161–8.

Luan, B., Huynh, T., and Zhou, R. 2016. Complete wetting of graphene by biological lipids. *Nanoscale* 8 (10): 5750–4.

Malathi, B., Mona, S., Thiyagarajan, D., and Kaliraj, P. 2015. Immunopotentiating nano-chitosan as potent vaccine carter for efficacious prophylaxis of filarial antigens. *Int J Biol Macromol* 73: 131–7.

Manukumar, H.M., Umesha, S., and Kumar, H.N.N. 2017. Promising biocidal activity of thymol loaded chitosan silver nanoparticles (T-C@AgNPs) as anti-infective agents against perilous pathogens. *Int J Biol Macromol* 102: 1257–65.

Matsuhashi, S. and Kume, T. 1997. Enhancement of antimicrobial activity of chitosan by irriadiation. *J Sci Food Agric* 73: 237–41.

Maya, S., Indulekha, S., Sukhithasri, V., Smitha, K.T., Nair, S.V., Jayakumar, R. et al. 2012. Efficacy of tetracycline encapsulated O-carboxymethyl chitosan nanoparticles against intracellular infections of Staphylococcus aureus. *Int J Biol Macromol* 51 (4): 392–9.

Moreno, E., Schwartz, J., Larrea, E., Conde, I., Font, M., Sanmartín, C. et al. 2015. Assessment of β-lapachone loaded in lecithin-chitosan nanoparticles for the topical treatment of cutaneous leishmaniasis in L. major infected BALB/c mice. *Nanomedicine* 11 (8): 2003–12.

Morens, D.M., Folkers, G.K., and Fauci, A.S. 2008. Emerging infections: A perpetual challenge. *Lancet Infect Dis* 8: 710–9.

Mukhopadhyay, A. and Basu, S.K. 2003. Intracellular delivery of drugs to macrophages. *Adv Biochem Eng Biotechnol* 84: 183–209.

Muñoz, P., Bouza, E., Cuenca-Estrella, M., Eiros, J.M., Pérez, M.J., Sánchez-Somolinos, M., Rincón, C., Hortal, J., and Peláez, T. 2005. Saccharomyces cerevisiae fungemia: an emerging infectious disease. *Clin Infect Dis* 40 (11): 1625–34.

Noinaj, N., Kuszak, A.J., Gumbart, J.C., Lukacik, P., Chang, H., Easley, N.C. et al. 2013. Structural insight into the biogenesis of β-barrel membrane proteins. *Nature* 501 (7467): 385–90.

O'Gorman, S.M., Britton, D., and Collins, P. 2015. Anuncommon dermatophyte infection: Two cases of cutaneous infection with Trichophyton verrucosum. *Clin Exp Dermatol* 40 (4): 395–8.

Park, Y., Kim M.H., Park, S.C, Cheong, H., Jang, M.K. Nah, J.W., and Hahm, K.S. 2008 Investigation of the antifungal activity and mechanism of action of LMWS-chitosan. *J Microbiol. Biotechnol* 18: 1729–34.

Piras, A.M., Maisetta, G., Sandreschi, S., Gazzarri, M., Bartoli, C., Grassi, L. et al. 2015. Chitosan nanoparticles loaded with the antimicrobial peptide temporin B exert a long-term antibacterial activity in vitro against clinical isolates of Staphylococcus epidermidis. *Front Microbiol* 6: 372.

Pornpattananangkul, D., Zhang, L., Olson, S., Aryal, S., Obonyo, M., Vecchio, K, et al. 2011. Bacterial toxin-triggered drug release from gold nanoparticle stabilized liposomes for the treatment of bacterial infection. *J Am Chem Soc* 133: 4132–9.

Raafat, D. and Sahl, H.G. 2009. Chitosan and its antimicrobial potential-a critical literature survey. *Microb Biotechnol* 2 (2): 186–201.

Rabea, E.I., Badawy, M.E.T., Stevens, C.V., Smagghe, G., and Steurbaut, W. 2003. Chitosan as antimicrobial agent: Applications and mode of action. *Biomacromolecules* 4: 1457–65.

Rai, J., Randhawa, G.K., and Kaur, M. 2013. Recent advances in antibacterial drugs. *Int J Appl Basic Med Res* 3: 3–10.

Rhoades, J. and Roller, S. 2000. Chitosan disrupts the barrier properties of the outer membrane of Gram-negative bacteria. *Int J Food Microbiol* 171: 235–244.

Ribeiro, T.G., Franca, J.R., Fuscaldi, L.L., Santos, M.L., Duarte, M.C., and Lage, P.S. 2014. An optimized nanoparticle delivery system based on chitosan and chondroitin sulfate molecules reduces the toxicity of amphotericin B and is effective in treating tegumentary leishmaniasis. *Int J Nanomedicine* 9: 5341–53.

Salouti, M. and Ahangari, A. 2014. Nanoparticle based drug delivery systems for treatment of infectious diseases. In: Sezer, A.D. (Ed.), *Application of Nanotechnology in Drug Delivery*. Intech.

Schnadig, V.J. and Woods, G.L. 2009. *Histopathology of fungal infections in clinical mycology*. In: Anaissie, E.J., McGinnis, M.R., and Pfaller, M.A (Eds.), *Clinical Mycology*. 2nd ed., pp. 79–108. Churchill Livingstone, Elsevier.

Shahnaz, G., Edagwa, B.J., McMillan, J., Akhtar, S., Raza, A., Qureshi, N.A. et al. 2017. Gendelman HE. development of mannose-anchored thiolated amphotericin B nanocarriers for treatment of visceral leishmaniasis. *Nanomedicine (Lond)* 12 (2): 99–115.

Silva, N.C., Silva, S., Sarmento, B., and Pintado, M. 2015. Chitosan nanoparticles for daptomycin delivery in ocular treatment of bacterial endophthalmitis. *Drug Deliv* 22 (7): 885–93.

Singla, A.K. and Chawla, M. 2001. Chitosan: Some pharmaceutical and biological aspects – an update. *J Pharm Pharmaco* 153: 1047–67.

Sobhani, Z., Mohammadi Samani, S., Montaseri, H., and Khezri, E. 2017. Nanoparticles of chitosan loaded ciprofloxacin: Fabrication and antimicrobial activity. *Adv Pharm Bull* 7 (3): 427–432.

Song, J., Remmers, S.J., Shao, J., Kolwijck, E., Walboomers, X.F., and Jansen, J.A. et al. 2016. Antibacterial effects of electrospun chitosan/poly(ethylene oxide) nanofibrous membranes loaded with chlorhexidine and silver. *Nanomedicine* 12 (5): 1357–64.

Sotelo-Boyás, M., Correa-Pacheco, Z., Bautista-Baños, S., and Gómez, Y. 2017. Release study and inhibitory activity of thyme essential oil-loaded chitosan nanoparticles and nanocapsules against foodborne bacteria. *Int J Biol Macromol* 103: 409–14.

Stewart, P.S. 2002. Mechanisms of antibiotic resistance in bacterial biofilms *Int J Med Microbiol* 292 (2): 107–13.

Tripathi, P., Dwivedi, P., Khatik, R., Jaiswal, A.K., Dube, A., Shukla, P. et al. 2015. Development of 4-sulfated N-acetyl galactosamine anchored chitosan nanoparticles: A dual strategy for effective management of Leishmaniasis. *Colloids Surf B Biointerfaces* 136: 150–9.

Tripathy, S., Chattopadhyay, S., Dash, S.K., Chowdhuri, A.R., Das, S., Sahu, S.K. et al. 2015. Chitosan conjugated chloroquine: Proficient to protect the induction of liver apoptosis during malaria. *Int J Biol Macromol* 74: 585–600.

Tripathy, S., Das, S., Dash, S.K., Mahapatra, S.K., Chattopadhyay, S., Majumdar, S. et al. 2014. A prospective strategy to restore the tissue damage in malaria infection: Approach with chitosan-trypolyphosphate conjugated nanochloroquine in Swiss mice. *Eur J Pharmacol* 737: 11–21.

Ulanski, P., Pajak, A., Rosiak, J., and Sonntag, C.2000. Radiolysis and sonolysis of chitosan – two convenient techniques for a controlled reduction of the molecular weight. *Adv Chitin Sci* 4: 429–435.

Upadhayay, P., Kumar, M., and Pathak, K.2016. Norfloxacin loaded pH triggered nanoparticulate in-situ gel for extraocular bacterial infections: Optimization, ocular irritancy and corneal toxicity. *Iran J Pharm Res* 15 (1): 3–22.

Vårum, K.M., Myhr, M.M., Hjerde, R.J.N., and Smidsrød, O. 1997. In vitro degradation rates of partially N-acetylatedchitosans in human serum. *Carbohydr Res* 299: 99–101.

Wang, L., Hu, C., and Shao, L. 2017. The antimicrobial activity of nanoparticles: Present situation and prospects for the future. *Int J Nanomedicine* 12: 1227–1249.

Wazed Ali, S., Joshi, M., and Rajendran, S. 2010. Modulation of size, shape and surface charge of chitosan nanoparticles with reference to antimicrobial activity. *Adv Sci Lett* 3: 452–60.

Williamson, B., Tudzynski, B., Tudzynski, P., and van Kan, J.A. 2007. Botrytiscinerea: The cause of grey mould disease. *Mol Plant Pathol* 8: 561–80.

World Health Organization (WHO). *Anti-microbial resistance, global report on surveillance.* 2014. Summary, WHO Press.

Xu, Y., Wei, M.T., Ou-Yang, H.D., Walker, S.G., Wang, H.Z., Gordon, C.R. et al. 2016. Exposure to TiO_2nanoparticles increases *Staphylococcus aureus* infection of HeLa cells. *J Nanobiotechnology* 14: 34.

Yang, W., Shen, C., Ji, Q., An, H., Wang, J., Liu, Q., and Zhang, Z. 2009. Food storage material silver nanoparticles interfere with DNA replication fidelity and bind with NA. *Nanotechnology* 20 (8): 085102.

Zakharova, O.V., Godymchuk, A.Y., Gusev, A.A., Gulchenko, S.I., Vasyukova., I.A., and Kuznetsov, D.V. 2015. Considerable variation of antibacterial activity of Cu nanoparticles suspensions depending on the storage time, dispersive medium, and particle sizes. *Biomed Res Int* 2015: 412530.

Zaki, N.M. and Hafez, M.M. 2012. Enhanced antibacterial effect of ceftriaxone sodium-loaded chitosan nanoparticles against intracellular Salmonella typhimurium. *AAPS PharmSciTech* 13 (2): 411–21.

Zapalski, M.K. and Hubert, B.L.M. 2011. First fossil record of parasitism in devonian calcareous sponges (stromatoporoids). Parasitology 138: 132–8.

Zhang, N., O'Donnell, K., Sutton, D.A., Nalim, F.A., Padhye, A.A., and Geiser, D.M. 2006. Members of the Fusarium solani species complex that cause infections in both humans and plants are common in the environment. *J Clin Microbiol* 44: 2186–2190.

Zhang, Y., Liang, R.J., Xu, J.J., Shen, L.F., Gao, J.Q., and Wang, X.P. et al. 2017. Efficient induction of antimicrobial activity with vancomycin nanoparticle-loaded poly(trimethylene carbonate) localized drug delivery system. *Int J Nanomedicine* 12: 1201–14.

Zhao, L., Zhu, B., Jia, Y., Hou, W., and Su, C. 2013. Preparation of biocompatible carboxymethyl chitosan nanoparticles for delivery of antibiotic drug. *Biomed Res Int* 2013: 236469.

5 Heparin and Its Derivatives-Based Nanoparticles for Cancer Therapy

Amit Kundu, Prasanta Dey, Subham Banerjee, Pradipta Sarkar, Arnab De, Amit Maity, and Hyung Sik Kim

CONTENTS

5.1 INTRODUCTION

Cancer is a major cause of mortality and possesses a significant public health threat in the 21st century. The global report of the IARC (International Agency for Research on Cancer) showed around 14.1 million people were diagnosed with cancer, where 8.2 million died and 32.6 million people survived with various types of cancer (based on five years of diagnosis reports) in 2012 (Torre et al. 2015). According to Thun et al. the mortality rate is about 17 million people per year. By 2030, it is expected that there will be 26 million around the globe who will have suffered with this deadly disease (Thun et al. 2010).

Chemotherapy is the most popular method for management of cancer. However, drawbacks in the use of chemotherapeutic agents, such as non-specific systemic distribution, inadequate drug concentrations reaching the tumor site, non-specific toxicity, limited ability to monitor therapeutic responses, and the development of multiple drug resistances, leads to inadequate therapeutic efficacy (Das et al. 2009; Parveen and Sahoo 2006; Parveen and Sahoo 2008).

Mother nature provides different ailments to prevent or cure various diseases. Traditional healers from various parts of the world use their knowledge to cure different diseases with the help of natural products (Karuna et al. 2018; Dey and Bhakta 2012). Researchers have also focused on different synthetic methodologies for the betterment of the therapeutic regime. Interestingly, nanotechnology offers magnificent benefits for overcoming the drawbacks associated with conventional chemotherapy through the proper entrapment of many potential antineoplastic drugs to ensure better tumor targeting. Such technology also provides a prolonged release of the drugs either by active or passive diffusion to the main site of action. In addition, this can be effectively delivered through various routes of drug administration such as oral, nasal, transdermal, parenteral, perioral, etc., with the aim of improving therapeutic intervention at the desired site of action via minimizing the drug-associated adverse effects (Dey and Bhakta 2012; Dey and Das 2013)

That is why nanotechnology is the best approach over conventional dosage from having poor patient compliance in cancer management.(Reichert and Wenger 2008; Zou 2005). The development of nanotechnology has shown remarkable results in the delivery of chemotherapeutic agents and provides remarkable prevention against cancer. For better treatment of cancer, synthetic and natural compounds have been introduced with nanocarrier-mediated delivery systems. Synthesis of bio-nanoparticles can be prepared using various kinds of protein and/or polysaccharide-based materials. Proper selection of materials for matrix fabrication is generally dependent on three important parameters: (1) NPs size, shape, surface charge, and diffusivity across the biological membrane; (2) drug solubility, permeability, and stability; (3) particle biodegradability, biocompatibility, toxicity, release kinetics, and particle antigenicity (Bera et al. 2016).

The most-applied polysaccharide nanoparticles contain: chitosan, hyaluronic acid, dextran, heparin, and pullulan alginate. The polysaccharide components are highly biocompatible, non-toxic, non-immunogenic, and biodegradable in nature, which are being introduced in the development of modern nanoformulation (Gorain et al. 2014; Aider 2010). Heparin, a highly sulfated carbohydrate polymer, is a member of the glycosaminoglycan family with a variably acidic mammalian polysaccharide (Mizrahy and Peer 2012; Bentolila et al. 2000). The most common disaccharide unit consists of a 2-O-sulfated iduronic acid and 6-O-sulfated, N-sulfated glucosamine, IdoA(2S)-GlcNS(6S) (Gatti et al. 1979).

Animal tissues like porcine intestine and bovine lung are used as a source of heparin. Heparine has been approved as an anticoagulant since 1935. Despite its anticoagulant action, it has other biological functions such as an anti-inflammatory effect. Heparin was used as a carrier in gold and silver nanoparticles which exhibited important biological activities (Boddohi et al. 2009). The heparin coating increases the hydrophilic property of the magnetic nanoparticles that help to attach the cells to the surface of the nanoparticles. To detect a tumor in a patient by using magnetic resonance imaging (MRI), heparin-immobilized magnetic nanoparticles (MNPs) have been designed as a novel biomarker (Saravanakumar et al. 2012). More examples of heparin-based nanoformulations are summarized in Table 5.1.

It has been shown that nanoparticles produce strong antiangiogenic and antitumor activity. They also acted as an apoptosis inducer agent on a 4T1 breast tumor model (Hou et al. 2012).

Adsorption or encapsulation gives nanocarriers promising advantages over others in the field of drug delivery. Nanocarrier-based drug delivery approaches have significant advantages in the prevention of cancer which include: better pharmacokinetic index, target specificity, both passive and active targeting approaches, suitable biodegradability, excellent drug release rate, better safety profile, and satisfactory therapeutic efficacy.

TABLE 5.1

Examples of Drug-Loaded Heparin Nanoparticles and their Mechanism of Action

Drug	Cell Line Studied	Mechanism of Action	Reference
Docetaxel	MDAMB 231	Inhibits cell proliferation Inhibits tumor growth in xenograft mice	(Kim et al. 2014)
Anthranoid conjugates	HepG2	Inhibits cell proliferation	(Durdureanu-Angheluta et al. 2014)
Taurocholic acid and docetaxel	Caco-2 and MDAMB231	Inhibits cell proliferation Reduces tumor volume in xenograft mice	(Khatun et al. 2014)
Doxorubicin	4T1	Reduces tumor volume in xenograft mice	(She et al. 2013)
Paclitaxel and all-trans retinal	N/A	Reduces tumor volume in xenograft mice	(Hou et al. 2012)

5.2 LIMITATIONS OF CONVENTIONAL ANTICANCER THERAPY

Different nanoformulations, such as mesoporous silica nanoparticles, nanoparticulated poloxamer, solid lipid nanoparticles, magnetic nanoparticles, nanoparticulated chemo sensitizer, and polymeric nanoparticles, change the scenario of the multidrug resistance phenomenon common in cancer chemotherapy. Nanocrystals, albumin-based nanoparticles, liposomal formulation, polymeric micelles, cyclodextrin, and chitosan-based nanoparticles help to overcome the poor aqueous solubility and low bioavailability of chemotherapeutics due to their hydrophobic nature.

Conventional chemotherapeutic agents do not only destroy the neoplastic cells but also damage normal healthy cells (Zhao and Rodriguez 2013). This unwanted side effect is due more to the non-specificity of the target, and may result in myelosuppression, mucositis, alopecia, organ dysfunction, and thrombocytopenia (Nguyen 2011; Coates et al. 1983). Sometimes anti-neoplastic agents are unable reach the core of solid tumors and as a result cancerous cells remain alive (Tannock et al. 2002).

Engulfment of active agents by macrophages in blood circulation limits the therapeutic activity of chemotherapeutic agents due to an insufficient concentration in cancer tissue. Poor solubility and low bioavailability is a major problem in conventional drug therapy. The physicochemical properties of a drug should be evaluated by performing *in vitro* and *in vivo* experiments to overcome the above drawbacks (Maity et al. 2016). Even in cancer therapies the drug did not show a better efficacy after administration.

However, orthodox chemotherapy has a few boundaries: (a) poor aqueous solubility: most plant-derived or synthetic chemotherapeutics suffer from inadequate hydrophilicity and require diluents or solvents to frame the desired dosage form which may be responsible for other adverse effects. To increase the solubility, hydrophobic drugs can be encapsulated in micelles (Patri et al. 2005); (b) inadequate selectivity of anticancer drugs: the poor selectivity profile of most chemotherapeutics cause noteworthy impairments to rapidly multiplying normal cells; and (c) multidrug resistance (MDR): efflux pumps such as P-glycoprotein (Pgp) in the cell membrane contributes advantageous multidrug resistance properties to cancerous cells by transporting anticancer drugs out of the cells (Kwon 2003; Luo and Prestwich 2002; Stavrovskaya 2000). A novel approach was made in which vincristine-loaded solid lipid nanoparticles were tagged with an anti P-glycoprotein monoclonal antibody (MRK-16) in order to restrict the P-glycoprotein-mediated drug efflux phenomenon. This showed remarkable results in improving cytotoxocity in a resistant human myelogenous leukemia cell line compared to non-tagged lipid nanoparticles (Matsuo et al. 2001).

MDR is the main problem in chemotherapy which can be avoided by administering mesoporous silica nanoparticles, solid lipid nanoparticles, polymeric nanoparticles, and magnetic nanoparticles.

5.3 THE CURRENT SCENARIO IN CANCER THERAPEUTICS AND DRUG DEVELOPMENTS

In developing countries, the development of pharmaceuticals and products is limited to the manufacture of generic medicines. (Suggitt and Bibby 2005; Talmadge et al. 2007; Lu et al. 2015; Merris 2005). Over the last two decades, drug discovery, development, and manufacture has been in a bottleneck stage. Insufficient investment in research and development, unqualified manpower, and lack of proper rules and regulations decelerate the development process day by day.(Merris 2005). Profit for mass production has fallen. Developed countries like the United States, the United Kingdom, and others have invested US$1–2 billion in cancer treatment, which may boost the development of cancer treatments (Merris 2005; Ruggeri et al. 2014). There is still more clinical practice required for improving treatments, especially those for cancer metastasis (Mina and Sledge 2011; Lu and Lu 2010; Lu et al. 2012; Lu et al. 2013; Lu et al. 2016; Fidler 1990; Fidler 2003; Gupta and Massague 2006; Talmadge and Fidler 2010; Valastyan and Weinberg 2011; Herter-Sprie et al. 2013; Sava and Bergamo 1999; Kessenbrock et al. 2010; Taraboletti and Margosio 2001). Hence, the exploration of anticancer drugs has been challenging with unfavorable conditions for development and manufacturing worldwide (Lu and Lu 2010; Lu et al. 2012; Lu et al. 2013; Lu et al. 2016; Fidler 1990; Fidler 2003; Gupta and Massague 2006; Talmadge and Fidler 2010).

5.4 EMERGENCE AND NOVEL APPROACHES OF ANTICANCER DRUG DELIVERY

Since the beginning of the modern era of chemotherapy, a novel drug delivery system to deliver anticancer treatment has been in much demand. An ideal novel delivery system carries the anticancer agents to the targeted tumor tissue without any harmful effect on normal tissue and accumulates at the tumor site for a prolonged time and promotes therapeutic efficacy. There are so many advantages of this delivery system, due to the small particle size of nanoparticles. Small particle size improves surface area as well as the rate of absorption and encapsulation. The penetration properties of nanosized formulation systems is much better and allows more treatment deeper into the tumor tissue, than other types of delivery system. The cell uptake rate is also very high compared to other delivery systems. The application of biodegradable nanoparticles provides additional advantages by reducing the toxicity of chemotherapeutic agents to healthy tissues. However, nanoparticulate systems are being focused on globally to boost up drug efficiency and to diminish toxicity.

There are some beneficial effects of non-therapeutic anticancer drug delivery systems such as a prolonged shelf life, easier to deliver lipophilic and lyophobic drugs, multi delivery routes through oral, nasal, parenteral, intraocular, etc., a better bio distribution of cancer drugs, more convenient control and sustained release of the drugs, and the intercellular concentration is higher than other conventional dosage forms due to the enhanced permeability and retention effect (EPR) (Cho et al. 2008; Mohanraj and Chen 2006).

Formulation is designed to achieve and increase the permeability and retention (EPR) effect (Matsumura and Maeda 1986; Gerlowski and Jain 1986), the FDA has approved liposomal doxorubicin (Doxil™/Caelyx™) which stands as the first anticancer nanomedicine since 1995 (Gabizon et al. 2003; Barenholz 2012; Goebel et al. 1996; Robert et al. 2004). For better therapy and safety Doxil™/Caelyx™ shows a differential distribution of doxorubicin (Solomon and Gabizon 2008). Doxil™ has reached about a 300-fold increase in bioavailability compared to free doxorubicin (Gabizon et al. 2003). The new nanomedicine has been approved based on therapeutic outcome, safety index, and better effects than the standard treatment (O'Brien et al. 2004). Synthetic chemistry is one of the auspicious tools for the innovation and development of novel anticancer drugs. Many synthetic compounds have already been reported on which possess positive anticancer activity (Jeon et al. 2017; Jeong et al. 2017; Jeong et al. 2017). Many good anticancer drugs have proved themselves pre-clinically but are yet to be reviewed clinically (Venditto and Szoka 2013). Some more examples of heparin-based anticancer drugs and their clinical status are summarized in Table 5.2. For a long time nanocarriers have possessed an important role in cancer therapy. These novel formulation systems act on an active as well as a passive mechanistic approach toward tumor-based targeting therapy. However, further research is required for the development of nanocarrier system from their current nascent stage to the better treatment of cancer.

5.5 ADVANTAGES OF HEPARIN IN CANCER NANOTECHNOLOGY

Heparin basically shows four types of advantages: (1) Being an endogenous polysaccharide heparin is a non-toxic agent in nature. (2) The anticancer activity of heparin via angiogenesis and metastasis has unique features compared to other polysaccharides. (3) Based on the good affinity to various protein, heparin may help to develop a platform for delivering active pharmaceuticals by encapsulating the active moiety. 4) Since heparin exhibited very high-affinity to some proteins which may control tumors growth by regulating angiogenesis, this characteristic can be utilized in targeted drug delivery system (Park et al. 2007; Borsig 2010; Bobek and Kovarik 2004; Lapierre et al. 1996; Lever and Page 2002; Mousa and Petersen 2009). Several scientific reports demonstrated that heparin had a significant effect on animal models at metastasis. (Lever and Page 2002; Alonso et al. 1996; Zacharski et al. 2000; Hettiarachchi et al. 1999).

In most cells, heparin sulfate chains are broken down by heparinase (Lever and Page 2002). After the activation of endoglycosidase in tumors accelerates, the degeneration of the extracellular matrix (as a result of extravasation) takes place in tumor cells. Based on this phenomenon, heparinase can be inhibited following the interaction between heparin and heparinase, resulting in a mitigated metastasis.

Several reports revealed that heparin can suppress the effect of P- and L-selectins, which are stimulating agents in the metastasis stage of a tumor (Borsig 2010; Borsig et al. 2001). Heparin also prevents angiogenesis co-administration with fibroblast growth factors (FGF) and vascular endothelial growth factor (VEGF) (Mousa and Petersen 2009).

Phosphormannopentaose (PI-88) an oligosaccharide which has shown a strong preventive effect against angiogenesis, metastasis, and tumor growth, is now under phase III clinical trials (Parish et al. 1999; Ferro et al. 2007).

Current research claims that heparin acts as a potent inducer to apoptotic cell death via interaction with transcription factors (Linhardt 2004; Yu et al. 2007). For drugs delivery, a coating material or as a backbone of nanocarriers, heparin is an all-rounder in multidisciplinary bio field research. Due to an excellent affinity toward tumors, heparin can be recommended as a targeting functional moiety (Chung et al. 2010; Yuk et al. 2011).

Unfractionated heparin (UFH) and low molecular weight heparins (LMWHs) are applied in venous thrombosis associated cancer therapy. Angiogenesis induced by FGF was suppressed by both UFH and LMWH in humans, using an *in vitro* angiogenesis model (Collen et al. 2000). A human dose of UFH can increase plasma concentration of growth factors such as FGF (D'Amore 1992; Folkman et al. 1989).

Various reports suggest that heparin derivatives also showed good response in clinical trial of cancer patients (Cosgrove et al. 2002; Kakkar and Williamson 1999; Zacharski and Ornstein 1998; Goger et al. 2002). Based on these clinical outcomes further studies were completed on various animal models for screening tumor invasion and metastasis (Smorenburg and Van Noorden 2001). Heparin showed an inhibitory effect on heparanase and prevented the polysaccharide barrier to metastasis. It also exhibited an inhibitory effect on pro-angiogenic factors. Based on efficacy heparin also acts as a good anticancer agent in rodent cancer models (Zetter 1998; Bentolila et al. 2000).

TABLE 5.2

Examples of Anticancer Nanomedicines in Clinical Trials or on the Market

Nanomedicine Type	Drug	Product Name/Company	Indication	Clinical Phase
Liposomes	Doxorubicin	Myocet™/Teva UK	Metastatic breast cancer	Approved
		Doxil™/Janssen	Kaposi's sarcoma Ovarian cancer (post-first line failure) Multiple myeloma	Approved
	Vincristine	2B3–101/2-BBB Medicines BV	Brain metastases Glioma	Phase II
		Marqibo™/Spectrum Pharmaceuticals	Acute lymphoblastic leukemia	Phase II
	Daunorubicin	DaunoXome™/Galen	HIV-related Kaposi's sarcoma	Approved
	Cytarabine	Depocyt™/Pacira Pharmaceuticals	Lymphomatous meningitis	Approved
	Irinotecan	Onivyde™/Merrimack Pharmaceuticals	Metastatic pancreatic cancer (2nd line)	Approved
	Cytarabine: daunorubicin 5:1 fixed ratio	CPX-351/Celator	Acute myeloid leukemia	Phase III
	Cisplatin	Lipoplatin/Regulon	Non-small cell lung cancer	Phase III
		SPI77/ALZAPharmaceuticals	Ovarian cancer	Phase II
	Oxaliplatin	MBP-426/Mebiopharm	Gastrointestinal adenocarcinoma	Phase II
	Paclitaxel	LEP—ETU/Insys	Breast cancer	Phase II
	SN-38	LE-SN38/Neopharm	Metastatic colorectal cancer	Phase II
	Irinotecan: Floxuridine 1:1 ratio	CPX-1/Celator	Colorectal cancer	Phase II
Polymeric conjugates	Camptothecin	CRLX101 (cyclodextrin adamantane)/Cerulean	Renal cancer Small cell lung cancer Ovarian cancer	Phase II
	Asparaginase	Oncaspar™ (PEG)/Baxalta	Acute lymphoblastic leukemia	Approved
	Paclitaxel	Opaxio™ (Polyglycerol adipate)/CTI Biopharma	Ovarian cancer	Phase III maintenance
	Irinotecan	NKTR102 (PEG)/Nektar	Small cell lung cancer (Woman)	Phase III
	Camptothecin	CRLX101 (nanoparticle)/Cerulean	Renal cell carcinoma (3rd/4th line)	Phase II

(Continued)

TABLE 5.2 (CONTINUED)

Examples of Anticancer Nanomedicines in Clinical Trials or on the Market

Nanomedicine Type	Drug	Product Name/Company	Indication	Clinical Phase
Polymeric nanoparticles	Docetaxel + Prostate-Specific Membrane Antigen (PSMA)	BIND-014 (Accurin™)/BIND Therapeutics	Cholangiocarcinoma, Cervical cancer, Bladder cancer, Head and neck cancer, Non-small cell lung cancer subtypes	Phase II
	AZD2811 (AZD1152 hydroxyquinazoline pyrazol anilide; Aurora-B Kinase Inhibitor)	AZD2811 (Accurin™) nanoparticle/ AstraZeneca	Advanced solid tumors	Phase I
Polymeric micelles	Paclitaxel	Genexol-PM™/Samyang Biopharmaceuticals	Breast cancer, Non-small cell lung cancer, Ovarian cancer	Approved
		NK105/NanoCarrier™	Stomach cancer	Phase II
	DACH-platin	NC-4016/NanoCarrier™	Solid tumors	Phase I
		Nanoxel™/Samyang Biopharmaceuticals	Advanced breast cancer	Phase I
		NC-6004 Nanoplatin™/NanoCarrier™	Pancreatic cancer	Phase III
Other	Irinotecan	HA-irinotecan HyACT™/Alchemia	Colorectal cancer	Phase II
			Lung cancer	Phase III
	Tumor Necrosis Factor (TNF)	CYT-6091/CytImmune	Non-small cell lung cancer	Phase II
	Paclitaxel	Abraxane™/Celgene	Advanced breast cancer, Advanced non-small cell lung cancer, Advanced pancreatic cancer	Approved

Source: (Hare et al. 2017).

The expression rate of heparanase is very high in the case of angiogenic and metastatic cancer cells, whereas negligible in normal tissue (Vlodavsky et al. 2002). Expression of heparanase was detected in humans associated with progressive disorders, like metastasis in breast cancer (Maxhimer et al. 2002), colon cancer (Friedmann et al. 2000), ovary cancer (Ginath et al. 2001) bladder cancer (Gohji et al. 2001), pancreas cancer (Koliopanos et al. 2001), acute myeloid leukemia (Bitan et al. 2002), non-small cell lung cancer (Takahashi et al. 2004), and myeloma (Yang et al. 2005).

A report also revealed that heparin and its derivatives suppresses heparanase activity in tumor cells (Irimura et al. 1986; Vlodavsky et al. 1994; Yoshitomi et al. 2004; Sciumbata et al. 1996; Ono et al. 2002; Nakajima et al. 1988; Parish et al. 1987; Vlodavsky et al. 1999; Poggi et al. 2002) that are associated with a lower metastatic potential (Irimura et al. 1986; Vlodavsky et al.1994; Nakajima et al. 1988; Parish et al. 1987; Miao et al. 1999). Based on the above attractive beneficial effects, heparin-based nanocarriers, like nanogels, polyelectrolyte nanoparticles, and heparin-coated nanoparticles can be used as a potential tool in cancer therapy.

5.6 SYNTHETIC APPROACH OF HEPARIN DERIVATIVES BY COVALENT ADAPTATION

Before application of heparin in the formulation of nanoparticles they should be synthesized with several derivatives with unique features. Carboxylic, amino, and 16 hydroxyl groups of heparin are responsible for derivatization by chemical method. Sometimes heparin based on amide derivatives, has been modified by association with carboxylic groups of heparin and amino groups of other compounds. For example, aminated deoxycholic acid (DOCA) is covalently bound to heparin in presence of 1-ethyl-3-(3-dimethylaminopropyl) carbodiimide hydrochloride (EDAC). Hydrophobically modified heparin chains were used as a potent carrier for hydrophobic drugs or quantum dots (Park et al. 2004; Khatun et al. 2012).

By the same phenomena, heparin could be linked with biocin (Osmond et al. 2002; Yang et al. 1995), fluorescent amines (Fernandez et al. 2006), aminated folic acid (FA) (Tran et al. 2013), aminated retinoic acid, aminated lithocholic acid (Park et al. 2008), tyramine (Kim et al. 2013), polyethylenimine (PEI) (Gou et al. 2010; Wei et al. 2011), and so on. For the synthesis of heparin derivative, several sensitive functional moieties are inserted into the heparin backbone. These phenomena show advantages for nanogels formulations by using heparin derivatives. It has been shown that the molar ratio of the diamine and carboxyl groups of heparin is more than 1/1, diamine attached with a pendant group and a free amino group again connected with several lipophilic fragments to form amphiphiles. Hydrogel formation takes place at a ratio of less than 1/1. After the addition of azido groups into the heparin chain, the amidation reaction takes place with N-(tert-Butoxycarbonyl)-N-(4-azido butyl)-ethylenediamine (She et al. 2013). Additionally, a similar method was applied in end-thiol-modified heparin for hyaluronic acid modification (Tae et al. 2007).

Sometimes thiol groups are inserted into the heparin chain via reductive amination reaction (Bae et al. 2008). These end-thiol groups associated with heparin derivatives have been utilized in the synthesis of nanogels (crosslinked) with disulfide bonds. Carboxyl group in heparin is more important than hydroxyl group for the modification of heparin base delivery. (Wang et al. 2009; Wang et al. 2011; Peng et al. 2011; Wang et al. 2009).

For example, succinylated heparin was synthesized thorough an interaction between the succinic anhydride and hydroxyl part of heparin under O-acylation reaction conditions (Wang et al. 2009). The anticoagulant action of succinylated heparin was altered probably due to its conformational change (Peng et al. 2011). Pluronic F127 (MW 12.6 kDa) was synthesized through the use of urethane linkage and formation took place in the primary amine group of heparin and the terminal hydroxyl group of F127 (Chung et al. 2010).

5.7 HEPARIN AND ITS DERIVATIVES AS A FRAMEWORK FOR NANOCARRIERS

Heparin/heparin derivative chains are one of the most important tools for formulation of nanoparticles. In different studies it was been shown that there are two types of conjugation reaction that takes place which are: heparin-drug consolidate and heparin-based polymeric conjugate (Figure 5.1) (Yang et al. 2015) These nanoparticles are mainly formulated by heparin derivatives based on hydrophobic force. Drugs have been inserted in these nanocarriers by physical encapsulation or chemical conjugation. For insoluble drugs such types of nanocarriers exhibit a significant potential in drug delivery.

Hydrophilic nanogels with a three-dimensional porous network, act as drug reservoirs as well as stability enhancers by protecting from environmental degradation.

Several types of heparin nanoparticles and their derivatives (polycation, polyelectrolyte complex) were manufactured in general circumstances for appropriate biological functions (Figure 5.1) (Yang et al. 2015).

5.7.1 HEPARIN-DRUG COMPLEX

Heparin-drug conjugates are one of the outstanding formulations in drug delivery systems. Heparin is one of the best water-soluble polysaccharides. The significant advantages can be achieved by modifying the hydrophilic backbone of the heparin chain. Amphiphilic copolymers are synthesized by inserting hydrophobic chains into heparin. These copolymers accumulate into micelle-like nanoparticles dependent on the intermolecular relation between lipophilic components upon connection with the aqueous media.

The hydrophobic drugs are mainly encapsulated into nanoparticles to enhance the dissolution property of the molecule, ensuring uniform drug diffusion. Hydrophobic drugs are attached to

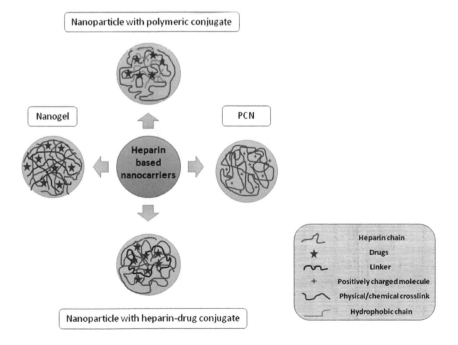

FIGURE 5.1 Backbone of heparin and its derivatives. Heparin-based nanoparticle encapsulated with the drug. Polyelectrolyte complex nanoparticles (PCNs) conjugation between polyanion heparin and polycations as a result polyelectrolyte are produced. Drug-loaded nanogel with a three-dimensional network constructed by physical and chemical reaction. Heparin drug-conjugated nanoparticle with hydrophobic drug.

heparin chains and formulated as a heparin-drug conjugate. After polymeric conjugate formation drugs are condensed inside hydrophobic cores (Figure 5.2) (Yang et al. 2015).

The advantages of such types of formulation is that 1) enhanced solubility of the lipophobic drugs; 2) increased bioavailability and the half-life of the drugs are extended; 3) protection of the drugs from degradation 4) improved distribution *in vivo* due to EPR; and 5) prompted release rate, directly in correlation with the pH or enzyme. Such types of conjugation are especially advantageous for cancer treatments due to their suitable size. Tumors packed with leaky and irregular blood vessels, caused by rapid angiogenesis, may lead to accumulation of nanoparticles into tumor tissues (Bertrand et al. 2014). The drug-heparin complex was used for target-specific delivery by attaching ligands on heparin (Wang et al. 2011; Wang et al. 2009).

Paclitaxel (PTX) was attached and condensed into nano-dualistic PTX-loaded heparin-PTX nano-complexes (Wang et al. 2009). Hypothetically, it was predicted that target specificity of the nanoparticles toward positive tumors sites increases after the fusion of FA. Though *in vivo* reports revealed that there are irrelevant changes in xenograft tumors experiments (48 h treatment) after the application of heparin folate-PTX and heparin-PTX nanoparticles (Wang et al. 2009).

Based on this phenomenon the authors wanted to verify whether the nanoparticles were accrued on the outer or inner surface of the tumor cells with the help of fluorescence microscopy (Wang et al. 2009). In this case it was revealed that the heparin-folate-PTX nanoparticles were stored inside the tumor cells by endocytosis that assured the anticancer activity.

It was suggested that the heparin backbone may be a good potential candidate for antitumor activity (Wang et al. 2011). To approve this phenomenon, a matrigel-based capillary tube development assay was implemented to detect the production of tubes. It clearly showed that tube development was decreased by PTX-heparin-folate-based nanoparticles (Wang et al. 2011). Even after inhibition of tube formation, there was no major change observed between the control and PTX-treated group (Wang et al. 2011). The inducing property of heparin has already been reported in the inhibition of angiogenesis, but now it can also be used as a potent carrier of chemotherapeutic agent in cancer treatment (Miao et al. 1999; She et al. 2013).

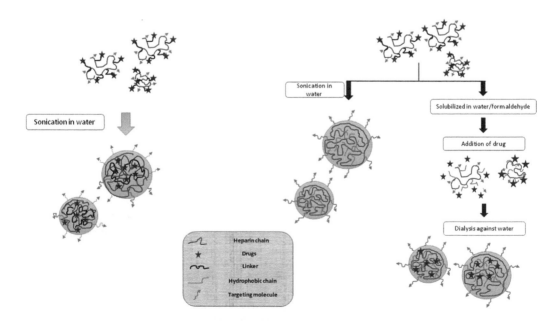

FIGURE 5.2 Association of two types of amphiphilic conjugation. Heparin-drug complex self-assembles into nanoparticles in water having targeted the molecule on the surface. Encapsulation of a heparin-based polymeric conjugate with a drug can be achieved in the hydrophobic part by the application of dialysis.

Conjugation of heparin takes place directly only for a few drugs but in other cases linkers can be used. Simple linkers and small molecules with short chemical structures were applied for conjugation of the drug and heparin. To make drug-heparin conjugate, linkers with a simple and short chemical structure (such as ethylenediamine) were used. For other, linkers also form pH-labile hydrazine bonds, which enables them to develop a stimuli-responsive drug delivery system.

In the tumor sites, pH value may decrease to 6.5 or less due to the presence of acidic metabolites including carbon dioxide (CO_2) and lactic acid. The anticancer conjugates transform gradually to lysosomes at a pH range of between 4.5 and 5 (Ohkuma and Poole 1978).

This type of nanosystem is not familiar with an acidic atmosphere, it shows better therapeutic efficiency for cancer in normal tissues (pH 7.4). This is why a special focus has been created in heparin-drug associates including pH-labile hydrazone linkers (Li et al. 2014; She et al. 2013). Dexamethasone (DEX) and doxorubicin (DOX) based on a heparin derivative is one of the most important combinatorial deliverables. The *in vitro* evaluation test of both DEX and DOX at pH 5.0 revealed that in the first three days, the cumulative release rate was extremely higher than in pH 6.0 and pH 7.4 (Li et al. 2014).

5.7.2 Heparin Polymeric Conjugates as a Drugs Carrier

In polymeric conjugation, hydrophobic chains like poly(β-benzyl-L-aspartate) (PBCA) (Li et al. 2012; Li et al. 2011) polycaprolactone (PCL) and DOCA (Park et al. 2004; Park et al. 2006; Park et al. 2007) have an important role in the conjugation of heparin and polymers from heparin and heparin-based polymeric complexes. After they are synthesized they accumulate into nanoparticles. The hydrophilic shells of these combinations protect interactions between nanoparticles and proteins and confirms firmness and increases the half-life. Insoluble drugs accumulate at hydrophobic cores via hydrophobic interactions (Lu and Park 2013). The main important criteria is that hydrophobic core material must always be non-immunogenic and non-toxic and the drug should be compatible with the core material. The compatibility is dependent on the nature of the drugs polarity and hydrophobicity (Lu and Park 2013). Various heparin-based polymeric conjugate nanoparticles have been regularly modified to target tumor sites via both passive and active targeting.

The concept of photodynamic therapy (PDT) in cancer treatment was merged with heparin-based nanoparticles. PDT is one type of clinical treatment, where cancer cells are destroyed with the help of specific drugs and photosensitizers (PSs). Photosensitizers are stimulated by light at a particular wavelength and produce a reactive oxygen species which can cause the death of tumor cells (Del Burgo et al. 2014).

The utility of PDT is limited due to the poor tumor selectivity of the photosensitizers. Nanocarriers may be combined with three-dimensional controlled light systems to increase the target specific ability toward tumors (Del Burgo et al. 2014). When photosensitizers are used along with nanovehicles, solubility increases. Such as pheophorbide A (PhA) attached to heparin-PBCA derivative which may lead them to accumulate in the cancer cell (Li et al. 2011).

For increasing the efficiency rate of PhA toward the target, a ternary amphiphilic base heparin-folate-retinoic acid bioconjugates by associating with hydrophobic retinoic acid, FA, to heparin complex (Tran et al. 2013).

5.7.3 Nanogels

Nanogel is one of the most important nanoparticles to have been used for its hydrophilicity and three-dimensional structure. The small particle size (50–200 nm) of this crosslinked polymeric nanoparticle provides high stability and a better drug delivery (Nguyen et al. 2011). The porous property of crosslinked networks provides protection for the drugs from environmental degradation (Yallapu et al. 2011). Due to presence of a nanoscaled structure, nanogels provide the desired response promptly in cancer therapy (Raemdonck et al. 2009).

Depending on the development of mechanistic approaches, nanogels are categorized into physical and chemical crosslinked nanogels (Hennink and van Nostrum 2012). Heparin has been widely used in both cases of the nanogels development process. Biological drugs like protein and nucleic acid are delivered by a physical crosslinked process, under a mild and simple synthetic method. There are various kinds of non-covalent attractive forces used in physical crosslinked nanogel formation. For example, to deliver the ribonuclease A (RNase A) protein, heparin-pluronic F127 nanogel conjugates by hydrophobic interaction (Choi et al. 2010). Hydrophilic poly(ethylene oxide) (PEO), hydrophobic polyvinyl toluene (PPO) and F127 could accumulate into micelles and form into an amphiphilic tri-block via hydrophobic interactions. As a result, the temperature will increase and the biological drugs will be incapable of encapsulating. These problems could be overcome by using heparin due to its attraction with positive charged drugs.

On the other hand, chemically crosslinked nanogels are created with a heparin backbone for the construction of chemical bonds like disulfide and amide bonds (Gou et al. 2010; Wei et al. 2011; Bae et al. 2008; Liu et al. 2014).

For example, as in the gene therapy of cancer, crosslinked heparin/polyethylenimine (PEI) nanogels are developed through amide bonds. Due to the negative charge of heparin, it fails to condense and deliver the gene. Several reports revealed that the development of gene carriers could be possible after the linking of heparin to a PEI/gene (Gou et al. 2010; Liu et al. 2012). Since 1995, cationic PEI has acted as a potential agent for genomic study. PEI 25K (MW 25,000 Da) is one of the important PEI derivatives applied as a "gold standard" worldwide (Gou et al. 2010; Lungwitz et al. 2005; Neu et al. 2005).

The degree of cytotoxicity depends on the length of the PEI chains (Gou et al. 2010; Kunath et al. 2003). For reducing the unwanted effect of PEI nanogel formulation, chains should be shortened and fixed into longer chains with the biodegradable heparin (Gou et al. 2010; Liu et al. 2014). After application of heparin into PEI, circulation time as well as therapeutic potential increases. Gou et al. formulated a nanogel through amidation interaction with heparin and PEI (Gou et al. 2010).

It was shown that the cytotoxicity is lower in PEI 25K, compared with PEI 2K. Various *in vivo* experimental data shows that colon carcinoma was significantly inhibited by the nanogel formulation. Nanogels based on PEI/heparin complex have shown satisfactory effects and less toxicity in the case of colon cancer via plasmid expressing vesicular stomatitis virus matrix protein (pVSVMP) gene vectors (Liu et al. 2014; Xie et al. 2011).

It produces a complex that has potent activity in CT26 (colon cancer cells), and is able to target the lungs (Wei et al. 2011). For advance redox-responsive nanosystems, heparin-based nanogels have an important role in the release of drugs intracellularly. This nanosystem was buildup by disulfide bonds, which were susceptible to being carved into thiol groups in the intracellular region; as a result, encapsulated agents were released out from the cytosol. Such types of oxidation and reduction reaction depends on expression levels of glutathione (GSH). Glutathione is present in cytosol (2–10 μM) and plasma (2–10 mM) (Li et al. 2012; Schafer and Buettner 2001; Balendiren et al. 2004) The concentration of GSH content is distinctly higher compared to normal tissue that is excellent for cancer therapy (Li et al. 2012; Kuppusamy et al. 2002).

For inserting the disulfide bonds into a heparin-modified gel formulation, two methods have been recommended generally (Figure 5.3) (Yang et al. 2015). The disulfide linkages were designed by thiol groups, existing in the heparin chain. In some cases crosslinking takes place in nanogels. Such a type of phenomena via disulfide linkages is found in facile and ultrasonic treatments which generate free radicals and therefore accelerate the oxidation phenomena associated with thiols.

Bae et al. (2008) revolutionized intracellular transfer of heparin (which might induce apoptotic cell death) by preparing heparin-based nanogels formulation in dual steps. They did this by producing disulfide links between adjacent thiolated heparin chains through dissolving the thiolated heparin in DMSO with PEG as a condensing agent, followed by ultrasonication. This heparin redox-sensitive nanogels was primarily established on the subsequent deliberations.

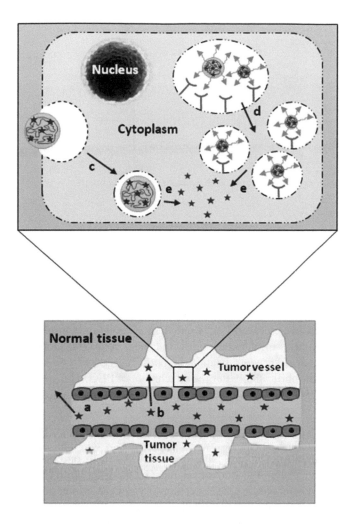

FIGURE 5.3 Active and passive targeting mechanism. Drug accumulation rate increases toward the tumor for the EPR effect. Nanoparticles reuptake into tumor cells were facilitated by receptor through fluid-phase pinocytosis followed by drug release in cytoplasm.

Primarily, the nanoparticulate form was more favored for transmembrane conveyance paralleled to free heparin. Additionally, redox-dependent cleavage of disulfide bonds enable the nanogels to be quickly degraded and released free heparin within cells. This nanogel formulation shows better apoptotic activity.

Nanogel is potent when it is used in a combined form for tumor therapy, some reports show that the thiol group of the heparin chain is responsible for modifying the disulfide linkages. Insertion of a disulfide bond into a nanogel formulation depends on their capacity for the crosslinking to become stable and deliver the RNase intracellularly (Figure 5.4) (Nguyen et al. 2011; Yang et al. 2015).

5.7.4 POLYELECTROLYTE COMPLEX NANOPARTICLES

The principle of polyelectrolyte complex nanoparticles (PCNS) synthesis depends on the electrostatic interaction of reversely charged polyelectrolytes under a favorable state (Ishihara et al. 2011).

Polyanion heparin and polycations, such as proteins and chitosan, are conjugated together and as a result polyelectrolytes are produced for biological application (Mori et al. 2010). Many reports suggest that heparin/protamine PCNs are also synthesized comparatively (Bae et al. 2009).

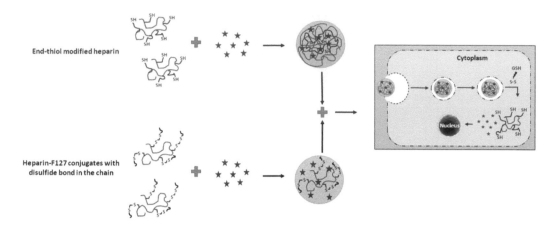

FIGURE 5.4 Uptake and destruction of nanogels intracellularly. Disulfide bonds are connected to nanogel by crosslinked interaction with thiol groups. Disulfide bonds are an essential part of heparin-F127 derivative. Formation of overload amount of GSH in cells may cause breakdown of disulfide bonds, demolition of nanogels, and drug release intracellularly.

Bae et al. suggest that PCNs, chitosan-g-poly (ethylene glycol), and chitosan-g-polyethylene glycol (PEG) micelles significantly stimulated apoptosis in cancer cells (Bae et al. 2009).

Micelles were created after neutralization of both charges of chitosan-g-PEG and heparin. Chitosan produces a hydrophilic shell after the attachment of PEG. The apoptosis inducing capacity of PCNs in cancer cells depend on the uptake rate of heparin intracellularly in micelles.

5.8 NANOPARTICLES ADAPTED WITH HEPARIN AND ITS DERIVATIVES

For 50 years, heparin and its derivatives have been used as anti-thrombogenic agents in blood. For better cancer therapy, heparin and its derivatives must be modified with time.

The most important advantages are (1) better stability rate; (2) protection of the nanoparticles by the reticuloendothelial system (RES) cells; (3) target-specific delivery to tumor sites; (4) developing the drug loading of nanoparticles; (5) multipurpose pharmacological activity of heparin (e.g., anti-inflammatory, anti-angiogenesis, antitumor cell proliferation properties); (6) high cellular uptake capacity.

Being a micelle-like structure of particles, heparin acts as a potent modifying agent. In nanoparticles formulations, electrostatic interaction is applied for the grafting of heparin with core nanoparticles via covalent bonds.

5.8.1 HEPARIN-BASED INORGANIC NANOPARTICLES

5.8.1.1 Heparin-Inspired Magnetic Nanoparticles

Due to the presence of the attractive characteristics of the magnetic field, magnetic nanoparticles have different functions like imaging, cell tagging, drug delivery, gene therapy, and malignant hyperthermia (Xie et al. 2011).

Due to existence of some internal defects of magnetic nanoparticles, immediate steps are mandatory to promote stability and compatibility, which allows for the specific target capacity and drug filling potency of the magnetic nanoparticles. Heparin was applied as a coating agent in magnetic nanoparticles for satisfactory biocompatibility. Iron oxide nanoparticles coated with heparin have been prepared with the help of chemical and physical modification methods (Khurshid et al. 2009; Liu et al. 2007).

Liu et al. shows an example where heparin was grafted covalently with polyvinyl alcohol (PVA) shell magnetic nanoparticles through amino tri methoxy silane (ATMS) and 4,4-diphenyl methane diisocyanate (HMDI) (Liu et al. 2007).

Through the beneficial effect of the electrostatic interactions among heparin and positively charged poly(L-lysine) (PLL), PLL-coated iron oxide nanoparticles were used as a coating material for heparin (Khurshid et al. 2009). Such types of studies have revealed that a heparin coating develops biocompatibility and particle magnetization affecting it targeting specific tumor sites and regulating the metastasis.

Magnetic iron oxides are dense and solid in nature. Due to this major drawback, drug delivery capability is very low. Therefore, surface modification of iron oxide is a basic requirement. Heparin-modified PEGylated iron oxide magnetic nanoparticles are used for the induction of a tumor through the transportation of protamine subcutaneously, which is a clinical advantage of such formulation (Zhang et al. 2013).

The binding and interaction capacity of magnetic nanoparticles containing heparin, depends on the concentration of fibrinogen derivative in normal tissue and solid tumors (Niers et al. 2007; Irimura et al. 1986).

5.8.1.2 Heparin-Revised Gold Nanoparticles

Due to presence of multiple distinctive characteristics such as less toxicity, good biocompatibility, a large surface area, and simple formulation, gold nanoparticles act as an important tool among the other nanocarriers in the field of cancer nanotechnology (Ghosh et al. 2008). Multifunctional gold nanoparticles were established and modified by heparin, acting as an apoptosis inducing agent of metastatic cancer cells (Lee et al. 2010).

For accomplishing the fluorescence resonance energy transfer (FRET), end-thiol-modified heparin binds with the external part of the gold nanoparticles through gold-thiol complexation. A quenching property of gold nanoparticles was exhibited by FRET at a specific distance between the dye and the nanoparticles (Kalita et al. 2014).

Due to over-expression of the heparin-cleavage enzyme under metastasis conditions, it can be used as a good diagnostic agent in advanced cancer. Heparin released intracellularly depends on redox sensitive properties. Arginine-glycine-aspartic acid was grafted with nanoparticles for a target-specific delivery. As per research by Li et al. conjugation of nanoparticles with gold nanoparticles can act as an energy quencher and a heparin coating material (Li et al. 2013).

Generally gold nanoparticles with a 40 nm size are used for formulation through a conjugation reaction via a gold-thiol interaction. Photoactivation (PhA) is incapable of producing fluorescent and photoactivity during circulation because of potent photoquenching via FRET of gold nanoparticles after the excitation at 405 nm. Then it was bounded into tumor sites and adopted into the tumor cells. GSH assisted the release of PhA by breakdown of the gold-thiol interlink and enhancing the photo activation properties. By the application of a photo radiation associated mechanistic pathway, photo activation has antitumor activity. *In vivo* effects depict that the novel nanoparticles potentially decrease tumor volume in mice (A549) which ensures the production of cytotoxic singlet oxygen in the tumor.

5.9 HEPARIN-CUSTOMIZED ORGANIC NANOPARTICLES

During circulation, opsonization takes place due to the fast clearance rate of nanoparticles by the reticuloendothelial system (RES) cells existing in the liver and spleen. To overcome this drawback, neutral hydrophilic polymers are used for modification with the help of electronic theory (Passirani et al. 1998a,b).

The effect of heparin has two types in nature. First, heparin coating is represented as a biomimetic method because glycosaminoglycan is used as a coating agent in both cases (the surface of cells and the pathogens). This is a vital method for facilitating the phagocytosis of the RES (Passirani et al. 1998a). Second, nanoparticles modified with heparin molecules maintain a dense brush-like structure. Such types of structure was familiar with protecting the interaction with proteins in the blood. As with, Han et al. a conjugation reaction between negatively charged heparin and DOX-loaded cationic liposomes via hatching liposomes in heparin solution for 2 h, may result in the zeta potential changing from 14 mV to 70 mV (Han et al. 2006). The half-life of DOX encapsulated into heparin-liposomes was found to be significantly higher than the control liposomes.(Passirani et al. 1998a,b). Passirani et al. showed that, heparin-based amphiphilic formulation conjugated with heparin-poly(methyl methacrylate) (PMMA) can aggregate in an aqueous medium using nanoparticles with a diameter of approximately 80 nm (Passirani et al. 1998b).

A published report revealed that heparin-poly(methyl methacrylate)/N-vinyl carbazole (PMMA/NVC) nanoparticles were significantly improved compared with PMMA nanoparticles in respect of half-life (from 3 min to more than 5 h). Heparin and its derivatives possess a higher binding affinity and permeability toward vascular endothelial cells, which are rich at the target site (tumor).

5.10   CONCLUSIONS AND IMMINENT APPROACHES

Compared to other polysaccharides, heparin possesses outstanding pharmacological features like anti-angiogenesis and anti-metastasis which justifies its potential for anticancer therapy. Drug delivery to the endothelial cells by heparin-based nanoformulations is a better focus of interest. Due to the presence of distinctive characteristics, a special focus has been given in assimilating heparin into nanoformulations for cancer therapy. Interestingly, heparin is extremely hydrophilic in nature and present within sufficient adaptable functional groups on its chain that make it suitable for amphiphilic drug delivery systems. Polyelectrolyte complex nanoparticles are prepared using heparin in a simple condition for its electronegativity nature. Comparatively, by utilizing chemical modification or electrostatic interaction, heparin can be popularized worldwide and applied in multidisciplinary fields. These attractive nanocarriers have been applied not only for research purposes but also in magnetic therapy, photodynamic therapy, and the gene therapy of cancer, securing its therapeutic ground in a competitive therapeutic field. The type of flexible design of heparin-based nanocarriers make it a deserving focus in the nano-research field. The toxic complication viz. the hemorrhagic complexity of heparin and its analogs can be overcome by chemical modification keeping the anticancer activity preserved.

With the depth of knowledge on quantitative structure-activity relationships (QSAR) one can precisely separate the anticancer and anticoagulant activity of heparin in the discovery and development of the heparin-based nanoformulations pipeline. To maintain the quality of heparin-based nanoformulations, valid evaluation methods should be established.

ACKNOWLEDGMENTS

Amit Kundu and Subham Banerjee are both highly thankful to Sungkyunkwan University, Republic of Korea and Shoolini University, India respectively for providing access to necessary literature resources and essential library facilities for writing this book chapter. Acknowledgment is also extended to all the authors of papers, books, and websites, and all other published sources listed in the references that were used to prepare the contents of this chapter.

DISCLOSURES

The authors declare no known conflicts of interest.

ABBREVIATIONS

ATMS	Aminotrimethoxysilane
DEX	Dexamethasone
DOCA	Desoxycortosterone acetate.
DOX	Doxorubicin
EDAC	1-ethyl-3-(3-dimethylaminopropyl) carbodiimide hydrochloride
EPR	Enhanced permeability and retention
FA	Folic acid
FGF	Fibroblast growth factors
FRET	Fluorescence resonance energy transfer
GSH	Glutathione
HMDI	4, 4-diphenyl methane diisocyanate
IARC	International Agency for Research on Cancer
LMWHs	Low molecular weight heparins
MDR	Multidrug resistance
MNPs	Magnetic nanoparticles
PBCA	Poly(β-benzyl-L-aspartate)
PCL	Polycaprolactone
PCNs	Polyelectrolyte complex nanoparticles
PDT	Photodynamic therapy
PEI	Polyethylenimine
PEG	Polyethylene glycol
PEO	Poly(ethylene oxide)
PLL	Poly(L-lysine)
PMMA	Poly(methyl methacrylate)
PMMA/NVC	Poly(methyl methacrylate)/N-vinyl carbazole
PPO	Polyvinyl toluene
PSs	Photosensitizers
PTX	Paclitaxel
pVSVMP	Plasmid expressing vesicular stomatitis virus matrix protein
RES	Reticuloendothelial system
QSAR	Quantitative structure–activity relationship
UFH	Unfractionated heparin

CELL LINE DETAILS

4T1	Tumor cell line
Caco-2	Colon carcinoma
CT26	Colon cancer cells
HEPG2	Liver cancer cell line
MDAMB 231	Breast cancer cell line
MRK-16	Colorectal carcinoma cell lines

REFERENCES

Aider, M. 2010. Chitosan application for active bio-based films production and potential in the food industry: Review. *LWT - Food Sci. Technol* 43: 837–42.

Alonso, D., Bertolesi. G., Farias, E., Eijan, A., Joffe. E., and DeCidre, L. 1996. Antimetastatic effects associated with anticoagulant properties of heparin and chemically modified heparin species in a mouse mammary tumor model. *Oncol Rep* 3: 219–22.

Bae, K.H., Mok, H., and Park, T.G. 2008. Synthesis, characterization, and intracellular delivery of reducible heparin nanogels for apoptotic cell death. *Biomaterials* 29: 3376–83.

Bae, K.H., Moon, C.W., Lee, Y., and Park, T.G. 2009. Intracellular delivery of heparin complexed with chitosan-g-poly(ethylene glycol) for inducing apoptosis. *Pharm Res* 26: 93–100.

Balendiran, G.K., Dabur, R., and Fraser, D. 2004. The role of glutathione in cancer. *Cell Biochem Funct* 22: 343–52.

Barenholz, Y. 2012. Doxil(R)—the first FDA-approved nano-drug: Lessons learned. *J Control Release* 160: 117–34.

Bentolila, A., Vlodavsky, I., Haloun, C., and Domb, A.J. 2000. Synthesis and heparin-like biological activity of amino acid-based polymers. *Polym. Adv Tech.*11: 377–87.

Bentolila, A., Vlodavsky, I., Ishai-Michaeli, R., Kovalchuk, O., Haloun, C., and Domb, A.J. 2000. Poly(N-acryl amino acids): A new class of biologically active polyanions. *J Med Chem* 43: 2591–600.

Bera, R., Kundu, A., Sen, T., Adhikari, D., and Karmakar, S. 2016. In vitro metabolic stability and permeability of gymnemagenin and its in vivo pharmacokinetic correlation in rats—A pilot study. *Planta Med* 82: 544–50.

Bertrand, N., Wu, J., Xu, X., Kamaly, N., and Farokhzad, O.C. 2014. Cancer nanotechnology: The impact of passive and active targeting in the era of modern cancer biology. *Adv Drug Deliv Rev* 66: 2–25.

Bitan, M., Polliack, A., Zecchina, G. et al. 2002. Heparanase expression in human leukemias is restricted to acute myeloid leukemias. *Exp Hematol* 30: 34–41.

Bobek, V. and Kovařík, J. 2004. Antitumor and antimetastatic effect of warfarin and heparins. *Biomed Pharmacother* 58: 213–19.

Boddohi, S., Moore, N., Johnson, P.A., and Kipper, M.J. 2009. Polysaccharide-based polyelectrolyte complex nanoparticles from chitosan, heparin, and hyaluronan. *Biomacromolecules* 10: 1402–9.

Borsig, L. 2010. Antimetastatic activities of heparins and modified heparins. Experimental evidence. *Thromb Res* 125:S66–S71.

Borsig, L., Wong, R., Feramisco, J., Nadeau, D.R., Varki, N.M., and Varki, A. 2001. Heparin and cancer revisited: Mechanistic connections involving platelets, P-selectin, carcinoma mucins, and tumor metastasis. *Proc Natl Acad Sci U S A* 98: 3352–57.

Cho, K., Wang, X., Nie S., Chen, Z.G. and Shin, D.M. 2008. Therapeutic nanoparticles for drug delivery in cancer. *Clin Cancer Res* 14: 1310–16.

Choi, J.H., Jang, J.Y., Joung, Y.K., Kwon, M.H., and Park, K.D. 2010. Intracellular delivery and anti-cancer effect of self-assembled heparin-Pluronic nanogels with RNase A. *J Control Release* 147: 420–27.

Chung, Y.I., Kim, J.C., Kim, Y.H. et al. 2010. The effect of surface functionalization of PLGA nanoparticles by heparin- or chitosan-conjugated Pluronic on tumor targeting. *J Control Release* 143: 374–82

Coates, A., Abraham, S., Kaye, S.B. et al. 1983. On the receiving end patient perception of the side-effects of cancer chemotherapy. *Eur J Cancer Clin Oncol* 19: 203–8.

Collen, A., Smorenburg, S.M., Peters, E. et al. 2000. Unfractionated and low molecular weight heparin affect fibrin structure and angiogenesis in vitro. *Cancer Res* 60: 6196–200.

Cosgrove, R.H., Zacharski, L.R., Racine, E., and Andersen, J.C. 2002. Improved cancer mortality with low-molecular-weight heparin treatment: a review of the evidence. *Semin Thromb Hemost.* 28: 79–87.

D'Amore, P.A. 1992. Capillary growth: A two-cell system. *Semin Cancer Biol* 3: 49–56.

Das, M., Mohanty, C., and Sahoo S.K. 2009. Ligand-based targeted therapy for cancer tissue. *Expert Opin Drug Deliv* 6: 285–304.

Del Burgo, L. Saenz, Pedraz, J.L., and Orive, G. 2014. Advanced nanovehicles for cancer management. *DrugDiscovToday* 19: 1659–70.

Dey, P. and Bhakta, T. 2012. Evaluation of in-vitro anticoagulant activity of *Molineriarecurpata* leaf extract. *J. Nat. Prod. Plant Resour* 2: 685–88.

Dey, P. and Das, N. 2013. Carbon nanotubes: It's role in modern health care. *Int J Pharm Pharm Sci* 5: 9–13.

Dey, P. and Bhakta, T. 2012 Nanotechnology for the delivery of poorly water soluble drugs. *Global J Pharmaceut Res* 1: 225–50.

Durdureanu-Angheluta, A., Uritu, C.M., Coroaba, A. et al. 2014. Heparin-anthranoid conjugates associated with nanomagnetite particles and their cytotoxic effect on cancercells. *J Biomed Nanotechnol* 10: 131–42.

Fernandez, C., Hattan, C.M., and Kerns, R.J. 2006. Semi-synthetic heparin derivatives: Chemical modifications of heparin beyond chain length, sulfate substitution pattern andN-sulfo/N-acetyl groups. *Carbohydr Res* 341: 1253–65.

Ferro, V., Dredge, K., Liu, L. et al. 2007. PI-88 and novel heparan sulfate mimetics inhibit angiogenesis. *Semin Thromb Hemost* 33: 557–68.

Fidler, I.J. 1990. Critical factors in the biology of human cancer metastasis: Twenty-eight GHA Clowes memorial awards lecture. *Cancer Res* 50: 6130–38.

Fidler, I.J. 2003. The pathogenesis of cancer metastasis: The "seed and soil" hypothesis revisited. *Nat Rev Cancer* 3: 453–58.

Folkman, J., Weisz, P.B., Joullie, M.M., Li, W.W., and Ewing, W.R. 1989. Control of angiogenesis with synthetic heparin substitutes. *Science* 243: 1490–3.

Friedmann, Y., Vlodavsky, I., Aingorn, H. et al. 2000. Expression of heparanase in normal, dysplastic, and neoplastic human colonic mucosa and stroma. Evidence for its role in colonic tumorigenesis. *Am J Pathol* 157: 1167–75.

Gabizon, A., Shmeeda, H., and Barenholz, Y. 2003. Pharmacokinetics of pegylated liposomal doxorubicin: Review of animal and human studies. *Clin Pharmacokinet* 42: 419–36.

Gatti, G., Casu, B., Hamer, G.K., and Perlin, A.S. 1979. Studies on the conformation of heparin by1H and13C NMR spectroscopy. *Macromol* 12: 1001–07.

Gerlowski, L.E. and Jain, R.K. 1986. Micro vascular permeability of normal and neoplastic tissues. *Microvasc Res* 31: 288–305.

Ghosh, P., Han, G., De, M., Kim, C., and Rotello, V. 2008. Gold nanoparticle in delivery applications. *Adv Drug Deliv Rev* 60: 1307–15.

Ginath, S., Menczer, J., Friedmann, Y. et al. 2001. Expression of heparanase, Mdm2, and erbB2 in ovarian cancer. *Int J Oncol* 18: 1133–44.

Goebel, F.D., Goldstein, D., Goos, M., Jablonowski, H., and Stewart J.S. 1996. Efficacy and safety of stealth liposomal doxorubicin in AIDS related Kaposi's sarcoma. The International SL-DOX Study Group. *Br J Cancer* 73: 989–94.

Goger, B., Halden., Y., Rek A. et al. 2002. Different affinities of glycosaminoglycan oligosaccharides for monomeric and dimeric interleukin-8: A model for chemokine regulation at inflammatory sites. *Biochemistry* 41: 1640–6

Gohji, K., Hirano, H., Okamoto, M. et al. 2001. Expression of three extracellular matrix degradative enzymes in bladder cancer. *Int J Cancer* 95: 295–301.

Gorain, B., Choudhurya, H., Kundu A. et al. 2014. Nanoemulsion strategy for olmesartan medoxomil improves oral absorption and extended antihypertensive activity in hypertensive rats. *Colloids Surf B Biointerfaces* 115: 286–94.

Gou, M., Men, K., Zhang, J. et al. 2010. Efficient inhibition of C-26 colon carcinoma by VSVMP gene delivered by biodegradable cationic nanogel derived from polyethylcneimine. *Acs Nano* 4: 5573–84.

Gupta, G.P. and Massague, J. 2006. Cancer metastasis: Building a framework. *Cell* 127: 679–95.

Han, H.D., Lee, A., Song, C.K. et al. 2006. In vivo distribution and antitumor activity of heparin-stabilized doxorubicin-loaded liposomes. *Int J Pharm* 313: 181–8.

Hare, I.J, Lammers, T., Marianne, B., Puri, S., Storm, G., and Barry, T.S. 2017. Challenges and strategies in anti-cancer nanomedicine development: An industry perspective. *Adv Drug Deliv Rev*108: 25–38

Hennink, W.E. and van Nostrum, C.F. 2012. Novel crosslinking methods to design hydrogels. *Adv Drug Deliv Rev* 64: 223–36.

Herter-Sprie, G.S., Kung, A.L., and Wong, K.K. 2013. New cast for a new era: Preclinical cancer drug development revisited. *J Clin Invest* 123: 3639–45.

Hettiarachchi, R.J., Smorenburg, S.M., Ginsberg, J., Levine, M., Prins, M.H., and Büller, H.R. 1999. Do heparins do more than just treat thrombosis? The influence of heparins on cancer spread. *Thromb Haemost* 82: 947–52.

Hou, L., Yao, J., Zhou, J. and Zhang, Q. 2012. Pharmacokinetics of a paclitaxel-loaded low molecular weight heparin-all-trans-retinoid acid conjugate ternary nanoparticulate drug delivery system. *Biomaterials* 33: 5431–40.

Irimura, T., Nakajima, M., and Nicolson, G.L. 1986. Chemically modified heparins as inhibitors of heparan sulfate specific endo-beta-glucuronidase (heparanase) of metastatic melanoma cells. *Biochemistry* 9: 5322–28.

Ishihara, M., Kishimoto, S., Takikawa, M., Mori, Y., Nakamura, S., and Fujita, M.J. 2011. Low-molecular-weight heparin and protamine-based polyelectrolyte nano complexes for protein delivery. *J Biomater Nanobiotechnol* 2: 500–9.

Jeon, M., Park, J., Dey, P. et al. 2017. Site-selective Rhodium(III)-catalyzed C–H amination of 7-azaindoles with anthranils: Synthesis and anticancer evaluation. *Adv Synth Catal* 359: 1–9.

Jeong, T., Lee, S.H., Mishra, N.K. et al. 2017. Synthesis and cytotoxic evaluation of N-Aroylureas through Rhodium (III)-catalyzed C–H functionalization of indolines with isocyanates. *Adv Synth Catal* 359: 1–9.

Jeong, T., Mishra, N.K., Dey, P. et al. 2017. C (sp 3)–H amination of 8-methylquinolineswith azodicarboxyl-
    ates under Rh (iii) catalysis: Cytotoxic evaluation ofquinolin-8-ylmethanamines. *Chem Commun* 53:
    11197–200.
Kakkar, A.K. and Williamson, R.C. 1999. Antithrombotic therapy in cancer. *BMJ* 318: 1571–72.
Kalita, M., Balivada, S., Swarup, V.P. et al. 2014. A nanosensor for ultrasensitive detection of oversulfated
    chondroitin sulfate contaminant in heparin. *J Am Chem Soc* 136: 554–57.
Karuna, D.S., Dey, P., Das, S., Kundu A., and Bhakta, T. 2018. In vitro antioxidant activities of root extract of
    AsparagusracemosusLinn. *J Tradit Complement Med* 8: 60–5.
Kessenbrock, K., Plaks, V., and Werb, Z. 2010. Matrix metallopoteinases: Regulator of the tumor microenvi-
    ronment. *Cell* 141: 52–67.
Khatun, Z., Nurunnabi, Cho, K.J., Byun, Y., Bae, Y.H., and Lee, Y.K. 2014 Oral absorption mechanism and
    anti-angiogenesis effect of taurocholic acid-linked heparin-docetaxel conjugates. *J Control Release* 177:
    64–73.
Khatun, Z., Nurunnabi, M., Cho, K.J., and Lee, Y.K. 2012. Imaging of the GI tract by QDs loaded heparin–
    deoxycholic acid (DOCA) nanoparticles. *Carbohydr Polym* 90: 1461–68.
Khurshid, H., Kim, S.H., Bonder, M.J. et al. 2009. Development of heparin-coated magnetic nanoparticles for
    targeted drug delivery applications. *J Appl Phys*105: 07B308.
Kim, B.Y., Bae, J.W., and Park, K.D. 2013. Enzymatically in situ shell cross-linked micelles composed of
    4-arm PPO–PEO and heparin for controlled dual drug delivery. *J Control Release* 172: 535–40.
Kim, D.H., Termsarasab, U., Cho, H.J. et al. 2014. Preparation and characterization of self-assembled nanopar-
    ticles based on lowmolecular- weight heparin and stearylamine conjugates for controlled delivery of
    docetaxel. *Int J Nanomed* 8: 5711–27.
Koliopanos, A., Friess, H., Kleeff, J. et al. 2001. Heparanase expression in primary and metastatic pancreatic
    cancer. *Cancer Res* 61: 4655–9.
Kunath, K., von Harpe, A., Fischer, D. et al. 2003. Low-molecular-weight polyethylenimine as a non-viral
    vector for DNA delivery: comparison of physicochemical properties, transfection efficiency and in vivo
    distribution with high-molecular-weight polyethylenimine. *J Control Release* 89: 113–25.
Kuppusamy, P., Li, H., Ilangovan, G. et al. 2002. Noninvasive imaging of tumor redox status and its modifica-
    tion by tissue glutathione levels. *Cancer Res* 62: 307–12.
Kwon, G.S. 2003. Polymeric micelles for delivery of poorly water-soluble compounds. *Crit Rev Ther Drug
    Carrier Syst* 20: 357–403.
Lapierre, F., Holme, K., Lam, L. et al. 1996. Chemical modifications of heparin that diminish its antico-
    agulant but preserve its heparanase-inhibitory, angiostatic, anti-tumor and anti-metastatic properties.
    Glycobiology 6: 355–66.
Lee, K., Lee, H., Bae, K.H., and Park, T.G. 2010. Heparin immobilized gold nanoparticles for targeted detec-
    tion and apoptotic death of metastatic cancer cells. *Biomaterials* 31: 6530–6.
Lever, R. and Page, C.P. 2002. Novel drug development opportunities for heparin. *Nat Rev Drug Discov* 1:
    140–48.
Li, J., Huo, M., Wang, J. et al. 2012. Redox-sensitive micelles self-assembled from amphiphilic hyaluronic
    acid-deoxycholic acid conjugates for targeted intracellular delivery of paclitaxel. *Biomaterials* 33:
    2310–20.
Li, L., Kim, J.K., Huh, K.M., Lee, Y.K., and Kim, S.Y. 2012. Targeted delivery of paclitaxel using folate-
    conjugated heparin-poly (β-benzyl-l-aspartate) self-assembled nanoparticles. *Carbohydr Polym* 87:
    2120–8.
Li, L., Moon, H.T., Park, J.Y. et al. 2011. Heparin-based self-assembled nanoparticles for photodynamic ther-
    apy. *Macromol. Res.* 19: 487–94.
Li, L., Nurunnabi, M., Nafiujjaman, M., Lee, Y.K., and Huh, K.M. 2013. GSH mediated photoactivity of
    pheophorbide a conjugated heparin/gold nanoparticle for photodynamic therapy. *J Control Release* 171:
    241–50.
Li, N.N., Lin, J., Gao, D., and Zhang, L.M. 2014. A macromolecular prodrug strategy for combinatorial drug
    delivery. *J Colloid Interface Sci* 417: 301–9.
Linhardt, R.J. 2004. Heparin-induced cancer cell death. *Chem Biol* 11: 420–22.
Liu, L., Gou, M., Yi, T., Bai, Y., Wei, Y., and Zhao, X. 2014. Antitumor effects of heparin-polyethyleneimine
    nanogels delivering claudin-3-targeted short hairpin RNA combined with low-dose cisplatin on ovarian
    cancer. *Oncol Rep* 31: 1623–8.
Liu, T.Y., Huang, L.Y., Hu, S.H., Yang, M.C., and Chen, S.Y. 2007. Core–shell magnetic nanoparticles of
    heparin conjugate as recycling anticoagulants. *J Biomed Nanotechnol* 3: 353–9.

Lu, D.Y., Chen, E.H., and Lu, T.R. 2015. Anticancer drug development, a matter of money or a matter of idea? *Metabolomics* 5: e134.

Lu, D.Y. and Lu, T.R. 2010. Antimetastatic activities and mechanisms of bisdioxopiperazine compounds. *Anticancer Agents Med Chem* 10: 564–70.

Lu, D.Y., Lu, T.R., Wu, H.Y., and Cao, S. 2013. Cancer Metastasis treatments. *Curr Drug Therapy* 8: 24–9.

Lu, D.Y., Lu, T.R., and Cao, S. 2012. Cancer metastases and clinical therapies. *Cell Dev Biol* 1: 110.

Lu, D.Y., Lu, T.R., Xu, B. et al. 2016. Cancer metastasis, a clinical dilemma for therapeutics. *Curr Drug Therapy* 11: 163–9.

Lu, Y. and Park, K. 2013. Polymeric micelles and alternative nanonized delivery vehicles for poorly soluble drugs. *Int J Pharm.* 453: 198–21.

Lungwitz, U., Breunig, M., Blunk, T., and Göpferich, A. 2005. Polyethylenimine-based non-viral gene delivery systems. *Eur J Pharm Biopharm* 60: 247–66.

Luo, Y. and Prestwich, G.D. 2002 Cancer-targeted polymeric drugs. *Curr Cancer Drug Targets.* 2: 209–26.

Maity, S., Kundu, A., Karmakar, S., and Sa, B. 2016. In vitro and in vivo correlation of colon-targeted compression-coated tablets. *J Pharm* 2016: 1–9.

Matsumura, Y. and Maeda, H. 1986. A new concept for macromolecular therapeutics in cancer chemotherapy: Mechanism of tumoritropic accumulation of proteins and the antitumor agent smancs. *Cancer Res* 46: 6387–92.

Matsuo, H., Wakasugi, M., Takanaga, H. et al. 2001. Possibility of the reversal of multidrug resistance and the avoidance of side effects by liposomes modified with MRK-16, amonoclonal antibody to P-glycoprotein *J Control Release* 77: 77–86.

Maxhimer, J.B., Quiros, R.M., Stewart, R. et al. 2002. Heparanase-1 expression is associated with the metastatic potential of breast cancer. *Surgery* 132: 326–33.

Merris, J. 2005. Productivity counts-but the definition is key. *Science* 309: 726–7.

Miao, H.Q., Elkin, M., Aingorn, E., Ishai-Michaeli, R., Stein, C.A., and Vlodavsky, I. 1999. Inhibition of heparanase activity and tumor metastasis by laminarin sulfate and synthetic phosphorothioate oligodeoxynucleotides. *Int J Cancer* 83: 424–31.

Mina, L.A. and Sledge, G.W. 2011. Rethinking the metastatic cascade as a therapeutic target. *Nat Rev Clin Oncol* 8: 325–32.

Mizrahy, S. and Peer, D. 2012. Polysaccharides as building blocks for nanotherapeutics. *Chem Soc Rev* 41: 2623–40.

Mohanraj, V.J. and Chen, Y. 2006. Nanoparticles—A review. *Trop J Pharm Res* 5: 561–73.

Mori, Y., Nakamura, S., Kishimoto, S. et al. 2010. Preparation and characterization of low-molecular-weight heparin/protamine nanoparticles (LMW-H/P NPs) as FGF-2 carrier. *Int J Nanomedicine* 5: 147–55.

Mousa, S.A. and Petersen, L.J. 2009. Anti-cancer properties of low-molecular-weight heparin: Preclinical evidence. *Thromb Haemost* 102: 258–67.

Nakajima, M., Irimura, T., and Nicolson, G.L. 1988. Heparanases and tumor metastasis. *J Cell Biochem* 36: 157–67.

Neu, M., Fischer, D., and Kissel., T. 2005. Recent advances in rational gene transfer vector design based on poly(ethylene imine) and its derivatives. *J Gene Med.* 7: 992–1009.

Nguyen, D.H., Choi, J.H., Joung, Y.K., and Park, K.D. 2011. Disulfide-crosslinked heparin-pluronic nanogels as a redox-sensitive nanocarrier for intracellular protein delivery. *J Bioact Compat Polym* 26: 287–300.

Nguyen, K.T. 2011. Targeted nanoparticles for cancer therapy: promises and challenges. *J Nanomed Nanotechnol* 2: 1–2.

Niers, T.M., Klerk, C.P., DiNisio, M. et al. 2007. Mechanisms of heparin induced anti-cancer activity in experimental cancer models. *Crit Rev Oncol Hematol* 61: 195–207.

O'Brien, M.E., Wigler, N., Inbar, M. et al. 2004. Reduced cardiotoxicity and comparable efficacy in a phase III trial of pegylated liposomal doxorubicin HCl (CAELYX/Doxil) versus conventional doxorubicin for first-line treatment of metastatic breast cancer. *Ann Oncol* 15: 440–49.

Ohkuma, S. and Poole, B. 1978. Fluorescence probe measurement of the intralysosomal pH in living cells and the perturbation of pH by various agents. *Proc Natl Acad Sci USA* 75: 3327–31.

Ono, K., Ishihara, M., Ishikawa, K. et al. 2002. Periodate-treated, nonanticoagulant heparin-carrying polystyrene (NAC-HCPS) affects angiogenesis and inhibits subcutaneous induced tumour growth and metastasis to the lung. *Br J Cancer* 86: 1803–12.

Osmond, R.I., Kett, W.C., Skett, S.E., and Coombe, D.R. 2002. Protein-heparin interactions measured by BIAcore 2000 are affected by the method of heparin immobilization. *Anal Biochem* 310: 199–207.

Parish, C.R., Coombe, D.R., Jakobsen, K.B., Bennett, F.A., and Underwood, P.A. 1987. Evidence that sul-
phated polysaccharides inhibit tumour metastasis by blocking tumour-cell-derived heparanases. *Int J Cancer* 15: 511–8.

Parish, C.R., Freeman, C., Brown, K.J., Francis, D.J. and Cowden, W.B. 1999. Identification of sulfated oligo-
saccharide-based inhibitors of tumor growth and metastasis using novel in vitro assays for angiogenesis
and heparanase activity. *Cancer Res* 59: 3433–41.

Park, K., Kim, K., Kwon, I.C. et al. 2004. Preparation and characterization of self-assembled nanoparticles of
heparin-deoxycholic acid conjugates. *Langmuir* 20: 11726–31.

Park, K., Lee, G.Y., Kim, Y.S. et al. 2006. Heparin–deoxycholic acid chemical conjugate as an anticancer drug
carrier and its antitumor activity. *J Control Release* 114: 300–6.

Park, K., Kim, Y.S., Lee, G.Y. et al. 2007. Antiangiogenic effect of bile acid acylated heparin derivative.
Pharm Res 24: 176–85.

Park, K., Kim, Y.S., Lee, G.Y. et al. 2008. Tumor endothelial cell targeted cyclic RGD-modified heparin
derivative: Inhibition of angiogenesis and tumor growth. *Pharm Res* 25: 2786–98

Park, K., Lee, S.K.; Park, A.S.H. et al. 2007. The attenuation of experimental lung metastasis by a bile acid
acylated-heparin derivative. *Biomaterials* 28: 2667–76.

Parveen, S. and Sahoo, S.K. 2006. Nanomedicine: Clinical applications of polyethylene glycol conjugate proteins and drugs. *Clin Pharmacokinet* 45: 965–88.

Parveen, S. and Sahoo, S.K. 2008. Polymeric nanoparticles for cancer therapy. *J Drug Target* 16: 108–23.

Passirani, C., Barratt, G., Devissaguet, J.P., and Labarre, D. 1998a. Interactions of nanoparticles bearing
heparin or dextran covalently bound to poly(methyl methacrylate) with the complement system. *Life
Sci* 62: 775–85.

Passirani, C., Barratt, G., Devissaguet, J.P., and Labarre, D. 1998b. Long-circulating nanoparticles bearing
heparin or dextran covalently bound to poly(methyl methacrylate). *Pharm Res* 15: 1046–50.

Patri, A.K., Kukowska-Latallo, J.F., and Baker, J.R. 2005. Targeted drug delivery with dendrimers: Comparison
of the release kinetics of covalently conjugated drug and non-covalent drug inclusion complex. *Adv
Drug Deliv Rev* 57: 2203–14.

Peng, X.H., Wang, Y., Huang, D. et al. 2011. Targeted delivery of cisplatin to lung cancer using ScFvEGFR-
heparin-cisplatin nanoparticles. *ACS Nano* 5: 9480–93.

Poggi, A., Rossi, C., Casella, N. et al. 2002. Inhibition of B16-BL6 melanoma lung colonies by semisynthetic
sulfamino heparosan sulfates from E. coli K5 polysaccharide. *Semin Thromb Hemost* 28: 383–92.

Raemdonck, K., Demeester, J., and De Smedt, S. 2009. Advanced nanogel engineering for drug delivery. *Soft
Matter* 5: 707–15.

Reichert, J.M. and Wenger, J.B. 2008. Development trends for new cancer therapeutics and vaccines. *Drug
Discov Today* 13: 30–7.

Robert, N.J., Vogel, C.L., Henderson, I.C. et al. 2004. The role of the liposomal anthracyclines and other systemic therapies in the management of advanced breast cancer. *Semin Oncol* 31: 106–46.

Ruggeri, B.A., Camp, F., and Miknyoczki, S. 2014. Animal models of disease: Preclinical animal models of
cancer and their applications and utility in drug discovery. *Biochem Pharmacol* 87: 150–61.

Saravanakumar, G., Jo, D.G., and Park, J.H. 2012. Polysaccharide-based nanoparticles: A versatile platform
for drug delivery and biomedical imaging. *Curr Med Chem* 19: 3212–29.

Sava, G. and Bergamo, A. 1999. Drug control of solid tumour metastases: A critical view. *Anticancer Res* 19:
1117–24.

Schafer, F.Q. and Buettner, G.R. 2001. Redox environment of the cell as viewed through the redox state of the
glutathione disulfide/glutathione couple. *Free Radic Biol Med* 30: 1191–212.

Sciumbata, T., Caretto, P., Pirovano, P. et al. 1996. Treatment with modified heparins inhibits experimental metastasis formation and leads, in some animals, to long-term survival. *Invasion Metastasis* 16:
132–43.

She, W., Li, N., Luo, K. et al. 2013. Dendronized heparin_doxorubicin conjugate based nanoparticle as pH-
responsive drug delivery system for cancer therapy. *Biomaterials* 34: 2252–64.

Smorenburg, S.M. and Van Noorden, C.J. 2001. The complex effects of heparins on cancer progression and
metastasis in experimental studies. *Pharmacol Rev* 53: 93–106.

Soloman, R. and Gabizon, A.A. 2008. Clinical pharmacology of liposomal anthracyclines: Focus on pegylated
liposomal doxorubicin. *Clin Lymphoma Myeloma* 8: 21–32.

Stavrovskaya, A.A. 2000. Cellular mechanisms of multidrug resistance of tumor cells. *Biochemistry (Mosc)*
65: 95–106.

Suggitt, M. and Bibby M.C. 2005. 50 years of preclinical anticancer drug screening: Empirical to target-
driven approaches. *Clin Cancer Res* 11: 971–81.

Tae, G., Kim, Y.J., Choi, W.I., Kim, M., Stayton, P.S., and Hoffman, A.S. 2007. Formation of a novel heparin-based hydrogel in the presence of heparin-binding biomolecules. *Biomacromolecules* 8: 1979–86.

Takahashi, H., Ebihara, S., Okazaki, T. et al. 2004. Clinical significance of heparanase activity in primary resected non-small cell lung cancer. *Lung Cancer* 45: 207–14.

Talmadge, J.E. and Fidler, I.J. 2010. The biology of cancer metastasis: Historical perspective. *Cancer Res* 70: 5649–69.

Talmadge, J.E., Singh, R.K., Fidler, I.J., and Raz, A. 2007 Murine models to evaluate novel and conventional therapeutic strategies for cancer. *Am J Pathol* 170: 793–804.

Tannock, I.F., Lee, C.M., Tunggal, J.K., Cowan, D.S.M., and Egorin, M.J. 2002. Limited penetration of anticancer drugs through tumor tissue: A potential cause of resistance of solid tumors to chemotherapy. *Clin Cancer Res* 8: 878–84.

Taraboletti, G. and Margosio, B. 2001. Antiangiogenic and antivascular therapy for cancer. *Curr Opin Pharmacol* 1: 378–84.

Thun, M.J., DeLancey, J.O., Center, M.M., Jemal, A., and Ward, E.M. 2010. The global burden of cancer: Priorities for prevention. *Carcinogenesis* 31: 100–10.

Torre, L.A., Bray, F., Siegel, R.L., Ferlay, J., Lortet-Tieulent, J., and Jemal, A. 2015. Global cancer statistics, 2012. *CA Cancer J Clin* 65: 87–108.

Tran, T.H., Bae, B.C., Lee, Y.K., Na, K., and Huh, K.M. 2013. Heparin-folate-retinoic acid bioconjugates for targeted delivery of hydrophobic photosensitizers. *Carbohydr Polym* 92: 1615–24.

Valastyan, S. and Weinberg, R.A. 2011. Tumor metastasis: Molecular insights and evolving paradigms. *Cell* 147: 275–92.

Venditto, V.J. and Szoka Jr., F.C. 2013. Cancer nanomedicines: So many papers and so few drugs!. *Adv Drug Deliv Rev* 65: 80–8.

Vlodavsky, I., Friedmann, Y., Elkin, M. et al.1999. Mammalian heparanase: Gene cloning, expression and function in tumor progression and metastasis. *Nat Med* 5: 793–802.

Vlodavsky, I., Goldshmidt, O., Zcharia, E. et al. 2002. Mammalian heparanase: Involvement in cancer metastasis, angiogenesis and normal development. *Semin Cancer Biol* 12: 121–9.

Vlodavsky, I., Mohsen, M., Lider, O. et al. 1994. Inhibition of tumor metastasis by heparanase inhibiting species of heparin. *Invasion Metastasis* 14: 290–302.

Wang, X., Li, J., Wang, Y. et al. 2009. HFT-T, a targeting nanoparticle, enhances specific delivery of paclitaxel to folate receptor-positive tumors. *ACS Nano* 3: 3165–74.

Wang, X., Li, J., Wang, Y. et al. 2011. A folate receptor-targeting nanoparticle minimizes drug resistance in a human cancer model. *ACS Nano* 5: 6184–94.

Wang, Y., Xin, D., Liu, K., Zhu, M., and Xiang, J. 2009. Heparin-paclitaxel conjugates as drug delivery system: Synthesis, self-assembly property, drug release, and antitumor activity. *Bioconjug Chem* 20: 2214–21.

Wei, W., Mu, Y., Li, X. et al. 2011. Adenoviral vectors modified by heparin-polyethyleneimine nanogels enhance targeting to the lung and show therapeutic potential for pulmonary metastasis *in vivo*. *J Biomed Nanotechnol* 7: 768–75.

Xie, C., Gou, M.L., Yi, T. et al. 2011. Efficient inhibition of ovarian cancer by truncation mutant of FILIP1L gene delivered by novel biodegradable cationic heparin-polyethyleneimine nanogels. *HumGeneTher* 22: 1413–22.

Xie, J., Liu, G., Eden, H.S., Ai, H., and Chen, X. 2011. Surface-engineered magnetic nanoparticle platforms for cancer imaging and therapy. *Acc Chem Res* 44: 883–92e

Yallapu, M.M., Jaggi, M., and Chauhan, S.C. 2011. Design and engineering of nanogels for cancer treatment. *Drug Discov Today* 16: 457–63.

Yang, B.H., Yang, B.L., and Goetinck, P.F. 1995. Biotinylated hyaluronic acid as a probe for identifying hyaluronic acid-binding proteins. *Anal Biochem* 228: 299–306.

Yang, X., Du, H., Liu, J., and Zhai, G. 2015. Advanced nanocarriers based on heparin and its derivatives for cancer management. *Biomacromolecules* 16: 423–36.

Yang, Y., Macleod, V., Bendre, M. et al. 2005. Heparanase promotes the spontaneous metastasis of myeloma cells to bone. *Blood* 105: 1303–9.

Yoshitomi, Y., Nakanishi, H., Kusano, Y. et al. 2004. Inhibition of experimental lung metastases of Lewis lung carcinoma cells by chemically modified heparin with reduced anticoagulant activity. *Cancer Lett* 207: 165–74.

Yu, M.K., Lee, D.Y., Kim, Y.S., et al. 2007. Antiangiogenic and apoptotic properties of a novel amphiphilic folate-heparin-lithocholatederivative having cellular internality for cancer therapy. *Pharm Res* 24: 705–14.

Yuk, S.H., Oh, K.S., Cho, S.H., et al. 2011. Glycol chitosan/heparin immobilized iron oxide nanoparticles with a tumor-targeting characteristic for magnetic resonance imaging. *Biomacromolecules* 12: 2335–43.

Zacharski, L.R. and Ornstein, D.L. Heparin and cancer. 1998. *Thromb Haemost* 80: 10–23.

Zacharski, L.R., Ornstein, D.L., and Mamourian, A.C. 2000. Low-molecular-weight heparin and cancer. *Semin Thromb Hemost* 26: 69–77.

Zetter, B.R.1998. Angiogenesis and tumor metastasis. *Annu Rev Med.* 49: 407–24.

Zhang, J., Shin, M.C., David, A.E. et al. 2013. Long-circulating heparin-functionalized magnetic nanoparticles for potential application as a protein drug delivery platform. *Mol Pharm* 10: 3892–902.

Zhao, G. and Rodriguez, B.L. 2013. Molecular targeting of liposomal nanoparticlesto tumor microenvironment. *Int J Nanomedicine* 8: 61–71.

Zou, W. 2005. Immunosuppressive networks in the tumor environment and their therapeutic relevance. *Nat Rev Cancer* 5: 263–74.

6 Delivery of Biomolecules to the Central Nervous System Using a Polysaccharide Nanocomposite

Anroop B. Nair, Shah Jigar, Chavda Vishal, Shah Hiral, and Patel Snehal

CONTENTS

6.1   INTRODUCTION

The delivery of biomolecules to the central nervous systems (CNS) is one of the biggest challenges to drug delivery scientists owing to the existence of the blood brain barrier (BBB) that controls the diffusion of therapeutic and diagnostic agents. The conventional therapy in treating brain diseases and disorders remains ineffective, invasive, short acting, and creates problems for the patients. Neuroscientists have recognized that effective delivery of biomolecules into the CNS can be more realistic with better knowledge of the physiology of the BBB and its components, the permeability mechanisms of the BBB in a normal and pathological state, the effect of physical and chemical stimuli on the BBB, and also availability of different transporters or receptor expression at the BBB. At present, better understanding of the structure of the BBB, knowledge of various receptors and their mechanisms of function, development in medical technologies, and the discovery of novel approaches based on nanotechnology has led to many new effective therapies in treating various CNS diseases. These therapies developed for the effective treatment of CNS disorders include direct or indirect transport of therapeutic actives to the brain. In addition, the neuroscientists were successful in uncovering some new avenues of exploration for the treatment of brain diseases through delivering and or replacing various biomolecules. In this context, nanoparticulate carrier systems have been assessed for their potential for delivering therapeutics or biomolecules to the CNS. This chapter provides a general description of neurological disorders and approaches for their treatment with an emphasis on polysaccharide nanocomposites.

6.2   NEUROPHYSIOLOGY

Humans are high caliber and unique because of the distinctive anatomy and physiology of the nervous system that they possess. Humans remain a superior race as a result of the wonderful and brilliant mental power produced from their cortex. The weight of the brain (~1.5 kg) is roughly 1%–2% of the complete body weight but its oxygen occupying capacity is 70%–80% more than all the other organs. Typically, the nervous system is anatomically constituted in the CNS (brain and spinal cord) and the peripheral nervous system (ganglia, cranial nerves, and spinal nerves). The CNS is involved and is accountable to various composite neuronal processing. The two divisions of the peripheral nervous system are the somatic and autonomic nervous system, wherein the former is accountable for body movement while the latter regulates the automated responses. The neurons require a persistent supply of oxygen so as to make adenosine triphosphate (ATP) as preserved energy. Neurons are cells that need glucose as a fuel along with oxygen to make storable energy and to maintain their cell cycle. However, the neuronal cells are unable to make use of lipids, proteins, fats or cholesterol as a reserved raw material for ATP production. Moreover, they do not contain any tissue as a reservoir of glucose and hence the neuronal cells need a permanent and constant supply of both oxygen and glucose. In addition, the concentration of glucose in the blood is critical and needs to be carefully regulated for normal brain physiological functions as it regulates the physiology of the whole body. Brain damage may result in the permanent loss of neurons and loss of neuronal functions (Lo et al. 2001; De Boer and Gaillad 2007).

The brain is mainly divided into six parts (cerebrum, hypothalamus, midbrain, cerebellum, pons, and medulla oblongata) in terms of its physiological functions (Lo et al. 2001; Banks 1999). The functional tissues consisting of neurons and glial cells in the brain are denoted as brain parenchyma. Neurons, the basic cells of the brain-structural and functional unit consist of three main parts (cell body, dendrites, and axons). The function of dendrites is to receive message from other neurons while axons transmit information to different neurons, muscles, and glands. An excited neuron conveys or sends particulars to other neurons by producing an electrical impulse, with the specific information of the task to be done. Thus, the produced signals further spread like waves and get transformed to chemical signals through the synapses, which is described as neuronal signaling or neuronal firing (Banks 1999). The neuronal firing is the most important step in performing any specific task. As soon as the impulse reaches the axon terminals, the neurotransmitter molecules will get released. The cerebrum is divided into four lobes to perform a variety of physiological functions of the brain. The frontal lobe is the most efficient part of the brain concerned with higher intellectual functions as it is associated with maximum neuronal signals and mostly involved in the neurobehavioral activities. It is also responsible for certain inhibitory primitive behaviors. The epithalamus, thalamus, and hypothalamus have a specific role in sleep physiology. Various sensory and motor functions are controlled and regulated by the thalamus. The hypothalamus acts as a regulator of body functions, which involves controlling and regulating different functions of the body. Midbrain plays a major and vital role in the cranial reflexes and visual pathways. The cerebellum which is also called the "little brain" is associated with the controls of postural reflexes of muscles in the body and in the production of skilled movements which are responsible for learning memory. The medulla oblongata is the actual second major part of brain which regulates a variety of visceral or vital centers. Moreover, the additional physiological centers for sneezing, coughing, hiccupping, swallowing, and vomiting are also regulated and maintained by the medulla oblongata. This brain part continues with another unit of the nervous system—the spinal cord. The delicate neural tissue of the brain covered and protected by the bones of the skull, vertebral column, cranial, and spinal meninges.

Cerebrospinal fluid (CSF) is the major transformer which flows between central canals of the brain. It serves as a transfer medium between the blood and the nervous tissues. The main physiological function of CSF in neurophysiology is to act as a liquid buffer and to absorb mechanical shocks to the brain. CSF is constantly formed, circulated, and absorbed. The circulation of CSF includes the whole brain and all the brain hemisphere too. CSF production, absorption, and reproduction are most essential for normal brain physiology and neurophysiological functions (Abbott 2004; Dickson 1995). Any variation in the production or flow of CSFs generally causes enlargement of the cranium, cerebral edema, or increase in intracranial pressure. These factors could lead to serious neuropathological conditions and brain infections, occasionally resulting in mortality.

The BBB, an extremely selective semipermeable membrane, divides the blood from the brain's extracellular fluid and is designed to protect the brain from infection and neurotoxins. Typically, it is composed of brain endothelial cells, which are linked by tight junctions around capillaries that are absent in other parts of the circulatory system. Endothelial cells restrict the diffusion of large hydrophilic molecules but allow certain small molecules which are mostly hydrophobic. In addition to the endothelial cells, the brain's vasculature is supported by an extracellular base membrane, along with major cells like pericytes, astrocytes, and microglia. The close contact and functional interaction between all these cells leads to a well-designed unit namely a neurovascular unit (Rustenhoven et al. 2017) (Figure 6.1).

6.2.1 Neuropathology

Neurotransmitters play an important role in normal neuronal signaling and routine functioning. Variation or change in normal neurotransmission creates a pathology or abnormality in normal brain physiology. Epilepsy is a hyper excitation state due to an imbalance of excitatory amino acids such as glutamate, α-amino-3-hydroxy-5-methyl-4-isoxazole propionic acid, N-methyl-D-aspartate, and inhibitory amino acids such as gamma-aminobutyric acid, glycine, etc. (Meldrum 2000). Parkinsonism is the imbalance of acetylcholine and dopamine receptors which regulates the skeletal responses. Other neurotransmitters are also involved in neuropathology like schizophrenia, bipolar disorders, psychosis, etc. Thus, overall it is necessary to maintain normal neurotransmission via natural neurotransmitters (Abbott 2004; Dickson 1995; Meldrum 2000). On the other hand, it is imperative to understand the normal physiology when applying therapeutics via the BBB (a protective physiological barrier that permits the passage of only certain molecules into the brain) in various brain delivery systems to neuropathologies. Moreover, the possible therapy in raised or non-regulated intracranial pressure is to remove unregulated cell growth preferably by surgery

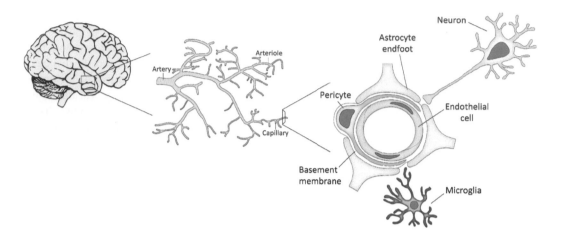

FIGURE 6.1 Schematic representation of the brain, neurovascular unit, and blood brain barrier (Reprinted from *Trends Pharmacol Sci* 38, Rustenhoven, J., Jansson, D., Smyth, L.C., and Dragunow, M. Brain pericytes as mediators of neuroinflammation, 291–304, Copyright 2017, with permission from Elsevier.)

or draining CSF from the ventricles, or using certain pharmacotherapeutics like steroids, osmotic dehydrating agents, and barbiturates (Abbott 2013; Misra et al. 2003).

The common neuropathologies, which are described below, are a result of dysfunction of normal brain physiology (Lo et al. 2001; De Boer and Gaillad 2007; Banks 1999; Abbott 2013).

- Brain oncology: brain tumors (systemic pathologies: glioblastoma, meningioma)
- Causative viral infections and associated encephalitis (active immunological response)
- Cerebrovascular stroke (altered or stopped arterial, venous blood brain flow into the brain resulting in oxygen deprivation to the neurons and neurodegeneration)
- Gray-white matter pathologies: e.g. multiple sclerosis
- Hyper excitation stage: status epileptics (due to up regulation of inhibitory and excitatory neurotransmitters)
- Metabolic encephalopathy, metabolic disorder (ketoacidosis), hetero pathology, hormonal or metabolic diseases due to associated brain pathologies
- Neurodegenerative disorders: Alzheimer's disease, Parkinsonism, dementia, cognitive decline, psychomotor sleep disorders, depressive disorders
- Neuromuscular disorders: myopathy, myasthenia gravis, etc.
- Neuropathies (retinopathy, diabetic neuropathy, hyperalgesia)
- Spinal cord malformation or dysfunction: myelopathy
- Traumatic brain injury and followed cognitive decline (depressive or altered behavior) due to systemic pathologies, e.g. diabetes, hypertension

There are other types of neuropathologies which transmit with the help of microorganisms. Bacteria tends to reach the brain primarily by traveling through the bloodstream. They often do not penetrate into the brain, but they will cause a purulent inflammation in the meninges, which affects function. So, most bacterial infections of the CNS are meningitis. There are several viruses that have neurons or other nervous system cells as their specific target. Rabies, a deadly virus, spreads in humans due to a dog bite or scratch. The rabies virus grows in the brain and salivary glands. Similarly, there are several fungi from the environment that can gain access to the body and may settle down in the brain. However, there are no fungi that are specific to the brain. Moreover, toxoplasma is a common infection among all mammalian species due to parasite infection.

Nutrition also plays an important role in CNS disorders. For instance, thiamine is essential for metabolism in many organs, including the brain. Its deficiency in the body leads to death of neurons in the cerebral cortex. The lesion is often called polioencephalomalacia (Lo et al. 2001; Abbott 2013; De Lange et al. 2005). The imbalance in glucose signaling throughout the brain causes diabetes associated macro and microvascular complications along with cognitive impairment (Abbott 2013; De Lange et al. 2005; Neuwelt et al. 2008). Copper deficiency will cause inadequate development of white matter (Abbott 2013).

Many toxins also affect CNS functions. For example, *Clostridium botulinum* produces one of the most powerful toxins currently known. Even a very small amount of ingested toxin will cause paralysis. The toxin acts by preventing the release of acetylcholine from the end of the axon onto the motor endplate. Lead poisoning causes toxicity to neurons and astrocytes, so the damage is primarily in the cerebral cortex. Similarly, excessive accumulation of ammonia in hepatic encephalopathy causes degeneration of astrocytes, which leads to brain edema.

6.3 TRANSPORT ROUTES OF DRUGS ACROSS THE BBB

It is well established that the movement of molecules into and across any biological membrane is primarily influenced by the physical and chemical properties of the molecule as well as the physiological properties of the membrane (Al-Dhubiab et al. 2015; 2016). The BBB manages essential brain homeostasis; however, it considerably restricts the delivery of biomolecules to the brain. Transport pathways of biomolecules include the para-cellular pathway, transcellular diffusion, carrier-mediated transport, receptor-mediated transcytosis, adsorptive-mediated transcytosis, and efflux pumps (Kasinathan et al. 2015). Various transport mechanisms by which biomolecules move across the BBB are depicted in Figure 6.2. In the para-cellular pathway, the tight junctions prevent movement of large hydrophilic substances and are ideal for water soluble molecules with a low molecular size. In transcellular diffusion, the lipophilic molecules (MW <500 Da) move with a concentration gradient into and through the cell. In a carrier-mediated transport system, the binding of various endogenous solutes (glucose, amino acids, purines, etc.) to specific protein molecules (transporter) on the outer side of membrane triggers changes in protein structure, resulting in the transport of these substances according to a concentration gradient, or it may follow an active transport mechanism in some cases. Receptor-mediated transcytosis provides the selective uptake of macromolecules. Endothelial cells contain receptors that

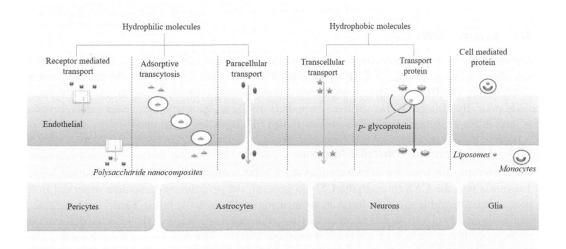

FIGURE 6.2 Schematic representation of transport pathways across the blood brain barrier.

are specialized in the plasma membrane known as coated pits or endosome and form vesicles after binding with ligands such as insulin. After acidifications of these endosomes, the ligands dissociate and move across the membrane. Transferrin receptors, insulin receptors, insulin-like growth factors, lipoprotein receptors, glutathione transporters, scavenger receptors, and diphtheria toxin receptors etc., expressed on endothelial cells are responsible for endocytosis and exocytosis transport mechanisms. Adsorptive transcytosis, also termed pinocytosis, is activated by an electrostatic interaction between the positive charges of peptides such as cationic protein or cell-penetrating peptides and the negative charges of plasma membrane surfaces such as heparan sulfate proteoglycans. This transport system involves movement of cationic proteins or peptides. Pinocytosis has a lower affinity but higher capacity than receptor-mediated transcytosis. In cell-mediated transcytosis, transportation depends on the functioning of immune cells like monocytes and macrophages. It is a unique transport system and can be used for any materials, molecules, and particulate carrier systems. The efflux pumps like P-glycoprotein, multi-drug resistance-associated proteins, etc., expels drugs and xenobiotics and rejects the entry of molecules.

Due to the unique properties of tight junctions, the parameters considered for the transport of drug molecules by passive diffusion across the BBB are (Kasinathan et al. 2015):

- Unionized form
- Molecular weight - <400–500 Da
- Log p value near to 2 (1.5–2.7)
- Basic (more preferable than acidic counterparts to enter into the brain as the cell membrane is negatively charged)
- Cumulative hydrogen bonding <10 (more the number of hydrogen bonds, less permeability across the BBB)

6.4 APPROACHES FOR TREATMENT OF CNS DISORDERS

Brain drug delivery has received greater attention and has been investigated more extensively in the last few decades. However, finding an effective way to transport therapeutic molecules through the BBB, or bypassing it in brain disorders, remains a formidable challenge. A few approaches have been identified and developed by scientists for supplying drug molecules into the brain. Currently, the following approaches are used (Gabathuler 2010).

6.4.1 INVASIVE APPROACH

Invasive methods involve injecting or infusing the therapeutic drug molecules directly into the brain, the cerebro-ventricles or CSF or intranasal cavity. This approach works on the principle of overcoming the BBB and delivering drugs directly into the brain. However, major limitations include poor distribution of therapeutic compounds into brain parenchyma, lesser safety, invasiveness, and a short residence time. This approach uses the following techniques:

6.4.1.1 Intra-Cerebroventricular Infusion

In this technique, the injection of therapeutics straight into cerebral lateral ventricles causes delivery of materials into the CNS through the CSF. In general, the pharmacokinetic data observed in this approach is comparable to a slow intravenous infusion of drugs in the brain (Pardridge 2005). To be pharmacologically effective, it is necessary to have the target receptors of the selected drug situated near the ependymal surface of the brain (Pardridge 2007b). The major limitation associated with this approach is the poor delivery of the drug in the brain parenchyma when the target is not near to the ventricles.

6.4.1.2 Convection Enhanced Delivery

The convection enhanced delivery procedure involves a minor surgical process and implanting a catheter into the brain parenchyma. The drug is actively pumped through the inserted catheter (stereotactically guided) and enters into the interstitial space. The drug infusion is continued for days and weeks and at the end of treatment the catheters are removed. The parameters considered in this approach are mainly two: the site where the catheter is placed and the infusion criteria for delivery of the drug at a proper location in the brain parenchyma. The major constraint in this approach is the limited permeation of infusate to certain areas of brain. So, by knowledge of proper placement of catheters and infusion parameters, accurate drug delivery can be possible (Vandergrift et al. 2006).

6.4.1.3 Intra-Cerebral Injection or Implants

The diffusion of the drug from the administration site to the disease target site is the most prevalent mechanism for intracerebral injection or placement of a biodegradable implants. The distribution of the drugs in the brain by a diffusion process decreases exponentially as distance increases. The precise identification of the injection site ensures a good efficacy of administered drugs and also overcomes the issues related to the diffusion of therapeutic actives in the brain parenchyma.

6.4.2 DISRUPTION OF THE BBB

Disruption of the BBB by loosening of tight junctions between the endothelial cells of the brain capillaries, gives the drug components open access to the brain. There are various mechanisms by which tight junctions can be disrupted such as osmotic-based disruption (Fortin et al. 2007), magnetic resonance imaging guided BBB disruption (Kinoshita et al. 2006), and the application of bradykinin-analogue (Borlongan and Emerich 2003). The limitations of this approach are many: high cost, necessity of medical supervision, and poor patient compliance. Additionally, in the case of cancer treatment, these techniques may cause spreading of the cancerous cells due to disruption of the BBB. Finally, neurons could be affected permanently because of uncontrolled flow of blood components in the brain.

6.4.3 PHARMACOLOGICAL APPROACH

Molecules like alcohol, nicotine, and benzodiazepine can enter into the brain easily. As mentioned earlier, the transport of molecules through the BBB is primarily influenced by the molecular size, charge on molecule, and degree of lipophilicity (Kasinathan et al. 2015; Lipinski et al. 2001). In this approach, knowledge of medicinal chemistry is used to modify a molecule which is effective against a CNS target and make it possible to enter the BBB. Modification in the structure of the drugs can make them suitable to cross the BBB. For example, either a decrease in the number of polar groups or an increase in lipophilicity of molecules, increases the transport of a drug across the BBB. But sometimes, these modifications also result in reduction of the desired CNS therapeutic activity. Also, an increase in the lipoidal nature of a molecule makes it a substrate for the efflux pump P-glycoprotein.

6.4.4 PHYSIOLOGICAL APPROACH

Some of the essential substances like glucose, insulin, growth hormone, low density lipoprotein, etc., are required for the metabolism and the existence of brain cells. For these substances to be transported to the brain, there are special transport mechanisms where the specific receptors recognize these substances and transport them into the brain. Normally, every brain neuron has its own capillary, so the brain comprises of large number of capillaries which are highly perfused (Pardridge 2005; Pardridge 2007a). This in turn makes these capillaries the most efficient pathway for transporting therapeutic drug molecules via selective transporters or specific internalizing receptors present in capillaries. Therefore, various strategies have been worked under this approach either by modifying the drugs which can utilize basic BBB nutrient transport systems or by linking to ligands that identify receptors present at the BBB. Finally, after receptor-mediated transcytosis, these molecules are carried through the BBB. But here also multiple factors need to be considered for successful transport across the BBB, such as: a) the kinetics involved in the transfer of drug molecules; b) the structural specificity or binding mechanisms of the transporter; c) the modification of the therapeutic molecule to ensure that it does not only bind but also remains active and shows its therapeutic effect *in vivo*; and d) actually get transported into the brain, as opposed to binding to the transporter (Gabathuler 2010).

6.4.5 PRODRUGS

Various transport mechanisms such as passive diffusion, carrier-mediated, or receptor-mediated transport have been used for the successful delivery of pseudo-nutrient prodrugs across the BBB. For example, the prodrug L-DOPA (L-3,4-dihydroxyphenylalanine) used to treat Parkinson's disease (Rautio et al. 2008). It is designed to target a carrier-mediated transport system, i.e. the L-amino acid transporter which can transport a large number of neutral amino acids (Gynther et al. 2008).

6.4.6 INTRANASAL DRUG DELIVERY

As one of the non-invasive drug delivery techniques, it can bypass the BBB using the olfactory nerves as a route of drug delivery. A study of the intranasal administration of methotrexate for brain cancer, confirmed the reduction in weight of a brain tumor by 80% (Shingaki et al. 2010). This delivery is easy and safe for administration which makes it the best alternative option for brain drug delivery. However, only a very limited amount of molecules can diffuse through the olfactory epithelium.

6.5 THE NEED FOR ALTERNATIVE THERAPY

The BBB imposes an obstruction to delivery of therapeutic compounds such as antibiotics, anticancer drugs, and neuropeptides to transport through the endothelial capillaries to the CNS (Kinoshita 2006). Nevertheless, many drug delivery methodologies or techniques have been identified and used for transportation of therapeutics to brain related diseases or disorders. However, the majority of these are lacking target specificity while being invasive in nature. These methods are restricted for the delivery of some selected therapeutics which had suitable structure-activity relationship properties or proper drug-receptor interactions, and also an intact structure-transport relationship (Jones and Shusta 2007). However, there is urgent need to deliver various biological compounds including therapeutic biomolecules across the biological membrane along with keeping normal body functions intact (Senel et al. 2001). Thus, it is of the utmost importance to develop new approaches/ technologies which are non-invasive and capable of carrying therapeutics using any of the transport mechanisms to cross the BBB, allow an uniform distribution in the brain, and finally provide rapid and target site exposure to the brain cells (Gabathuler 2010). Moreover, it is also necessary to select an appropriate drug amongst the hundreds of new compounds through proper justification or rationale of the drug design along with high throughput screening for receptor-ligand interactions.

In addition to molecular size, charge on molecules, lipophilicity, the other important parameters which influence drug delivery to CNS are drugs binding to non-transporters (ineffective), enzymatic action (converting the drug in an inactive form or cause the formation of non-therapeutic/ inactive intermediate drug form), surface activity of molecules, etc. Consequently, active transport, structure-activity protection, safe delivery, availability, and the therapeutic action of the drug at the target site are highly essential for the treatment of brain related disorders and diseases. Moreover, drug–receptor interactions with various neurons, structural activity relationships, and structure–transport relationships are essential parameters which need to be evaluated to ensure the successful delivery of any biomolecules into the brain. By understanding the physiology of the brain, the BBB, and various transport mechanisms (Kasinathan et al. 2015), one may design and optimize a suitable drug delivery system for the brain without disrupting the BBB. The lists of various non-invasive approaches that are under investigation to deliver biomolecules across the BBB without damaging it are listed below:

- Nanocomposites
- Modifying solubility of the drug
- Using the principle of the chimeric peptide
- Peptidomimetics approach
- Trojan approach
- Inhibition of efflux transportation of active drug molecules

The aforementioned methods are generally considered as a safe and non-invasive way of delivering biomolecules. Among these, nanoparticulate delivery systems provide a better and favorable alternative to target biomolecules to the CNS.

6.6 NANOCOMPOSITES

Nanostructured compounds are more interactive with cell membranes and proteins. The nanoparticles assist as an excellent carrier for the transport of both micro and macromolecules such as proteins, peptides, genes, and vaccines to the site of interest. Indeed, the physical (size, geometry/shape) and chemical properties (charge on the surface, composition, nature, etc.), as well as *in vivo* behavior, drug release characteristics etc., influence the overall efficacy of the nanoparticles (Kamaly et al. 2012). Incorporation of site specific ligands on these nanocomposites generally overcome the major toxic issues and cross the multifaceted *in vivo* barriers which in turn deliver the therapeutic actives to the site of action. Various nanoparticles and their biophysiochemical features which influence their performance both *in vitro* and *in vivo* are illustrated in Figure 6.3.

Due to advancements in the fields of material science and nanoengineering, biocompatible nanocomposites such as nanoparticles, nanocapsules, and conjugates have been developed for the CNS delivery of biomolecules. On the other hand, there are instances (e.g. treatment of disorders like brain tumors) wherein the delivery of macromolecules in a controlled concentration across the BBB is necessitated. For such cases, nanocomposites could be a promising method when compared to the other methods available. Hence, well-designed nanoparticle systems with sophisticated tools are necessary for treatment of brain tumors and viral and neurodegenerative diseases. In addition, these nanocomposites are labeled as favorable drug delivery carriers due to properties like versatility in formulation, biocompatibility with various cells/tissues in the body, and sustained release capacity (Mahapatro and Singh 2011). Beside polymeric nanoparticles, other carriers like liposomes, dendrimers, carbon nanotubes, and micelles are also evaluated for their role in the delivery of biomolecules to the brain. The effective delivery of camptothecin and paclitaxel by solid lipid nanoparticles to the brain is also reported (Kamboj et al. 2010). Indeed, these nanocarriers have demonstrated their potential to transport into and through the BBB and deliver the therapeutically relevant amount of biomolecules to a specific site and also reduce the problems associated with other invasive techniques. Transport pathways such as receptor-mediated transcytosis as well as adsorptive-mediated transcytosis are used by nanoparticles to cross the BBB and enter the brain. Specific transport mechanisms for nanoparticles are: a) open tight junctions or improved permeabilization of the BBB (either free drug or conjugate with nanoparticles) (Gao et al. 2014; Choi et al. 2010); b) pass through endothelial cells by transcytosis (Wiley et al. 2013); c) first transport through endothelial cells by endocytosis, followed by exocytosis in the

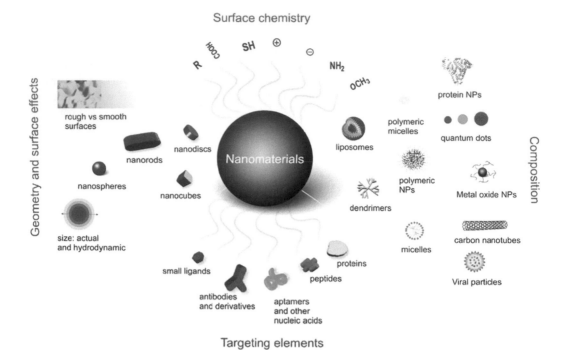

FIGURE 6.3 Various nanoparticles and their biophysiochemical characteristics which affect their perfor-mance both *in vitro* and *in vivo*. (Reprinted from *Chem Soc Rev* 41, Kamaly, N., Xiao, Z., Valencia, P.M., Radovic-Moreno, A.F., and Farokhzad, O.C. Targeted polymeric therapeutic nanoparticles: Design, develop-ment, and clinical translation, 2971–3010, Copyright 2012, Royal Society of Chemistry.)

endothelium abluminal side (Kong et al. 2012); d) increased retention of nanoparticles in capillar-ies with adsorption to capillary walls, which create concentration gradients (Yemişci et al. 2015); e) use of a coating agent to inhibit an efflux system like P-glycoprotein; and f) a combination of several mechanisms. For a transcytosis mechanism, various receptors are targeted by nanocom-posites which includes transferrin receptors (Yemişci et al. 2015) and low-density lipoprotein receptors (Song et al. 2014; Koffie et al. 2011). In general, the targeting is mostly achieved by the physical or chemical modification of nanocomposites prepared using peptides (Song et al. 2014; Zhang et al. 2014), proteins (Koffie et al. 2011), or antibodies (Yemişci et al. 2015).

The choice of transport mechanism across the BBB for nanoparticles is mostly dependent on its physicochemical properties (Grabrucker et al. 2016). There are various factors which are respon-sible for the ability of nanoparticle systemic circulation, BBB transport, and cellular delivery. In many studies, it was observed that there was an opposite relation between nanoparticle size and BBB penetration. Particles in a nanosize range (between 50 nm to 100 nm) were extensively used for the treatment of stroke, Alzheimer's disease, and Parkinson's disease. Similarly, the shapes of nanoparticles also affect brain distribution and cellular uptake. Among spherical, cubic, rod-like, and many other forms, the spherical forms are easy to prepare while nanorods have greater adhesion properties. Nanoparticles with moderate and high positive and negative zeta potentials are able to cross the BBB and show efficient brain delivery (Saraiya et al. 2016). The existence of ligands on the nanoparticles surface, their numbers, and their receptor affinity also affect BBB penetration. For the success of nanoparticulate brain delivery, along with improvements in brain penetration, it is also important to clear nanoparticles slowly from the bloodstream. Hence, for effective clearance, the charge and morphology of nanoparticles are very important. The neutral and zwitterionic nanopar-ticles have a longer circulation time than negative or positive charge nanoparticles. Also, short-rod nanoparticles show a greater clearance rate than their long-rod counterparts because the latter are held in the spleen and have a low clearance rate.

The development of new strategies for the effective delivery of nanoparticles to the brain depends on the interactions between the nanoparticles, the BBB, and their intracellular transport pathways. Many nanomaterials like gold, titanium dioxide, and silica can cross the BBB and accumulate in the brain without any known functionalization. For adsorptive-mediated transcytosis, the mechanism is through functionalization of the nanoparticles surface which causes electrostatic interaction with the luminal surface of the BBB. To promote this electrostatic interaction, usually a positive charge is introduced on the nanoparticles surface which in turn reacts with the negative charged endothelial cells of the brain. In receptor-mediated transcytosis, the normal strategy is to use the specific receptors on luminal cells' surface which can transport macromolecules using transcytosis. Transcytosis in endothelial cells starts with internalization of extracellular macromolecular cargo into the cell by vesicular carriers. The uptake of macromolecules starts either through clathrin-coated pits or caveolae-like membrane domains, etc. The nanoparticles intracellular uptake or transport depends on the particle surface characteristics for a given size. Exploring more and more receptors for receptor dependent endocytosis is providing efficient delivery of nanoparticles to the brain because these mechanisms are devoid of lysosomal degradation. The breaking of the BBB in neuroinflammatory diseases allows nanoparticles to open tight junctions transiently and reversibly and increase their permeability at the BBB and other sites. Beside this, some newer strategies such as infiltration of the monocytes/macrophages in the CNS and nanoparticles mimicking activated monocytes might be effective in brain related disorders.

Drug targeting to an area of interest within the body increases the therapeutic potency, increases safety, and reduces toxicity. Indeed, both passive and active targeting strategies are widely investigated for brain targeting. However, targeting in an active approach requires a specific expression of the target molecule on the cell of interest. The various approaches used in drug targeting to the CNS system include; administration through systemic therapy, injecting through CSF path, and direct administration into the brain. Moreover, there are many advantages which enhance the scope and interest of targeted brain drug delivery and are listed below:

- Increases therapeutic treatment efficacy
- Increases specific localization
- Produces controlled biodistribution
- Decreases toxic side effects
- Reduces dose dependent organ toxicity
- Reduces the problem with bioavailability
- Improves patient compliance

Nanocomposites have received a lot of attention from neuroscientists in the effective treatment of CNS diseases/disorders in recent years, owing to their potential to target various organs/tissues. Thus, nanocomposites are considered as the current research interest in targeted brain drug delivery. Different nanosized carriers have been assessed to target endothelial cells for increasing brain uptake in various disorders (Alzheimer's disease, malignant glioma, stroke, cerebral ischemia, etc.). Indeed, targeting is mainly achieved by conjugating with ligands such as vascular cell adhesion molecule-1 binding peptide, polysorbate 80, anti-transferrin receptor monoclonal antibody, cyclic Arg-Gly-Asp peptide, folate, transferrin, angiopep-2, insulin, choline derivate, dermorphin, etc. (Zhang et al. 2016). It has been established that those ligands with a specific affinity for receptors in the BBB (choline transporter, transferrin receptor, integrin $\alpha v\beta 3$, insulin, etc.) interact with endothelial transporters and help receptor-mediated transcytosis. After crossing the BBB, these nanocarriers are generally taken up through an activated microglia, infiltrating macrophage, or tumor-associated microglia/macrophage through clathrin-mediated endocytosis or phagocytosis. The incorporation of additional targeting ligands in these nanoparticles eventually leads to the specific uptake by neurons (ligands such as ten-eleven translocation methylcytosine dioxygenase 1, rabies virus glycoprotein peptide). Similarly, the targeting of glioma using nanoparticles with a tumor targeting ligand is also reported. A few attempts have also been made to target astrocytes, brain cancer cells, and neurons based on the pathology of a disease following intravenous administration.

Injectable nanocomposites are available for the targeted brain drug delivery for Alzheimer's disease in the form of hydrogel-based gold or silver nanotubes or nanoparticles. Iontophoresis and liquid ion delivery have also been assessed for nanomaterial-based targeted brain delivery (Arruebo et al. 2007; Sun et al. 2016; Liu et al. 2016). Diseases related to the BBB are targeted using nanocomposites through various pathways as well as delivery systems such as drug-loaded nanoparticles, halloysite nanotubes, etc. Halloysite nanotubes are promising nanoparticulate systems due to their unique nanosize, hollow lumen, good biocompatibility, and low cost. These nanocarrier systems have a great potentiality for targeted delivery and a good platform for tumor therapy. The potential of these nanotubes in successfully delivering gamma-aminobutyric acid to the brain in epilepsy-induced rat was demonstrated (Kırımlıoğlu et al. 2015). In addition, glucose is the most transparent and permeable molecule which can easily cross the BBB and, if incorporated with lipid nanotubes, could be the most helpful material for brain drug delivery and targeting.

Drug release from nanocarriers is generally influenced by various factors such as formulation components (polymer, drug, and additives), their concentrations, interaction between the ingredients, method of preparation, etc. Major mechanisms for the drug release from such nanocarriers can be diffusion-controlled release, solvent-controlled release, polymer degraded release, or pH sensitive release (Son et al. 2017). After the successful delivery of biomolecules, its availability and accumulation at the target site is highly essential in the treatment of pathogenesis related brain diseases (Bian-Sheng et al. 2013). However, delivery of more therapeutics than required in the brain causes many difficulties like osmotic imbalances and also affects membrane permeability, and limits or sometimes stops the supply of nutrients. Also, irreversible loosening of tight junctions may result in seizures and eventually compromise brain functions because homeostasis of the brain is disturbed (Secko 2006).

6.7 POLYSACCHARIDES AS A CARRIER FOR DELIVERY OF BIOMOLECULES TO THE CNS

Biomaterials are substances that have applications in therapeutic or diagnostic preparations and generally act together with the components of a living system (Williams 2009). Various synthetic polymers and metals, or even ceramics, are used for such applications because of their reproducible nature and improved performance. However, several limitations have restricted their use and hence natural polymers have been tapped for their potential. The ideal properties of biomaterials used in CNS delivery should be inert and non-interactive with the living systems. Polysaccharides are naturally derived polymers, originating from various plants and organisms. The abundant availability of these polysaccharides makes them an inexhaustible resource for developing carriers to deliver biomolecules. The production cost of these polymers is generally very low and also found to be easily processable. Typically, they are carbohydrate molecules which consist of long chains of monosaccharide units. As they are from natural resources, they possess good biocompatibility, biodegradability, and are non-toxic. Further, their unique structure, special characteristics, and versatile modification properties also make them suitable candidates in other fields. Polysaccharides can be classified based on their structural and storage properties. Dependent on the presence of the monosaccharide unit, polysaccharides again can be classified further as possessing a linear or branched architecture. Along with the structural variability, polysaccharides have many numbers of functional groups, like hydroxyl, amino, and carboxylic acid, which indicate the chances for chemical modification (Zhang et al. 2013), enhanced bioadhesion with biological tissues, and forming non-covalent bonds, which is a useful strategy for improving the bioavailability of drugs (Lee et al. 2000). These unique characteristics and other properties like biodegradability and biocompatibility, solubility, molecular weight variability, ability for alteration, and bioactivity make them ideal for drug delivery systems including CNS delivery.

6.7.1 CHARACTERISTICS OF POLYSACCHARIDES

6.7.1.1 Biodegradability and Biocompatibility

Polysaccharides being natural polymers attained from plants and organisms, are biodegradable and biocompatible in nature (Zhang et al. 2013). For instance, dextrans are biopolymers made of glucose with potential branching at different linkages and they exhibit a low toxicity as well as high biocompatibility. They are also subject to enzymatic degradation which could eventually help in releasing the therapeutic actives (Mehvar 2003).

6.7.1.2 Solubility

The various functional groups present in polysaccharide backbones, like carboxylic acid groups, amine groups, and hydroxyl groups, etc., have greater water solubility. Further, the solubility could be also changed by various approaches to modification of a monomer, etc.

6.7.1.3 Ease of Modification

The majority of polysaccharides are easy to modify. Due to the presence of a large number of free reactive hydroxyl groups, glucose-based polysaccharides such as amylose, amylopectin, and cellulose, etc., they are always ready to modify. In addition, the polysaccharides having both hydroxyl and carboxylic acid moieties can also be freely altered.

6.7.1.4 Bioactivity

Several polysaccharides own inherent bioactivity, mainly mucoadhesive, antimicrobial, and anti-inflammatory properties. Chitosan, one of the most widely explored polysaccharides possesses a positive charge and can easily bind to a negatively charged membrane. Many polysaccharides also have antimicrobial and anti-inflammatory properties. The bactericidal effects of chitosan are based on the reaction between protonated amines with the negatively charged bacterial cell wall. Heparin, another polysaccharide can bind to the lysine-rich region of anti-thrombin and further help in the inhibition of the process of blood clotting.

6.7.2 POLYSACCHARIDE-BASED NANOCOMPOSITES FOR DELIVERY OF BIOMOLECULES TO CNS

Most brain diseases have been associated with inability in the functioning of proteins or enzymes and, therefore, their delivery is one of the current research interests. The surface multifunctionalization properties of nanocomposites make them suitable either for the targeting of the BBB or helping to transport through it. Many of the special features of nanocomposites such as good chemical and biological stability, incorporation of hydrophilic and hydrophobic molecules, ability to administer by various routes (Petkar et al. 2011), and feasibility to conjugate with several ligands (antibodies, proteins, aptamers, etc.) make them attractive for targeting specific tissues. Indeed, the wide surface area of nanoparticles allows numerous copies of a ligand to be attached (Montet et al. 2006). Many applications of polysaccharide nanocomposites are reported including drug delivery and tissue engineering (Zheng et al. 2015).

Polysaccharides have been extensively studied for formulating nanocomposites for delivery of therapeutic actives. Due to their chemical modification ability, these carbohydrate polymers help to fine tune the properties of nanoparticles. In addition, owing to their role as polyelectrolytes and cell surface receptors, these polysaccharides can be used in the design of targeted nanoparticulate delivery systems (Lalatsa and Barbu 2016). Polysaccharide-based formulations used in the delivery of various biomolecules to the CNS are summarized in Table 6.1. Indeed, low affinity for plasma

TABLE 6.1

Polysaccharide Nanocomposites for Delivery of Biomolecules to the Brain

Polysaccharides	Nanocomposite Form	Biomolecules	Effect on Target Cells of Brain	References
Albumin	Nanoparticles	Apolipoprotein E	Enhancing BBB passage *in vivo*	Michaelis et al. 2006; Zensi et al. 2009
Alginate	Nanoparticles	Protein-anti-p15E-immuno-stimulatory proteins	Showed inhibition of tumor cell growth, significant longer survival	Lang et al. 1995
Chitosan	Nanocarriers	Rabies virus glycoprotein	Specific target of peptide to brain	Kim et al. 2013
	Nanoparticles	Caspase inhibitor	Transport across the BBB	Yemişci et al. 2012
	Nanoparticles	Neuropeptides	Successfully delivered growth factors and peptides to brain	Yemişci et al. 2015
	Nanoconjugated particles	Hormone	Effective delivery to neurocompartments	Upadhyay 2014
	Nanoparticles	siRNA	Successful delivery to hippocampus, thalamus, hypothalamus, and Purkinje cells in cerebellum 4 h postnasal delivery	Lalatsa and Barbu 2016
	Nanoparticles	Piperine	Successfully tailored for effective, safe, and non-invasive piperine delivery with 20-folds decrease in oral dose	Elnaggar et al. 2015
Dextran	Nanoparticles	Rhodamine B	Enhanced permeation in brain endothelial cell monolayers	Toman et al. 2015
Glycol chitosan	Nanoparticles	Dopamine	Increased dopamine content in the ipsilateral striatum following intranasal delivery	Di Gioia et al. 2015
Hyaluronic acid	Implant	Polyclonal antibody	Repair the defects and support neural regeneration in the brain	Ma et al. 2007
N-palmitoyl-N-monomethyl-N,N-dimethyl-N,N,N-trimethyl-6-O-glycolchitosan	Nanofibers	Leucine(5)-enkephalin	Enables the peptide to escape liver uptake, avoid enzymatic degradation, prolonged half-life and enhanced brain delivery	Lalatsa et al. 2015

(Continued)

TABLE 6.1 (CONTINUED)

Polysaccharide Nanocomposites for Delivery of Biomolecules to the Brain

Polysaccharides	Nanocomposite Form	Biomolecules	Effect on Target Cells of Brain	References
N-Trimethyl Chitosan	Nanoparticles	Leucine-enkephalin	Permeability of neurotransmitter improved from nasal mucosa; significant improvement in antinociceptive effect	Kumar et al. 2013
Pullulan	Nanogel	Cholesterol	Detection and treatment of Alzheimer's disease	Nazem and Mansoori 2008
Quaternary ammonium palmitoyl glycol chitosan	Nanofibers	Leucineenkephalin	*In vivo* oral and IV administration, increase leucine encephalin levels, and enhanced antinociceptive effects	Lalatsa et al. 2012
Thiolated chitosan	Nanoparticles	Buspirone	The brain concentration achieved after intranasal administration of thiolated chitosan nanoparticles was significantly high	Bari et al. 2015

protein binding as well as fewer uptakes by the mononuclear phagocyte system for polysaccharide-coated nanocomposites makes them the best carriers for intravenous delivery to the brain (Lalatsa et al. 2015). In addition, these carriers generally experience less uptake by the liver, avoid enzyme-based degradation to non-active forms and offer a longer plasma half-life. On the other hand, it is very difficult to deliver proteins or enzymes, due to their delicate nature in the biological environment and the existence of various barriers in the body, including those in circulation (Lalatsa and Barbu 2016). The most widely used polysaccharides in CNS drug delivery are chitosan, alginate, hyaluronic acid, cyclodextrin, pullulan, dextrans, etc.

Chitosan-based formulations are widely assessed to deliver drug molecules to CNS diseases/disorders (Sarvaiya and Agrawal 2015). The cationic charge in chitosan is primarily due to the free amino groups. This polymer exhibits a positive charge in physiological conditions and can easily interact with opposite charged epithelial cells in the BBB. The phenomenal adhesion of chitosan to the endothelial cells in the BBB has been demonstrated following the systemic delivery of nanoparticles prepared using it. Several molecules (amyloid-beta sub-fragments, dopamine, and caspase inhibitors) have been effectively transported to the CNS following parenteral administration of drug-loaded chitosan nanoparticles (Patel et al. 2012). In addition, the potential of uncharged chitosan nanoparticles to modify tight junctions has also been demonstrated. The efficiency of chitosan nanocomposites to deliver estradiol to the CNS was also demonstrated following intranasal application. Moreover, the prospective of PEGylated chitosan nanoparticles to deliver small interfering RNA (siRNA) to the brain segments targeting neurodegenerative diseases following intranasal application has been confirmed (Lalatsa and Barbu 2016). In another attempt, Leucine-enkephalin was effectively delivered through the intranasal route by preparing N-trimethyl chitosan nanoparticles (Kumar et al. 2013). Furthermore, the chitosan nanocomposites are conjugated or surface-modified with specific ligands to provide site specific targeting in the CNS, while overcoming the BBB (Patel et al. 2012). Yemişci et al. (2015) have demonstrated enhanced BBB permeation of chitosan nanoparticles containing peptides by targeting endothelial cells using transferrin (a targeting ligand) following intravenous administration in a mouse model of stroke.

Hyaluronic acid, another polysaccharide, possesses several distinct properties which are ideal for drug delivery. This hydrophilic polymer can easily form hydrogels. A recent study indicates that a cationic liposome-hyaluronic acid hybrid nanocomposite has been evaluated for vaccine delivery via nasal route (Fan et al. 2015). Further, a drug-polymer conjugate prepared using this polymer has been explored for targeting biomolecules in brain tumors, wherein the BBB is partially compromised (Chang et al. 2016).

Alginate-based nanocomposite has also been investigated for their potential for CNS delivery, primarily because of its mucoadhesive characteristics as well as its potential to diminish the drug degradation and improve permeability. In addition, this anionic polysaccharide is combined with chitosan and evaluated for its potential in delivering biomolecules to the CNS. The combined effect of these polymers have demonstrated significant enhancement in the bioavailability of venflaxine when administered intranasally (Haque et al. 2014).

Maltose-based polysaccharide polymer, pullulan, has received a great deal of attention in the treatment of CNS diseases, particularly Alzheimer's. Both nanocomposite and hydrogel formulations have been prepared using pullulan and were widely investigated. In one attempt, pullulan-based nanogel formulation containing cholesterol showed a greater efficiency in a cortical cell culture, which demonstrates its prospects in treating neurological disorders (Nazem and Mansoori 2008).

Dextran is probably one of the most promising polysaccharides with excellent physicochemical properties. Indeed, this polymer is important because of its greater physiological acceptance (Toman et al. 2015). In few instances, dextran was used as a coating agent for polymeric/lipid nanocomposites or as a stabilizer for other formulations aimed at CNS delivery. However, modified dextran-based nanocomposite with rhodamine B showed a greater permeability in brain endothelial cell monolayers (Toman et al. 2015).

Cyclodextrin, produced from starch has also been assessed for delivering biomolecules in CNS disorders. This polysaccharide has the potential to encapsulate pharmaceutical actives of appropriate size in its hydrophobic cavities. Various cyclodextrin derivatives have also been utilized by drug delivery scientists while preparing nanocomposite formulations for the delivery of drugs to the CNS (Godinho et al. 2013).

Cellulose nanocrystals, an alternative drug delivery vector, have also been investigated for their prospective in CNS therapy. Normally, these polysaccharide-based carriers are elongated, possess large surface areas (in a nanosize range), and can be easily surface-modified. Importantly, the presence of a long axial geometry and a greater number of hydroxyl groups on the nanocrystal surface enables the coupling of various moieties for imaging, targeting, and therapeutic agents to the surface. The coupling further makes the nanoparticle surface hydrophilic, which delays its systemic clearance as well as ensures its targeting to the brain. Moreover, they did not show any toxicity in the human brain endothelial cells, while they saw significantly higher uptake in folate receptor-positive rat C6 brain tumor cells (Dong et al. 2014).

Scientific literature also indicates the utility of metal-polysaccharide nanocomposites, metal oxides, and inorganic compound nanocomposites with polysaccharides, structured carbon-polysaccharide nanocomposites, biomolecule-polysaccharide nanocomposites, functional polymer-polysaccharide nanocomposites, and polysaccharide-polysaccharide nanocomposites with different applications (Zheng et al. 2015). Various polysaccharides are also been combined with other polymers to effectively deliver therapeutic actives to the brain and some are listed in Table 6.2. Polysaccharides have also been used to modify the rheology, stability of emulsion, and surface characteristics of nanocomposites.

6.7.3 Methods for Preparation of Polysaccharide Nanocomposites

Various methods are listed in the literature on how to prepare nanocomposites. The most commonly used methods are electrospinning, film casting, dip coating, physically mixing, layer-by-layer assembly, ionotropic gelation, colloidal assembly, co-precipitation, in situ preparation, and covalent coupling. The basic mechanisms involved in these methods are hydrogen-bonding, coulombic interactions, hydrophobic effects, and electrostatic-ionic interactions (Zheng et al. 2015).

6.7.3.1 Electrospinning

In this method, the extrusion process is involved where polymer solution containing dispersed nanomaterial is extruded through a syringe needle under a high voltage field. There are different types of the electrospinning method such as wet-dry electrospinning, wet-wet electrospinning, and co-axial electrospinning, etc. In the wet-dry electrospinning method, the nanocomposite is spun and the volatile solvent evaporates while in the wet-wet electrospinning method, a non-volatile solvent is spun into a second solvent which is collected in a receiver dish which is located between spinneret and collection plate. The newest technology, i.e. the third method, co-axial electrospinning can develop specific fibers (having core-sheath structure) simultaneously from two varieties or different types of components. Room temperature ionic liquids, which are non-volatile, salt-based, organic solvents, with a high thermal stability and broad electrochemical window, are used for certain polysaccharides which are crystalline in nature. Cellulose solutions can be electrospun in ethanol or a water bath to obtain nanofibers using simple wet-wet spinning (Viswanathan et al. 2006). Co-spinning a polysaccharide with a second polysaccharide is also possible.

6.7.3.2 Film Casting, Dip Coating, and Physical Mixing

These methods are widely used to prepare polysaccharide nanocomposites. Polysaccharide multi-walled carbon nanotubes were successfully prepared by the thermal chemical vapor deposition method (Pushparaj et al. 2007). For example, cellulose dissolved in room temperature ionic liquids and then filtered into the multi-walled carbon nanotubes form a thin uniform cast film of

TABLE 6.2

Polysaccharides with Other Polymers for Delivery of Biomolecules to Brain

Polysaccharides	Polymers	Biomolecules	Therapeutic Applications/ Prominent Features	References
Alginate	Polycaprolactone	Neurotropic protein S 100	Composite scaffolds showed progressive human mesenchymal stem cells growth and resulted in higher amount of DNA content	Shelke et al. 2016
Chitosan	Poly(n-butylcyanoacrylate)	Quercetin	Significantly improved oral bioavailability and increased biodistribution in the brain	Bagad and Khan 2015
	Poly- γ-glutamic acid	Hydrophobic drugs	Trehalose as cryoprotectant in formulation and chitosan as permeation enhancer.	Sung and Tu 2011
	Gelatin	Hyaluronic acid and Heparin	Nanocomposite scaffolds were suitable for neural cells' adhesion, survival, and growth and could be used for neural tissue engineering applications	Guan et al. 2013
	Polyethylene Glycol	Hydralazine	Targeted damaged nerves and improved cellular oxidative metabolism	Youngnam et al. 2011
	Polyethylene Glycol	-	Brain uptake of OX26-conjugated nanoparticles was significantly higher than of unmodified nanoparticles	Monsalve et al. 2015
	Polyethylene Glycol Pluronic 127	β-galactosidase	Administration of nanocomposite resulted in greater β-galactosidase activity in the whole brain regions	Kim et al. 2013
	Polyethylene Glycol	Si-RNA	Successful delivery of siRNA to hippocampus, thalamus, hypothalamus, and Purkinje cells in cerebellum 4 h postnasal delivery	Malhotra et al. 2014
	Different lipids	Dyes	The nanostructured lipid carriers demonstrated efficient brain delivery of the particles with no toxicity after intranasal administration	Gartziandia et al. 2015

(Continued)

TABLE 6.2 (CONTINUED)
Polysaccharides with Other Polymers for Delivery of Biomolecules to Brain

Polysaccharides	Polymers	Biomolecules	Therapeutic Applications/ Prominent Features	References
Hyaluronic acid/ Chitosan	Polyethylene Glycol	Curcuminoid and lactoferrin	Nanoparticles could effectively target and accumulate within the gliomas after enhanced permeation through BBB	Xu et al. 2017
N-Trimethyl Chitosan	Polyethylene Glycol	Nucleic acid and Rabies Virus Glycoprotein peptide	Acetylcholine receptor mediated transfection of SiRNA to neuro-2a cells achieved	Tongying et al. 2013
	Poly (lactide co-glycolide)	Quantum dots	Fluorescent nanoparticles administered in animals to detect and characterize lesions within the body	Sung and Tu 2013
Pullulan	Spermine	Gene	Promising method for delivering DNA to brain endothelial cells	Thomsen et al. 2011

cellulose-multi-walled carbon nanotubes which has excellent electrical properties. The cast films of glycerol with pullulan and nanofibrillated cellulose show excellent thermal and mechanical properties (Trovatti et al. 2012). Polysaccharide-based polyelectrolyte complex nanoparticles using chitosan, heparin, and hyaluronic acid can be prepared by dissolving them in an acetate buffer (Boddohi et al. 2009).

6.7.3.3 Layer-By-Layer Assembly

This method involves a layer-by-layer structure and forms polyanions or polycations complexes. For example, the layer-by-layer structure of a polysaccharide film of alginate and chitosan-coated cellulose nanofibers was prepared by electrospinning in presence of layered silicate (Deng et al. 2011).

6.7.3.4 Colloidal Assembly, Ionotropic Gelation, and Co-Precipitation

Colloidal assembly, between polysaccharides and certain synthetic polymers to form ionically stabilized biomimetic nanocomposites has been reported (Wang et al. 2011). Another example is the emulsion solvent diffusion of poly(lactide co-glycolide), heparin, and pluronic gives heparin nanoparticles (Chung et al. 2006). The ionotropic gelation of chitosan nanoparticles have been prepared for the delivery of monoclonal antibodies (Vongchan et al. 2011). The co-precipitation method is used to prepare heparin-coated iron oxide nanoparticles containing the anticancer drugs (Javid et al. 2014).

6.7.3.5 In Situ Nanoparticle Preparation

The synthesis of in situ nanoparticles of calcium carbonate with cellulose fibers can be made by adding a sodium hydroxide solution slowly to calcium chloride and dimethylcarbonate (Vilela et al. 2010). Similarly, the in situ formation of zinc oxide nanoparticles using alginate was also reported (Trandafilovic et al. 2012).

6.7.3.6 Covalent Coupling

Covalent coupling can be carried out through the coupling of bioactive ligands to nanomaterial. In this method, various techniques are used such as: (i) activation chemistry using carbodiimides or dehydrative as coupling reagents; and (ii) ligand activation using isothiocyanates, cyanogen bromide, epoxides, schiff-based chemistry, silanization, and grafting or by co-synthesis (Zheng et al. 2015).

6.8 CONCLUSION

Currently, nanotechnology represents the most innovative, successful, and promising approach for drug transport to the CNS. Various types of nanoparticles having special features and applications can be used for the delivery of different neuroactive compounds like drugs, proteins and peptides, growth factors, genes, and cells to the brain. There are significant advantages of using nanoparticles such as a reduced drug dose, less side effects, greater transport across the BBB, increased drug half-life, site specific targeting, etc. The mechanism of nanoparticle-based molecule transport into the CNS has been shown to be mostly receptor-mediated transcytosis. To reduce the risk associated with the physicochemical dependent toxicity of nanoparticles, biodegradable biomaterials should be ideal for brain drug delivery. Polysaccharides acquired from nature are the ideal candidates for this challenge owing to their unique characteristics and structural advantages. The prospective of polysaccharide-based nanoparticles in delivering biomolecules across the BBB, by an active as well as passive approach, has been demonstrated by several researchers. Some preclinical studies have also demonstrated that chitosan-mediated nanoparticles can achieve an effective therapeutic level for many drugs, proteins, peptides, and genetic materials in the brain. Beside chitosan, the other polysaccharides like dextran, pullulan, cellulose nanocrystals, etc., have the potential for overcoming the BBB and can be used in emerging technologies. Unfortunately, no clinical trials are reported for drug delivery using polysaccharide nanocomposites to target the CNS. In this perspective, it is important to assess the prospect of the clinical translation of potentially validated preclinical data to meet the demands of the growing prevalence of neurological disorders.

REFERENCES

Abbott, N.J. 2004. Evidence for bulk flow of brain interstitial fluid: Significance for physiology and pathology. *Neurochem Int* 45: 545–52.

Abbott, N.J. 2013. Blood–brain barrier structure and function and the challenges for CNS drug delivery. *J Inherit Metab Dis* 36: 437–49.

Al-Dhubiab, B.E., Nair, A.B., Kumria, R., Attimarad, M., and Harsha, S. 2015. Formulation and evaluation of nano based drug delivery system for the buccal delivery of acyclovir. *Colloids Surf B Biointerfaces* 136: 878–84.

Al-Dhubiab, B.E., Nair, A.B., Kumria, R., Attimarad, M., and Harsha, S. 2016. Development and evaluation of buccal films impregnated with selegiline-loaded nanospheres. *Drug Deliv* 23: 2154–62.

Arruebo, M., Fernandez-Pacheco, R., Ibarra, M.R., and Santamaria, J. 2007. Magnetic nanoparticles for drug delivery. *Nano Today* 2: 22–32.

Bagad, M. and Khan, Z.A. 2015. Poly (n-butylcyanoacrylate) nanoparticles for oral delivery of quercetin: Preparation, characterization, and pharmacokinetics and biodistribution studies in Wistar rats. *Int J Nanomedicine* 10: 3921–35.

Banks, W.A. 1999. Physiology and pathology of the blood-brain barrier: Implications for microbial pathogenesis, drug delivery and neurodegenerative disorders. *J Neurovirol* 5: 538–55.

Bari, N.K., Fazil, M., Hassan, M.Q., Haider, M.R., Gaba, B., Narang, J.K., Baboota, S., and Ali, J. 2015. Brain delivery of buspirone hydrochloride chitosan nanoparticles for the treatment of general anxiety disorder. *Int J Biol Macromol* 81: 49–59.

Bian-Sheng, J., Cen, J., Liu, L., and He L. 2013. *In vitro* and *in vivo* study of dodichyl phosphate on the efflux of P-glycoprotein at the blood brain barrier. *Int J Dev Neurosci* 31: 828–35.

Boddohi, S., Moore, N., Johnson, P.A., and Kipper, M.J. 2009. Polysaccharidebased polyelectrolyte complex nanoparticles from chitosan, heparin, and hyaluronan. *Biomacromolecules* 10: 1402–9.

Borlongan, C.V. and Emerich, D.F. 2003. Facilitation of drug entry into the CNS via transient permeation of blood–brain barrier: Laboratory and preliminary clinical evidence from bradykinin receptor agonist. *Brain Res Bull* 60: 297–306.

Chang, M., Zhang, F., Wei, T. et al. 2016. Smart linkers in polymer–drug conjugates for tumor-targeted delivery. *J Drug Target* 24: 475–91.

Choi, C.H.J., Alabi, C.A., Webster, P., and Davis, M.E. 2010. Mechanism of active targeting in solid tumors with transferrin-containing gold nanoparticles. *Proc Natl Acad Sci U S A* 107: 1235–40.

Chung, Y., Tae, G., and Yuk, S.H. 2006. A facile method to prepare heparin-functionalized nanoparticles for controlled release of growth factors. *Biomaterials* 27: 2621–26.

De Boer, A.G. and Gaillard, P.J. 2007. Drug targeting to the brain. *Annu Rev Pharmacol Toxicol* 47: 323–55.

de Lange, E.C., Ravenstijn, P.G., Groenendaal, D., and van Steeg, T.J. 2005. Toward the prediction of CNS drug-effect profiles in physiological and pathological conditions using microdialysis and mechanism-based pharmacokinetic-pharmacodynamic modeling. *AAPS J* 7: E532–E543.

Deng, H., Wang, X., Liu, P. et al. 2011. Enhanced bacterial inhibition activity of layer-by-layer structured polysaccharide film-coated cellulose nanofibrous mats via addition of layered silicate. *Carbohydr Polym* 83: 239–45.

Di Gioia, S., Trapani, A., Mandracchia, D. et al. 2015. Intranasal delivery of dopamine to the striatum using glycol chitosan/sulfobutylether-β-cyclodextrin based nanoparticles. *Eur J Pharm Biopharm* 94: 180–93

Dickson, D.W. 1995. Apoptosis in the brain. Physiology and pathology. *Am J Pathol* 146: 1040–4.

Dong, S., Cho, H.J., Lee, Y.W., and Roman, M. 2014. Synthesis and cellular uptake of folic acid-conjugated cellulose nanocrystals for cancer targeting. *Biomacromolecules* 15: 1560–7.

Elnaggar, Y.S., Etman, S.M., Abdelmonsif, D.A., and Abdallah, O.Y. 2015. Intranasal piperine-loaded chitosan nanoparticles as brain-targeted therapy in Alzheimer's disease: Optimization, biological efficacy, and potential toxicity. *J Pharm Sci* 104: 3544–56.

Fan, Y., Sahdev, P., Ochyl, L.J., Akerberg, J.J., and Moon, J.J. 2015. Cationic liposome-hyaluronic acid hybrid nanoparticles for intranasal vaccination with subunit antigens. J *Control Release* 208: 121–9.

Fortin, D., Gendron, C., Boudrias, M., and Garant, M.P. 2007. Enhanced chemotherapy delivery by intraarterial infusion and blood–brain barrier disruption in the treatment of cerebral metastasis. *Cancer* 109: 751–60.

Gabathuler, R. 2010. Approaches to transport therapeutic drugs across the blood-brain barrier to treat brain disease. *Neurobiol Dis* 37: 48–57.

Gao, X., Qian, J., Zheng, S. et al. 2014. Overcoming the blood– brain barrier for delivering drugs into the brain by using adenosine receptor nanoagonist. *ACS Nano* 8: 3678–89.

Gartziandia, O., Herran, E., Pedraz, J.L., Carro, E., Igartua, M., and Hernandez, R.M. 2015. Chitosan coated nanostructured lipid carriers for brain delivery of proteins by intranasal administration. *Colloids Surf B Biointerfaces* 134: 304–13.

Godinho, B.M., Ogier, J.R., Darcy, R., O'Driscoll, C.M., and Cryan, J.F. 2013. Self-assembling modified β-cyclodextrin nanoparticles as neuronal siRNA delivery vectors: Focus on Huntington's disease. *Mol Pharm* 10: 640–9.

Grabrucker, A.M., Ruozi, B., Belletti, D. et al. 2016. Nanoparticle transport across the blood brain barrier. *Tissue Barriers* 4: e1153568.

Guan, S., Zhang, X.L., Lin, X.M., Liu, T.Q., Ma, X.H., and Cui, Z.F. 2013. Chitosan/gelatin porous scaffolds containing hyaluronic acid and heparan sulfate for neural tissue engineering. *J Biomater Sci Polym Ed* 24: 999–1014.

Gynther, M., Laine, K., Ropponen, J. et al. 2008. Large neutral amino acid transporter enables brain drug delivery via prodrugs. *J Med Chem* 51: 932–36.

Haque, S., Md, S., Sahni, J.K., Ali, J., and Baboota, S. 2014. Development and evaluation of brain targeted intranasal alginate nanoparticles for treatment of depression. *J Psychiatr Res* 48: 1–12.

Javid, A., Ahmadian, S., Saboury, A.A., Kalantar, S.M., and Rezaei-Zarchi, S. 2014. Novel biodegradable heparin-coated nanocomposite system for targeted drug delivery. *RSC Adv* 4: 13719–28.

Jones, A.R. and Shusta, E.V. 2007. Blood-brain barrier transport of therapeutics via receptor-mediation. *Pharm Res* 24: 1759–71.

Kamaly, N., Xiao, Z., Valencia, P.M., Radovic-Moreno, A.F., and Farokhzad, O.C. 2012. Targeted polymeric therapeutic nanoparticles: Design, development and clinical translation. *Chem Soc Rev* 41: 2971–3010.

Kamboj, S., Bala, S., and Nair, A.B. 2010. Solid lipid nanoparticles: An effective lipid based technology for poorly water soluble drugs. *Intl J Pharm Sci Rev Res* 5: 78–90.

Kasinathan, N., Jagani, H.V., Alex, A.T., Volety, S.M., and Rao, J.V. 2015. Strategies for drug delivery to the central nervous system by systemic route. *Drug Deliv* 22: 243–57.

Kim, J.Y., Choi, W.I., Kim, Y.H., and Tae, G. 2013. Brain targeted delivery of protein using chitosan- and RVG peptide conjugated, pluronic-based nano-carrier. *Biomaterials* 34: 1170–9.

Kinoshita, M. 2006. Targeted drug delivery to the brain using focused ultrasound. *Top Magn Reson Imaging* 17: 209–15.

Kinoshita, M., McDannold, N., Jolesz, F.A., and Hynynen, K. 2006. Targeted delivery of antibodies through the blood–brain barrier by MRI-guided focused ultrasound. *Biochem Biophys Res Commun* 340: 1085–90.

Kırımlıoğlu, G.Y., Yazan, Y., Erol, K., and Ünel, Ç.Ç. 2015. Gamma-aminobutyric acid loaded halloysite nanotubes and in vitro-in vivo evaluation for brain delivery. *Int J Pharm* 495: 816–26.

Koffie, R.M., Farrar, C.T., Saidi, L.-J., William, C.M., Hyman, B.T., and Spires-Jones, T.L. 2011. Nanoparticles enhance brain delivery of blood–brain barrier-impermeable probes for *in vivo* optical and magnetic resonance imaging. *Proc Natl Acad Sci USA* 108: 18837–42.

Kong, S.D., Lee, J., Ramachandran S. et al. 2012. Magnetic targeting of nanoparticles across the intact blood–brain barrier. *J Control Release* 164: 49–57.

Kumar, M., Pandey, R.S., Patra, K.C. et al. 2013. Evaluation of neuropeptide loaded trimethyl chitosan nanoparticles for nose to brain delivery. *Int J Biol Macromol* 61: 189–95.

Lalatsa, A. and Barbu, E. 2016. Carbohydrates nanoparticles for brain delivery. *Int Rev Neurobiol* 130: 115–53.

Lalatsa, A., Lee, V., Malkinson, J.P., Zloh, M., Schätzlein, A.G., and Uchegbu, I.F. 2012. A prodrug nanoparticle approach for the oral delivery of a hydrophilic peptide, leucine5-enkephalin, to the brain. *Mol Pharm* 9: 1665–80.

Lalatsa, A., Schatzlein, A.G., Garrett, N.L. et al. 2015. Chitosan amphiphile coating of peptide nanofibres reduces liver uptake and delivers the peptide to the brain on intravenous administration. *J Control Release* 197: 87–96.

Lang, M.S., Hovenkamp, E., Savelkoul, H.F.J., Knegt, P., and Ewijk, W.V. 1995. Immunotherapy with monoclonal antibodies directed against the immunosuppressive domain of p15E inhibits tumour growth. *Clin Exp Immunol* 102: 468–75.

Lee, J.W., Park, J.H., and Robinson, J.R. 2000. Bioadhesive-based dosage forms: the next generation. *J Pharm Sci* 89: 850–66.

Lipinski, C.A., Lombardo, F., Dominy, B.W., and Feeney, P.J. 2001. Experimental and computational approaches to estimate solubility and permeability in drug discovery and development settings. *Adv Drug Deliv Rev* 46: 3–26.

Liu, J., Luo, Z., Zhang, J. et al. 2016. Hollow mesoporous silica nanoparticles facilitated drug delivery via cascade pH stimuli in tumor microenvironment for tumor therapy. *Biomaterials* 83: 51–65.

Lo, E.H., Singhal, A.B., Torchilin, V.P., and Abbott, N.J. 2001. Drug delivery to damaged brain. *Brain Res Rev* 38: 140–8.

Ma, J., Tian, W.M., Hou, S.P. et al. 2007. An experimental test of stroke recovery by implanting a hyaluronic acid hydrogel carrying a Nogo receptor antibody in a rat model. *Biomed Mater* 2 (4): 233–40.

Mahapatro, A. and Singh, D.K. 2011. Biodegradable nanoparticles are excellent vehicle for site directed invivo delivery of drugs and vaccines. *J Nanobiotechnology* 9: 55.

Malhotra, M., Tomaro-Duchesneau, C., Saha, S., and Prakash, S. 2014. Intranasal delivery of chitosan–siRNA nanoparticle formulation to the brain. *Methods Mol Biol* 1141: 233–47.

Mehvar, R. 2003. Recent trends in the use of polysaccharides for improved delivery of therapeutic agents: Pharmacokinetic and pharmacodynamic perspectives. *Curr Pharm Biotechnol* 4: 283–302.

Meldrum, B.S. 2000. Glutamate as a neurotransmitter in the brain: Review of physiology and pathology. *J Nutr* 130 (4S Suppl): 1007S–15S.

Michaelis, K., Hoffmann, M.M., Dreis, S. et al. 2006. Covalent linkage of apolipoprotein E to albumin nanoparticles strongly enhances drug transport into the brain. *J Pharmacol Exp Ther* 317: 1246–53.

Misra, A., Ganesh, S., Shahiwala, A., and Shah, S.P. 2003. Drug delivery to the central nervous system: A review. *J Pharm Sci* 6 (2): 252–73.

Monsalve, Y., Tosi, G., Ruozi, B. et al. 2015. PEG-g-chitosan nanoparticles functionalized with the monoclonal antibody OX26 for brain drug targeting. *Nanomedicine (Lond)* 10: 1735–50.

Montet, X., Funovics, M., Montet-Abou, K., Weissleder, R., and Josephson, L. 2006. Multivalent effects of RGD peptides obtained by nanoparticle display. *J Med Chem* 49: 6087–93.

Nazem, A. and Mansoori, G.A. 2008. Nanotechnology solutions for Alzheimer's disease: Advances in research tools, diagnostic methods and therapeutic agents. *J Alzheimers Dis* 13: 199–223.

Neuwelt, E., Abbott, N.J., Abrey, L. et al. 2008. Strategies to advance translational research into brain barriers. *Lancet Neurol* 7: 84–96.

Pardridge, W.M. 2005. The blood–brain barrier: bottleneck in brain drug development. *NeuroRx* 2: 3–14.

Pardridge, W.M. 2007a. Blood–brain barrier delivery. *Drug Discov Today* 12: 54–61.

Pardridge, W.M. 2007b. Drug targeting to the brain. *Pharm Res* 24: 1733–44.

Putel, T., Zhou, J., Plepmeier, J.M., and Saltzman, W.M. 2012. Polymeric nanoparticles for drug delivery to the central nervous system. *Adv Drug Deliv Rev* 64: 701–5.

Petkar, K.C., Chavhan, S.S., Agatonovik-Kustrin, S., and Sawant, K.K. 2011. Nanostructured materials in drug and gene delivery: A review of the state of the art. *Crit Rev Ther Drug Carrier Syst* 28: 101–64.

Pushparaj, V.L., Shaijumon, M.M., Kumar, A. et al. 2007. Flexile energy storage devices based on nanocomposite paper. *Proc Natl Acad Sci U S A* 104: 13574–7.

Rautio, J., Laine, K., Gynther, M., and Savolainen, J. 2008. Prodrug approaches for CNS delivery. *AAPS J* 10: 92–102.

Rustenhoven, J., Jansson, D., Smyth, L.C., and Dragunow, M., 2017. Brain pericytes as mediators of neuroinflammation. *Trends Pharmacol Sci* 38: 291–304.

Saraiva C, Praça C, Ferreira R, Santos T, Ferreira L, and Bernardino L. 2016. Nanoparticle-mediated brain drug delivery: Overcoming blood-brain barrier to treat neurodegenerative diseases. *J Control Release* 235: 34–47.

Sarvaiya, J. and Agrawal, Y.K. 2015. Chitosan as a suitable nanocarrier material for anti-Alzheimer drug delivery. *Int J Biol Macromol* 72: 454–65.

Secko, D. 2006. Breaking down the blood–brain barrier. *CMAJ* 174: 448.

Senel, S., Kremer, M., Nagy, K., and Squier, C. 2001. Delivery of bioactive peptides and proteins across oral (Buccal) mucosa. *Curr Pharm Biotechnol* 2 (2): 175–86.

Shelke, N.B., Lee, P., Anderson, M., Mistry, N., Nagarale, R.K., Ma, X.M., Yu, X., and Kumbar, S.G. 2016. Neural tissue engineering: nanofiber-hydrogel based composite scaffolds. *Polym Adv Technol* 27(1): 42–51.

Shingaki, T., Inoue, D., Furubayashi, T. et al. 2010. Transnasal delivery of methotrexate to brain tumors in rats: A new strategy for brain tumor chemotherapy. *Mol Pharm* 7: 1561–8.

Son, G.H., Lee, B.J., and Cho, C.W. 2017. Mechanisms of drug release from advanced drug formulations such as polymeric-based drug-delivery systems and lipid nanoparticles. *J Pharm Invest* 47: 287–96.

Song, Q., Huang, M., Yao, L. et al. 2014. Lipoprotein-based nanoparticles rescue the memory loss of mice with Alzheimer's disease by accelerating the clearance of amyloid-beta. *ACS Nano* 8: 2345–59.

Sun, Z., Worden, M., Thliveris, J.A. et al. 2016. Biodistribution of negatively charged iron oxide nanoparticles (IONPs) in mice and enhanced brain delivery using lysophosphatidic acid (LPA). *Nanomedicine* 12: 1775–84.

Sung, H.W. and Tu, H. 2011. Nanoparticles for protein drug delivery. *US Patent* 7,910,086.

Sung, H.W. and Tu, H. 2013. Pharmaceutical composition of nanoparticles. *US Patent* 8,449,915.

Thomsen, L.B., Lichota, J., Kim, K.S., and Moos, T. 2011. Gene delivery by pullulan derivatives in brain capillary endothelial cells for protein secretion. *J Control Release* 151: 45–50.

Toman, P., Lien, C.F., Ahmad, Z. et al. 2015. Nanoparticles of alkylglyceryl-dextran-graft-poly(lactic acid) for drug delivery to the brain: Preparation and in vitro investigation. *Acta Biomater* 23: 250–62.

Tongying, J., Siling, W., and Kun, G.Y. 2013. Trimethyl chitosan-graft-polyethylene glycol/nucleic acid brain-targeting micellar and preparation method thereof. Chinese Patent 103182087 A.

Trandafilovic, L.V., Bozanic, D.K., Dimitrijevic-Brankovic, S., Luyt, A.S., and Djokovic, V. 2012. Fabrication and antibacterial properties of ZnO–alginate nanocomposites. *Carbohydr Polym* 88: 263–9.

Trovatti, E., Fernandes, S.C.M., Rubatat, L. et al. 2012. Pullulan–nanofibrillated cellulose composite films with improved thermal and mechanical properties. *Compos Sci Technol* 72: 1556–61.

Upadhyay, R.K. 2014. Drug delivery systems, CNS protection, and the blood brain barrier. *Biomed Res Int* 2014: 869269.

Vandergrift, W.A., Patel, S.J., Nicholas, J.S., and Verma, A.K. 2006. Convection-enhanced delivery of immunotoxins and radioisotopes for treatment of malignant gliomas. *Neurosurg Focus* 20: E13.

Vilela, C., Freire, C.S., Marques, P.A., Trindade, T., Neto, C.P., and Fardim, P. 2010. Synthesis and characterization of new CaCO3/cellulose nanocomposites prepared by controlled hydrolysis of dimethylcarbonate. *Carbohydr Polym* 79: 1150–6.

Viswanathan, G., Murugesan, S., Pushparaj, V., Nalamasu, O., Ajayan, P.M., and Linhardt, R.J. 2006. Preparation of biopolymer fibers by electrospinning from room temperature ionic liquids. *Biomacromolecules* 7 (2): 415–8.

Vongchan, P., Wutti-In, Y., Sajomsang, W., Gonil, P., Kothan, S., and Linhardt, R.J. 2011. N, N, N-Trimethyl chitosan nanoparticles for the delivery of monoclonal antibodies against hepatocellular carcinoma cells. *Carbohydr Polym* 85: 215–20.

Wang, M., Olszewska, A., Walther, A. et al. 2011. Colloidal ionic assembly between anionic native cellulose nanofibrils and cationic block copolymer micelles into biomimetic nanocomposites. *Biomacromolecules* 12: 2074–81.

Wiley, D.T., Webster, P., Gale, A., and Davis, M.E. 2013. Transcytosis and brain uptake of transferrin-containing nanoparticles by tuning avidity to transferrin receptor. *Proc Natl Acad Sci U S A* 110: 8662–67.

Williams, D.F. 2009. On the nature of biomaterials. *Biomaterials* 30: 5897–909.

Xu, Y., Asghar, S., Yang, L., Li, H., Wang, Z., Ping, Q., and Xiao, Y. 2017. Lactoferrin-coated polysaccharide nanoparticles based on chitosan hydrochloride/hyaluronic acid/PEG for treating brain glioma. *Carbohydr Polym* 157: 419–28.

Yemişci, M., Caban, S., Gürsoy-Özdemir, Y. et al. 2015. Systemically administered brain-targeted nanoparticles transport peptides across the blood–brain barrier and provide neuroprotection. *J Cereb Blood Flow Metab* 35: 469–75.

Yemişci, M., Gürsoy-Özdemir, Y., Caban, S., Bodur, E., Capan, Y., and Dalkara, T. 2012. Transport of a caspase inhibitor across the blood–brain barrier by chitosan nanoparticles. *Methods Enzymol* 508: 253–69.

Youngnam, C.H.O., Shi, R., Ivanslevic, A., and Borgens, R. 2011. Repairing damaged nervous system tissue with nanoparticles. *US Patent Application* 12/863: 357.

Zensi, A., Begley, D., Pontikis, C. et al. 2009. Albumin nanoparticles targeted with Apo E enter the CNS by transcytosis and are delivered to neurons. *J Control Release* 137: 78–86.

Zhang F, Lin Y-, Kannan S, and Kannan RM. 2016. Targeting specific cells in the brain with nanomedicines for CNS therapies. *J Control Release* 240: 212–26.

Zhang, C., Wan, X., Zheng, X. et al. 2014. Dual-functional nanoparticles targeting amyloid plaques in the brains of Alzheimer's disease mice. *Biomaterials* 35: 456–65.

Zhang, N., Wardwell, P.R., and Bader, R.A. 2013. Polysaccharide-based micelles for drug delivery. *Pharmaceutics* 5: 329–52.

Zheng, Y., Monty, J., and Linhardt, R.J. 2015. Polysaccharide-based nanocomposites and their applications. *Carbohydr Res* 405: 23–32.

7 Polysaccharide-Based Nanoparticles for the Enhanced Delivery of Poorly Soluble Drugs

Prithviraj Chakraborty, Urmi Chaurasia, Debarupa Dutta Chakraborty, and Indranil Chanda

CONTENTS

7.1 INTRODUCTION

One of the most common and preferred routes of administration for the delivery of drugs is through the oral route as it is simple, convenient, and acceptable to patients, particularly in chronic therapies requiring a repeated dosage (Sant et al. 2005). Oral products cover 60% of marketed drugs (Masaoka et al. 2006). However, formulation of a therapeutic agent for administration through the oral route is not an easy task. The two most important parameters viz. solubility and permeability govern the bioavailability of oral drugs. On the basis of these parameters, the biopharmaceutic classification system (BCS) classifies the drugs into four categories. Therapeutic entities, existing and new, fall into either BCS class II (low solubility and high permeability) or BCS class IV (low solubility and low permeability).

In the drugs discovered, candidates possessing poor water solubility have the problems of poor and variable bioavailability associated with them. It is projected that about 70% of new chemical entities show poor aqueous solubility while many are poorly soluble in an organic medium. About 40% of immediate-release drugs for oral administration, available on the market, are practically insoluble (solubility less than 100 µg/mL) in water (Wei et al. 2013). Low solubility causes limitations in the rate at which the drug dissolves and this often results in the decreased bioavailability of the oral drug. Dose escalation studies of the drug have often been carried out to achieve the required therapeutic concentration in the target sites (Monjazeb et al. 2012). However, this may result in increased toxicity leading to decreased patient compliance, and therefore it is undesirable. Also, the high drug load of pharmaceutical products often causes difficulties in completion of the study.

Some of the possible strategies that have been used to bring about an increase in the bioavailability of poorly soluble drugs are solid dispersions, ionized salts addition, micronization, and soft gel technology. However, these techniques have some inherent limitations associated with them, such as drug-load capacity, toxicity, biodegradability, large dosages, and environmental considerations. In recent years, nanotechnology has arisen as a promising field to address these issues.

This branch of nanotechnology involves the preparation of nanoscale materials with dimensions ranging from 1–100 nm because due to their minute size these materials show unique properties. Nanomaterials were earlier made up of "hard" materials like metals and carbon-only nanostructures, such as carbon nanotubes (CNTs) or buckyballs but currently "soft" nanomaterials, which is made up of synthetic polymers and biopolymers, are gaining importance so as to avoid nano toxicity and environmental issues (Zheng et al. 2015).

Nanoparticles, which have well-defined size distributions, possess the potential to release large fractions of their drug-load into the small intestine in the first few hours, maybe due to their large surface area. A number of polymeric materials that have been used for this purpose are poly(lactic acid), poly(glycolic acid), polycaprolactone, polysaccharides, the poly(acrylic acid) family, proteins, and polypeptides (e.g., gelatin).

Since matter in a nano-state exhibits unique properties, understanding these new properties will pave the way for new avenues of exploration. Therefore, nanotechnology has been of great scientific interest and much research has been carried out since the middle of the 20th century, with still so much remaining to be discovered (Tibbals 2010). Nanotechnology has found application in various areas of technology and has been found to have a large prospective in the field of medicine, and this concept has taken the shape of nanomedicine. The National Institute of Health refers to nanomedicine as the applications of nanotechnology for treatment, diagnosis, monitoring, and control of biological systems (Moghimi et al. 2005).

7.2 A BRIEF ABOUT NANOTECHNOLOGY

Nanomedicine has been defined in many ways in literature, however, in simple terms, it can be referred to as "applying nanotechnology to medicine".

In contrast with other therapies, nanomedicine uses sophisticated approaches that result in either killing specific cells or repairing them one cell at a time. This approach also offers possibilities toward developing personalized medicine (Gurwitz and Livshits 2005).

The primary aim and focus of nanomedicine is on the treatment of certain diseases such as non-infectious diseases, especially cancer, and on degenerative diseases in order to characterize them in the increasingly sedentary and aging populations of the wealthiest countries that lead medical research (Martinez et al. 2012). Nanoparticles are the most essential and promising tools employed in nanomedicine for medical applications. They are solid, colloidal particles consisting of macro molecular substances that vary in size from 10 nm to 1000 nm. Particles >200 nm are not of much use in nanomedicine, which often employs devices <200 nm (i.e., the width of micro capillaries). Nanospheres or nanocapsules can be prepared by employing different techniques and methods, which are selected so as to give different properties and release characteristics to increase the delivery or encapsulation of the therapeutic agent (Martinez et al. 2012). One of the advantages of nanovector nanoparticles is their knack for overcoming various biological barriers and to localize to the target tissue. The nanovectors that are presently used and explored may be classified into three major groups or "generations" (Sakamoto et al. 2007). First generation nanovectors get localized in the target site and comprise of a passive delivery system. In the case of a tumor, the system passes through the fenestrations in the adjacent neovasculature and reaches the tumor. The circulation time is substantially prolonged as it is normally decorated by a "stealth" layer in order to avoid uptake by the phagocytic blood cells. Particle size is the main driving force to target the tumor site, but not the specific recognition of the tumor or neovascular targets. For example, particles based on albumin-paclitaxel which have been approved by the FDA recently for their use in metastatic breast cancer (Kratz 2008). Second generation nanosystems include additional functionalities that allow for molecular recognition of the target tissue or for active or triggered release of the payload at the disease site. These include ligands, aptamers, and small peptides that bind to specific target-cell surface markers or surface markers expressed in the disease microenvironment (Kang et al. 2008). Responsive systems, like the pH-sensitive polymers, are included in this category. The FDA has not yet approved the second generation nanosystems, however, there are numerous ongoing clinical trials which involve targeted nanovectors, particularly in cancer applications. Third-generation nanovectors focus on successfully overcoming the natural barriers that the vector needs to bypass to efficiently deliver the drug to the target site. This goal will only be reached by a "multistage" approach, and such a system has only recently been reported (Martinez et al. 2012).

Nanotechnology has emerged as a promising field for addressing the issues relating to drug-load capacity, toxicity, biodegradability, large dosages, and environmental considerations. Many polymeric materials have been used, and among these polysaccharides are recently the most popular nanoparticle material for drug delivery.

7.2.1 Reasons for the Solubility Increments in Nanoparticles

An increase within the exposed surface area (or surface area-to-volume ratio) via particle size reduction causes a rise in the dissolution rate and influences oral bioavailability (Jog and Burgess 2016). Additionally, in keeping with the Kelvin equation, the saturation solubility (in terms of vapor pressure) of the drug relies on the drug particle size (which interprets the curvature effect). In theory, reduction in particle size can cause a rise in drug solubility. However, the particular increase in saturation solubility for "nanocrystalline suspensions" (colloidal sizes vary between 100 and 1000 nm) is marginal, around 2%–10% compared to unmilled particles. Thus, nanosized crystalline powders might not be a helpful approach for solubility-limited drugs (i.e., solubility is rate limiting for oral bioavailability). In the case of amorphous formulations, the solubility of the drug is higher than that of the crystalline form as a result of its high energy (higher Gibbs' free energy). Instead, amorphous formulations are unstable and can transform into stable crystalline form over pharmaceutically pertinent timescales.

The major formulation challenge related to amorphous nanoparticles is their stability, which depends on their active pharmaceutical ingredient (API) properties such as melting temperature (T_m), T_m/T_g ratio, and consequently, the properties of the polymer or stabilizer is exploited. Mostly, there are two basic strategies for manufacturing nanoparticles: (1) a "top-down approach" (i.e., milling/grinding of the particles to realize the desired size) and (2) a "bottom-up approach" (i.e., precipitation of the drug from a solvent system).

Although the bottom-up approach is less time consuming, which frequently results in amorphous particles, the quick evaporation of the solvent in the process results in precipitation of the API as amorphous particles. The mechanism by which nanoparticles improve the dissolution rate and bioavailability of poorly soluble APIs (BCS category II and II/IV) is the increased extent of surface-to-volume ratio as delineated by the Noyes-Whitney equation. Using the Noyes-Whitney equation, dissolution rate J is given in the subsequent equation as (7.1).

$$J = \frac{DA}{h}\left(C_S - C\right) \tag{7.1}$$

where:

J is the dissolution rate
D the diffusion coefficient of drug
A the extent of the dissolving solid
h the thickness of the diffusion layer
Cs the saturation solubility of the compound within the dissolution medium
C the concentration of the drug within the medium at different time points throughout dissolution.

Increases within the surface-to-volume ratio, and therefore the dissolution rate of nanoparticles, improves their pharmacokinetic properties in terms of accumulation rates and the extent of release and absorption, fast onset of action, reduced side effects, and improved clinical performance.

7.3 POLYSACCHARIDES

Polysaccharides are complex carbohydrate polymers which consist of more than two monosaccharides that are linked together covalently by glycosidic linkages in a condensation reaction. Cellulose is the most abundant polysaccharide found in nature. It is a linear polymer consisting of 6-member ether rings (D-glucose or dextrose) linked together covalently by ether groups, the so-called glycosidic bonds. The cellulose polymer is usually made up of many thousand repeat glucose units. Cellulose derivatives are chosen as they are open to chemical modification and are also biologically compatible, and their derivatives like carboxymethyl cellulose acetate butyrate, N-trimethyl chitosan (TMC) have been shown to improve the amount of drug solubilized (Mazumder et al. 2017).

7.3.1 SOME NATURALLY OCCURRING POLYSACCHARIDES

7.3.1.1 Chitosan

Chitosan is the generic name for a group of strongly polycationic subsidiaries of poly-N-acetyl-D-glucosamine (chitin). It is present inside the exoskeletons of shellfish like crabs, shrimps and microorganisms (Tombs and Harding 1998; Mao et al. 2010). The N-acetyl aggregate in chitosan (Figure 7.1) is either absolutely or mostly replaced by NH causing the level of acetylation to fluctuate from DA = 0 (completely deacetylated) to DA = 1 (completely acetylated, i.e., chitin). Acetylated monomers (GlcNAc; A-unit) and deacetylated monomers (GlcN; D-unit) are considered to be distributed randomly or blockwise (Varum et al. 1991a,b, 1994)

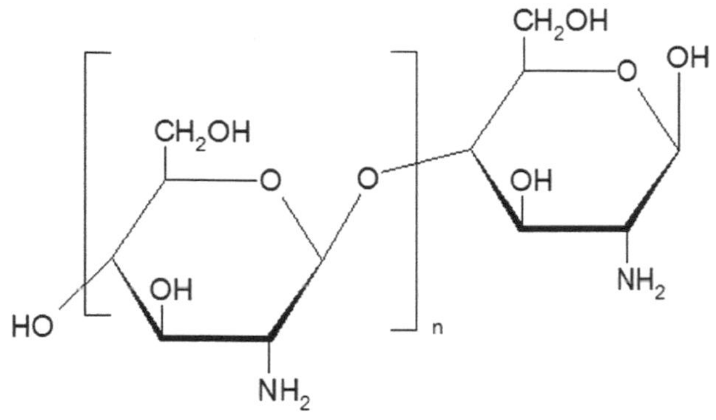

FIGURE 7.1 Chemical structure of chitosan.

Chitosan is biodegradable, non-dangerous, non-immunogenic, and biocompatible (Terbojevich and Muzzarelli 2000; Muzzarelli 2009), and the normally occurring polycationic polymer chitosan and its subordinates have applications in the food, cosmetic, and pharmaceutical industries. Essential applications incorporate water and waste treatment, antitumor, antibacterial, and anticoagulant properties (Muzzarelli 2009; Illum 1998). Being a semicrystalline polymer, it displays a level of polymorphism. In an aqueous acidic condition, it is quickly solubilized, because of the acetyl moieties being removed in the amine functional group. However, its solubility is restricted to inorganic acids in contrast to natural acids. Solubilization occurs as a result of the protonation of $-NH_2$ functional groups on the C-2 position of D-glucosamine residues (Morris et al. 2010). Chitosan, a weak base, possesses pKa values from 6.2 to 7 and, at a physiological pH of 7.4 or higher, bears low solubility (Park et al. 1983). However, its ability to go into solution depends on the dispersion of its acetyl gatherings and its molecular weight (Kubota and Eeguchi 1997). The increase in DA increases its solubility in water (Varum et al. 1994). Salting out may be seen with an increase in electrolyte amount, bringing about the development of chitosan chlorhydrate (Rinaudo 2006). Salting out can likewise be utilized to regain chitosan from solution, and the salting out efficiency of anions depends on the Hofmeister arrangement $SO_4^{-2} -> H_2PO_4 \sim HPO_4^{2-} > NO_3^-$ (Lehoux and de Puis 2007). The addition of electrolytes reduces the inter-chain repulsion and induces a more random coil-like conformation in the molecule as it counteracts the repelling effect of each positively charged deacetylated unit (Terbojevich and Muzzarelli 2000).

7.3.1.2 Starch

Starch is made out of two sorts of polymers: amylose and amylopectin. Amylose is a straight homopolymer of -1,4-connected glucose, having a low level of stretching with a 1,6-linkage (Martinez et al. 2012). Amylose makes up ~35% of starch. In arrangement, it shapes hydrogen bound with other amylase atoms to yield unbending gels. Then again, amylopectin is a remarkable branch type of amylose. Here, the straight -1,4-connected glucose spine is spread at ~20 buildups by a -1,6-linkage which is stretched out by -1,4-connected linkages (Della Valle et al. 1998).

7.3.1.3 Alginate

Alginate, a well-known polysaccharide, is isolated from characteristic sources, which incorporates its extraction from cell dividers and intercellular spaces of marine green growth, and furthermore by its generation from microbes. It may be portrayed as an anionic copolymer whose synthetic structure depends on a backbone of 1,4-connected-D-mannuronic acid (M units) and -L-guluronic acid (G units) of differing structure and arrangement, relying upon the source of the alginate and resulting in a blockwise example of GG, MG, and MM pieces. This molecule has a variable molecular weight which depends on the enzymatic control during its production and the degree of depolymerization caused by its extraction. The business alginates have a normal sub-atomic weight of approx. 200,000 Da, however, values as high as 400,000–500,000 Da are likewise accessible (Martinez et al. 2012).

The physico-chemical properties of alginate are observed to be profoundly influenced by the M/G proportion and additionally by the structure of the substituting zones, which may be controlled by enzymatic pathways (Yang et al. 2011). The alginate organization's effect on the adaptability of the polysaccharide chain was first announced by Smidsrod, who suggested that the expansion of the alginate chain was subject to its creation, with the characteristic adaptability of the blocks diminishing in the order MG>MM>GG (Smidsrod 1973). M piece sections had indicated straight and adaptable compliance due to the (1→4) linkages. Additionally, the guluronic acid offers ascendance to (1→4) linkages, which serve to present a steric obstacle around the carboxylic gatherings, and give collapsing and unbending basic adaptations that are in charge of an articulated firmness of the sub-atomic chains (Sujata 2002).

Alginate is a biopolymer and a polyelectrolyte which is thought to be biocompatible, non-immunogenic, non-lethal, and biodegradable. Alginate is a biopolymer and a polyelectrolyte that is thought to be biocompatible, non-immunogenic, non-lethal, and biodegradable. As calcium salts form, alginate with a high substance of guluronic acid block can be delivered crosslinked, thus stabilizing the structure of the polymer in an unbending gel frame. This provides answers to process alginates being divided into the type of films, globules, and wipes (Sujata 2002). In any case, high mannuronic acid alginate capsules are basic for cell transplantation and for bio hybrid organs, because of their consistency.

Compositional alterations of regular alginates are obtained by mannuronan C-5 epimerases delivered by alginate-creating microbes, for example, *A. vinelandii*. As of late, the blend of various epimerases has been used as a key apparatus for making particular engineered alginates with any desired block length and construction (Rehm 2009). In addition, alginate, with a vast number of free hydroxyl and carboxyl gatherings conveyed along the spine, is exceedingly responsive to the possibility of suitable alteration by chemical functionalization. Accordingly, properties, for example, solvency, hydrophobicity, physicochemical, and organic qualities may be adjusted for potential applications. Such changes have been accomplished utilizing procedures which contain, oxidation, sulfation, esterification, amidation, or joining techniques (Yang et al. 2011).

Because of its wealth, low cost, and safety, alginate has been utilized as a part of various enterprises; for example, it's utilized as an added substance and thickener in the serving of salad dressings and desserts in the food business (Nair and Laurencin 2007). Additionally, its biocompatibility and usefulness makes it a great biopolymer material for biomedical applications, for example, frameworks for tissue design, immobilization of cells, and controlled medication discharge gadgets. Applications in nanomedicine have likewise been widely examined, where it has been utilized as a medication conveyance gadget allowing the rate of medication discharge to be altered, varying the drug polymer assembly, and by the chemical immobilization of the medication in the polymer spine utilizing the receptive carboxylate groups. Aside from its simple functionalization, there are many different focal points and properties which makes it valuable in the utilization of medication conveyance (Della Valle et al. 1998).

It is a characteristic polymer, compatible with a large assortment of substances, that doesn't require sophisticated medication incorporation methods or processes. Besides, it is mucoadhesive and biodegradable, and therefore, it can be utilized as a part of controlled medication delivery frameworks with upgraded sedate bioavailability (Nair and Laurencin 2007). Along these lines, the biocompatibility, accessibility, and adaptability of this polysaccharide make it a vital and confident device in the field of nanomedicine, particularly in the preparation of nanoparticulate drug delivery systems.

7.3.1.4 Hyaluronic Acid

Hyaluronic acid (HA), also called sodium hyaluronic or hyaluronan, is a polysaccharide with rehashing disaccharide units of D-glucuronic acid and N acetyl D-glucosamine connected by (1–3) and (1–4) glycosidic bonds (Figure 7.2) (Martinez et al. 2012; Cafaggi et al. 2011). Changes to this

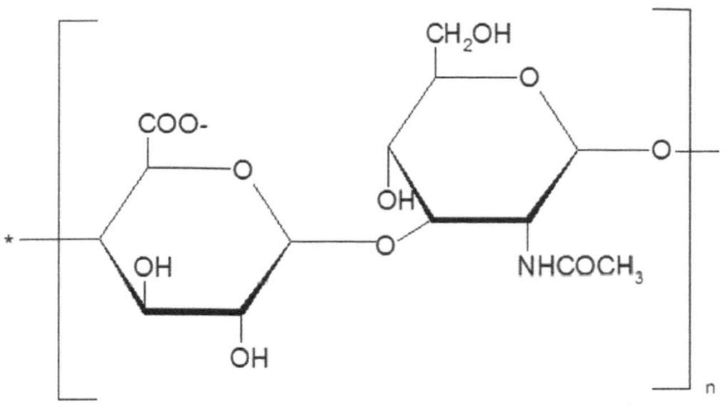

FIGURE 7.2   Chemical structure of hyaluronic acid.

polysaccharide may help to improve modifying properties which incorporate alterations prompting hydrophobicity and organic movement. Three useful gatherings where compound change may occur, incorporate glucuronic acid, carboxylic acid, essential and optional hydroxyl gatherings, and the N-acetyl gathering (Burdick and Prestwich 2011).

This class of polysaccharide has an atomic weight that can reach as high 107 Da. It has a place with in a group of substances known as glycosaminoglycans. It is the most basic among them, the one not covalently connected with a center protein, and also the special case that is non-sulphated. Since hyaluronan is a physiological substance, it is broadly circulated in the extracellular network of vertebrate tissues. It is primarily blended in the extracellular matrices of vertebrates for its useful viscoelastic and rheological properties. It is a noteworthy and essential segment of ligament, skin, and synovial liquid (Martinez et al. 2012).

HA is normally connected to different biopolymers within a lifeform, and a few separation methodologies are applied, keeping in mind the end goal is to get the unadulterated compound, for example, protease absorption, HA particle match precipitation, layer ultrafiltration, HA non-dissolvable precipitation, as well as lyophilization. With these strategies, HA from 200,000 Da up to 2.5 MDa can be acquired. However, a few microorganisms discharged HA with a molar mass in the scope of a few MDa, for example, weakened strains of *Streptococcus zooepidemicus*, *S. Equi.*, and *Bacillus subtilis* has been as of late hereditarily adjusted to culture an exclusive recipe to yield hyaluronans (Mendichi and Soltes 2002).

HA is a biodegradable, bioactive, non-immunogenic, non-cytotoxic, and adversely charged polysaccharide (Oh et al. 2010) that has been related with a few cell forms, including angiogenesis and the control of aggravation. Among its applications, it is generally used as a covering for the surface alteration of different biomaterials utilized for prosthetic ligament, vascular join, guided nerve recovery, and medication conveyance (Li et al. 2006).

Like different glycosaminoglycans, hyaluronan can fill in as a vehicle for the conveyance of chemotherapeutic specialists to harmful tissues, as many tumors over express the hyaluronan CD44 and RHAMM receptors. As a medication conveyance transporter, HA has a few points of interest, including negligible non-specific connection with serum parts because of its polyanionic attributes and the profoundly productive directed conveyance toward the liver tissues with HA receptors (Martinez et al. 2012).

Recently, HA has been perceived as an imperative building hinder for the production of new biomaterials with utility in tissue design and regenerative prescriptions (Allison and Grande-Allen 2006). Additionally, it has been demonstrated that HA ties to cells and successfully advances new bone arrangements. Balazs grouped the biomedical uses of HA and its subordinates into the regions: vicosurgery, viscoaugmentation, viscoseparation, viscosupplementation, and viscoprotection (Balazs 2004). Thus, along these lines, there is a wide number of utilizations for HA in pharmaceutical and beauty care products, for example, ophthalmology, orthopaedic surgery and rheumatology, otolaryngology, wound mending, pharmacology, and medication conveyance, which indicates HA is a fruitful as a part of various fields of biomedicine.

7.3.1.5 Pullulan

Pullulan is a direct bacterial homopolysaccharide created from starch by growing *Aureobasidium pullulans*. The spine is framed with glycosidic linkages between -(1→6) D-glucopyranose and -(1→4) D-glucopyranose units in a 1:2 proportion (Figure 7.3). The atomic weight of pullulan ranges from 1,000 to 2,000,000 Da depending on the development conditions (Rekha and Chandra 2007).

The backbone structure of pullulan has a tendency to carry on as an irregular extended adaptable curl in an aqueous solution with modeling studies demonstrating that this adaptability is bestowed by the (1→6) linkage. This could be the motivation behind why pullulan is biodegradable and has high bond, basic adaptability, and solvency (Leathers 2003). Pullulan can likewise be effectively derivatized keeping in mind the end goal to bestow new physico-compound properties, e.g., to expand the dissolvability in natural solvents or to present responsive gatherings.

This polysaccharide has various utilizations: in sustenance and refreshments as a filler; as an eatable, for the most part, boring polymer, the main business utilization of pullulan is in the fabricate of consumable movies that are utilized as a part of different breath fresheners or oral cleanliness items; in pharmaceuticals as a covering specialist; in assemblies and gadgets it is utilized in light of its film- and fiber-shaping properties. It is important that pullulan films, framed by drying pullulan solutions, are clear and profoundly oxygen-impermeable and have fantastic mechanical properties.

Because it is hemocompatible, non-immunogenic, non-cancer-causing, the FDA have approved it for an assortment of uses (Coviello et al. 2007). As of late, pullulan has been examined for being utilized as a part of different biomedical applications, for example, medication and gene delivery (Rekha and Chandra 2007), tissue building (Thebaud et al. 2007), and wound recuperating (Bae et al. 2011).

Various papers examine pullulan hydrogels as medication delivery frameworks, especially as miniaturized scale and nanogels. Pullulan is not a characteristic gelling polysaccharide; suitable compound derivatization of its spine can really prompt a polymeric structure fortified for shaping hydrogels. The investigation of nanogels has been increased in the course of the most recent decade because of the related potential applications in the improvement and usage of new ecologically responsive or shrewd materials, biomimetics, biosensors, counterfeit muscles, tranquillize conveyance frameworks, and synthetic partitions (Coviello et al. 2007).

Keeping in mind the end goal is to acquire nanostructures that have the ability to deliver various medications, the spine structure of pullulan is altered with hydrophobic atoms, bringing about a particle of hydrophobized pullulan that self-gathers in water arrangements. Cholesterol, hexadecanol, or vitamin H are a few atoms that are joined to the structure of pullulan with the goal of producing micelles in the water arrangement (Adams 2010).

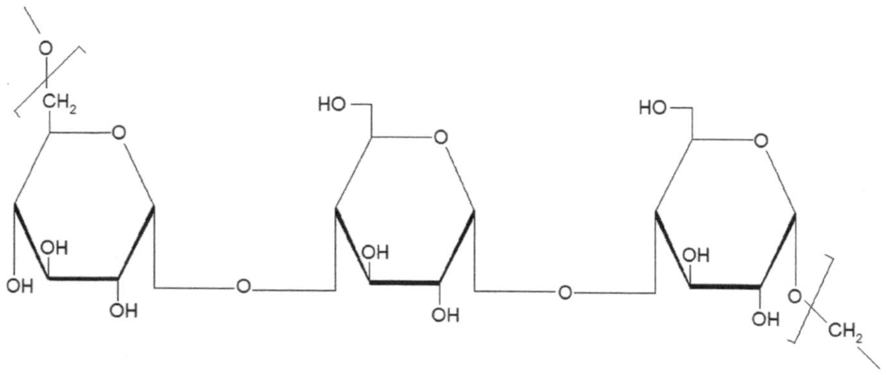

FIGURE 7.3   Chemical structure of pullulan.

7.3.1.6 Guar Gum

Guar gum, a water dissolvable polysaccharide is removed from the seeds of *Cyamopsistetragonoloba*. Likewise called guaran, it is a non-ionic characteristic polysaccharide obtained from guar beans. Its spine comprises of direct chains of 1,4-D-mannopyranosyl units with -D-galactopyranosyl units joined by 1,6-linkages (Figure 7.4), shaping short side-branches (Sarmah et al. 2011).

Guar gum hydrates in icy water to frame an exceptionally gooey arrangement in which the single polysaccharide chains collaborate with each other impressively (Barbucci et al. 2008). Its nine hydroxyl bunches are accessible for the arrangement of hydrogen bonds with different atoms. However, it remains impartially charged because of the non-appearance of dissociable utilitarian gatherings. Extraordinary pH and high-temperature conditions (e.g., pH 3 at 50°C) degrade its structure (Tiraferri et al. 2008). It stays stable in arrangements over pH 5–7. Solid acids cause hydrolysis and loss of thickness, and salts in solid focus additionally have a tendency to lessen consistency. It is insoluble in most hydrocarbon solvents.

It's generally connected in numerous mechanical fields because of its ease, simple accessibility, and non-poisonous nature. It is ordinarily utilized as a thickening specialist in beautifying agents and in sauces, salad dressings, and frozen yogurts in the food industry (Barbucci et al. 2008). In pharmaceuticals, it's utilized as a binder in tablet formulation and as a disintegrant, as a hydrophilic grid, for planning oral controlled-release measurement frames (Sarmah et al. 2011). Guar gum has been broadly utilized for colon conveyance because of its medication discharge hindering properties and defenselessness to microbial debasement in the digestive organs (Soumya et al. 2010). Guar gum artificially adjusted by chemical modification can be utilized with the aim of changing its inherent attributes of dissolvability, thickness, and rheological conduct.

In the case of biomedical or pharmaceutical fields, for example, 3D platforms for cell culture, fillers for tissue building, and transporters for drugs, the physically cross-connected material is gotten through a spacer arm between the polymer chains and allows the acquisition of an insoluble compound in a broad range of pH with a decent mechanical security (Barbucci et al. 2008).

Little data is accessible concerning the likelihood of utilizing guar gum-based nanosized materials as medication bearers because of its dissolvability in water, which makes it hard to utilize as it is not adsorbent in fluid conditions. A few scientists have joined its structure with mixes like silica, so as to get insoluble mixes which could act as adsorbents in fluid media (Martinez et al. 2012) Additionally, guar gum-based nanosystems have been set up through nanoprecipitation and cross-connecting techniques (Soumya et al. 2010). An alternate use of this polysaccharide has been found as a stabilizer of nanosuspensions, where the nearness of guar gum during the combination procedure permits the accomplishment of a superior solidness of the nanoparticles (Tiraferri et al. 2008).

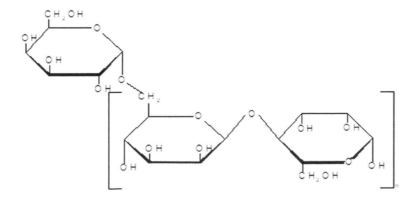

FIGURE 7.4 Chemical structure of guar gum.

7.3.1.7   Dextran

Dextran, a polysaccharide, is made up of numerous glucose atoms made from chains of changing lengths. It has a significant number of α-(1→6) glucosidic linkages in its primary chain (Figure 7.5), and a variable measure of α-(1→2), α-(1→3), and α-(1→4) stretched linkages (Misaki et al. 1980).

The bacterial strain that incorporates it decides the degree and type of expansion it undergoes. Its normal sub-atomic weight is as high as 10^7–10^8 Da but might be diminished by acidic hydrolysis when acquiring sub-atomic weight portions. The characteristic structure of dextran can be changed by reacting different molecules (such as hydrophobic atoms) with diverse hydroxyl groups (Heinze et al. 2006).

Numerous amphiphilic dextran derivates have been acquired by shifting the reacting atoms (fragment rings, aliphatic, or cyclic hydrocarbons) and the quantity of hydrophobic gatherings per 100 gluco-pyranose units or the level of substitution (Sinha and Kumria 2001).

Dextran is neutral, soluble in water, biocompatible, and biodegradable. Its characteristics may vary upon the atomic mass and additionally the passage, type of branches, and the level of fanning, which relies on the bacterial combination or post-blend responses to frame subsidiaries.

Dextran is synthetized by a wide variety of bacterial strains. *Leuconostoc mesenteroides* produces dextran from sucrose and *Gluconobacter oxydans* produces dextran from maltodextrin. *Streptococcus mutans* additionally creates dextran from sucrose. It can be likewise be acquired enzymatically utilizing a sans cell culture supernatant. Aside from these techniques, dextran can be additionally created by substance blend, building up a cationic ring-opening polymerization of levoglucosan (Martinez et al. 2012).

It has wide applications in various areas such as the pharmaceutical, substance, clinical, and food industries. Dextran is utilized as a medication (as a blood plasma volume expander), adjuvant, emulsifier, bearer, stabilizer, and a thickener of jam and frozen yogurt. Also, it is generally utilized for the detachment and sanitization of proteins in view of size rejection chromatography with a lattice of cross-connected dextran gel layers. Its subordinates even have different applications depending on the qualities that auxiliary changes give them.

Both dextran and its subsidiaries have potential application in the planning of altered medication conveyance (Coviello et al. 2007).

It appears that dextran is an exceptionally valuable device in the field of nanomedicine, demonstrating great accessibility, biocompatibility, and biodegradability, and being assigned by many specialists as a biomaterial for use in nanosystems.

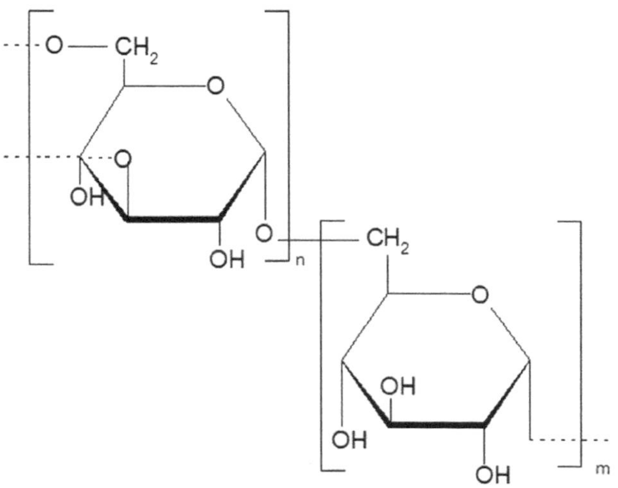

FIGURE 7.5   Chemical structure of dextran.

7.3.1.8　Pectin

Pectin is a basic polysaccharide acquired from the cell mass of all plants, where it is ensnared in cell adhesion. It has a heterogeneous compound structure in view of a lot of poly(D-galacturonic acid) fortified by means of $(1 \rightarrow 4)$ glycosidic linkage (Figure 7.6). Pectin has a 200 to around 1,000 building pieces for each particle, with a normal atomic weight of around 50,000–180,000 Da (Sinha and Kumria 2001). The carboxyl gatherings are mostly in the methyl ester shape with various levels of esterification and amidation, deciding the content of carboxylic acid in pectin chains.

Previously, pectin has mainly been used in the food industry, as a gelling or thickening operator, yet recently has begun to be utilized as an excipient for pharmaceutical purposes. Some of its uses have moved into biomedical applications including, the conveyance of particular groupings of amino acids, anti-inflammatories, anti-coagulants, and wound-recuperating substances to tissue locales.

Pectin stays unbroken in the physiological condition of the stomach and small digestive system; however, it does get tainted by pectinases. Due to these properties, it is very conceivable that pectin could work as a conveyance vehicle to escort protein and polypeptide drugs from the mouth to the colon. Pectin-based composites can be shaped into layers, microspheres, platforms, or injectable gels (Sinha and Kumria 2001; Martinez et al. 2012).

The most positive property of pectin for mechanical applications is its gelling movement. Parameters such as the type and conjunction of (DE, DA) of pectin, the change of hydroxyl gatherings, the pH, the temperature, and the presence of cations decide the gel procedure. For instance, a high DE of pectin produces the gel arrangement, expanding the measures of hydrophobic regions, and diminishing the dissolvability of pectin. On the other hand, when the DE is less than half, pectin is extremely water soluble, and gel development is at very low pH, or within the sight of divalent cations, which cross-interface the galacturonic acids of the primary polymer chain (Liu et al. 2003). Likewise, it is conceivable to lessen the hydrophilic property with a greater tendency to shape gels by the presentation of amide bunches in low-DE pectin.

7.4　PREPARATION OF NANOPARTICLES USING POLYSACCHARIDES TO OVERCOME SOLUBILITY ISSUES: RELEVANT CASE STUDIES

In the last decade, more polysaccharide-based nanoparticles have been developed, which have extraordinarily improved the flexibility of nanoparticle transporters as far as structure and capacity are concerned. As indicated by auxiliary attributes, these nanoparticles are arranged essentially by four components, in particular, covalent crosslinking, ionic crosslinking, polyelectrolyte complexation, and the self-assembly of hydrophobically modified polysaccharides (Figure 7.7) (Liu et al. 2008).

7.4.1　Covalently Crosslinked Polysaccharide Nanoparticles

The early evolution of polysaccharide nanoparticles were made via methods of covalent crosslinking. Among the different polysaccharides, chitosan is the most abundantly utilized to get nanoparticles.

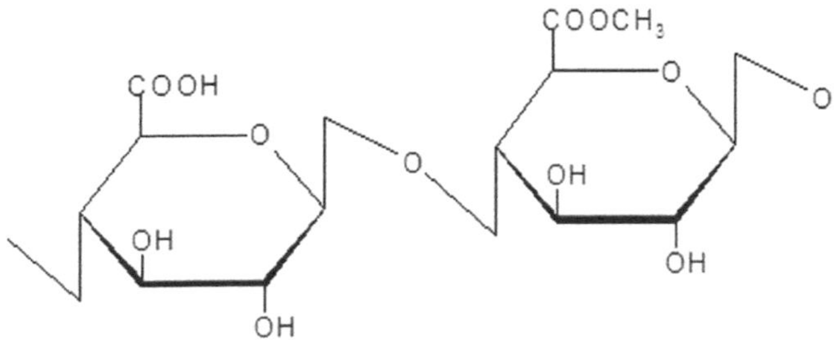

FIGURE 7.6　Chemical structure of pectin.

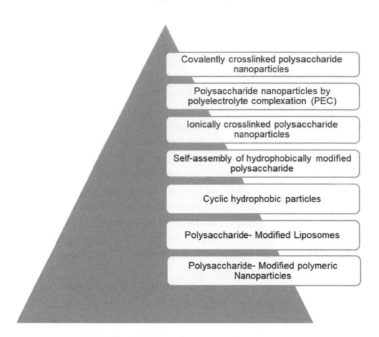

FIGURE 7.7 Methods of preparation of nanoparticles with polysaccharides.

As a standard crosslinker, glutaraldehyde was used to crosslink chitosan-based nanoparticles. As of late, some chitosan nanoparticles were still crosslinked with glutaraldehyde (Zhi et al. 2005; Liu et al. 2007). Tragically, the danger of glutaraldehyde on cellular suitability constrains its utility in the field of drug delivery. Alongside the utilization of biocompatible crosslinkers, biocompatible covalent crosslinking is promising. With the aid of water-soluble condensation, reaction, specially in carbodiimide, natural di- and tricarboxylic acids, including succinic acid, malic acid, tartaric acid, and citrus acid, find their place in being utilized for the intermolecular crosslinking of chitosan nanoparticles (Bodnar et al. 2005a,b). The condensation reaction was performed between the carboxylic group of characteristic acids and the pendant amino group of chitosan, through which biodegradable chitosan nanoparticles were obtained. This strategy permits the development of polycations, polyanions, and polyampholyte nanoparticles. The developed nanoparticles were stable in the aqueous medium at a low pH, neutral, and mild alkaline atmosphere. In a swollen state, the normal size of the particles were found to be 270–370 nm depending on the pH.

7.4.2 Ionically Crosslinked Polysaccharide Nanoparticles

Contrasted with covalent crosslinking, ionic crosslinking has more preferences: gentle conditions of preparation and straightforward methodology. For charged polysaccharides, the low MW of polyanions and polycations could act as ionic crosslinkers for the polycationic and polyanionic polysaccharides, individually. To date, the most utilized polyanion crosslinker is tripolyphosphate (TPP). Calvo et al. first created TPP crosslinked chitosan nanoparticles in 1997 (Calvo et al. 1997a,b). TPP is non-harmful and has multivalent anions. It can shape a gel by the ionic connection between positively charged amino groups of chitosan and adversely charged counterions of TPP (Jain and Banerjee 2008). From that point on, TPP-chitosan nanoparticles have been broadly used to transport different drugs and macromolecules (Lu et al. 2006a,b; Zhang et al. 2004).

Recently, water-soluble chitosan derivatives were likewise ionically crosslinked with nanoparticles. Contrasted with chitosan itself, its derivatives can, without much stretch, break down in neutral aqueous media while maintaining a strategic distance from the potential poisonous quality of the acids, and subsequently secure the bioactivity of loaded biomacromolecules. Xu et al. incorporated water-soluble chitosan derivatives, N-(2-hydroxyl) propyl-3-trimethyl ammonium chitosan chloride via a response between glycidyl-trimethyl-ammonium chloride and chitosan (Xu et al. 2003). Nanoparticles of 110–180 nm were shaped based on the ionic gelation procedure of the derivatives and TPP. Bovine serum albumin, as a model protein drug, was fused into the nanoparticles with an encapsulation efficiency of up to 90%. Furthermore, Amidi et al. arranged N-trimethyl chitosan nanoparticles by ionic crosslinking of N-trimethyl chitosan with TPP and assessed their potential as a carrier for the nasal delivery of the protein, ovalbumin (Amidi et al. 2006). The nanoparticles had a normal size of around 350 nm and a positive zeta potential. They demonstrated a loading efficiency of up to 95% and a loading limit up to 50% (w/w). Ovalbumin was found intact in the preparation. In 2007, Sandri et al. assessed the assimilation properties of N-trimethyl chitosan/TPP nanoparticles utilizing them as a part of *in vitro* (caco-2 cells) and *ex vivo* (extracted rodent jejunum) models. Shi et al. developed carboxymethyl chitosan nanoparticles (200–300 nm and in limited distribution) through ionic gelation with calcium ions and assessed the capability of the nanoparticles as transporters for the anticancer drug, doxorubicin. Impacts of the degree of substitution (DS) and MW of carboxymethyl chitosan on doxorubicin delivery were talked about.

In addition, calcium-crosslinked negatively charged polysaccharide nanoparticles have recently been discovered as having utility as drug transporters. A few polysaccharides bearing carboxylic groups on molecular chains can be crosslinked by bivalent calcium ions to shape nanoparticles. You et al. arranged Ca-crosslinked alginate nanoparticles through a water-in-oil reverse microemulsion technique in 2004. To inspect the strength of the nanoparticles for gene delivery, green fluorescent protein-encoding plasmids were embodied in the nanoparticles to explore the level of endocytosis by NIH 3T3 cells and the resulting transfection rate. Results demonstrated that Ca-alginate nanoparticles with a normal size of around 80 nm were extremely efficient gene bearers. Zahoor et al. additionally designed Ca-alginate nanoparticles (235.5±0 nm) by ion initiated gelification (Zahoor et al. 2005). Drug encapsulation efficiencies in the nanoparticles were 70%–90% for isoniazid and pyrazinamide, and 80%–90% for rifampicin. The relative bioavailability of all medications encapsulated was significantly higher than oral free drugs. The utilized drugs were identified in organs (the lungs, liver, and spleen) over the minimum inhibitory concentration for 15 days post-nebulization, while free drugs remained up to 1 day. These inhalable nanoparticles could be used as a perfect carrier for the controlled release of anti-tubercular drugs.

Also, Kim et al. encapsulated retinol into chitosan nanoparticles and reconstituted it into aqueous media for restorative and pharmaceutical applications. The solvency of retinol can increment more than 1600-fold by encapsulating it into chitosan nanoparticles (Kim et al. 2006). It was recommended that retinol was encapsulated into chitosan nanoparticles by ion complex because of the electrostatic cooperation between the amine group of chitosan and hydroxyl group of retinol.

7.4.3 Polysaccharide Nanoparticles by Polyelectrolyte Complexation (PEC)

Polyelectrolyte polysaccharides can shape PEC with oppositely charged polymers by an intermolecular electrostatic interaction. Polysaccharide-based PEC nanoparticles can be acquired by methods of altering the MW of component polymers in a specific range. In principle, any polyelectrolyte could cooperate with polysaccharides to manufacture PEC nanoparticles. In any case, these polyelectrolytes are limited to those water-soluble and biocompatible polymers in the perspective of safety. In this sense, chitosan is the main natural polycationic polysaccharide that satisfies the requirements. There are many negative polymers complexed with chitosan to shape PEC nanoparticles, which can be partitioned into polysaccharides, peptides, the polyacrylic acid family, etc.

7.4.3.1 Negative Polysaccharides

Cui et al. utilized carboxymethyl cellulose to complex chitosan to frame stable cationic nanoparticles and explored the topical use of these nanoparticles containing plasmid DNA as a potential way to deal with hereditary immunization (Cui and Mumper 2001). Plasmid DNA was coated on pre-framed cationic chitosan/carboxymethylcellulose nanoparticles. The chosen plasmid DNA-covered nanoparticles (with plasmid DNA up to 400 mg/ml) were stable within the serum. A few diverse chitosan-based nanoparticles containing plasmid DNA brought about both recognizable and quantifiable levels of luciferase articulation in mouse skin 24 h after topical application and a significant antigen-specific IgG titer to communicated ß-galactosidase at 28 days.

Chen et al. in 2003, created a chitosan/dextran sulfate nanoparticle delivery system by utilizing a straightforward coacervation process. The examination researched the impact of the weight proportion of the two polymers on particle size, surface charge, capture efficiency, and release qualities of an anti-angiogenesis peptide. Particles of 223 nm mean breadth were delivered under ideal conditions with a zeta potential of around −32.6 mV. The physicochemical and release qualities of the nanoparticles could be balanced by changing proportions of two ionic polymers. Tiyaboonchai et al. built a nanoparticulate delivery system for amphotericin B with chitosan and dextran sulfate together with zinc sulfate as a crosslinking and solidifying agent (Tiyaboonchai and Limpeanchob 2007). The nanoparticles acquired had a mean molecule size of 600–800 nm with a polydispersity index of 0.2, demonstrating a tight size distribution. The deliberate zeta potential of the nanoparticle surface was roughly −32 mV, showing a solid negative charge at the particle's surface. Drug association efficacy of up to 65% was accomplished. Sarmento et al. 2006 contemplated dextran sulfate or alginate complexation with chitosan on mean particle size, insulin association efficiency, loading limit, and release profile (Sarmento et al. 2006). Nanoparticles were shaped by ionotropic complexation and coacervation between polyanions (dextran sulfate and alginate) and chitosan. Mean nanoparticle width ran from 423 to 850 nm, insulin association efficiency from 63% to 94% and loading limit from 5% to 13%. Dextran sulfate/chitosan nanoparticles gave the most elevated insulin association efficiency and maintenance of insulin in gastric simulated conditions. In 2006, Sarmento et al. arranged insulin-combined nanoparticles by the ionotropic pre-gelation of alginate with calcium chloride after complexation amongst alginate and chitosan. A similar group tested the basic integrity of insulin subsequent to being intertwined with chitosan/alginate nanoparticles (Sarmento et al. 2007). The results confirmed that no significant conformational changes of insulin happened as far as a-helix and ß-sheet content. Alonso-Sande et al. (2006) utilized two distinct sorts of glucomannan (non-phosphorylated and phosphorylated) and two diverse ways to deal with developing nanoparticles. This methodology included the interaction of chitosan and glucomannan in the presence or non-appearance of sodium tripolyphosphate, which was used as an ionic crosslinking agent for chitosan. Contingent upon the formulation conditions, it was conceivable to get nanoparticles with measurements from 200 to 700 nm and a zeta potential from −2 to +39 mV. The nanoparticles displayed an extraordinary limit with regards to insulin with the immunomodulatory protein P1, achieving association efficiency esteems as high as 89%. Du et al. arranged carboxymethyl konjac glucomannan/chitosan nanoparticles under extremely mild conditions by means of polyelectrolyte complexation (Du et al. 2004, 2005). Bovine serum albumin, as a model protein drug, was fused into the nanoparticles and the encapsulation efficiency and *in vitro* release profile of bovine serum albumin were determined. The nanoparticles showed pH-responsive properties, as well as delicate ionic quality properties. Liu et al. 2007, arranged heparin/chitosan nanoparticles by polyelectrolyte complexation. Entrapment investigations of the nanoparticles were led utilizing bovine serum albumin as a model protein. Specifically, the impacts of the pH estimation of chitosan solution, chitosan MW, chitosan concentration, heparin fixation, and the protein content on the nanoparticle measure, the nanoparticle yield, and the protein encapsulation were examined in detail. Li et al. arranged quaternized chitosan/alginate nanoparticles in a neutral condition for the oral delivery of protein (Li et al. 2007). The diameter of the nanoparticles with a positive surface charge was around 200 nm.

7.4.3.2 Negative Peptides

Lin et al. arranged poly-γ-glutamic corrosive/chitosan nanoparticles utilizing an ionic-gelation technique (Lin et al. in 2005). Assessment of the arranged nanoparticles in improving intestinal paracellular transport was researched *in vitro* in caco-2 cell monolayers. It was discovered that the nanoparticles with chitosan on the surfaces could adequately diminish the transepithelial electrical resistance of caco-2 cell monolayers and opened the tight intersections between caco-2 cells and permitted the transport of the nanoparticles by means of the paracellular pathways. Additionally, the nanoparticles were utilized transdermally for gene delivery. Contrasted with this, chitosan/DNA, chitosan/poly-γ-glutamic acid/DNA saw enhanced entrance into the mouse skin and upgraded gene expression. These perceptions might be credited to the way that chitosan/poly-γ-glutamic acid/DNA were more compact in their interior structures and had a more prominent density than their chitosan/DNA partners, in this way having a bigger force to enter into the skin boundary (Lee et al. 2008).

Zheng et al developed chitosan/glycyrrhetic acid nanoparticles by polyelectrolyte complexation and concentrated on glycyrrhetic acid encapsulation efficiency and *in vitro* release (Zheng et al. 2006). Stoilova et al. designed PEC nanoparticles amongst chitosan and poly(2-acryloylamido-2-methylpropanesulfonic acid) by blending an aqueous solution of its parts or by free radical polymerization on a chitosan template (Stoilova et al. 1999). The nanoparticles (mean breadth 250 nm and monomodal distribution) were steady in an acidic and neutral medium and separated at pH 8. Zheng et al. arranged anionic or cationic nanoparticles in view of chitosan and polyaspartic acid sodium salt (Zheng et al. 2007). A hydrophilic drug, 5-fluorouracil, was loaded into the nanoparticles.

Moreover, the nanoparticle shaped by complexation between chitosan or its derivatives and DNA or RNA is an uncommon kind of delivery system, which has been very much contemplated (Thanou et al. 2002; Kim et al. 2007; Tan et al. 2007). It is important is that the classification of this sort of nanoparticle will ceaselessly increment since: (1) chitosan has a considerable positively charged subsidiaries, for example, glycol chitosan, N-trimethyl chitosan and N-triethyl chitosan, which can be utilized as polycation rather than chitosan; (2) more biocompatible negative polymers will be thought of, specifically, different polyanionic polysaccharides.

7.4.4 Self-Assembly of Hydrophobically Modified Polysaccharides

At the point when hydrophilic polymeric chains are joined with hydrophobic fragments, amphiphilic copolymers are blended. Upon contact with an aqueous media, polymeric amphiphiles precipitously frame micelles or micelle-like aggregates by means of experiencing intra- or intermolecular association between hydrophobic moieties, which fundamentally limits interfacial free energy. These polymeric micelles show one of a kind attributes, contingent upon hydrophilic/hydrophobic constituents, for example, an unordinary rheological component, little hydrodynamic radius (not exactly microsize) with center shell structure, and thermodynamic steadiness. Specifically, polymeric micelles have been perceived as a promising drug transporter, since their hydrophobic area, encompassed by a hydrophilic external shell, can fill in as a preservatory for different hydrophobic drugs (Letchford and Burt 2007). As of late, various examinations have been done to research the combination and the use of polysaccharide-based self-aggregate nanoparticles as drug carrier systems. Generally, these hydrophobic molecules can be isolated into straight, cyclic hydrophobic particles, hydrophobic drug, polyacrylate family, and so forth.

Opanasopit et al. integrated amphiphilic joined copolymers, N-phthaloylchitosan-grafted poly(ethylene glycol) methyl ether (Opanasopit et al. 2007). These copolymers could shape micelle-like nanoparticles. The CMC of these nanoparticles in water was comparative (28 μg/ml). The nanoparticles showed a general circular shape with core-shell structure with sizes in the measure of 100–250 nm. Camptothecin as a model medication was stacked into the inward center of the micelles. Hu et al. incorporated stearic acid grafted chitosan oligosaccharide by 1-ethyl-3-(3-dimethylaminopropyl) carbodiimide-intervened coupling response (Hu et al. 2006). The CMC of the copolymer was around 0.06, 0.04, 0.01 mg/ml, individually. To build the steadiness of the micelle *in vivo* and the controlled release profile, the shells of micelles were cross-connected by glutaraldehyde. Paclitaxel was utilized as a model drug to be loaded into the micelles, and the surfaces of the micelles were further crosslinked by glutaraldehyde to frame drug-loaded and shell cross-connected nanoparticles. Higher drug encapsulation efficiencies (over 94%) were seen in all cases. Gref et al. and Lemarchand et al. blended amphiphilic dextran by coupling it between a carboxylic function exhibited on preformed PCL monocarboxylic acid and the hydroxyl bunches on dextran (Gref et al. 2002; Lemarchand et al. 2003a,b). The comb-like copolymers (dextran-PCL) comprised of a dextran spine onto which preformed PCL blocks were joined. Nanoparticles of under 200 nm were effectively arranged by utilizing the new materials. Further, bovine serum albumin and lectin were consolidated in the nanoparticles.

7.4.5 CYCLIC HYDROPHOBIC PARTICLES

Conjugating hydrophobic cholesterol to hydrophilic polysaccharides may shape amphiphilic copolymers which may additionally frame self-gathering nanoparticles in a watery environment. Wang et al. combined cholesterol-modified chitosan conjugate with succinyl linkages (Wang et al. 2007). The CMC was 1.16×10^{-2} mg/ml in 0.1 M acetic acid solution. The conjugates framed monodisperse self-aggregated nanoparticles with a generally circular shape and a mean diameter of 417.2 nm via probe sonication in fluid media. Epirubicin, as a model anticancer medication, was physically entangled inside the nanoparticles by the remote stacking technique. Epirubicin-stacked nanoparticles were practically spherical, and their size expanded from 338.2–472.9 nm with the epirubicin-stacking content expanding from 7.97% to 14%. Epirubicin release rate diminished with the pH increment of the dissolution media. In PBS pH 7.4, the epirubicin discharge was moderate, and the aggregate release was around 24.9% out of 48 h. Wang et al. likewise set self-aggregated nanoparticles of cholesterol-modified O-carboxymethyl chitosan and examined the response between bovine serum albumin and self-aggregated nanoparticles (Wang et al. 2007).

Lee et al. covalently conjugated deoxycholic acid to chitosan by means of a carbodiimide-intervened response to produce self-accumulated nanoparticles. Adriamycin was physically entangled inside the self-aggregates (Lee et al. 1998a; Lee et al. 1998b). The most extreme measure of entrapped adriamycin achieved was 16.5 wt. % of the self-aggregate, recommending an entrapment efficiency of 49.6 wt. %. The extent of adriamycin-stacked self-aggregate expanded while expanding the loading content of adriamycin. Adriamycin was gradually discharged from the self-aggregates in pH 7.2 PBS (Lee et al. 2000).

Poly(methyl methacrylate) and poly(isobutyl cyanoacrylate) (PIBCA) all have a place within the polyacrylate family and are generally utilized for biomaterials. Containing carboxylic ester bunches in their structures, they are hydrophobic. Yang et al. arranged PIBCA-chitosan nanoparticles by the emulsion polymerization of IBCA within the sight of chitosan as a polymeric stabilizer at a low pH (Yang et al. 2000). Nimodipine as a model medication was effectively joined into the nanoparticles with a mean molecule breadth of 31.6 nm and a positive charge.

In addition to being a significant constituent of colloidal nanoparticles, polysaccharides have conjointly been accustomed to modify other colloidal drug carriers (such as liposomes and polymeric nanoparticles), to enhance their physical and biological stability, and to permit them to focus on specific organs and cells (Saravanakumar et al. 2012). A list of hydrophobic drugs recently being delivered through polysaccharide-based nano formulations is summarized in Table 7.1.

7.4.6 POLYSACCHARIDE-MODIFIED LIPOSOMES

Liposomes, that have vesicular structures made of lipoid bilayers, are initial generation nanocarriers that are widely studied as vehicles for a broad range of medication due to the solubility of each hydrophilic and oleophilic drugs in the aqueous core and lipid bilayer. Liposomal formulations of DOX have already been approved by the US Food and Drug Administration (FDA) for the treatment of certain types of cancer, such as ovarian cancer (Torchilin 2005). In general, liposomes are coated with polysaccharides through simple surface assimilation of natural polysaccharides or

TABLE 7.1
Some Other Examples of Solubility/Bioavailability Enhancement through NPs Using Polysaccharide

SL. No.	Drug	Polysaccharide	Method of Preparation of NPs	References
1.	Perphenazine	dextran sulfate	millifluidics and bulk mixing	Dong and Hadinoto 2017
2.	Paclitaxel	chitosan	polystyrene nanospheres (PS) as templates	Jiang et al. 2017
3.	Fenofibrate and Itraconazole	fine sub-50µm lactose (GranuLac® 200)	fluidized bed coated with nanosilica,	Azad et al. 2016
4.	Curcumin	soy-soluble polysaccharides (SSPS)	core-shell complex nanoparticles	Chen et al. 2016
5.	Griseofulvin	pullulan films, with xanthan gum (XG)	wet-stirred media milling (WSMM)	Krull et al. 2016
6.	Camptothecin	cationic aminocellulose	Micelles	Songsurang et al. 2015
7.	Naproxen	HPMC	precipitation-ultrasonication	Mishra et al. 2015
8.	Propofol	modified alginate (carboxylic group of alginate is grafted to octanol, Alg-C8)	Encapsulated nanoparticles	Najafabadi et al. 2015
9.	Amorphous ibuprofen	cationic dextran	controlled electrostatic self-assembly	Abioye et al. 2015
10.	Ciprofloxacin	dextran sulfate (DXT) and carrageenan	electrostatic complexation	Cheow et al. 2015
11.	Itraconazole	dextran sulfate as the polyelectrolyte and hydroxypropylmethylcellulose as the surface stabilizer	drug-polyelectrolyte complexation and pH-shift precipitation	Cheow et al. 2014
12.	Near-infrared fluorescent dye IR-775 chloride with Lactoferrin	β-cyclodextrin (β-CD)	drug polymer conjugation via the heterobifunctional polyethyleneglycol (PEG) linker NHS-PEG-MAL	Ye et al. 2013
13.	Aripiprazole	hydroxypropylcellulose (HPC)	coprecipitation and nanomilling	Abdelbary et al. 2014
14.	Carvedilol	chitosan	spherical nanosilica matrix	Sun et al. 2013

integration (anchoring) of hydrophobized polysaccharides into the liposomal bilayer. Liposomes, coated using the adsorption methodology, were found to be thermodynamically unstable as a result of the easy, natural process of the polysaccharides from the liposomal surface. In distinction, polysaccharide-anchored liposomes, prepared using hydrophobized polysaccharides, showed improved stability against harsh conditions. Wang et al. demonstrated that cholesterol succinyl (CS)-anchored liposomes exhibited better physical storage stability and sustained drug release characteristics than blank or CS-coated liposomes obtained through electrostatic interactions (Wang et al. 2010).

In another study, the improved stability of O-palmitoyl scleraglucan-anchored liposomes loaded with leuprolide in stimulated gastric fluid (SGF) or bile acid solution was demonstrated (Zhang et al. 2004).

7.4.7 POLYSACCHARIDE-MODIFIED POLYMERIC NANOPARTICLES

Many colloidal polymeric nanoparticles, ready from artificial polymers like PLA and PLGA, are physically or chemically changed with polysaccharides to confer the attributes of bioadhesivity, targetability, and extended circulatory ability to the nanoparticles. Varied ways are adopted to switch polysaccharides on the surfaces of polymeric nanoparticles, together with emulsion-solvent evaporation, nanoprecipitation, and spray drying (Sun et al. 2013). For instance, Guo and Gemeinhart prepared CS-coated PLGA nanoparticles using an emulsion-solvent evaporation methodology and studied the adsorption mechanism of CS onto PLGA nanoparticles (Guo and Gemeinhart 2008). They found that a rise in the concentration of CS resulted in associate augmented particle size and zeta potential as a result of higher CS adsorption. They attributed the adsorption of CS onto the PLGA nanoparticles to the cationic nature and microporous non-uniform surface of the PLGA nanoparticles. With the aid of chemically modified HA-PLGA, nanoparticles demonstrated higher colloidal stability and specific uptake in CD44 expressing human carcinoma cells than the unadapted nanoparticles. Nanoparticles supported poly(methyl methacrylate) have conjointly been changed with polysaccharides like HEPA and dextran to decrease the uptake of the particles by the mononuclear phagocyte system (MPS) (Passirani et al. 1998).

7.5 CONCLUSION AND FUTURE PROSPECTS

In the last decade, there has been a great deal of interest in the use of polysaccharides, as they show variability and versatility, due to their complex structure, which is difficult to replicate with synthetic polymers. Thus, inherent polysaccharides and their derivatives have emerged in the last few years as one of the most used biomaterials in the field of nanomedicine, especially as carriers to be used in the preparation of nanoparticulate drug delivery systems, which may lead to an increase in the solubility of low soluble drugs. As reviewed in this chapter, a wide diversity of preparation methods for the nanoparticles has been established, and three features have marked the progress of these methods: the need for less toxic agents, simplification of the procedures, and optimization to improve yield and entrapment efficiency. Now it is possible to choose the best method of preparation and the best suitable polymer to accomplish an efficient encapsulation of the drug, taking into account the drug features in the selection. As manifested in various studies, simple ionic complexation of mucoadhesive polysaccharides such as chitosan with fragile proteins and peptides can be used to obtain nanosized formulations that have amplified *in vivo* residence times with added ability to protect their payloads from degradation and enhance absorption across the epithelial barrier. Similarly, hydrophobic drugs, including anticancer drugs, have been successfully delivered to targeted sites such as tumor tissues using various self-assembled amphiphilic polysaccharide nanoparticles via the Enhanced Permeation and Retention (EPR) effect. Nanoparticles based on polysaccharides with target-specific properties have been shown to passively target tumor tissue and effectively deliver their therapeutic payloads intracellularly through receptor-mediated endocytosis.

In addition, coating other colloidal drug carriers using polysaccharides has been shown to enhance the *in vivo* circulation half-life of these drug carriers and to improve their targeting efficacy. As time goes on, more polysaccharide-based nanoparticles emerge, which greatly enriches the versatility of nanoparticle carrier agents in terms of category and function. Deeper studies, such as the assessment of interaction between cells, tissues, and organs, as well as how the administration of these systems can affect metabolism, need to be carried out. In fact, more and more nanoparticle systems are emerging and these necessary studies will be focused on in the near future, completing the evaluation of these hopeful polysaccharide-based nano systems.

REFERENCES

Abdelbary, A.A., Li, X., and El-Nabarawi, M. 2014. Comparison of nanomilling and coprecipitation on the enhancement of *in vitro* dissolution rate of poorly water-soluble model drug aripiprazole. *Pharm Dev Technol* 19: 491–500.

Abioye, A.O. and Kola-Mustapha, A. 2015. Controlled electrostatic self-assembly of delivery tool for poorly soluble drugs. *Pharm Res* 32: 2110–31.

Allison, D.D. and Grande-Allen, K.J. 2006. Hyaluronan: A powerful tissue engineering tool. *Tissue Eng* 12: 2131–40.

Alonso-Sande, M., Cuna, M., and Remunan-Lopez, C. 2006. Formation of new glucomannan– chitosan nanoparticles and study of their ability to associate and deliver proteins. *Macromolecules* 39: 4152–8.

Amidi, M., Romeijn, S.G., Borchard, G. et al. 2006. Preparation and characterization of protein-loaded N-trimethyl chitosan nanoparticles as nasal delivery system. *J Control Release* 111: 107–16.

Azad, M., Moreno, J., Bilgili, E. et al. 2016. Fast dissolution of poorly water soluble drugs from fluidized bed coated nanocomposites: Impact of carrier size. *Int J Pharm* 513: 319–31.

Bae, H., Ahari, A.F., and Shin, H. 2011. Cell-laden microengineered pullulan methacrylate hydrogels promote cell proliferation and 3D cluster formation. *Soft Matter* 7: 1903–11.

Balazs E.A. 2004. Viscoelastic properties of hyaluronan and its therapeutics use. In: H.G. Garg and C.A. Hales (Eds.), *Chemistry and Biology of Hyaluronan*, pp. 415–455. Amsterdam: Elsevier.

Barbucci, R., Pasqui, D., Favaloro, R. 2008. A thixotropic hydrogel from chemically cross-linked guar gum: Synthesis, characterization and rheological behaviour. *Carbohydr Res* 343: 3058–65.

Bodnar, M., Hartmann, J.F., and Borbely, J. 2005a. Nanoparticles from chitosan. *Macromol Symp* 227: 321–26.

Bodnar, M., Hartmann, J.F., and Borbely, J. 2005b. Preparation and characterization of chitosanbased nanoparticles. *Biomacromolecules* 6: 2521–27.

Burdick, J.A. and Prestwich, G.D. 2011. Hyaluronic acid hydrogels for biomedical applications. *Adv Mater* 23: H41–H56.

Cafaggi, S., Russo, E., Stefani, R. et al. 2011. Preparation, characterisation and preliminary antitumour activity evaluation of a novel nanoparticulate system based on a cisplatin-hyaluronate complex and N-trimethyl chitosan. *Invest New Drugs* 29: 443–55.

Calvo, P., Remunan Lopez, C., VilaJato, J.L. et al. 1997a. Novel hydrophilic chitosanpolyethyleneoxide nanoparticles as protein carriers. *J Appl Polym Sci* 63: 125–32.

Calvo, P., Remunan Lopez, C., VilaJato, J.L. et al. 1997b. Chitosan and chitosan ethylene oxide propylene oxide block copolymer nanoparticles as novel carriers for proteins and vaccines. *Pharm Res* 14: 1431–6.

Carafa, M., Marianecci, C., Annibaldi, V. 2006. Novel o-palmitoyl scleroglucan-coated liposomes as drug carriers: Development, characterization and interaction with leuprolide. *Int Pharm* 325: 155–62.

Chan, J.M., Valencia, P.M., Zhang, L. et al. 2010. Polymeric nanoparticles for drug delivery. In: S. Grobmyer and B. Moudgil (Eds.), *Cancer Nanotechnology*, pp. 163–175. New York: Humana Press.

Chen, F.P., Ou, S.Y., and Tang, C.H. 2016. Core-shell soy protein-soy polysaccharide complex (Nano) particles as carriers for improved stability and sustained release of curcumin. *J Agric Food Chem* 64: 5053–9.

Chen, Y., Mohanraj, V.J., and Parkin, J.E. 2003. Chitosan-dextran sulfate nanoparticles for delivery of an anti-angiogenesis peptide. *Lett Pept Sci* 10: 621–9.

Cheow, W.S., Kiew, T.Y., and Hadinoto, K. 2015 Amorphous nanodrugs prepared by complexation with polysaccharides: Carrageenan versus dextran sulfate. *Carbohydr Polym* 117: 549–58.

Cheow, W.S., Kiew, T.Y., and Yang, Y. 2014. Amorphization strategy affects the stability and supersaturation profile of amorphous drugnanoparticles. *Mol Pharm* 11: 1611–20.

Coviello, T., Matricardi, P., Marianecci, C. et al. 2007. Polysaccharide hydrogels for modified release formulations. *J Control Release* 119: 5–24.

Cui, Z.R. and Mumper, R.J. 2001. Chitosan-based nanoparticles for topical genetic immunization. *J Control Release* 75: 409–19.

Della, Valle., G., Buleon, A., Carreau, P.J et al. 1998. Relationship between structure and viscoelastic behavior of plasticized starch. *J Rheol* 42: 507–25.

Dong, B. and Hadinoto, K. 2017. Direct comparison between millifluidic and bulk-mixing platform in the synthesis of amorphous drug-polysaccharidenanoparticle complex. *Int J Pharm* 523: 42–51.

Du, J., Sun, R., and Zhang, S. 2004. Novel polyelectrolyte carboxymethyl konjac glucomannan–chitosan nanoparticles for drug delivery. *Macromol Rapid Commun* 25: 954–58.

Du, J., Sun, R., Zhang, S. et al. 2005. Novel polyelectrolyte carboxymethyl konjac glucomannan-chitosan nanoparticles for drug delivery. I. Physicochemical characterization of the carboxymethyl konjac gluco-mannan– chitosan nanoparticles. *Biopolymers* 78: 1–8.

Du, J., Zhang, S., Sun, R. et al. 2005. Novel polyelectrolytecarboxymethyl konjac glucomannan–chitosan nanoparticles for drug delivery. II. Release of albumin *in vitro*. *J Biomed Mater Res Part B-Appl Biomat* 72B: 299–304.

Gref, R., Rodrigues, J., and Couvreur, P. 2002. Polysaccharides grafted with polyesters: Novel amphiphilic copolymers for biomedical applications. *Macromolecules* 35: 9861–7.

Guo, C. and Gemeinhart, R.A. 2008. Understanding the adsorption mechanism of chitosan onto poly (lactide-co-glycolide) particles. Eur J Pharm Biopharm 70: 597–604.

Gurwitz, D. and Livshits, G. 2006. Personalized medicine Europe: Health, genes and society. *Eur J Hum Genet* 14: 376–80.

Heinze, T., Liebert, T., Heublein, B. et al. 2006. Functional polymers based on dextran. *Adv Polym Sci* 205: 199–291.

Hu, F.Q., Ren, G.F., and Yuan, H. 2006. Shell cross-linked stearic acid grafted chitosan oligosaccharide self-aggregated micelles for controlled release of paclitaxel. *Colloids Surf B* 50: 97–103.

Illum, L. 1998. Chitosan and its use as a pharmaceutical excipient. *Pharm Res* 15: 1326–31.

Jain, D. and Banerjee, R. 2008. Comparison of ciprofloxacin hydrochloride-loaded protein, lipid, and chitosan nanoparticles for drug delivery. *J Biomed Mater Res* 86B: 105–12.

Jiang, J., Liu, Y., Wu, C. et al. 2017. Development of drug-loaded chitosan hollownanoparticlesfor delivery of paclitaxel to human lung cancer A549 cells. Drug Dev Ind Pharm 43: 1304–13.

Jog, R. and Burgess, D.J. 2016. Pharmaceutical amorphous nanoparticles. *J Pharm Sci* 106: 39–65

Kang, J., Lee, M.S., Copland, J.A. et al. 2008. Combinatorial selection of a single stranded DNA thioaptamer targeting TGF-beta1 protein. *Bioorg Med Chem Lett* 18: 1835–9.

Kim, D.G., Jeong, Y.I., Choi, C. et al. 2006. Retinolencapsulated low molecular water-soluble chitosan nanoparticles. *Int J Pharm* 319: 130–8.

Kim, T.H., Jiang, H.L., Jere, D. et al. 2007. Chemical modification of chitosan as a gene carrier *in vitro* and *in vivo*. *Prog Polym Sci* 32: 726–53.

Kratz, F. 2008. Albumin as a drug carrier: Design of prodrugs, drug conjugates and nanoparticles. *J Control Release* 132: 171–83.

Krull, S.M., Ma, Z., Li, M. 2016. Preparation and characterization of fast dissolving pullulan films containing BCS class II drugnanoparticlesfor bioavailability enhancement. *Drug Dev Ind Pharm*42: 1073–85.

Kubota, N. and Eeguchi, Y. 1997. Facile preparation of water-soluble n-acetylated chitosan and molecular weight dependence of its water-solubility. *Polym J* 29: 123–7.

Leathers, T.D. 2003. Biotechnological production and applications of pullulan. *Appl Microbiol Biotechnol* 62: 468–73.

Lee, K.Y., Jo, W.H., Kwon, I.C. et al. 1998. Structural determination and interior polarity of self-aggregates prepared from deoxycholic acid-modified chitosan in water. *Macromolecules* 31: 378–83.

Lee, K.Y, Kim, J.H., Kwon, I.C. et al. 2000. Self-aggregates of deoxycholic acid modified chitosan as a novel carrier of Adriamycin. *Colloid Polym Sci* 278: 1216–9.

Lee, K.Y., Kwon, I.C., Kim, Y.H. et al. 1998. Preparation of chitosan self-aggregates as a gene delivery system. *J Control Release* 51: 213–20.

Lee, P.W., Peng, S.F., Su, C.J. et al. 2008. The use of biodegradable polymeric nanoparticles in combination with a low-pressure gene gun for transdermal DNA delivery. *Biomaterials* 29: 742–51.

Lehoux, J.G. and de Puis, G. 2007. Recovery of chitosan from aqueous acidic solutions by salting-out: Part 1. use of inorganic salts. *Carbohydr Polym* 68: 295–304.

Lemarchand, C., Couvreur, P., Besnard, M. et al. 2003a. Novel polyester polysaccharide nanoparticles. *Pharm Res* 20: 1284–92.

Lemarchand, C., Couvreur, P., Vauthier, C. et al. 2003b. Study of emulsion stabilization by graft copolymers using the optical analyzer Turbiscan. *Int J Pharm* 254: 77–82.

Letchford, K. and Burt, H. 2007. A review of the formation and classification of amphiphilic block copolymer nanoparticulate structures: Micelles, nanospheres, nanocapsules and polymersomes. *Eur J Pharm Biopharm* 65: 259–69.

Li, T., Shi, X.W., Du, Y.M. et al. 2007. Quaternized chitosan/alginate nanoparticles for protein delivery. *J Biomed Mater Res* 83A: 383–90.

Li, Y., Nagira, T. and Tsuchiya, T. 2006. The effect of hyaluronic acid on insulin secretion in HIT-T15 cells through the enhancement of gap-junctional intercellular communications. *Biomaterials* 27: 1437–43.

Lin, Y.H, Chung, C.K, Chen, C.T. et al. 2005. Preparation of nanoparticles composed of chitosan/poly-gamma-glutamic acid and evaluation of their permeability through Caco-2 cells. *Biomacromolecules* 6: 1104–12.

Liu, H., Chen, B., Mao, Z.W. et al. 2007. Chitosan nanoparticles for loading of toothpaste actives and adhesion on tooth analogs. *J Appl Polym Sci* 106: 4248–56.

Liu, L., Fishman, M.L., Kost, J. et al. 2003. Pectin-based systems for colon-specific drug delivery via oral route. *Biomaterials* 24: 3333–43.

Liu, Z., Jiao, Y., Wang, Y. et al. 2008. Polysaccharides-based nanoparticles as drug delivery systems. *Adv Drug Deliv Rev* 60: 1650–62.

Liu, Z.H, Jiao, Y.P., and Liu, F. 2007. Heparin/chitosan nanoparticle carriers prepared by polyelectrolyte complexation. *J Biomed Mater Res* 83A: 806–12.

Lu, B., Xiong, S.B., and Yang, H. 2006a. Mitoxantrone-loaded BSA nanospheres and chitosan nanospheres for local injection against breast cancer and its lymph node metastases-I: formulation and *in vitro* characterization. *Int J Pharm* 307: 168–74.

Lu, B., Xiong, S.B., Yang, H. et al. 2006b. Mitoxantrone-loaded BSA nanospheres and chitosan nanospheres for local injection against breast cancer and its lymph node metastases-II: tissue distribution and pharmacodynamics. *Int J Pharm* 307: 175–81.

Mao, S., Sun, W. and Kissel, T. 2010. Chitosan-based formulations for delivery of DNA and siRNA. *Adv Drug Deliv Rev* 62: 12–27.

Martínez, A., Fernández, A., Pérez, E. et al. 2012. Polysaccharide-based nanoparticles for controlled release formulations. In: A. A. Hashim (Ed.), *Delivery of Nanoparticles*, pp. 185–222. Croatia: InTech Europe.

Masaoka, Y., Tanaka, Y., Kataoka, M. et al. 2006. Site of drug absorption after oral administration: Assessment of membrane permeability and luminal concentration of drugs in each segment of gastrointestinal tract. *European J Pharm Sci* 29: 240–50.

Mazumder, S., Dewangan, A.K., and Pavurala, N. 2017. Enhanced dissolution of poorly soluble antiviral drugs from nanoparticles of cellulose acetate based solid dispersion matrices. *Asian J Pharm Sci* 12: 532–41.

Mendichi, R. and Soltes, L. 2002. Hyaluronan molecular weight and polydispersity in some commercial intra-articular injectable preparations and in synovial fluid. *Inflamm Res* 51: 115–16.

Misaki, A., Torii, M., Sawai, T. et al. 1980. Structure of the dextran of Leuconostoc mesenteroides B-1355. *Carbohydr Res* 84: 273–85.

Mishra, B., Sahoo, J., and Dixit, P.K. 2015. Formulation and process optimization of naproxen nanosuspensions stabilized by hydroxy propyl methyl cellulose. *Carbohydr Polym* 127: 300–8.

Moghimi, S.M., Hunter, A.C., and Murray, J.C. 2005. Nanomedicine: Current status and future prospects. *FASEB J* 19: 311–30.

Monjazeb, A.M., Ayala, D., Jensen, C. et al. 2012. A phase I dose escalation study of hypo fractionated IMRT field-in-field boost for newly diagnosed glioblastoma multiforme. *Int J Radiat Oncol Biol Phys* 82: 743–48.

Morris, G., Kök, S., Harding, S., and Adams, G. 2010. Polysaccharide drug delivery systems based on pectin and chitosan. *Biotechnol Genet EngRev* 27: 257–84.

Muzzarelli, R.A.A. 2009. Genipin-crosslinked chitosan hydrogels as biomedical and pharmaceutical aids. *Carbohydr Polym* 77: 1–9.

Nair, L.S. and Laurencin, C.T. 2007. Biodegradable polymers as biomaterial. *Prog Polym Sci* 6: 762–98.

Najafabadi, A.H., Azodi-Deilami, S., Abdouss, M. et al. 2015. Synthesis and evaluation of hydroponically alginate nanoparticles as novel carrier for intravenous delivery of propofol. *J Mater Sci Mater Med* 26: 145.

Namazi, H. and Dadkhah, A. 2008. Surface modification of starch nanocrystals through ring opening polymerization of epsilon-caprolactone and investigation of their microstructures. *J Appl Polym Sci* 110: 2405–12.

Oh, E.J., Park, K., and Kim, K.S. 2010. Target specific and long-acting delivery of protein, peptide, and nucleotide therapeutics using hyaluronic acid derivatives. *J Control Release* 141: 2–12.

Opanasopit, P., Ngawhirunpat, T., Rojanarata, T. et al. 2007. Camptothecin-incorporating N-phthaloylchitosan-g-mPEG self-assembly micellar system: effect of degree of deacetylation. *Colloids Surf B* 60: 117–24.

Pandey, R. and Ahmad, Z. 2011. Nanomedicine and experimental tuberculosis: Facts, flaws, and future. Nanomedicine 7: 259–72.

Park, J.W., Choi, K.H., and Park, K.K. 1983. Acid-base equilibria and related properties of chitosan. *Bull Korean Chem Soc* 4: 68–72.

Passirani, C., Barratt, G., and Devissaguet, J.P. 1998. Long-circulating nanoparticles bearing heparin or dextran covalently bound to poly (methyl methacrylate). *Pharm Res* 15: 1046–50.

Rehm, B.H.A. 2009. *Alginates: Biology and Applications.* India: Springer.

Rekha, M.R. and Chandra, P.S. 2007. Pullulan as a promising biomaterial for biomedical applications: A perspective. *Trends Biomat Artif Org* 20: 116–21.

Rinaudo, M. 2006. Chitin and chitosan: Properties and applications. *Prog Polym Sci* 31: 603–32.

Rotureau, E., Leonard, M., Dellacherie, E. et al. 2004. Amphiphilic derivatives of dextran: Adsorption at air/water and oil/water interfaces. *J Colloid Interface Sci* 279: 68–77.

Sakamoto, J., Annapragad,a A., Decuzzi, P. et al. 2007. Antibiological barrier nanovector technology for cancer applications. 2007. *Expert Opin Drug Deliv* 4: 359–69.

Sandri, G., Bonferoni, M.C., Rossi, S. et al. 2007. Nanoparticles based on N-trimethylchitosan: Evaluation of absorption properties using in vitro (Caco-2 cells) and ex vivo (excised rat jejunum) models. *Eur J Pharm Biopharm* 65: 68–77.

Sant, V.P., Smith D., and Leroux, J.C. 2005. Enhancement of oral bioavailability of poorly water-soluble drugs by poly (ethylene glycol)-block-poly(alkyl acrylate-co-methacrylic acid) self assemblies. *J Control Release* 104: 289–300.

Saravanakumar, G., Jo, D.G., and Park, J.H. 2012. Polysaccharide-based nanoparticles: A versatile platform for drug delivery and biomedical imaging. *Curr Med Chem* 19: 3212–29.

Sarmah, J.K., Mahanta, R., Bhattacharjee, S.K.2011. Controlled release of tamoxifen citrate encapsulated in cross-linked guar gum nanoparticles. *Int J BiolMacromol* 49: 390–6.

Sarmento, B., Ferreira, D., Veiga, F. et al. 2006. Characterization of insulin-loaded alginate nanoparticles produced by ionotropic pre-gelation through DSC and FTIR studies. *Carbohydr Polym* 66: 1–7.

Sarmento, B., Ferreira, D.C., and Jorgensen, L. 2007. Probing insulin's secondary structure after entrapment into alginate/chitosan nanoparticles. *Eur J Pharm Biopharm* 65: 10–17.

Sarmento, B., Martins, S., Ribeiro, A. et al. 2006. Development and comparison of different nanoparticulate polyelectrolyte complexes as insulin carriers. *Int J Pept Res Ther* 12: 131–38.

Sarmento, B., Ribeiro, A., Veiga, F. et al. 2006. Development and characterization of new insulin containing polysaccharide nanoparticles. *Colloids Surf B* 53: 193–202.

Sinha, V.R. and Kumria, R. 2001. Polysaccharides in colon-specific drug delivery. *Int J Pharm* 224: 19–38.

Songsurang, K., Siraleartmukul, K., and Muangsin, N. 2015. Mucoadhesive drug carrier based on functional-modified cellulose as poorly water-soluble drug delivery system. *J Microencapsul* 32: 450–9.

Soumya, R.S., Ghosh, S. and Abraham, E.T. 2010. Preparation and characterization of guar gum nanoparticles. *Int J Biol Macromol* 46: 267–9.

Stoilova, O., Koseva, N., Manolova, N. et al. 1999. Polyelectrolyte complex between chitosan and poly (2-acryloylamido-2-methylpropanesulfonic acid). *Polym Bull* 43: 67–73.

Sujata, V.B. 2002. *Biopolymers.* India: Springer.

Sun, L., Wang, Y., Jiang, T. et al. 2013. Novel chitosan-functionalized spherical nanosilica matrix as an oral sustained drug delivery system for poorly water-soluble drug carvedilol. *ACS Appl Mater Interfaces* 5: 103–13.

Tan, W.B., Jiang, S., and Zhang, Y. 2007. Quantum-dot based nanoparticles for targeted silencing of HER2/neu gene via RNA interference. *Biomaterials* 28: 1565–71.

Terbojevich, M. and Muzzarelli, R.A.A. 2000. Chitosan. In: G.O. Phillips and P.A. Williams (Eds.), *Handbook of Hydrocolloids,* 367–78. Cambridge: Woodhead Publishing.

Thanou, M., Florea, B.I., Geldof, M. et al. 2002. Quaternized chitosan oligomers as novel gene delivery vectors in epithelial cell lines. *Biomaterials* 23: 153–9.

Thebaud, N.B., Pierron, D., Bareille, R. et al. 2007. Human endothelial progenitor cell attachment to polysaccharide-based hydrogels: A pre-requisite for vascular tissue engineering. *J Mater Sci Mater Med* 18: 339–45.

Tibbals, H.F. 2012. *Medical Nanotechnology and Nanomedicine.* Boca Raton, FL: CRC Press.

Tiraferri, A, Chen, KL, Sethi, R, and Elimelech, M. 2008. Reduced aggregation and sedimentation of zero-valent iron nanoparticles in the presence of guar gum. *J Colloid Interface Sci* 324: 71–9.

Tiyaboonchai, W. and Limpeanchob, N. 2007. Formulation and characterization of amphotericin B-chitosan-dextran sulfate nanoparticles. *Int J Pharm* 329: 142–9.

Tombs, M.P. and Harding, S.E. 1998. *An Introduction to Polysaccharide Biotechnology*. London: Taylor & Francis.

Torchilin, V.P. 2005. Recent advances with liposomes as pharmaceutical carriers. *Nat Rev Drug Discov* 4: 145–60.

Varum, K.M., Anthonsen, M.W., Grasdalen, H. et al. 1991a. Determination of the degree of N-acetylation and distribution of N-acetyl groups in partially N-deacteylated chitins (chitosans) by high-field NMR spectroscopy. *Carbohydrate Res* 211: 17–23.

Varum, K.M., Anthonsen, M.W., Grasdalen, H. et al. 1991b. 13C NMR studies of the acetylation sequences in partially N-deacteylated chitins (chitosans). *Carbohydrate Res* 217: 19–27.

Varum, K.M., Ottoy, M.H., and Smidsrod, O. 1994. Water-solubility of partially N-acetylated chitosans as a function of pH: Effect of chemical composition and depolymerisation. *Carbohydr Polym* 25: 65–70.

Wang, Y., Tu, S., Li, R. et al. 2010. Cholesterol succinyl chitosan anchored liposomes: Preparation, characterization, physical stability, and drug release behavior. Nanomedicine 6: 471–77.

Wang, Y.S., Jiang, Q., Liu, L.R. et al. 2007. The interaction between bovine serum albumin and the self-aggregated nanoparticles of cholesterol-modified O-carboxymethyl chitosan. *Polymer* 48: 4135–42.

Wang, Y.S., Liu, L.R., Jiang, Q. et al. 2007. Self-aggregated nanoparticles of cholesterol-modified chitosan conjugate as a novel carrier of epirubicin. *Eur Polym J* 43: 43–51.

Wei, X., Peixue, L., and Tianmin, Z. 2013. Polymeric micelles, a promising drug delivery system toenhance bioavailability of poorly water-soluble drugs. *J Drug Deliv* 2013: 1–15

Xu, Y.M., Du, Y.M., Huang, R.H. et al. 2003. Preparation and modification of N-(2hydroxyl) propyl-3-trimethyl ammonium chitosan chloride nanoparticle as a protein carrier. *Biomaterials* 24: 5015–22.

Yang, J.S., Xie, Y.J., and He, W. 2011. Research progress on chemical modification of alginate: A review. Carbohydr Polym 84: 33–9.

Yang, S.C., Ge, H.X., Hu, Y. et al. 2000. Formation of positively charged poly (butyl cyanoacrylate) nanoparticles stabilized with chitosan. *Colloid Polym Sci* 278: 285–92.

Ye, Y., Sun, Y., Zhao, H. et al. 2013. A novel lactoferrin-modified β-cyclodextrin nanocarrier for brain-targeting drug delivery. *Int J Pharm* 458: 110–7.

You, J.O. and Peng, C.A. 2004. Calcium-alginate nanoparticles formed by reverse microemulsion as gene carriers. *Macromol Symp* 219: 47–153.

Zahoor, A., Sharma, S., and Khuller, G.K. 2005. Inhalable alginate nanoparticles as antitubercular drug carriers against experimental tuberculosis. *Int J Antimicrob Agents* 26: 298–303.

Zhang, H., Oh, M., Allen, C. et al. 2004. Monodisperse chitosan nanoparticles formucosal drug delivery. *Biomacromolecules* 5: 2461–68.

Zheng, Y., Monty, J., and Linhardt, R.J. 2015. Polysaccharide-based nanocomposites and their applications. *Carbohydrate Res* 405: 23–32.

Zheng, Y.L., Wu, Y., Yang, W.L. et al. 2006. Preparation, characterization, and drug release *in vitro* of chitosan-glycyrrhetic acid nanoparticles. *J Pharm Sci* 95: 181–91.

Zheng, Y.L., Yang, W., Wang, C.C. et al. 2007. Nanoparticles based on the complex of chitosan and polyaspartic acid sodium salt: Preparation, characterization and the use for 5-fluorouracil delivery. *Eur J Pharm Biopharm* 67: 621–31.

Zhi, J., Wang, Y.J., Luo, G.S. 2005. Adsorption of diuretic furosemide onto chitosan nanoparticles prepared with a water-in-oil nanoemulsion system. *React Funct Polym* 65: 249–57.

8 Development of Nanoparticles from Grafted Natural Polysaccharides for Drug Delivery

Anupam Roy, Sreyajit Saha, and Animesh Ghosh

CONTENTS

8.1 INTRODUCTION

Nanotechnology deals with nanosized materials offering several application utilities (Roy et al. 2015). Large surface-to-volume ratio (LSVR) provides unique properties to nanoparticles compared with macro counterparts, which widely varies with its counter bulk part. Nanoparticles become more reactive due to their LSVR and find applications in different fields (Roy et al. 2013). Application of nanotechnology in the fields of medicine, food, materials, energy and electronics, and environment and manufacturing has contributed significantly to the betterment of human civilization. Nanotechnological application provides solutions to several unsolved problems in the mentioned fields. In the perspective of medicine, most of the active ingredients face problems of solubility, bioavailability, reactivity, stability, target-specific delivery, and release. Processing parameters, i.e., temperature and pressure, may create negative impacts on the activity of the drugs while preparing them in different deliverable forms (such as capsules or gel). Even after packaging, drugs may suffer from issues of stability (i.e., thermal, oxidative) during handling and storage. Most interestingly, drugs which are basic or acidic in nature, or prone to enzymatic degradation, suffer in oral delivery. A wide variation of pH and the presence of myriad enzymes in the intestine provide challenges for oral delivery, and they become unavailable during target-specific delivery and release (Roy et al. 2016).

Bioactive ingredients or drugs are often delivered through a carrier matrix. The stability, target specific release, sustained release, and bioavailability of the drugs are solely dependent on the characteristics of the carrier matrix. This matrix is intended to provide stability for the active drugs from environmental conditions and protect it from thermal and oxidative damage. The carrier matrix is also intended to enhance the solubility, bioavailability, target-specific delivery, and release of the active drugs in the harsh operating conditions of the intestinal tract. Further, if the drugs have a high pH level or are easily degraded by enzymatic action they also need a special carrier system for intestinal delivery (Florek et al. 2017). Thus, the carrier has a significant role to fulfil in the activity of the drugs. The carrier often comes with inherent bioactivity, i.e., mucoadhesion, target specific reach, and an inflammatory response, which provides a positive influence on the activity of the drugs. The carrier prevents reduction of the drug's efficacy by providing adverse interactions with the inhibitors of its absorption (Garti 2008).

The drug release pattern from the carrier matrix is crucial for carrying out the required activity in the varying conditions. Both fast or slow/sustained release bears importance in application of its specific use (Omenn et al. 1996). Overloading of the drug molecules into the transport system may also show a negative impact, yielding undesirable excursions in plasma and tissue concentration (Faulks et al. 2008).The degree of release and bioavailability of the drugs are also correlated with the size and shape of the carrier matrix. Reactivity of the material is generally increased with an increase in the surface area. This increased surface area may be achieved with different nanoparticle-based carrier materials (Florek et al. 2017).

Polysaccharides are complex carbohydrates with long chains of monosaccharide units bound together by glyosidic linkages. They offer linear to branched structures. In the perspective of the human digestive system, polysaccharides exist in both digestible (i.e., starch, dextrin, and glycogen) and non-digestible form (i.e., cellulose, hemicelluloses, polydextrose, inulin, etc.). The structure of most commonly used polysaccharides in drug delivery systems are shown in Figure 8.1.

Non-digestible carbohydrates offer nominal changes in the intestinal tract. They absorb a good quantity of water, pass through the gut in an intact form, and maintain bowel regularity. They are sometimes fermentable in the colon and help to promote the growth of beneficial intestinal bacteria. Most of the polysaccharides are soluble in water and can act as carriers for insoluble drugs. Even more, they also offer slow digestion. These properties make polysaccharides an effective carrier agent for targeted delivery (Shibakami et al. 2015; Corona-Hernandez et al. 2013). The tissue-specific attraction features of polysaccharides makes them a unique carrier for tissue-specific drugs delivery (Freshour et al. 1996). Polysaccharides are mostly biocompatible and offer quick biodegradability. Some selected polysaccharides inherently offer bioactivity. Mucoadhesion properties of polysaccharides are a common feature that plays a crucial role in enhancing the bioavailability of poorly adsorbed drugs (Uccello-Barretta et al. 2013; Chayed and Winnik 2007). They also reduce the inflammatory response and can be well formulated for preventive treatments (Zhang et al. 2018; Paiva et al. 2011; Chen et al. 2015). Functional groups of the polysaccharide backbone make it easy to perform chemical modification. This offers a wide range of structurally unique polysaccharide nanoscale entities (Saravanakumar et al. 2012; Fathi et al. 2014) providing unique features in drug delivery. These polysaccharide-based nanoscale entities can be obtained by covalent crosslinking, ionic crosslinking, polyelectrolyte complex, and the self-assembly of hydrophobically modification of the polysaccharides (Liu et al. 2008). In graft polymerization, tailor-made specifications of natural polysaccharides are achieved imparting a variety of functional groups to the polymer backbone. This provides polysaccharides' unique structure-function relationship with added features in the delivery and controlled release of the drug.

The current chapter is an attempt to give a systematic review of nanoparticles from grafted polysaccharides with applications in a nanoscale drug delivery matrix. Here efforts have been made to introduce the latest developments in the field. Apart from use, the development strategies of polysaccharide-based nanoparticles have also been well addressed making it more attractive from a researcher's viewpoint.

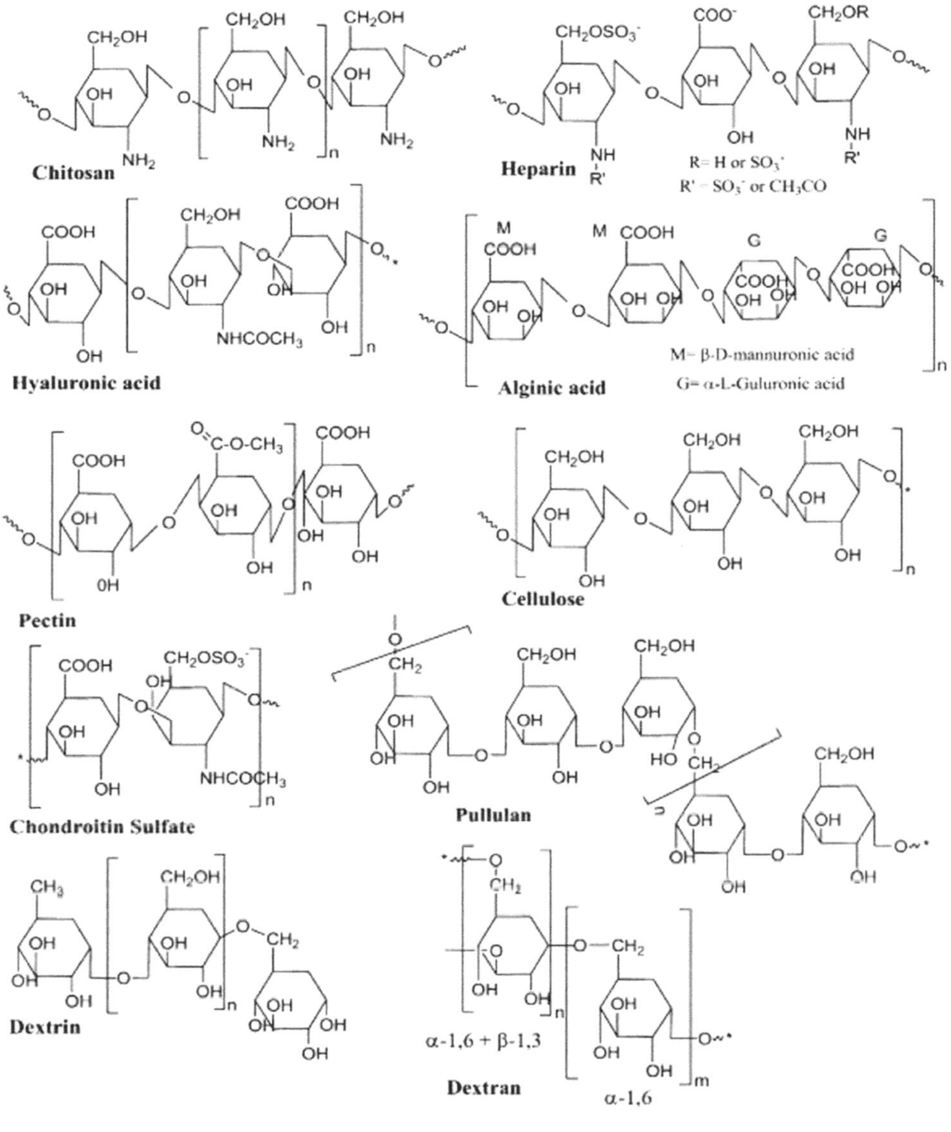

FIGURE 8.1 The structure of most commonly used polysaccharides in drug delivery systems. (Reprinted from *Mater Sci Eng C* 68, Debele, T.A., Mekuria, S.L., and Tsai, H.C. Polysaccharide-based nanogels in the drug delivery system: Application as the carrier of pharmaceutical agents, 964-81, Copyright 2016, with permission from Elsevier.)

8.2 IMPORTANCE OF NATURAL POLYSACCHARIDE GRAFTING

A drug delivery matrix should protect the drugs from the harsh environment. This environment is either of drug handling and storage or of the gastrointestinal tract. In drug handling and storage, thermal stability is crucial as it reduces the efficacy of the drugs. In the intestinal tract, the activity of the drugs is reduced due to a wide pH variation and enzymatic action. In most cases, the insoluble or sparingly soluble nature of the drugs influences functional activity. Sustained and targeted delivery is also important in accordance with the recent needs of drug delivery.

Natural polysaccharides are a recent research interest in drug delivery. Polar functional groups in natural polysaccharides come with a high molecular weight and a relatively rigid backbone. They directly impart the physical and chemical properties of the natural polysaccharides. Natural polysaccharides are stable to a high temp (~200°C). They also offer high melting and softening temperatures and high cohesive forces of interaction. They offer the unique properties of providing biodegradability, bioavailability, solubility, stability, functional activity, sustained, and target-specific drug release.

Individual natural polysaccharides comes with a set of properties that makes them unique in drug delivery. However, improvements in the natural polysaccharides properties are also important in gaining the desired drug-specific output. In some cases multiple functional properties (like sustained and target-specific drug release) are not obtained from a single natural polymer. Thus, successful modifications in the natural polymer backbone are important to obtain the desired characteristics.

Natural polysaccharide grafting is a method where monomers of other polymers are covalently bonded onto the existing polymer chain (Bhattacharya and Misra 2004). It improves the structure-function relationship of natural polysaccharides by imparting a variety of functional groups onto the backbone. The presence of hydroxyl groups in the natural polysaccharides makes it easy to perform structural modifications.

8.3 NATURAL POLYSACCHARIDE GRAFTING AND NANOPARTICLE FORMATION

Material that is nanosized can either be achieved by striping down the large entity or by assembling molecules and atoms to achieve supramolecular architectures (Zhang 2003). When large scale entities are broken down to achieve the nanosized objects it is called a top-down approach. In an opposite approach, smaller building blocks of structural units re-associate by chemical and structural compatibility to form supramolecular architecture by weak or covalent interactions. This approach is generally termed as a bottom up method of nanoparticle synthesis. Bottom-up approaches form nanosized organized structures or patterns from spontaneous re-association of the disordered system of preexisting components (Whitesides and Boncheva 2002). In between bottom up and top down, an intermediate approach is also used for nanoparticle synthesis where both the mentioned strategies are used to form a bulk nano-structured solid. These strategies are shown in Figure 8.2.

The concept of grafting allows structural modification on the primary polymer backbone. This is also true for the case of natural polysaccharides. This modification allows generation of active sites on the natural polysaccharide backbone which further facilitates addition of another polymer monomer. Natural polysaccharides have a specific structure with an exclusive shape and size. This shape and size of the natural polysaccharides is built in accordance to their function in the host system. Now, incorporation of the additional polysaccharide monomer will offer a change in the native structure of the natural polysaccharides, and will generate entities with different structures. In the perspective of drug delivery, development of the supramolecular entity maintaining the inherent functional properties of is much needed. The tailor-made synthesis thus focuses on developing a natural polysaccharide nanoentity effective for drug delivery.

8.4 TECHNIQUES OF NATURAL POLYSACCHARIDE GRAFTING

Natural polysaccharide grafting is a technique by which a variety of functional groups are imparted into the polysaccharide backbone to graft single or multiple polysaccharide monomers. Natural polysaccharides contain polar functional groups. They also come with a high molecular weight and relatively rigid backbone which directly contributes to the physical and chemical properties of the polysaccharides. Polysaccharides can withstand a wider range of temperatures and offer high glass transition (T_g) and softening temperatures. But their stiff backbone makes

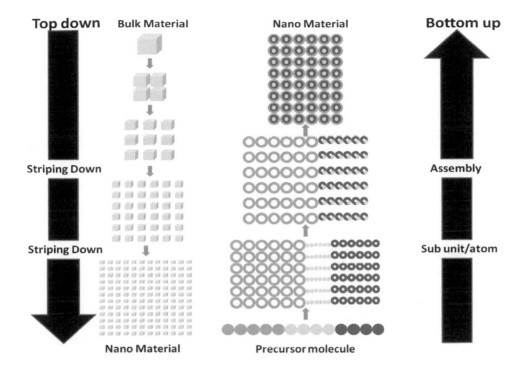

FIGURE 8.2 Top-down, intermediate, and bottom-up approaches to making bulk nanostructured solids.

polysaccharides brittle in nature with a high degree of crystallinity (Seidi et al. 2018). A high degree of crystallinity often makes polysaccharides insoluble in water and in common organic solvents. Thus, this produces a difficulty in polymer processing. Therefore, modification of the polysaccharides is often needed. Modification often delivers unique structural features providing suitability for drug delivery.

The process of natural polysaccharide grafting starts with the imparting of sufficient functional groups onto the existing polymer backbone. This facilitates the addition of other polymeric monomers in the main chain. The process is summarized in the following schematic diagram (Scheme 8.1). Imparting functional groups into the main polymeric chain is crucial for monomer grafting. Generation of free radicals or ions by chemical or physical means is important for polysaccharide grafting. The process of free radical polymerizations proceeds with initiation, propagation, chain transfer, and termination. Other strategies like grafting through living polymerization and enzymatic modification also play a crucial role and are mentioned herewith. The individual steps are also mentioned herewith.

8.4.1 GRAFTING THROUGH CHEMICAL USE

The chemical grafting method uses chemicals in the process of generating active sites on the existing polymer backbone (Surface Modification by Graft Polymerization 2009). The chemicals may generate free radicals or ions which specifically attack the polymer backbone. The chemicals responsible for generating free radicals are termed "initiators". These initiators or set of initiators produce free radicals from associated chemicals reactions. The generated free radicals react with the polymer backbone and propagate to generate active sites for the grafting of copolymers (monomers intended to be grafted over the polymer). The generated active side on the polymer backbone further results in monomer chain transfer. Finally, the reaction is terminated when the number of active sites is saturated within the monomer unit. Lewis acids, strong bases, and metal carbonyls are commonly used as a redox initiator in polymer grafting.

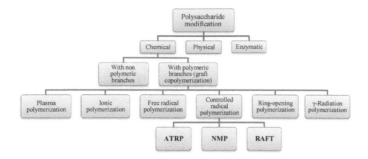

SCHEME 8.1 Different methods of polysaccharide modifications. (Reprinted from *Prog Polym Sci* 76, Seidia, F., Salimib, H., Shamsabadi, A.A., and Shabanian, M. Synthesis of hybrid materials using graft copolymerization on non-cellulosic polysaccharides via homogenous ATRP, 1–39, Copyright 2018, with permission from Elsevier.)

8.4.1.1 Grafting through Living Polymerization

There is a lack of control over chain transfer and termination during the chemical-based grafting of the polymer. Critical control over the initiation and chain transfer is necessary to gain the predetermined values of average molecular weight and narrow molecular weight distribution in polysaccharide-based graft polymerization (Cobo et al. 2015). To achieve this, numbers of initiator groups are set in accordance with the number of polymer chains that are to be produced. The polymerization will proceed until the active sites are filled within the monomer but the polymer chain ends remain active. These active sites will further facilitate polymerization once monomer units start getting added. This process is called living polymerization as this process retains the ability of polymerization or propagation leading to the attainment of maximum size.

Atom transfer radical polymerization (ATRP) also generates active sites over the polymer backbone. Inactive sites on the polymer backbone or dormant chains are initially capped with the halogen atom, which is then further transferred to metal complexes in lower oxidation states. This results in generation of transient growing radicals and complexes that further facilitate the monomer addition (Szwarc 1998; Krzysztof et al. 1997).

8.4.1.2 Grafting through Ionization or Radiation

Both the cation and anion have the potential to affect the structure of the polymer backbone and make it susceptible for copolymer addition (Scheme 8.2). The generation of ions is quite easy and different doses can be achieved through developed machineries. The radiation generates ions, which can be termed polymeric ions, that further react with the monomer and successfully add it into the

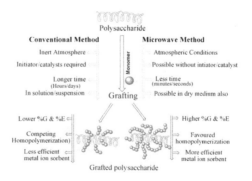

SCHEME 8.2 Schematic diagram of microwave-induced grafting of the polysaccharides. (Reprinted from *Prog Polym Sci* 37, Singh, V., Kumar, P., and Sanghi, R. Use of microwave irradiation in the grafting modification of the polysaccharides-A review, 340–64, Copyright 2012, with permission from Elsevier.)

polymer backbone (Vijan et al. 2012). Ionic grafting is a preferable choice as the reaction rate is quite high and can even be achieved at lower doses of radiation. Besides, the effective control over the numbers and lengths of the copolymers makes it unique for different applications X-rays, gamma rays, or accelerated electron beam radiations are mostly used for such purposes (Singh et al. 2012).

In a similar approach, plasma technology is also used for grafting. Plasma technology offers electron-induced excitation, ionization, and dissociation in the polymer entities. Energies cleave the bonds of the natural polymer and generate macromolecule radicals which in turn facilitate graft polymerization (Khelifa et al. 2016).

Other than high energy radiation (Huang et al. 1963), low energy radiation like UV and visible light can also generate the free radicals which in turn impart active sites in the polymer backbone and facilitate graft polymerization (Pillay et al. 2013).

8.4.2 Grafting through Physical Action

Polysaccharide grafting can also be achieved by physical treatments. Physical grafting does not require any additional crosslinking agents. Exposure to different temperature ranges, including thawing, freezing, freeze-thaw heating, and cold cycles, most often facilitate counterions on the polymer surface. Thus, physical grafting can be achieved through ionic interaction, crosslinking by crystallization, and hydrophobic modifications.

8.4.3 Grafting through Enzymatic Action

In some cases, enzymatic action facilitates the generation of active sites over the polymer backbone, which further facilitates the addition of different polymers. Grafting through enzymatic action requires milder reaction conditions and offers specific surface modifications in a non-destructive manner. Enzymes used for grafting are mostly biocompatible in nature, thus making them effective for drug delivery applications.

8.5 CARBOHYDRATE-BASED GRAFTED NANOSTRUCTURES

A compatible chemical nature as well as a biocompatible structure make polysaccharides a unique building block for drug delivery. In association with the inherent functional activity, the modification-friendly natural polysaccharide structures make it a unique medium for graft polymerization. Nanoparticles can be categorized as zero-dimensional, one-dimensional, two-dimensional, and three-dimensional (Cao and Wang 2011). Natural polysaccharide-specific nano-dimensional architectures are mentioned below. A summary list of the nanodimensional architectures from grafted natural polysaccharides intended for drug delivery are listed in Table 8.1.

8.5.1 Nanoparticles from Grafted Cellulose for Drug Delivery

The most abundant naturally occurring and renewable polysaccharide is cellulose. It is composed of thousands of linear chained D-glucose units linked by β-$(1\rightarrow4)$ linkage. Due an inability of digestion in the human digestive system, cellulose is not generally consumed by humans but used as animal fodder. Cellulose offers a linear ordered chain structure presenting semi crystalline behavior while having both crystalline and amorphous phases (Dima et al. 2017). Although it has hydrophilic hydroxyl groups, strong hydrogen bonding between cellulose chains makes it insoluble in water and other common solvents. The crystalline region in the cellulose structure comes from the hydrogen bonding in the cellulose chains and van der Waals forces between the glucose units (Chami and Robert 2013).

Cellulose-based graft polymerization offers a wide variety of nanostructures in drug delivery applications (Raus et al. 2011). The structure of the cellulose varies in accordance with structural changes. Microspheres or microfibers are commonly found in structures of cellulose which most

TABLE 8.1

Nanoparticles from Grafted Natural Polysaccharides

Natural Polymer	Existing form/Structure	Process of Grafting	Delivered Drug	Application	Structure	Reference
Cellulose	Microfibers	Free radical polymerization, and ATRP	Cephalexin	Controlled release of antibiotic	Microfibers	(Moghaddam et al. 2014)
	Nanofibril extracted bamboo cellulose	Free radical polymerization	Sodium salicylate	Universal carrier of drug	Nanofibril Aerogels	(Zhao et al. 2015)
	Microcrystal	ATRP	Betulinic acid	Delivery of anticancer drug	Nanosphere	(Dai and Si 2017)
	Ethyl cellulose	ATRP	Rifampicin	Delivery of antibiotic	Micelles	(D. Wang et al. 2011)
Starch	Native cassava starch	Free radical polymerization	Indomethacin	Delivery of anti-inflammatory drug	Amorphous particles of gelatinized starch	(Simi and Emilia Abraham 2007)
	Starch powder a	Atom transfer radical polymerization	Cephalexin	Delivery of antibiotic	Chain structure	(Avval et. al 2013)
	Potato, corn, and rice starches were	^{60}Co-gamma-radiation	Salicylic acid and theophylline	Universal carrier of drug	Nanoparticles	(Geresh et al. 2002)
	Maize Starch	Microwave irradiation	Aceclofenac	Delivery of anti-inflammatory drug	Microbead	(Setty et. al 2014)
Chitosan	Chitosan from crab shells with 88% of deacetylation	Physical grafting	Bovine serum albumin	Allowing proteins or drugs to be uniformly incorporated in the matrix structure with minimal or no denaturization.	Nanoparticle	(Bhattarai et al. 2006)
	Natural chitosan	Atom transfer radical polymerization	Plasmid DNA	Gene delivery	nanoparticles	(Choudhury et al. 2016)

(Continued)

TABLE 8.1 (CONTINUED)
Nanoparticles from Grafted Natural Polysaccharides

Natural Polymer	Existing form/Structure	Process of Grafting	Delivered Drug	Application	Structure	Reference
	Chitosan (viscosity = 200 CP, degree of deacetylation = 80%)	Atom transfer radical polymerization in association with ring-opening polymerization, and click chemistry	Doxorubicin	Temperature dependent drug delivery	micelles	(Yuan et al. 2011).
Dextran	Dextran from leuconostoc (MW 6 kDa),	Free radical polymerization	Therapeutic actives to the brain	to transport therapeutic actives to the brain	nanoparticles	(Toman et al. 2015).
	Dextran from Leuconostoc spp. (mol wt 6000 g/mol),	Atom transfer radical polymerization	Gene delivery	To offer lower cytotoxicity and better gene transfection yield	comb-shaped copolymers	(Wang et al. 2011).
	Dextran from Leuconostocmesenteroides (average molecular weights: 77,000),	Chemical method	Colonic drug	To be used as a colonic drug carrier	nanoparticles	(Jeong, et. al 2006).

often stays intact during graft polymerization. This structure remains unchanged or modifies after graft polymerization. Free radical polymerization and ATRP are commonly used in the preparation of cellulose-based grafted polymerization.

Moghaddam et al. used cellulose microfibers and further modified them via graft copolymerization of hydroxyethyl acrylate and acrylamide. They used both free radical polymerization and ATRP for the synthesis. The obtained grafted modified cellulose microfibers offered a controlled release of cephalexin drugs (Moghaddam et al. 2014).

In another study, cellulose nanofibrils were prepared from bamboo shoots. These cellulose nanofibrils were further modified and cellulose nanofibrils aerogels were prepared from polyethylenimine-grafted cellulose nanofibrils (CNFs-PEI). The free radical polymerization was used here to precede the synthesis. The developed nanofibrils can be used as versatile carrier for drug delivery. The developed material exhibited a high drug loading capability using water-soluble sodium salicylate as a model drug. The developed aerogels carrier also offered a pH and temperature dependent release of the loaded drug (Zhao et al. 2015).

The ATRP technique is also widely used to synthesize cellulose-grafted polymerization. Development of pH-responsive copolymers ethyl cellulose-graft- poly(2-(diethylamino) ethyl methacrylate (EC-g- PDEAEMA) micelles was achieved using ATRP. The developed micelles offered a higher release of the loaded drug rifampicin in a buffer solution at pH 6.6 compared to pH 7.4 (Wang et al. 2011).

In a recent study cellulose-graft-poly(methyl methacrylate) nanoparticles with a low polydispersity index was prepared by ATRP (Figure 8.3). The obtained cellulose-graft-poly(methyl

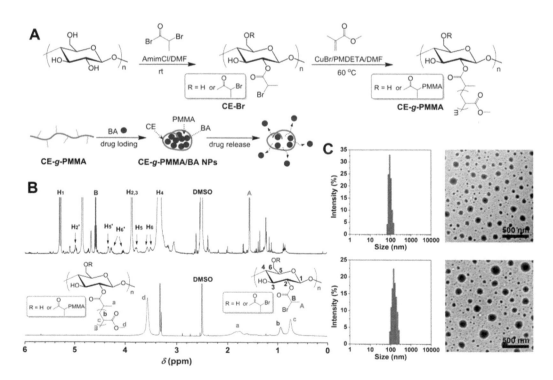

FIGURE 8.3 (A) Synthesis of CE-g-PMMA and illustration of CE-g-PMMA/BA NPs. (B) 1H NMR spectra of CE-Br and CE-g-PMMA. (C) Particle size of nanoparticles with different GR, particle size distribution and TEM of blank and BA-loaded nanoparticles. (Reprinted from *Mater Lett* 207, Dai, L., and Si, C.L. Cellulose-graft-poly(methyl methacrylate) nanoparticles with high biocompatibility for hydrophobic anticancer drug delivery, 213–6, Copyright 2017, with permission from Elsevier.)

methacrylate) nanoparticles offered high biocompatibility for hydrophobic anticancer drug delivery (Dai and Si 2017).

8.5.2 Nanoparticles from Grafted Starch for Drug Delivery

Starch is the second largest (next to cellulose) low-cost, abundantly found polysaccharide in nature. Structurally, starch is composed of a large number of glucose units joined by glycosidic bonds. The size of the starch molecules varies between 1 and 100 μm. It also exhibits heterogeneous behavior due to presence of both amorphous and crystalline regions. Starch is composed of amylose and amylopectin, two biopolymers associated with the starch structure. Amylose are the linear in nature and composed of D-glucose units joined by the α-1,4-glycosidic linkages. Amylose contributes 10%–30% to the starch network. It imparts amorphous behavior to starch. Amylopectin is a branched-chain polysaccharide composed of glucose units linked primarily by α-1,4-glycosidic bonds. In the polysaccharide backbone, the occasional presence of -1,6-glycosidic bonds are also seen which offers branching. Amylopectin contributes 70%–90% to the starch network and offers crystalline behavior. Starch is hydrophilic in nature and soluble in warm water. Due to its functional properties, starch is widely used in the food industry.

Generating nanoparticles from grafted starch for use in drug delivery is mostly achieved by free radical polymerization and ATRP. Synthesis of hydrophobic starch nanoparticles is achieved by free radical polymerization. Long chain fatty acids are used to impart hydrophobicity with potassium persulfate used as catalyst. The activity of the modified starch nanoparticles is further improved and stabilized by crosslinking it with sodium tripolyphosphate. The developed hydrophobic starch is used as an active carrier for the anti-inflammatory drug indomethacin (Simi and Emilia Abraham 2007).

ATRP is important for grafted starch preparation. Using this technique, successful grafting of acrylamide and hydroxyethylacrylate monomers over the starch backbone was achieved yielding carboxymethyl starch (CMS). Similarly, chloroacetylation also offers grafting over the starch. Both the cellulose-grafted polymers offer a biodegradable and superabsorbent nature. The developed grafted starch is used in the in vitro drug release of cephalexin antibiotic (Avval et al. 2013).

Radiation-induced grafting also finds application in the synthesis of grafted starch. ^{60}Co-gamma-radiation and ceric ammonium nitrate (CAN) redox-induced graft polymerization of acrylic monomers (acrylonitrile, acrylic acid, and methyl acrylate) to starch resulted in bioadhesive grafting (Geresh et al. 2002).

Microwave irradiation has also been used to prepare grafted starch. Different grades of hydrolyzed polyacrylamide grafted maize starch (HPam-g-MS) were synthesized by altering the microwave irradiation time. Using the grafted copolymers, aceclofenac-loaded microbeads were prepared via an ionic gelation method (Setty et al. 2014).

8.5.3 Nanoparticles from Grafted Chitosan Copolymers for Drug Delivery

Chitosan is another natural polysaccharide offering a linear structure. Shrimp and other sea crustaceans are the source of industrially used chitosan. A varying amount of (1–4)-glycosidic bonds linking N-acetyl-2-amino-2-deoxy-d-glucopyranose (glucosamine) and 2-amino-2-deoxy-d-glucopyranose (N-acetyl-glucosamine) are present in the chitosan structure (Ravi Kumar 2000; Agrawal et al. 2010). The "chitin" and "chitosan" represent a group of polymers with acetyl content. It is important to note that the degree of acetyl content determines whether the polysaccharide is termed as "chitin" or "chitosan". Molecular weight, degree of deacetylation, and the sequence of the amino and acetamido groups are the key parameters that determine the physical quality of chitin. The structure of chitin is interesting as it contains both cationic and hydrophobic sites. This renders chitin as an intrinsic polyelectrolyte, amphiphilic in nature. Acidic medium provides a positive charge to chitin. This happens due to the protonation of its amino groups in acidic medium, which provides a favorable environment for the chitin surface to become anionic. These bindings are mostly due to an electrostatic and hydrogen interaction. Oppositely charged biopolymers (i.e. xanthan, carrageenan, gum Arabic alginate, anionic lipids, and pectin) grafting can be thus easily be obtained (Huang 2012).

ATRP plays a crucial role in the process of chitosan grafting. A chitosan structure contains -NH2 and -OH groups, which offers ease of interaction with other reactive components. They make bridges via ATRP. The following schematic (Scheme 8.3) is a representation of the various synthetic strategies reported in the literature for preparation of chitosan-based graft copolymers by ATRP.

ATRP was successfully used to synthesize chitosan-graft-poly(methoxy polyethylene glycol methacrylate). Using this technique, vinyl monomers were grafted over the chitosan backbone. In the process of grafting, initially chitosan is reacted with 2-bromo-isobutyryl bromide in the presence of pyridine as a base, after the chitosan amino group had been protected by the imine (El Tahlawy and Hudson 2003).

In an another study of functionalization, chitosan yielded biodegradable cationic polymers having a chitosan backbone and poly((2-dimethyl amino) ethyl methacrylate) P (DMAEMA)) side chains of different length. The developed graft chitosan exhibited the ability to condense plasmid DNA (pDNA) into nanoparticles with a positive charge at nitrogen/phosphorus (N/P) ratios of 4 or higher. A biodegradable cationic polymer also protected the condensed DNA from enzymatic degradation by DNase I (Ping et al. 2010).

In a separate approach, ATRP in association with ring-opening polymerization and click chemistry offered amphiphilic chitosan graft copolymers-chitosan-g-poly(ε-caprolactone)-(g-poly(2-(2-methoxyethoxy)ethyl methacrylate)-co-oligo(ethylene glycol) methacrylate) (CS-g-PCL(-g-P(MEO2MA-co-OEGMA))) with double side chains of PCL and P(MEO2MA-co-OEGMA). The developed graft copolymers further assembled into a miceller structure. The thermo sensitivity properties and lower critical solution temperatures of the developed micelles depended upon the CS chains and the ratio of the PCL and P (MEO2MA-co-OEGMA) side chains. Drug release from the micelles was tested using doxorubicin as a model drug. Critical control over the operating temperature effectively controlled the drug release from the micelles (Yuan et al. 2011).

The grafting of chitosan with lactic acid was performed by physical grafting. Amide linkages were responsible for the grafting of lactic acid into the chitosan backbone. This resulted in a formation of nanoparticles ~10 nm in size. Grafting of chitosan exhibited a 92% drug encapsulation efficiency and a 28% release over a time span of 4 weeks. This grafting creates possibilities for preparing modified chitosan solution at a neutral pH. This is not possible for unmodified chitosan which is most often soluble in an acidic environment (Bhattarai et al. 2006).

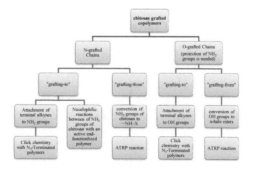

SCHEME 8.3   The various synthetic strategies reported in the literature for preparation of chitosan-based graft copolymers by ATRP. (Reprinted from *Prog Polym Sci* 76, Seidia, F., Salimib, H., Shamsabadi, A.A., and Shabanian, M. Synthesis of hybrid materials using graft copolymerization on non-cellulosic polysaccharides via homogenous ATRP, 1-39, Copyright 2018, with permission from Elsevier.)

8.5.4 Nanoparticles from Grafted Dextran for Drug Delivery

Dextran is a complex carbohydrate obtained from microbial origin. It is composed of a glucan unit (polysaccharide made of glucose). Dextran is composed of both straight and branched chains that attach to glucose molecules. Straight chains in the dextran (~95%) binds to glucose through α-1,6-glycosidic linkages, whereas branches (~5%) begin from α-1,3 linkages. The presence of variable quantities of α-1,2-, α-1,3-, and α-1,4-glycosidic bonds indicate the attachment position of side chains to the main chains. With structural uniqueness, several nanostructure entities are developed from dextran. Free radical polymerization and ATRP are also used to prepare grafted dextran. In an earlier study, chemical and enzymatic hydrolysis of a dextran formed water-insoluble modified dextrans. The synthesis was carried out reacting dextran with ethyl and butyl chloroformate using tertiary amines as a catalyst/acceptor systems and the DMF/LiCl system as a solvent (Chaves and Arranz 1985).

Core-shell type nanoparticles of a poly(DL-lactide-co-glycolide) (PLGA) grafted-dextran (DexLG) copolymer with a varying graft ratio of PLGA was synthesized using a chemical method. Grafted dextran offered nanoparticle formation (50 nm) in an aqueous medium with a self-aggregation process. Developed grafted dextran has been proposed for use as a colonic drug carrier (Jeong et al. 2006).

Dextran is functionalized via epoxide precursors of alkylglycerol and covalently linked to poly(lactic acid) using a carbodiimide crosslinker. This forms alkylglyceryl-modified dextran-graft-poly (lactic acid). Solvent displacement and electrospray allowed the grafted dextran to form nanoparticles with a unimodal size distribution profile of 100–200 nm. It offered good stability at a physiologically relevant pH and proposed for use as a carrier of therapeutic actives to the brain (Toman et al. 2015).

Using ATRP, well-defined comb-shaped copolymers composed of non-ionic hydrophilic dextran backbones and cationic poly((2-dimethyl amino) ethyl methacrylate) (or P(DMAEMA)) side chains were developed (Scheme 8.4). The synthesis was achieved by reacting hydroxyl groups of dextran with α-bromoisobutyric acid in the presence of 1,1'-carbonyldiimidazole yielding bromoisobutyryl-terminated dextran which further acted as multifunctional initiators for subsequent ATRP. Further quaternization of P-(DMAEMA) side chains in developed comb-shaped copolymers produced

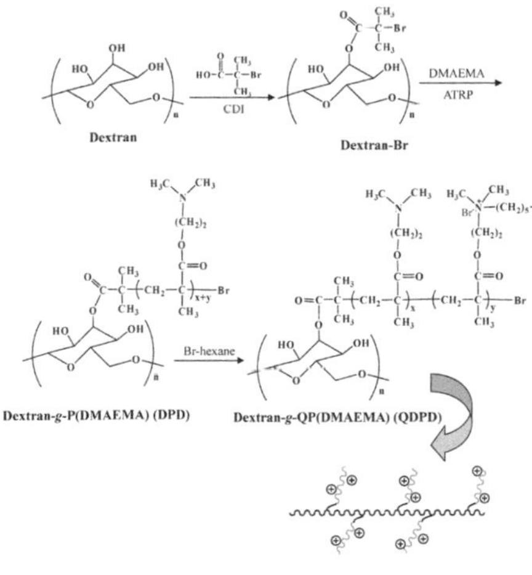

SCHEME 8.4 Schematic diagram illustrating the preparation processes of partially quaternized P(DMAEMA)-graft-dextran comb copolymers via atom transfer radical polymerization (ATRP) from 2-Bromoisobutyryl-terminated dextran. (Reprinted from *Macromolecules* 44, Wang, Z.H., Li, W.B., Ma, J., Tang, G.P., Yang, W.T., and Xu, F.J. Functionalized nonionic dextran backbones by atom transfer radical polymerization for efficient gene delivery, 230–9, Copyright 2010, with permission from American Chemical Society.)

quaternary ammonium comb-shaped copolymers. This further condensed pDNA into complex nanoparticles of 100–150 nm in size offering a lower cytotoxicity and better gene transfection yield (Wang et al. 2011).

8.6 CONCLUSION

The role of the carrier matrix is essential for drug delivery as the stability, release, and solubility of the drugs depend upon the properties of carrier matrix. Edible polysaccharides are now a recent popular choice as drug delivery carrier due to their functionality, bioavailability, and biodegradability. But the modification of the natural biopolymer is often required as a specific drug or group of drugs have particular delivery requirements. The grafted polymerization process easily achieves these natural biopolymer modifications. Grafting over the natural biopolymer modifies the polymer structures and develops novel polymeric carriers with unique properties for drug delivery. This method is a preferred choice of biopolymer modification due to the clean and convenient nature of synthesis that easily fulfils the drug-specific requirements. Grafting offers unique nanodimensional structural features to polysaccharides that provide additional benefits for drug delivery. Polysaccharide-based graft copolymers with their diversified properties can also be used for various other applications.

REFERENCES

Agrawal, P., Strijkers, G.J., and Nicolay, K. 2010. Chitosan-based systems for molecular imaging. *Adv Drug Deliv Rev* 62 (1): 42–58.

Avval, M.E., Moghaddam, P.N., and Fareghi, A.R. 2013. Modification of starch by graft copolymerization: A drug delivery system tested for cephalexin antibiotic. *Starch* 65 (7–8): 572–83.

Bhattacharya, A. and Misra, B.N. 2004. Grafting: A versatile means to modify polymers: Techniques, factors and applications. *Prog Polym Sci* 29 (8): 767–14.

Bhattarai, N., Ramay, H.R., Chou, S.-H. et al. 2006. Chitosan and lactic acid-grafted chitosan nanoparticles as carriers for prolonged drug delivery. *Int J Nanomed* 1 (2): 181–87.

Cao, G. and Wang, Y. 2011. *Nanostructures and Nanomaterials: Synthesis, Properties, and Applications.* World Scientific. Available at: https:// books. google. com/ books? id= cqaWjca5YeUC &pgis=1 (Accessed: 16 August 2015).

Chami Khazraji, A. and Robert, S. 2013. Self-assembly and intermolecular forces when cellulose and water interact using molecular modeling. *J Nanomater* 2013: 1–12.

Chaves, M.S. and Arranz, F. 1985. Water-insoluble dextrans by grafting, 2. Reaction of dextrans with n-alkyl chloroformates. Chemical and enzymatic hydrolysis. *Die Makromolekulare Chemie* 186 (1): 17–29.

Chayed, S. and Winnik, F.M. 2007. In vitro evaluation of the mucoadhesive properties of polysaccharide-based nanoparticulate oral drug delivery systems. *Eur J Pharm Biopharm* 65 (3): 363–70.

Chen, L., Liu, J., Zhang, Y., Dai, B. et al. 2015. Structural, thermal, and anti-inflammatory properties of a novel pectic polysaccharide from Alfalfa (Medicago sativa L.) Stem. *J Agric Food Chem* 63 (12): 3219–28.

Choudhury, A.J., Gogoi, D., Kandimalla, R. et al. 2016. Penicillin impregnation on oxygen plasma surface functionalized chitosan/Antheraea assama silk fibroin: Studies of antibacterial activity and antithrombogenic property. *Mater Sci Eng C* 60: 475–84.

Cobo, I., Li, M., Sumerlin, B.S. et al. 2015. Smart hybrid materials by conjugation of responsive polymers to biomacromolecules. *Nat Mater* 14 (2): 143–59.

Corona-Hernandez, R.I., Álvarez-Parrilla, E., Lizardi-Mendoza, J. et al. 2013. Structural stability and viability of microencapsulated probiotic bacteria: A review. *Comp Rev Food Sci Food Safety* 12 (6): 614–28.

Dai, L. and Si, C.-L. 2017. Cellulose-graft-poly(methyl methacrylate) nanoparticles with high biocompatibility for hydrophobic anti-cancer drug delivery. *Mater Lett* 207: 213–16.

Dima, S.-O., Panaitescu, D.-M., Orban, C. et al. 2017. Bacterial nanocellulose from side-streams of Kombucha beverages production: Preparation and physical-chemical properties. Polymers. *Multidisciplinary Digital Publishing Institute* 9 (8): 374.

El Tahlawy, K. and Hudson, S.M. 2003. Synthesis of a well-defined chitosan graft poly(methoxy polyethyleneglycol methacrylate) by atom transfer radical polymerization. *J Appl Polym Sci* 89 (4): 901–12.

Fathi, M., Martín, Á., and McClements, D.J. 2014. Nanoencapsulation of food ingredients using carbohydrate based delivery systems. *Trends Food Sci Technol* 39 (1): 18–39.

Faulks, R.M., Southon, S., and Ottaway, P.B. 2008. *Assessing the bioavailability of nutraceuticals*, 195–18. Woodhead Publishing Ltd.

Florek, J., Caillard, R., and Kleitz, F. 2017. Evaluation of mesoporous silica nanoparticles for oral drug delivery—current status and perspective of MSNs drug carriers. *Nanoscale* 9 (40): 15252–77.

Freshour, G., Clay, R.P., Fuller, M.S. et al. 1996. Developmental and tissue-specific structural alterations of the cell-wall polysaccharides of arabidopsis thaliana roots. *Plant Physiol* 110 (4): 1413–29.

Garti, N. 2008. *Delivery and Controlled Release of Bioactives in Foods and Nutraceuticals*. Elsevier.

Geresh, S., Gilboa, Y., Peisahov-Korol, J. et al. 2002. Preparation and characterization of bioadhesive grafted starch copolymers as platforms for controlled drug delivery. *J Appl Polym Sci* 86 (5): 1157–62.

Huang, Q. 2012. *Nanotechnology in the Food, Beverage and Nutraceutical Industries*. Elsevier Science.

Huang, R.Y.-M., Immergut, B., Immergut, E.H., and Rapson, W.H. 1963. Grafting vinyl polymers onto cellulose by high energy radiation. I. High energy radiation-induced graft copolymerization of styrene onto cellulose. *J Polym Sci Part A* 1 (4): 1257–70.

Jeong, Y.-I., Choi, K.-C., and Song, C.-E. 2006. Doxorubicin release from core-shell type nanoparticles of poly(DL-lactide-co-glycolide)-grafted dextran. *Arch Pharm Res* 29 (8): 712–19.

Khelifa, F., Ershov, S., Habibi, Y. et al. 2016. Free-radical-induced grafting from plasma polymer surfaces. *Chem Rev* 116 (6): 3975–4005.

Krzysztof, Matyjaszewski, Timothy, E., Patten, and Xia, J. 1997. *Controlled/"Living" radical polymerization. Kinetics of the homogeneous atom transfer radical polymerization of styrene*. American Chemical Society.

Liu, Z., Jiao, Y., Wang, Y. et al. 2008. Polysaccharides-based nanoparticles as drug delivery systems. *Adv Drug Deliv Rev* 60 (15): 1650–62.

Moghaddam, P.N., Avval, M.E., and Fareghi, A.R. 2014. Modification of cellulose by graft polymerization for use in drug delivery systems. *Colloid Polym Sci* 292 (1): 77–84.

Omenn, G.S., Goodman, G.E., Thornquist, M.D. et al. 1996. Effects of a combination of beta carotene and vitamin A on lung cancer and cardiovascular disease. *N Engl J Med* 334 (18): 1150–5.

Paiva, A.A., Castro, A.J., Nascimento, M.S., et al. 2011. Antioxidant and anti-inflammatory effect of polysaccharides from Lobophora variegata on zymosan-induced arthritis in rats. *Int Immunopharmacol* 11 (9): 1241–50.

Pillay, V., Seedat, A., Choonara, Y.E. et al. 2013. A review of polymeric refabrication techniques to modify polymer properties for biomedical and drug delivery applications. *AAPS Pharm Sci Tech* 14 (2): 692–11.

Ping, Y., Liu, C.-D., Tang, G.-P. et al. 2010. Functionalization of chitosan via atom transfer radical polymerization for gene delivery. *Adv Funct Mater* 20 (18): 3106–16.

Raus, V., Štěpánek, M., Uchman, M. et al. 2011. Cellulose-based graft copolymers with controlled architecture prepared in a homogeneous phase. *J Polym Sci A* 49 (20): 4353–67.

Ravi Kumar, M.,N. 2000. A review of chitin and chitosan applications. *React Funct Polym* 46 (1): 1–27.

Roy, A., Khanra, K., Mishra, A., and Bhattacharyya, N. 2013. Highly cytotoxic (PA-1), less cytotoxic (A549) and antimicrobial activity of a green synthesized silver nanoparticle using Mikania cordata L'. *Int J Adv Res* 1 (5): 193–98.

Roy, A., Shrivastava, S.L., and Mandal, S.M. 2016. Self-assembled carbohydrate nanostructures: Synthesis strategies to functional application in food. In: Grumezescu, A. (Ed.), *Novel Approaches of Nanotechnology in Food, Volume 1*. Elsevier Academic Press, pp. 133–64.

Roy, A., Shrivastava, S.L., Mandal, S.M., Roy, S.K., and Srivastava, S.K. 2015. Green synthesized 3 hexyne conjugated core–shell silver nanoparticles interferes peptidoglycan in inhibiting multidrug resistant pathogens. *Adv Sci Eng Med* 7 (6): 465–72.

Saravanakumar, G., Jo, D.-G., and Park, J.H. 2012. Polysaccharide-based nanoparticles: A versatile platform for drug delivery and biomedical imaging. *Curr Med Chem* 19 (19): 3212–29.

Seidi, F., Salimi, H., Shamsabadi, A.A., and Shabanian, M. 2018. Synthesis of hybrid materials using graft copolymerization on non-cellulosic polysaccharides via homogenous ATRP. *Prog Polym Sci* 76: 1–39.

Setty, C.M., Deshmukh, A.S., and Badiger, A.M. 2014. Hydrolyzed polyacrylamide grafted maize starch based microbeads: Application in pH responsive drug delivery. *Int J Biol Macromol* 70: 1–9.

Shibakami, M., Tsubouchi, G., Sohma, M., and Hayashi, M. 2015. Preparation of transparent self-standing thin films made from acetylated euglenoid β-1,3-glucans. *Carbohydr Polym* 133: 421–8.

Simi, C.K. and Emilia, Abraham, T. 2007. Hydrophobic grafted and cross-linked starch nanoparticles for drug delivery. *Bioprocess Biosyst Eng* 30 (3): 173–80.

Singh, V., Kumar, P., and Sanghi, R. 2012. Use of microwave irradiation in the grafting modification of the polysaccharides – A review. *Prog Polym Sci* 37 (2): 340–64.

Szwarc, M. 1998. Living polymers. Their discovery, characterization, and properties. *J Polym Sci Part A* 36 (1) 9–15.

Toman, P., Lien, C.-F., Ahmad, Z., et al. 2015. Nanoparticles of alkylglyceryl-dextran- graft -poly(lactic acid) for drug delivery to the brain: Preparation and in vitro investigation. *Acta Biomaterialia* 23: 250–62.

Uccello-Barretta, G., Balzano, F., Vanni, L., and Sansò, M. 2013. Mucoadhesive properties of tamarind-seed polysaccharide/hyaluronic acid mixtures: A nuclear magnetic resonance spectroscopy investigation. *Carbohydr Polym* 91 (2): 568–72.

Vijan, V., Kaity, S., Biswas, S. et al. 2012. Microwave assisted synthesis and characterization of acrylamide grafted gellan, application in drug delivery. *Carbohydr Polym* 90 (1): 496–506.

Wang, D., Tan, J., Kang, H. et al. 2011. Synthesis, self-assembly and drug release behaviors of pH-responsive copolymers ethyl cellulose-graft-PDEAEMA through ATRP. *Carbohydr Polym* 84 (1): 195–202.

Wang, Z.H., Li, W.B., Ma, J. et al. 2011. Functionalized nonionic dextran backbones by atom transfer radical polymerization for efficient gene delivery. *Macromolecules* 44 (2): 230–39.

Whitesides, G.M. and Boncheva, M. 2002. Beyond molecules: Self-assembly of mesoscopic and macroscopic components. *Proc Nat Acad Sci USA*, 99 (8): 4769–74.

Xu, Z., Wan,L., Huang, X. 2009. Surface modification by graft polymerization. Surface Engineering of Polymer Membrane. Springer, pp. 80–49.

Yuan, W., Li, X., Gu, S., Cao, A., and Ren, J. 2011. Amphiphilic chitosan graft copolymer via combination of ROP, ATRP and click chemistry: Synthesis, self-assembly, thermosensitivity, fluorescence, and controlled drug release. *Polymer* 52 (3): 658–66.

Zhang, K., Liu, Y., Zhao, X. et al. 2018. Anti-inflammatory properties of GLPss58, a sulfated polysaccharide from Ganoderma lucidum. *Int J Biol Macromol* 107 (Pt A): 486–93.

Zhang, S. 2003. Fabrication of novel biomaterials through molecular self-assembly. *Nat Biotechnol* 21 (10): 1171–8.

Zhao, J., Lu, C., He, X., et al. 2015. Polyethylenimine-grafted cellulose nanofibril aerogels as versatile vehicles for drug delivery. *ACS Appl Mater Interface* 7 (4): 2607–15.

9 Environmental Responsive Polysaccharide Nanocarriers for Controlled Drug Delivery

Yamini S. Bobde and Balaram Ghosh

CONTENTS

9.1 INTRODUCTION

Nature requires selectively designed molecular assemblies and interfaces to maintain biological function and sustain life, which provides a specific structure, particular function, and environment. Environmental responsive nanocarriers are nanostructures which are capable of bringing chemical and physical modifications for receiving internal or external stimuli. These changes are due to variations in physical and chemical polymer properties. The stimuli is obtained from changes in the environment of the materials, sucha as changes in pH, temperature, enzyme concentration, light or electric pulses, magnetic field, ultrasound intensity, etc. (Stuart et al. 2010). This environmental sensitivity is helpful in controlling the biodistribution of drugs and targeting diseased areas in the body. This is achieved through the development of environmental responsive nanocarriers which need the utilization of biocompatible materials that are capable of responding to particular stimuli, or which are able to undergo a hydrolytic cleavage, specific protonation, or change in the molecular conformational in response to a specific stimulus (Mura et al. 2013). Polysaccharides are one of the most popular polymeric materials for stimuli-responsive drug delivery systems (Cheng et al. 2013). The structure and property diversity of polysaccharides is due to their unique features such as their wide molecular weight range, reactive groups, and variability of chemical composition. Biochemically and chemically, polysaccharides can be modified easily due to the variable derivable groups present on their molecular chains, which lead to formation of various types of derivatives. Polysaccharides are safe, stable, non-toxic, and biodegradable (Liu et al. 2008). Polysaccharides like alginate, chitosan, dextran, hyaluronic acid, and carboxymethyl cellulose are environmental responsive polymers. Various factors like pH, temperature, and ionic strength of the medium affect conformation of polysaccharides chains. By the action of physical or chemical stimuli, trigger phase transitions of crosslinked and isolated chains can be exploited for sensitive conformation (Alvarez-Lorenzo et al. 2013). Polysaccharide can be affected by stimuli like the application of heat to increase the temperature or electric fields which alter charge distribution.(Brulé et al. 2011). The polysaccharides become attractive components of smart drug delivery systems (DDSs) because of their response to the variety of stimuli. Because of these smart responsive DDSs, the drug can be specifically released in the affected cells or tissues (Alvarez-Lorenzo and Concheiro 2008). In addition, most of the natural polysaccharides help with bioadhesion via non-covalent bonds which can form with biological tissues, mainly mucous membranes and epithelia. These non-covalent bonds form due to the presence of hydrophilic groups like carboxyl, hydroxyl, and amino groups. Both chitosan and alginate are good bioadhesive materials. These can prolong the time of residence and thus increase the absorption of loaded drugs (Wang et al. 2011). The recognition and binding to desirable surfaces can be facilitated by the polysaccharides through mimicking the surface of the bacteria, viruses, and eukaryotic cells (Liu et al. 2008). Thus, the novel environment-responsive, biocompatible, and even targetable DDSs can be obtained with the integration of the polysaccharides features (Hamidi et al. 2008). This review discusses the most significant progress in developing environment-responsive polysaccharide nanocarrier drug delivery systems in response to specific stimuli both endogenous and exogenous.

9.2   ENDOGENOUS AND EXOGENOUS STIMULI IN DRUG DELIVERY

Concentrations of specific analytes or enzymes, pH, and redox potential are endogenous stimuli. The variations in pH to control the delivery of drugs has been exploited in intracellular compartments like lysosomes, endosomes, or in specific organs like the vagina or gastrointestinal tract, and also in pathological conditions like inflammation or cancer. Two main strategies exist for this. First is the use of polymers (polyacids or polybases) that contain ionizable groups which undergo changes in solubility and/or conformation in response to environmental variation in pH; and second is polymeric system designs which contain acid liable bonds which can be cleaved allowing molecules to be released. Most anticancer DDSs are sensitive to variations in pH, such as pH values around 7.4 for healthy tissues and 6.5–7.2 for the microenvironment of solid tumors. This lower pH microenvironment of tumors is mainly because of the irregularity in angiogenesis in a fast-growing tumor which leads to a rapid deficiency of oxygen and nutrients, and thus glycolytic metabolism leads to the production of acidic metabolites in the tumor microenvironment. Hence, a sharp response to change in pH must be given by pH-sensitive systems. The alteration in specific enzyme expression like phospholipase, proteases, or glycosidases has been observed in conditions such as inflammation or cancer. This was explored to achieve drug release by an enzyme-mediated response. The redox sensitivity can be achieved by glutathione (GSH), which cleaves the disulfide bonds rapidly. The variation in GSH concentration, intracellular (~2–10 mM) and extracellular (~2–10 µM) compartments, and in tumor tissues compared with healthy ones has been exploited to control the release of the drug.

The temperature, ultrasounds, magnetic fields, electric fields, and light are the externally applied stimuli. Thermo-responsive drug delivery has been widely explored in oncology and investigated through stimuli-responsive strategies. A non-linear sharp change in temperature in one of the components of the nanocarrier results in the thermo-responsiveness and thus triggers the drug release. Ideally, thermo-responsive nanocarriers should be stable at body temperature (~37°C) and rapidly release the drug at (~40°C–42°C) within a locally heated tumor. Control of the drug release by ultrasounds is a spatiotemporal effective method. This is a non-invasive without radiation method. When a magnetic field is applied, the temperature increases thus it can be used to control the drug release. Electric signals which are weak (about 1 V) have been explored to achieve sustained or pulsed release of the drug via various actuation mechanisms. The structural modifications can be obtained by photo-responsiveness which leads to a particular drug release pattern from the nanocarriers (Mura et al. 2013).

9.3 ENVIRONMENTAL RESPONSIVE POLYSACCHARIDE NANOCARRIERS FOR CONTROLLED DRUG DELIVERY

Natural polysaccharides have received more attention in the new era of environmental responsive drug delivery. Polysaccharides are considered to be the most promising moiety in the nanometric carrier system. In this chapter, there will be a brief introduction of the different polysaccharides modulated with stimuli sensitivity.

9.3.1 ALGINATE AS AN ENVIRONMENTAL RESPONSIVE NANOCARRIER

Alginate is a polysaccharide which is linear and extracted from brown algae. The residues of 1,4-linked α-L-guluronic (G) and β-D-mannuronic (M) acid are present alternately in alginate as shown in Figure 9.1. Because of these carboxylic acid residues, alginate is pH-sensitive (Bazban-Shotorbani et al. 2017). The distribution and ratio of G and M blocks play an important role in the alginate's sensitivity to calcium ions and pH because of the different relative positions of the carboxylic acid group in each block (Bazban-Shotorbani et al. 2017). The pKa values of the carboxylic groups have been observed at 3.38 for mannuronic and 3.65 for guluronic acid monomers. Therefore, the pKa is around 3.5 for this acidic polysaccharide, alginate (Bazban-Shotorbani et al. 2017). Sodium ions exchange with divalent cations such as Ca^{2+} from the guluronic acid which leads to the gelation and crosslinking of alginate.

Alginate is useful in the design of controlled delivery systems because of its pH-sensitivity, bioadhesiveness, biocompatibility, and mild gelation conditions. In an oral delivery system, alginate beads have been used for the controlled release of macromolecules in a low pH solution (Bazban-Shotorbani et al. 2017). At a low gastric pH, the encapsulated drugs are not released because of shrinkage of alginate (George and Abraham 2006). A porous and insoluble alginic acid skin is formed from the hydrated sodium alginate in gastric fluid. After contact with the higher pH of the intestinal tract, a soluble viscous layer is obtained from the alginic acid skin. To customize the release profile, the pH-sensitive properties of alginate can be exploited. However, burst release of protein drugs may be observed due to rapid dissolution in the higher pH ranges of alginate matrices, and proteolytic enzymes may lead to denaturation of the protein drugs. Therefore, the physiochemical properties need to be modified for the controlled release of protein drugs (Bazban-Shotorbani et al. 2017).

In an early study, semisynthetic network alginate polymer (SNAP) was prepared. Reactive hydroxyls and carboxylic acid are present in the uronic acid monomer in alginate allowing for chemical modification. The preferred reaction targets were the hydroxyl functional groups because the carboxylate moieties were preserved for a greater pH-sensitive response. Glutaraldehyde consists of two terminal aldehydes therefore it is an effective chemical crosslinker with bifunctionality. In the presence of an acid catalyst, it reacted with four alcohols to yield two 1,1-geminal diethers, which are known as acetals, $R_2C(OR')_2$. Glutaraldehyde was used as crosslinking agent with alginate as shown in Figure 9.2. Cross-polarization magic-angle spinning ^{13}C solid state NMR was studied to confirm the hydrogel molecular structure. Gel equilibrium swelling was performed to study the reaction parameters which were affecting the polymer synthesis. The acetalization reaction was controlled thermodynamically which led to control of pore properties and gel swelling. Significant swelling was observed at alkaline pH and contraction in the acidic

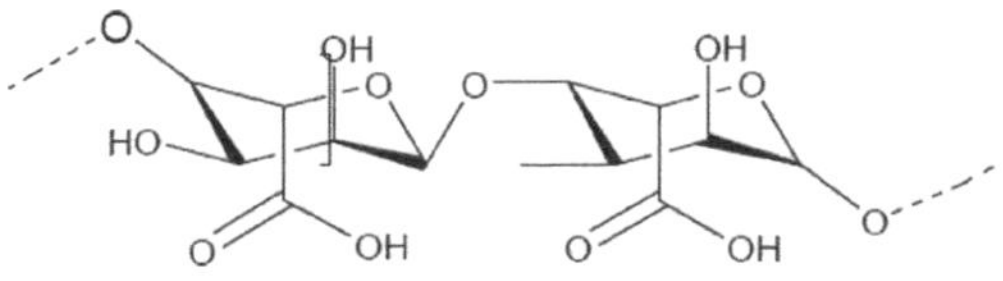

FIGURE 9.1 Chemical structure of alginate.

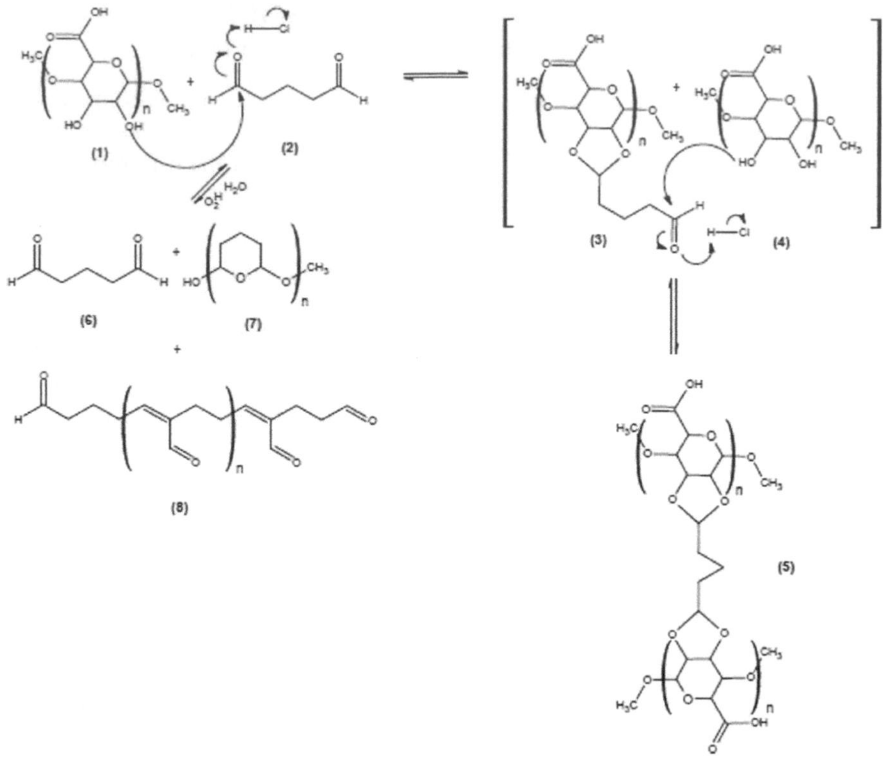

FIGURE 9.2 Semisynthetic network alginate polymer with glutaraldehyde as the crosslinker.

environment in response to pH-stimuli which yielded a potential vehicle for oral drug delivery. As a targeted delivery vehicle, a tissue scaffold can be developed by selecting optimum reaction conditions, pore size, gel swelling, and stimuli-responsive characteristics for regenerative medicine (Chan et al. 2009).

A similar study was been reported by Chan et al., who chemically modified alginate with dialdehyde with the help of an acid-catalyzed acetalization. Through equilibrium swelling of the networked polymer, the kinetics of acetalization were measured and it was found to follow a zero-order for alginate and second-order for dialdehyde. The rate constant and energy of activation were found be $19.06 \ \mu L \cdot mole^{-1} \cdot s^{-1}$ and $78.58 \ kJ \cdot mol^{-1}$ at 40°C respectively. By predictive estimation of formulation conditions and reagent concentration, the average pore size and gel swelling were controlled between 35 and 840 nm and 80–1,000-fold. This semisynthetic polymer can be used in protein therapeutics as stimuli-responsive exhibiting high water absorbency (Chan et al. 2008).

In another reported study, poly(ε-caprolactone)- block-(dimethylamino)ethyl methacrylate which is a six-arm block copolymer was used to load indomethacin incorporated into calcium alginate beads. The drug release from calcium alginate beads and alginate beads (without calcium) was studied and it was found that faster indomethacine release was observed from calcium alginate compared to alginate. Greater drug solubility was observed in the micelles. The diffusion from the beads was facilitated by the higher concentration gradient (Alvarez-Lorenzo et al. 2013).

In another study, novel dual-stimuli responsive (pH and thermosensitive) sodium alginate-grafted-PNIPAM copolymers (poly(N-isopropylacrylamide)) were synthesized. By radical polymerization, PNIPAAm-NH$_2$ was synthesized using $K_2S_2O_8$ (KPS) as initiator and AET HCl (2-aminoethane-thiol hydrochloride) as a redox coupling agent. Sodium alginate (AgA) was coupled with PNIPAAm using the condensing agent EDC (1-3-(3-dimethylaminopropyl)-3-ethyl-carbodiimide hydrochloride). Structural confirmation was done by an elemental analysis and a spectroscopic method like

1H NMR, FT-IR. The average molecular weights were varied from 100–690 kDa by light scattering measurements. With increasing AgA content, intrinsic viscosity linearly increases because of the increased alginate backbone contour length per total polymer unit mass mainly at low pH values. As the hydrophilic content increases, transition temperature increases which remains constant close to the lower critical solution temperature of PNIPAAm. The average size varied from 200 to 300 nm at low pH and 300–600 nm at high pH (Vasile and Nita 2011).

Brule and team proposed an innovative approach to achieve the combined effect of the efficient release of drugs and thermotherapy. In this study, the release of doxorubicin was triggered by magnetic nanoheaters in which alginate was embedded. The microemulsion method was used to synthesize the magnetic alginate microbeads by using a partially miscible organic solvent, 1-pentanol. A magnetic fluid was concentrated and encapsulated with a 8.6 mol L^{-1} high iron concentration (Figure 9.3). The diameter of iron oxide nanoparticles was 8 nm and composed of a maghemite-core (γ -Fe_2O_3) and synthesized by Massart's procedure with the help of alkaline co-precipitation of iron(II) (0.9 mol) and iron(III) (1.5 mol) salts. The nanoparticles were surface treated by citrate ions to improve compatibility and limit interactions. The diameter and polydispersity of the microbeads were found to be 50 μm and 0.32 μm respectively. The loading of doxorubicin and iron was 3.4 ± 0.4 μg per mg and 1.11 ± 0.16 mmol Fe per g of the bead respectively. When a magnetic field was applied to the microbeads, local temperature was increased to a plateau value of 53°C from 37°C. The release of doxorubicin was enhanced significantly by hyperthermia (45.3 μg mL^{-1}) compared to 20°C (25.9 μg mL^{-1}) from alginate microbeads. With an increase in release, the doxorubicin effect is also enhanced and the cell viability was found to be $5.7\% \pm 4.2\%$ in a MCF-7 breast cancer cell line (Brulé et al. 2011).

Electrodepositing at electrode surfaces has been observed for stimuli-responsive polysaccharides because of localized electrical signals. This is due to the induced pH gradients which leads to neutralization of the polymer in most of cases. In response to low pH, the acidic alginate was deposited at anode. In Figure 9.4 the electrodepositing mechanism for alginate films is represented. In this case, in sodium alginate solution insoluble CaCO3 is suspended. The localized solubilization of Ca^{2+} takes place due to a pH gradient which is generated by anodic electrolysis, and leads to induction for calcium alginate gels formation. The electrodeposition of polysaccharide gives it the important feature of co-deposition. Into the electro-deposited films, incorporation of suspended or dissolved materials in solution of polysaccharide can be carried out. This feature was used for the biosensor fabrication of glucose oxidase and gold nanoparticles. The composite surface coatings can also be generated with the help of co-deposition. In Ca^{2+} alginate films, bacterial cells which were viable were co-deposited using the mechanism illustrated in Figure 9.4. The bioprocessing capabilities of a Ca^{2+} alginate film were extended. The cells entrapped in the film were probed with immunoreagents which led to recognition of cell surface proteins (Yang et al. 2010).

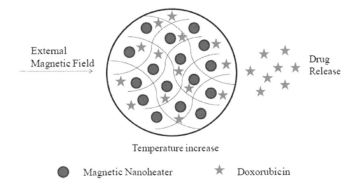

FIGURE 9.3 Representation of alginate microbeads loaded with doxorubicin and magnetic nanoheaters.

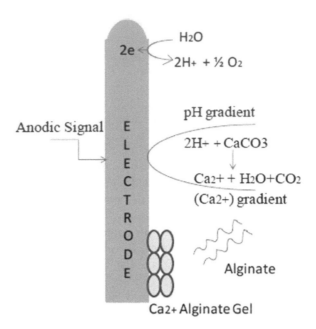

FIGURE 9.4 A calcium-alginate electrodeposition mechanism. A pH gradient was generated at anode by electrolysis that triggers the localized calcium release from insoluble CaCO3. The gelation of calcium alginate was induced by the localized solubilization of Ca2+ adjacent to the anode surface.

9.3.2 CHITOSAN AS AN ENVIRONMENTAL RESPONSIVE NANOCARRIER

Chitosan is a positively charged polysaccharide which is an N-deacetylation product of chitin. It consists of D-glucosamine units with N-acetyl-D-glucosamine units as shown in Figure 9.5. The pKa of chitosan is 6.3. The percentage of primary amine groups is determined by the deacetylation degree of this polymer, and this is responsible for its pH-sensitivity. Because of the protonation of amine groups, chitosan can be dissolved under acidic conditions and at a pH over 6.5, it precipitates due to hydrogen bonding between uncharged amine groups and hydroxyl groups (Bazban-Shotorbani et al. 2017). This versatile biopolymer has been widely used for pharmaceutical and biomedical applications.

A new class of hybrid nanogels based on chitosan was prepared via an in-situ immobilization technique. CdSe (cadmium-selenium) quantum dots (QDs) immobilized in the network of chitosan-poly(methacrylic acid-MAA) (chitosan-PMAA), as represented in Figure 9.6. The hybrid nanogels formed by the covalently crosslinked chitosan chains exhibited excellent structural and colloidal stability. In contrast, significant change in the composition and structure was observed upon physiological pH exposure when hybrid nanogels were formed by non-covalent physical association. Their mean diameter varied from 74.7 to 174.5 nm, when the ratio of MAA/chitosan changed from 0.53 to 2.10. Comparatively, a broader size distribution was observed in the chitosan-PMAA nanogel which

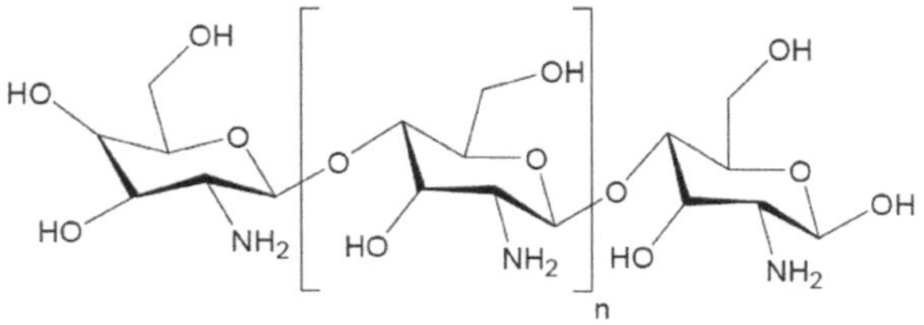

FIGURE 9.5 Structure of chitosan.

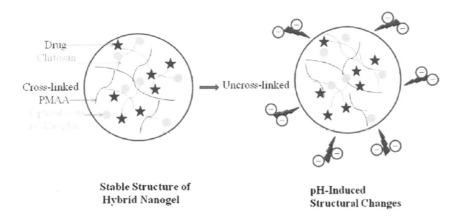

Stable Structure of Hybrid Nanogel

pH-Induced Structural Changes

FIGURE 9.6 Schematic illustration of the design of chitosan-PMAA-CdSe hybrid nanogel.

was formed by association of the physical chain. The negative surface charge was observed at pH ~5.0. As the MAA/chitosan ratio decreased, the zeta potential tended to be neutral. In a pH range of 5–7.4, the release of the anticancer drug was regulated for the covalently crosslinked hybrid nanogels. However, a non-reversible property of pH-sensitivity was exhibited by the physically associated hybrid nanogels and significant cytotoxicity was observed after 24 h treatment (Wu et al. 2010).

Through chitosan backbone modification with synthetic polymers, chitosan-based amphiphilic graft copolymers were obtained. A series of grafted copolymers of chitosan oligosaccharide were prepared. Its representation is shown in Figure 9.7. The self-organized nanoscale micelles (diameter <20 nm) of PCL-g-COs were formed in water with a PCL as core and COs as shell. A disulfide-containing bis-alkyne crosslinker was incorporated which can be degraded in response to redox stimuli. Due to the intracellular glutathione level, the release of an anticancer drug, doxorubicin, was exploited (Guerry et al. 2014). The addition of temperature-sensitive components for increasing the ability of controlled release of polysaccharides has been tested by several authors.

The polymers which undergo reversible phase transitions and particularly possess ionizable groups with a lower critical solution temperature are useful in controlling both the release rate of drugs and the site (Prabaharan and Mano 2006). A Thermosensitive NIPAAm polymer was used loaded with chitosan and caffeine and its characteristics were studied. Variables like crosslinking agent concentration and chitosan/NIPAAm weight ratio significantly influenced the loading of the caffeine. The amount of caffeine loaded was decreased at 20°C with the increase in crosslinking agent or increase in weight ratio of the chitosan/NIPAAm. The release of caffeine from the chitosan-g-NIPAAm copolymer was controlled by the swelling ratio and pore size at 37°C (Matsumura et al. 2008).

In another study on interpenetrating polymer networks (IPNs), PNIPAAm/chitosan release properties were reported. It has a greater affinity for the anionic drug, like diclofenac compared to the pure PNIPAAm hydrogels and sustain release of the drug was observed for more than 8 h in a pH 8 phosphate buffer, (Alvarez-lorenzo and Concheiro 2008).

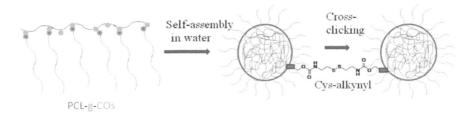

PCL-g-COs

Self-assembly in water

Cross-clicking

Cys-alkynyl

FIGURE 9.7 Self-assembly was formed by the grafted copolymer in aqueous solution and core cross-clicking of PCL-g-COs with the disulfide Cys-alkynyl.

Biomimetic smart thin coatings were developed through a layer-by-layer approach using a recombinant elastin-like recombinamer (ELR) and chitosan. Biomimetic smart thin coatings were developed through a layer-by-layer approach using a recombinant elastin-like recombinamer (ELR) and chitosan containing the cell attachment sequence arginine-glycine(aspartic acid) (RGD). Nanostructured, multilayered coatings can be formed by combining both polymers. Comparatively enhanced cell adhesion was observed. This smart coating could be used in control delivery systems and as smart biomimetic coatings for biomaterials (Costa et al. 2011).

Chitosan electrodeposits in response to induced pH gradients that neutralize the polymer. At the cathode surface, chitosan undergoes gel formation in response to a localized high pH which results in the formation of neutral amines from its cationic ammonium groups. The stimuli-responsive film-forming (Costa et al. 2011) chitosan was reported to allow the co-deposition of heparine (which is unable to deposit by itself) (Cheng et al. 2012).

Thermo- and pH-sensitive chitosan hydrogels were prepared. To provide reactive sites on the chitosan molecules, the modification of carboxymethyl chitosan (CMCH) was done with maleic anhydride to form maleilated CMCH. With the help of free-radical polymerization, the NIPAAm monomer was graft-copolymerized onto the maleilated CMCH in the presence of ammonium persulfate (APS) as the initiator and N,N,N,N-tetramethylene diamine (TEMED) as the accelerator, which led to the formation of the crosslinked hydrogel networks as shown in Figure 9.8. The magnetic iron oxide nanoparticles were embedded into the porous hydrogel networks which resulted in novel magnetic hybrid hydrogels. The magnetic iron oxide nanoparticles phase change was not observed. This magnetic hydrogel material was found to possess a potential magnetically assisted bio-separation application (Liang et al. 2007). A casting/solvent evaporation method can be used to form film composed of chitosan and polyethylene glycol, that promotes intermolecular hydrogen bonding. A faster release of ciprofloxacin was observed

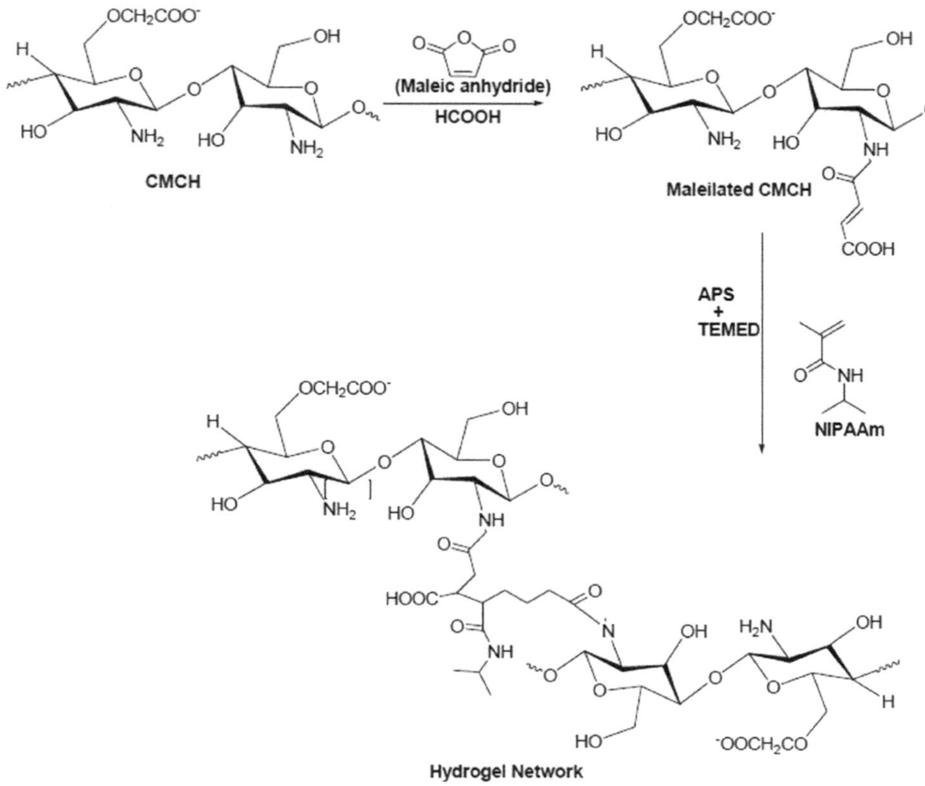

FIGURE 9.8 Synthesis of carboxymethyl chitosan and NIPAAm-based hydrogels.

when hydrogen bonds were broken in an acidic pH. Chitosan and poly(vinyl alcohol) (PVA) were crosslinked with glutaraldehyde and a faster release of 5-fluorouracil was observed at pH 2.1 than at pH 7.4. A network with an optimum crosslinking density plays an important role in pH-responsiveness (Alvarez-Lorenzo et al. 2013).

With the use of photo-sensitive functional groups, hydrogels can be developed. These reactive groups can be crosslinked with chitosan upon irradiation with UV light. This method is advantageous due to its ease of formation, safety, speed, low cost, etc., compared to conventional chemical methods like various reactive species, catalysts, and initiators. Ono and team developed a photo-crosslinked chitosan hydrogel as a biological adhesive. The polymer was functionalized in situ with azide groups (-N3). The reactive nitrene group was formed from the azide group after irradiation of UV. This reactive nitrene group binds to free amino groups of chitosan which cause gelation within 60 s. (Shiraki et al. 2010). In another study, photo-crosslinked chitosan hydrogels were developed for the controlled release of heparin and fibroblast growth factors which were found to be effective novel carriers through in vivo vascularization (Lin et al. 2009).

Another group developed a chitosan-based pH-responsive hydrogel film which was used for capping the pores of a silicon dioxide (SiO_2) layer (Figure 9.9). An electrochemically etched silicon wafer thermal oxidation was done to prepare the porous SiO_2 layer. The chitosan reaction with glycidoxypropyltrimethoxysilane (GPTMS) led to formation of the hydrogel film.

The insulin which is trapped in the porous layer of SiO_2 was released by the transition of the pH-dependent volume phase. The release of insulin was blocked from the top layer at pH 7.4 while insulin penetrated the swollen hydrogel layer at pH 6.0 which resulted in a steady release into the solution (Wu and Sailor 2009).

Zwitterionic chitosan (ZWC)-polyamidoamine (PAMAM) dendrimer complex nanoparticles were developed as pH-sensitive drug carriers by Liu and team. A small volume of PAMAM-methanol solution (40 mg/mL) was prepared by mixing in the ZWC solution. At pH 7.4, a stable electrostatic complex was formed. The surface of the PAMAM dendrimer was covered with ZWC as shown in Figure 9.10. The red blood cells were protected from the hemolytic activities and

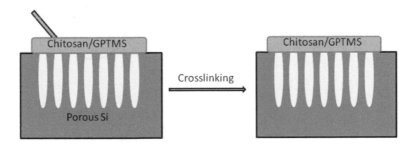

FIGURE 9.9 Illustration of capping porous SiO2 layers with GPTMS-crosslinked chitosan. An optical double layer is formed. The bottom layer is composed of open porous SiO2 and crosslinked chitosan on the top layer.

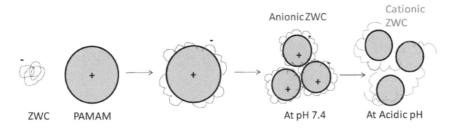

FIGURE 9.10 A pH-sensitive drug carrier for zwitterionic chitosan–polyamidoamine dendrimer complex nanoparticles.

fibroblast cells were protected from the cytotoxic activities of the PAMAM dendrimers because of the presence of the ZWC coating. The protective effect of the ZWC disappeared at a low pH due to the charge conversion of the ZWC which allowed PAMAM dendrimers to enter the cells. A surface coverage of the PAMAM dendrimers was provided by the ZWC in a pH-dependent manner. Thus, the PAMAM dendrimers can be used as a drug carrier in solid tumors because the microenvironment of tumors is acidic compared to normal cells (K.C. Liu and Yeo 2013).

The pH-responsive chitosan/heparin nanoparticles were developed for stomach-specific anti-*Helicobacter pylori* therapy. In this study, nanoparticles were produced instantaneously upon the addition of heparin solution to a chitosan solution with magnetic stirring at room temperature. The average particle size was 130–300 nm and the nanoparticles were stable at pH 1.2–2.5 with a positive surface charge, which protected the incorporated drug from the gastric juices which destroy the drug as shown in Figure 9.11 and 9.12 The nanoparticles had the ability to adhere to and infiltrate cell-cell junctions, and thus the drug could reach the *H. pylori* infected site (Lin et al. 2009).

The chitosan-based composite hydrogels were developed for the controlled release of tinidazole and theophylline. The free radical crosslink copolymerization of N,N-methylene bisacrylamide (MBA) and acrylic acid was performed in water with the presence of chitosan. Two vinyl (CH- CH) functional groups of one MBA monomer and two acrylic monomers were copolymerized and a three-dimensional network of crosslinked copolymer gel was formed. The characterization was done by ^{13}C NMR, FTIR, DTA-TGA, XRD, diffusion, and swelling characteristic and also network parameters. The in vitro release and loading were strongly influenced by the wt% of chitosan and MBA and the pH of the medium. The fastest rate of drug release was observed at a pH of 7.6 then at pH 1.5 (Samanta and Ray 2014).

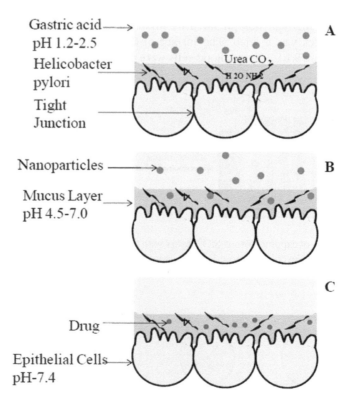

FIGURE 9.11   Representation of *H. pylori* locations in the stomach. (a) In gastric acid, nanoparticles are stable. (b) Nanoparticles adhere and infiltrate in the mucus layer. (c) Drug was released from nanoparticles after contact with *helicobacter pylori*.

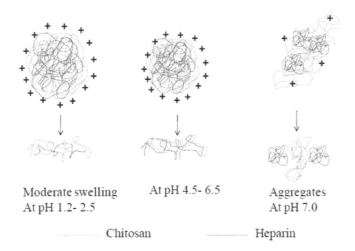

Moderate swelling   At pH 4.5- 6.5   Aggregates
At pH 1.2- 2.5   At pH 7.0

————— Chitosan   ————— Heparin

FIGURE 9.12 Representation of the physical structures of chitosan/heparin nanoparticles in specific pH environments.

For gadolinium neutron-capture therapy, gadopentetic acid-loaded chitosan nanoparticles were developed. Their release and retention properties in the tumor were found to be useful as intra-tumoral injectable devices for gadolinium neutron-capture therapy (Agnihotri et al. 2004).

Via ionic gelation of the positively charged chitosan, a cationic, hydrophilic molecule was entrapped into the nanoparticles. Doxorubicin (DOX) was masked by the positive charge through complexing it with dextran sulfate. The DOX encapsulation efficiency was doubled relative to the control group because of the modification with the loading of DOX up to 4.0 wt%. These nanoparticles were found to maintain cytostatic activity relative to the free DOX. This study reported good activity in cell culture. Also, nanoparticles were found to entrap and deliver DOX to cells in its active form (Janes et al. 2001).

From a literature survey, it was found that chitosan micro/nanoparticulate systems containing various drugs have a wide scope in controlled drug delivery and other therapeutic applications.

9.3.3 Dextran as Environmental Responsive Nanocarrier

Dextran is polysaccharide obtained from bacterial cultures. As Figure 9.13 shows, dextran contains 1,3- and 1,6-glucosidic linkages with D-glucopyranose residues (Kim and Chu 2000). Dextran has been used as a blood plasma substitute because of its good compatibility with the human body, and

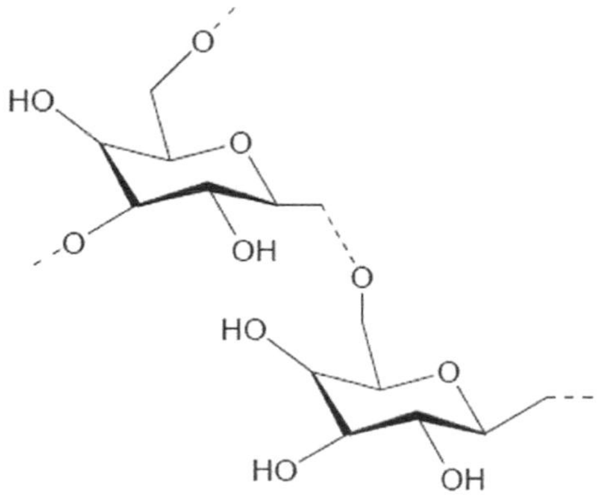

FIGURE 9.13 Chemical structure of dextran.

it has also used in drug delivery. Dextran is a non-toxic, inert, and biodegradable naturally occurring biopolymer. Dextran is stable in the stomach and small intestine therefore its commonly used in colon-specific delivery systems. It is degraded by dextranase which is produced by anaerobic gram-negative intestinal bacteria in the large intestine. Dextran is stable under mild acidic and basic environments and its properties are also extended to conjugation because of presence of a large number of hydroxyl groups (Crepon et al. 1991).

Dextran-methacrylated (MA) and thermal responsive poly(N-isopropylacrylamide) (PNIPAAm) particles were synthesized for controlled drug delivery. Smart hydrogel beads were produced using superhydrophobic surfaces. Several superhydrophobic surfaces were prepared from aluminum, poly-styrene and copper. The thermal responsive poly(N-isopropylacryla-mide) and photo-crosslinked dextran-methacrylated were mixed with a protein (albumin or insulin). The thermal responsive poly(N-isopropylacryla-mide) and photo-crosslinked dextran-methacrylated were mixed with a protein (albumin or insulin). These solutions were dropped on the superhydrophobic surfaces, and the obtained millimetric spheres were hardened in a dry environment under UV light. Within few minutes, non-sticky and spherical hydrogels particles were formed on the superhydrophobic surfaces with an almost 100% encapsulation yield. The homogeneous distribution of proteins were obtained in the particle network. Porosity, swelling, and protein release were exhibited by thermo-responsive dextran-MA/PNIPAAm hydrogels. These stimuli-responsive beads can potentially be used in various applications such as regenerative medicine and tissue engineering (Lima et al. 2011).

Long-circulating nanoparticles were covalently bound to poly(methyl methacrylate) (PMMA) and dextran and were developed by Passirani and team. In vivo studies were performed for dextran containing nanoparticles and compared with bare PMMA nanoparticles. A slow elimination rate was observed for over 48 h in the dextran nanoparticles and the PMMA nanoparticles were found to have only 3 min of half-life (Passirani et al. 1998).

The pH of cancerous tissues is ~6.8 which is comparatively lower than normal tissues (pH ~7.4). Thus, pH-sensitive drug delivery is advantageous for tumor targeted delivery. A Tumor-triggered drug release from supramolecular microcapsules (SMCs) was designed via host-guest interaction between carboxymethyl dextran-graft-β-CD (CMD-g-β-CD) and polyaldenhyde dextran-graft-adamantane (PAD-g-AD). These SMCs are pH-sensitive due to the presence of acid-sensitive hydrazone bonds in the PAD-g-AD. DOX was conjugated through hydrazone binding with adamantane and via host-guest interaction loaded onto the microcapsules. As illustrated in Figure 9.14, hydrazone bonds were cleaved under the weak acidic conditions at the tumor sites and thus DOX was removed from the PAD-g-AD, leading to SMCs destruction and DOX release. The released DOX was uptaken by the cancerous cells and targeted delivery was achieved (Luo et al. 2012).

Dextran-coated superparamagnetic iron oxide nanoparticles were found to have application in diagnostic imaging by positron emission tomography (PET) and magnetic resonance (MRI), and these nanoparticles also constitute a versatile platform for conjugation to targeting ligands. There are various methods for coupling dextran with different functional groups. A bioorthogonal [4+2] cycloaddition reaction between 1,2,4,5-tetrazene (Tz) and trans-cyclooctene (TCO) is a robust reaction for targeting ligands or labeling pre-targeted cells. Dextran-coated iron oxide nanoparticles containing poly(acrylic acid) (PAA) polymers were encapsulated in the chemotherapeutic drug Taxol with a near-infrared dye. Functionalization of this nanoparticle with folate allowed up-take into A549 lung cancer cells, Taxol release, and cell death (Tassa et al. 2011).

A novel magnetic drug-targeting carrier was synthesized and characterized through a core-shell structure. This core-shell carrier has the advantage of thermosensitivity and magnetic core properties, for example, an on-off mechanism responsive to external temperature change. The shell of the carrier was composed of dextran crosslinked and grafted with a poly(N-isopropylacryl-amide-co-N,N-dimethylacrylamide) (dextran-g-poly(NIPAAm-co-DMAAm)) with a core of superparamagnetic Fe_3O_4. Figure 9.15 represents the various steps involved in the synthesis of dextran-g-poly(NIPAAm-co-DMAAm). The diameter of the nanoparticles was ~8 nm with a 3 nm shell. The lower critical solution temperature (LCST) was found to be ~38°C determined by UV-vis

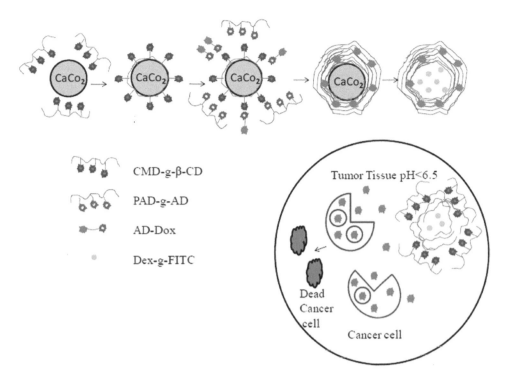

CMD-g-β-CD

PAD-g-AD

AD-Dox

Dex-g-FITC

Tumor Tissue pH<6.5

Dead Cancer cell

Cancer cell

FIGURE 9.14 Representation of drug-loaded microcapsules and pH-induced release of drug.

absorption spectroscopy. The composition of the carrier was confirmed by Fourier transform infrared spectroscopy (FTIR). This magnetic carrier system can be potentially used in magnetic resonance imaging and magnetic drug targeting delivery (Zhang, Srivastava, and Misru 2007).

Dextran grafted with poly(N-isopropylacrylamide) (PNIPAAm), dodecyl, and thiol end groups was synthesized by Lv et al using a RAFT polymerization process. Dodecyl-terminated polymers (DexPNI) can be self-assembled at room temperature through direct non-covalent interactions. Nanostructure collapsed as there was an increase in the environmental temperature due to the LCST phase transition of the PNIPAAm side chains, as represented in Figure 9.16.

It was found by turbidimetry that the phase transition behaviors of DexPNI were dependent on polymer concentration and PNIPAAm chain length, both lead to lower LCSTs and sharper phase transitions. By aminolysis of tri thio-carbonate groups, the dodecyl-terminated polymers were transformed by oxidation, into chemical (disulfide) crosslinked versions (SS-DexPNI). The sharper phase transitions were observed because of the "doubled" chain length of PNIPAAm. The self-assembly was observed in response to the external stimuli of either temperature or redox potential. These nanogels proved to be promising cargo for triggered intracellular delivery (Tan et al. 2011). For the layer-by-layer coating of dextran containing $CaCO_3$ microparticles, the carboxyl groups on the surface of gold nanoparticles (AuNP) were used with poly(allylamine hydrochloride) (PAH), followed by the dissolution of the $CaCO_3$ core. SEM, TEM, and confocal microscopy are used to characterize the hybrid nanoparticles/polyelectrolyte capsules. AuNPs is pH-sensitive because of the carboxyl groups on their surface. The pH-dependent swelling and deconstruction was exhibited by these microcapsules at a low and high pH. The amino groups of the PAH and the carboxyl groups of the AuNP were crosslinked by covalent bonding which was responsible for pH-responsive behavior. Activation of AuNPs can be done with the help of IR light, and because of this ability it can be used to enhance the detection and imaging of such capsules by Raman microspectrosopy, and also to release encapsulated material from the nanoparticles/polyelectrolyte capsules (De Geest et al. 2007). An incompatibility between polymers such as hydrophilic and hydrophobic groups is the inherent problem in the composition. The

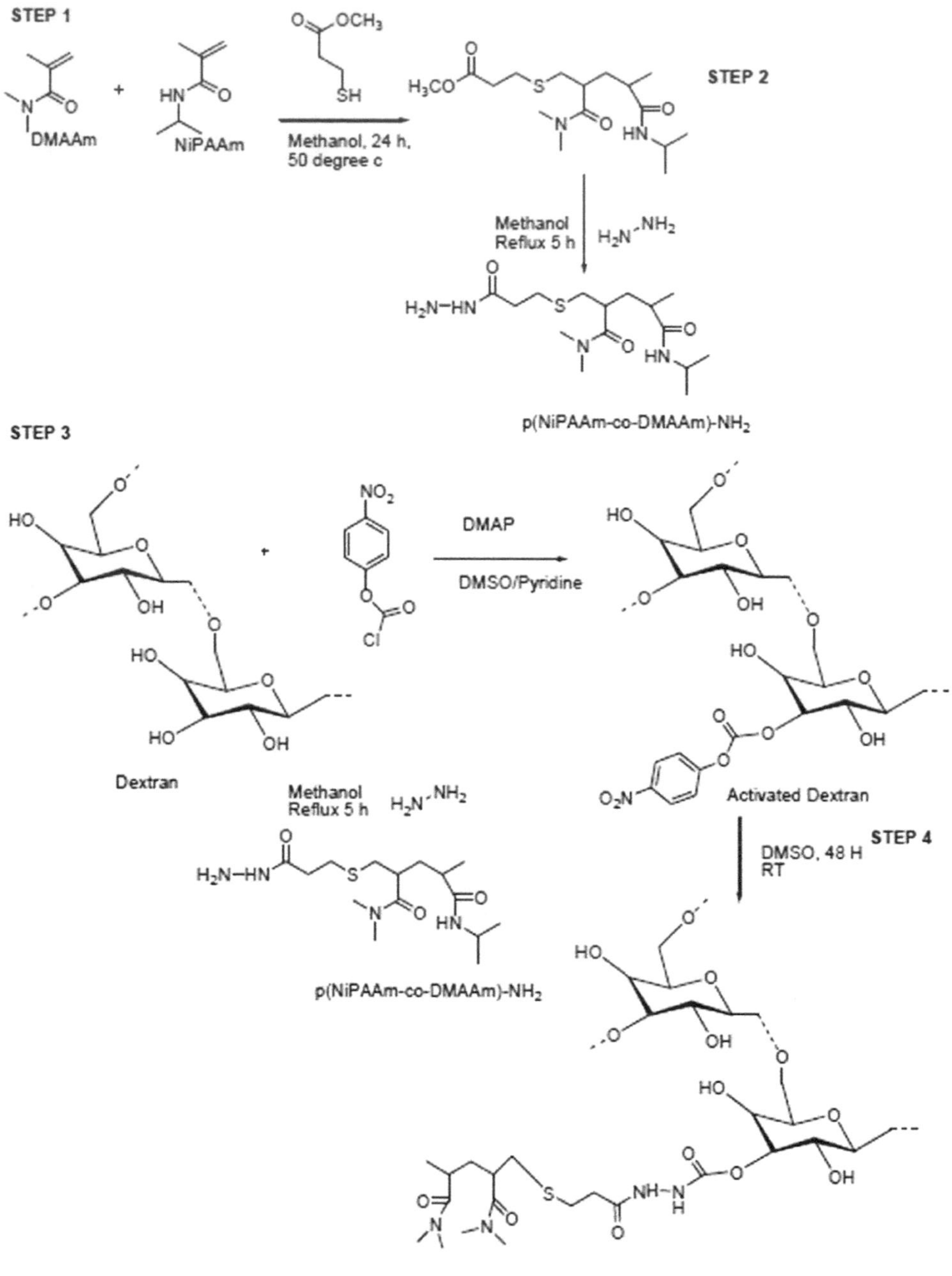

FIGURE 9.15 Synthesis of dextran grafted with poly(NIPAAm-co-DMAAm).

use of reactive compatibilizers was found to be beneficial in eliminating this problem. For example, the miscibility problem between PCL and dextran was solved with the addition of pNIPAM and the block copolymers of poly(2-dimethylamino ethyl) methacrylate (PDMA) or 7%–10% (w/w) PDMA and resulted in crosslinked gels with a precise composition. For controlling the release behavior of hydrophobic and hydrophilic drugs, the use of suitable amounts of these reactive compatibilizers was advantageous for inducing pH or both pH and temperature responsiveness, and the amphiphilic co-network (APCN) gels were synthesized. These gels were reported to have good degradability and exhibited good blood compatibility and cyto-compatibility. For tissue engineering scaffolds and sustained release of drugs, these kinds of gels were found suitable (Chandel et al. 2016).

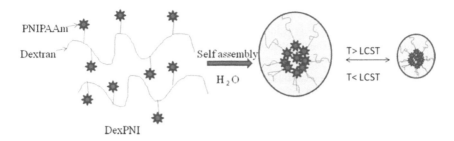

FIGURE 9.16 Schematic illustration of DexPNI nanogels and the self-assembly of DexPNI below and above LCST in water.

Dextran-DOX conjugate was encapsulated using chitosan nanoparticles for tumor targeted delivery. Dextran was conjugated with DOX, firstly dextran was allowed to react overnight with sodium periodate to form the polyaldehyde dextran (PAD). This PAD was dialyzed and then conjugated with DOX. The pure dextran-DOX conjugate was obtained through sephadex g-100 column purification. The chitosan nanoparticles were prepared by an emulsion method. The diameter size of the nanoparticles were 100 ± 10 nm. Thus, the enhanced permeability and retention effect (EPR) was favored as observed in most solid tumors. The anticancer activity of these nanoparticles were evaluated in J774A.1 macrophage tumor cells implanted in Balb/c mice. The reduced side effects and improved therapeutic efficacy was observed in the treatment of solid tumors (Mitra et al. 2001).

9.3.4 Hyaluronic Acid as an Environmental Responsive Nanocarrier

As depicted in Figure 9.17, hyaluronic acid is a linear polysaccharide obtained from animal sources. Hyaluronic acid consists of the disaccharide N-acetylglucosamine and D-glucuronic acid linked by alternating β-(1–3) and α-(14) bonds. The presence of hyaluronic acid can be found in the extracellular matrix of higher animals which helps with various functions like water retention, lubrication, adhesion, or proliferation affecting to cellular migration. It is non-immunogenic, biocompatible, and biodegradable (Alvarez-Lorenzo et al. 2013).

Because of its high affinity with CD44, Hyaluronic acid (HA) has received extensive attention (Yang et al. 2013). HA-based conjugates are widely used as passive targeting systems due to the presence of an enhanced permeation and retention (EPR) effect and the active targeting of CD44-bearing cancer cells, which does not require any additional targeting ligands. The efficacy of paclitaxel was improved in the brain metastases of breast cancer (HA MW 3–5 kDa) by conjugating with HA (Yang et al. 2013) in orthotopic HN5 xenograft models and OSC-19-luciferase models (HA MW 35 kDa) (Yang et al. 2013) and in mice bearing ovarian cancer (HAMW200 kDa) (Yang et al. 2013). The hydrogels were prepared by crosslinking HA with ethyleneglycol diglycidylether (EGDE). The release rate of negatively charged macromolecules from hyaluronic acid hydrogels crosslinked with EGDE was shown to decrease when an electric field was switched on. Hyaluronic acid hydrogels rapidly swell in water, but the swelling is hindered in the presence of ions. Similarly,

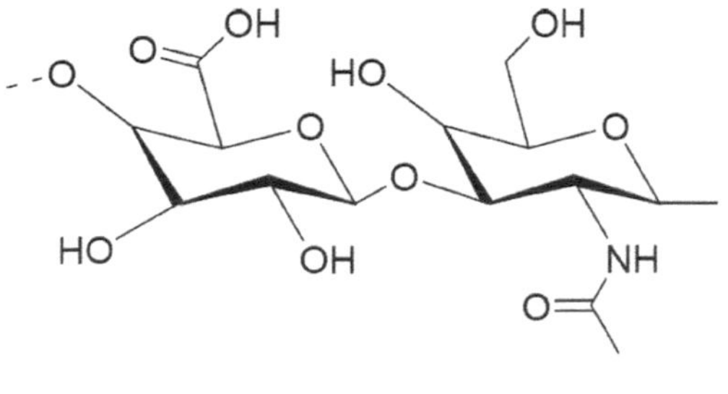

FIGURE 9.17 Structure of hyaluronic acid.

applying an electrical field dramatically reduced the swelling and, consequently, the release rate of poly (styrene sulfonic acid) and poly (glutamic acid, tyrosine) sodium salts. The rate of release was increased with the removal of the electric field (Alvarez-Lorenzo et al. 2013).

HA-ss-PTX conjugate was designed and synthesized by Yin et at and characterized for selective intracellular drug release and active tumor targeting. HA was covalently conjugated with paclitaxel in various sizes (MW 9.5, 35, 770 kDa). A disulfide bond was used in the crosslinking to shield drug leakage into blood circulation and to release the drug rapidly into the tumor cells in response to the glutathione. The drug loading, tumor targeting, and intracellular endocytosis was enhanced due to the incorporation of HA in comparison to mPEG. The molecular weight of HA was found to affect the properties and antitumor efficacy of the synthesized conjugates. Intracellular uptake of HA-ss-PTX was mediated by CD44-caveolae-mediated endocytosis toward MCF-7 cells. The improved tumor growth inhibition in vivo with a TIR of $83.27 \pm 5.20\%$ was demonstrated in HA9.5-ss-PTX compared with Taxol. HA9.5-ss-PTX was found to achieve the rapid intra-cellular release of PTX which improved its therapeutic efficacy. Therefore, it provides a platform for controlled intracellular release in chemotherapeutics and specific drug targeting (Yin et al. 2015).

For delivering paclitaxel (PTX) to tumors over-expressing CD44, paclitaxel-loaded coated with hyaluronic acid lipid carriers (HA-NLCs) were developed via electrostatic attraction. Via melt emulsion technology, cationic PTX-NLC was prepared. Then, as depicted in Figure 9.18, it was coated with HA. The dialysis method was used to evaluate the in vitro release of PTX. The release of PTX was more slowly from HA-NLC compared with Taxol. HA-NLC was investigated through in vitro MTT assay for cytotoxicity in CT26, B16, and CT26 cell lines. The cytotoxicity of HA-NLC was found superior to that of Taxol. In B16-bearing Kunming mice, the in vivo antitumor effect was evaluated to study the tissue distribution and the pharmacokinetics of HA-NLC. It was better tolerated with increased antitumor activity compared with Taxol. In addition to this, a prolonged circulation time in the blood was observed for PTX, with increased accumulation of PTX in the tumor. Therefore, the electrostatic attraction method used to prepare HA-NLC was found effective for delivering PTX to tumors overexpressing CD44 (Yang et al. 2013).

Natural HA and vinyl monomers were crosslinked and polymerized to entrap the natural polymers into the synthetic gel. As depicted in Figure 9.19, studies under an electric field (on-off switching) were performed and the rate of drug release was controlled by the gel. It was proved that electric-responsive drug releases were possible using hyaluronic acid entrapping gel. Factors such as crosslinkers and their density, degree of swelling, and the kind and composition of the vinyl monomer were found to affect the electro-responsiveness (Sutani et al. 2001).

Novel hydrogels with a polysaccharide-poly(amino acid) structure was prepared. In the first step, hyaluronic acid (HA) and α, β -poly(N-2-hydroxyethyl)-DL-aspartamide (PHEA) have been derivatized with methacrylic anhydride (AMA), thus obtaining HA-AMA and PHM derivatives, respectively. For the second step, irradiation of aqueous solutions of both these derivatives were

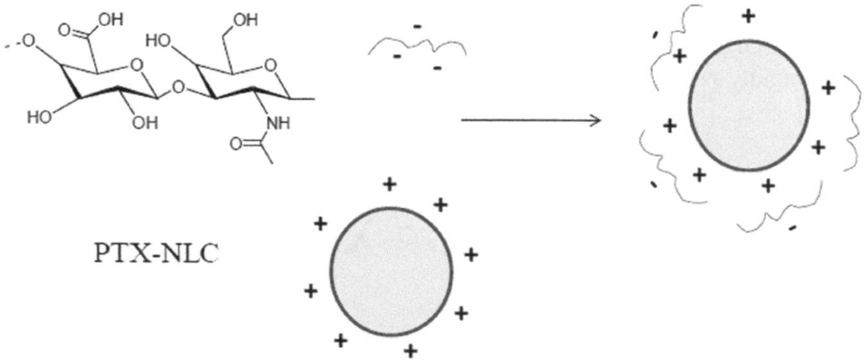

FIGURE 9.18   A schematic representation of the structure of HA-NLC.

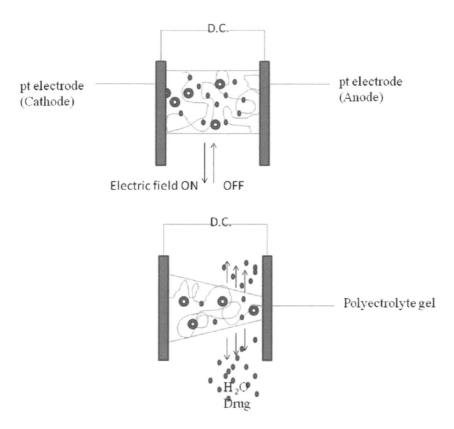

FIGURE 9.19 Scheme and the principle of device type signal responsive drug delivery system using gel actuator.

performed at 313 nm to obtain chemical hydrogels (Figure 9.20). The highest yield was obtained by irradiating 4% w/v of HA-AMA and 4% w/v of PHM for 15 min. It has pH-dependent swelling ability. In addition to this, a partial hydrolysis took place in the presence of enzymes such as hyaluronidase or esterase, but the degradation entity was found to be lower compared with HA-AMA alone. Thrombin was used as a model drug and the ability to entrap it in hydrogels was evaluated. In vitro release and platelet aggregation studies were performed. Thrombin was released in an active form from the HA-AMA/PHM hydrogel. Therefore, this hydrogel can be used in the treatment of hemorrhages (Pitarresi et al. 2006).

A pH-responsive hyaluronic acid-g-poly(L-histidine) (HA-PHis) copolymer was synthesized by conjugation of HA with poly(L-histidine). This conjugate showed tumor targeted activity and thus can be used as a carrier for anticancer drugs. The effect of the degree of substitution (DS) on the pH-responsive behavior of HA-PHis copolymer micelles was confirmed by studies of particles of different sizes. DOX was released in a pH-dependent manner from HA-PHis micelles as represented in Figure 9.21. The blank micelles were reported to be non-toxic and DOX-loaded micelles were cytotoxic, with low PHis. DS were highly cytotoxic, when evaluated against Michigan Cancer Foundation-7 (MCF-7) cells (over-expressed CD44 receptors) by MTT assay, which indicated that the carboxylic groups of HA are the active binding sites for CD44 receptors. The receptor-mediated endocytosis revealed that these pH-responsive HA-PHis micelles were uptaken in great amounts and delivery of DOX was efficiently observed in cytosol. The internalization of the HA-PHis micelles were studied by confocal images and endocytosis inhibition experiments which demonstrated that the micelles were internalized into cells mainly via clathrin-mediated endocytosis and also DOX triggered release into the cytoplasm. Therefore, HA-PHis micelles is a promising pH-responsive nanosystem for the targeted delivery of DOX (Qiu et al. 2014).

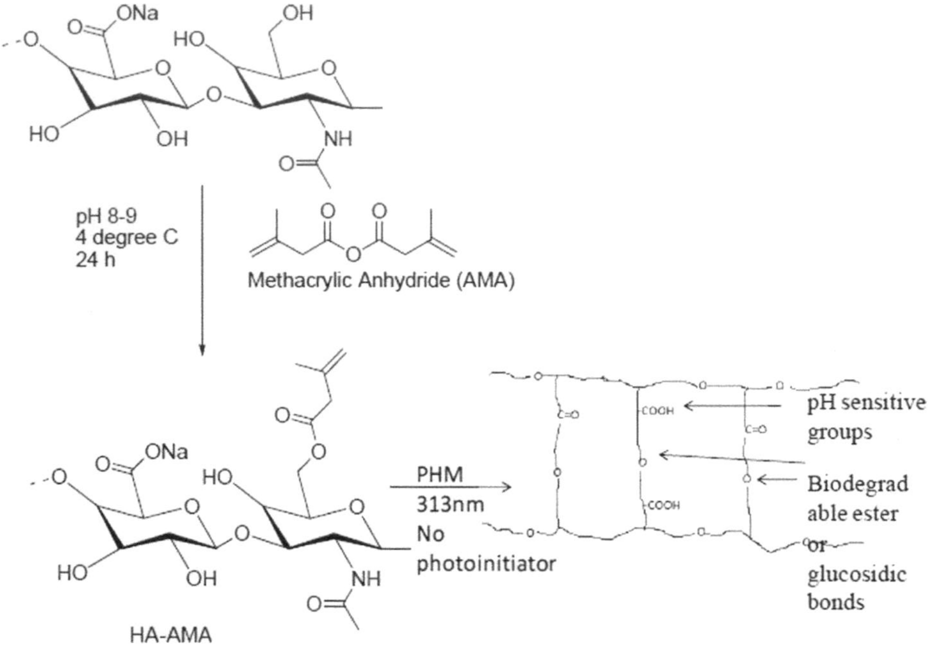

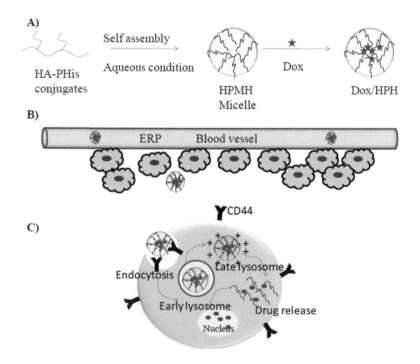

FIGURE 9.20   Reaction of hyaluronic acid (HA) with methacrylic anhydride (AMA) to form the HA-AMA derivative. After irradiation of HA-AMA and PHM, network of HA-AMA/PHM was formed.

FIGURE 9.21   Schematic representation of self-assembly HA-PHis micelles and pH- responsive intracellular drug delivery. (a) The DOX was encapsulated in HA-PHis copolymers micelles (b) Particles of suitable size were accumulated in tumor tissue by the EPR effect. (c) The micelles were selectively taken up by tumor cells via CD44 receptor-mediated endocytosis and delivered to the lysosomes, the release of DOX was triggered into the cytoplasm, improving intracellular drug release and increasing the antitumor efficacy.

For the treatment of liver fibrosis, a long-acting and target-specific hyaluronic acid (HA)-TRAIL conjugate was developed. A coupling reaction between the N-terminal amine group of TRAIL and aldehyde-modified HA was used to synthesize HA-TRAIL conjugate. In vitro anti-proliferation assay and caspase-3 expression was carried out in human colon cancer HCT116 cells. The target-specific delivery of near-infrared fluorescence dye-labeled HA-TRAIL conjugate was exhibited by the in vivo real-time bioimaging of the liver in mice. The HA-TRAIL conjugate was detected by pharmacokinetic studies after a single intravenous injection into Sprague-Dawley (SD) rats and it was detected for more than 4 days. Thus, the antifibrotic effect of HA-TRAIL conjugate was confirmed in an N-nitrosodimethylamine-induced liver fibrosis model SD rats (Yang et al. 2015).

9.4 APPLICATION OF ENVIRONMENTAL RESPONSIVE POLYSACCHARIDE NANOCARRIERS IN DIFFERENT DISEASES

Environmental responsive polysaccharide nanocarriers have wide biomedical and pharmaceutical applications, such as in tissue engineering, wound healing, and protein delivery systems for the treatment of lysosomal storage diseases. The stimuli-responsive properties of polysaccharides are being explored to target the microenvironment of tumors in various types of cancer. The acidic pH of the tumor environment has been targeted to deliver drugs to the tumor site. The pH-sensitive nanoconstructs containing polysaccharides, like alginate, chitosan, detxran, and hyaluronic acid, have been developed which deliver the drug to the tumor site. The higher glutathione concentration in cancer cells has been exploited to develop delivery systems for anticancer drugs which involve a redox cleavage of disulfide bonds. Nanocarriers containing polysaccharides crosslinked with redox-sensitive disulfide bonds have been developed. Thus, polysaccharides play an important role in environmental responsive nanocarrier development.

9.5 CONCLUSIONS

The design and development of environment-responsive smart biopolymers is increasing in in the application of drug delivery. The release mechanism, the design, and the application of a wide variety of stimuli-responsive polysaccharide-based drug carriers have been explored as is evident from the extensive literature presented. Drug loading ability, physicochemical properties, in vitro toxicity, and comparatively simple in vivo tests have been investigated. However, challenges such as stability, metabolism, excretion, interaction with the human organs, and clinical applications of these smart stimuli-responsive carriers still remain to be addressed. Collectively, the above literature shows that polysaccharide-based environment-responsive carriers have significant potential for controlled drug delivery and show great promise in the future of stimuli-sensitive nanomedicine.

NOTE

The authors declare no competing financial interests.

ACKNOWLEDGMENT

This work was supported by a SUN Pharma project grant to Dr. Balaram Ghosh. We also thank Dr. Tapan Kumar Giri and Dr. Bijaya Ghosh for his helpful advice in editing the manuscript.

REFERENCES

Agnihotri, S.A., Mallikarjuna, N.N., and Aminabhavi, T.M. 2004. Recent advances on chitosan-based micro- and nanoparticles in drug delivery. *J Control Release* 100 (1): 5–28.

Alvarez-Lorenzo, C., Blanco-Fernandez, B., Puga, A.M., and Concheiro, A. 2013. Crosslinked ionic polysaccharides for stimuli-sensitive drug delivery. *Adv Drug Deliv Rev* 65 (9): 1148–71.

Alvarez-Lorenzo, C. and Concheiro, A. 2008. Intelligent drug delivery systems: Polymeric micelles and hydrogels. *Mini Rev Med Chem* 8 (11): 1065–74.

Bazban-shotorbani, S., Hasani-sadrabadi, M.M., Karkhaneh, A., Serpooshan, V., Jacob, K.I., Moshaverinia, A., and Mahmoudi, M. 2017. Revisiting structure-property relationship of pH-responsive polymers for drug delivery applications. *J Controlled Release* 253: 46–63.

Brule, S., Levy, M., Wilhelm, C., Letourneur, D., Gazeau, F., Ménager, C., and Le-Visage, C. 2011. Doxorubicin release triggered by alginate embedded magnetic nanoheaters: A combined therapy. *Adv Mater* 23 (6): 787–90.

Chan, A.W., Whitney, R.A., and Neufeld, R.J. 2008. Kinetic controlled synthesis of pH-responsive network. *Biomacromolecules* 9: 2536–45.

Chan, A.W., Whitney, R.A., and Neufeld, R.J. 2009. Semisynthesis of a controlled stimuli-responsive alginate hydrogel. *Biomacromolecules* 10 (3): 609–16.

Chandel, A.K.S., Bera, A., Nutan, B., and Jewrajka, S.K. 2016. Reactive compatibilizer mediated precise synthesis and application of stimuli responsive polysaccharides-polycaprolactone amphiphilic co-network gels. *Polymer* 99: 470–9.

Cheng, R., Meng, F., Deng, C., Klok, H.A., and Zhong, Z. 2013. Biomaterials dual and multi-stimuli responsive polymeric nanoparticles for programmed site-specific drug delivery. *Biomaterials* 34 (14): 3647–57.

Cheng, Y., Luo, X., Payne, G.F., and Rubloff, G.W. 2012. Biofabrication: Programmable assembly of polysaccharide hydrogels in microfluidics as biocompatible scaffolds. *J Mater Chem* 22: 7659–66.

Costa, R.R., Custódio, C.A., Arias, F.J., Rodríguez-Cabello, J.C., and Mano, J.F. 2011. Layer-by-layer assembly of chitosan and recombinant biopolymers into biomimetic coatings with multiple stimuli-responsive properties. *Small* 7 (18): 2640–9.

Crepon, B., Jozefonvicz, J., Chytry, V., Řihová, B., and Kopeček, J. 1991. Enzymatic degradation and immunogenic properties of derivatized dextrans. *Biomaterials* 12: 550–4.

Geest, B.G.D., Skirtach, A.G., Beer, T.R.M.D., Sukhorukov, G.B., Bracke, L., Baeyens, W.R.G., Demeester, J., and Smedt, S.C.D. 2007. Stimuli-responsive multilayered hybrid nanoparticle/polyelectrolyte capsules. *Macromol. Rapid Commun* 28 (1): 88–95.

George, M. and Abraham, T.E. 2006. Polyionic Hydrocolloids for the intestinal delivery of protein drugs: Alginate and chitosan-a review. *J Control Release* 114: 1–14.

Guerry, A., Cottaz, S., Fleury, E., Bernard, J., and Halila, S. 2014. Redox-stimuli responsive micelles from DOX-encapsulating polycaprolactone-G-chitosan oligosaccharide. *Carbohydr Polym* 112: 746–52.

Hamidi, M., Azadi, A., and Rafiei, P. 2008. Hydrogel nanoparticles in drug delivery. *Adv Drug Deliv Rev* 60: 1638–49.

Janes, K.A., Fresneau, M.P., Marazuela, A., Fabra, A., and Alonso, M.J. 2001. Chitosan nanoparticles as delivery systems for doxorubicin. *J Controlled Release* 73: 255–67.

Kim, S.H. and Chu, C.C. 2000. Synthesis and characterization of dextran-methacrylate hydrogels and structural study by SEM. *J Biomed Mater Res* 49 (4): 517–27.

Liang, Y.Y., Zhang, L.M., Jiang, W., and Li, W. 2007. Embedding magnetic nanoparticles into polysaccharide-based hydrogels for magnetically assisted bioseparation. *Chem Phys Chem* 8 (16): 2367–72.

Lima, A.C., Song, W., Blanco-Fernandez, B., Alvarez-Lorenzo, C., and Mano, J.F. 2011. Synthesis of temperature-responsive dextran-MA/PNIPAAm particles for controlled drug delivery using superhydrophobic surfaces. *Pharm Res* 28 (6): 1294–305.

Lin, Y.H., Chang, C.H., Wu, Y.S., Hsu, Y.M., Chiou, S.F., and Chen, Y.J. 2009. Development of pH-responsive chitosan/heparin nanoparticles for stomach-specific anti- helicobacter pylori therapy. *Biomaterials* 30 (19): 3332–42.

Liu, K.C. and Yeo, Y. 2013. Zwitterionic chitosan–polyamidoamine dendrimer complex. *Mol Pharm* 10 (5): 1695–704.

Liu, Z., Jiao, Y., Wang, Y., Zhou, C., and Zhang, Z. 2008. Polysaccharides-based nanoparticles as drug delivery systems. *Adv Drug Deliv Rev* 60 (15): 1650–62.

Luo, G.F., Xu, X.D., Zhang, J., Yang, J., Gong, Y.H., Lei, Q. et al.2012. Encapsulation of an adamantane-doxorubicin prodrug in pH-responsive polysaccharide capsules for controlled release. *ACS Appl Mater Interfaces* 4 (10): 5317–24.

Matsumura, S., Hlil, A.R., Lepiller, C., Gaudet, J., Guay, D., Shi, Z. et al. 2008. Ionomers for proton exchange membrane fuel cells with sulfonic acid groups on the end-groups: Novel branched poly(ether-Ketone)s. *Macromolecules* 41 (2) 281–4.

Mitra, S., Gaur, U., Ghosh, P.C., and Maitra, A.N. 2001. Tumour targeted delivery of encapsulated dextran-doxorubicin conjugate using chitosan nanoparticles as carrier. *J Controlled Release* 74: 317–23.

Mura, S., Nicolas, J., and Couvreur, P. 2013. Stimuli-responsive nanocarriers for drug delivery. *Nature Mater* 12: 991–1003.

Passirani, C., Barratt, G., Devissaguet, J.P., and Labarre, D. 1998. Long-circulating nanoparticles bearing heparin or dextran covalently bound to poly(methyl methacrylate). *Pharm Res* 15: 1046–50.

Pitarresi, G., Pierro, P., Palumbo, F.S., Tripodo, G., and Farmaceutiche, T. 2006. Photo-cross-linked hydrogels with polysaccharide—poly (amino acid) structure: New biomaterials for pharmaceutical applications. *Biomacromolecules* 7: 1302–10.

Prabaharan, M. and Mano, J.F. 2006. Stimuli-responsive hydrogels based on polysaccharides incorporated with thermo-responsive polymers as novel biomaterials. *Macromol Biosci* 6: 991–1008.

Qiu, L., Li, Z., Qiao, M., Long, M., Wang, M., Zhang, X., Tian, C., and Chen, D. 2014. Self-assembled pH-responsive hyaluronic acid – G-poly (L-histidine) copolymer micelles for targeted intracellular delivery of doxorubicin. *Acta Biomaterialia* 10 (5): 2024–35.

Samanta, H.S. and Ray, S.K. 2014. Controlled release of tinidazole and theophylline from chitosan based composite hydrogels. *Carbohydr Polym* 106: 109–20.

Shiraki, T., Dawn, A., Tsuchiya, Y., and Shinkai, S. 2010. Thermo- and solvent-responsive polymer complex created from supramolecular complexation between a helix-forming polysaccharide and a cationic poly-thiophene. *J Am Chem Soc* 132: 13928–35.

Stuart, M.A., Huck, W.T., Genzer, J., Müller, M., Ober, C., and Stamm, M. et al. 2010. Emerging applications of stimuli-responsive polymer materials. *Nature Mater* 9: 101–13.

Sutani, K., Kaetsu, I., and Uchida, K. 2001. The synthesis and the electric-responsiveness of hydrogels entrapping natural polyelectrolyte. *Radiat Phys Chem* 61: 49–54.

Tan, J., Kang, H., Liu, R., Wang, D., Jin, X., Li, Q., and Huang, Y. 2011. Dual-stimuli sensitive nanogels fabricated by self-association of thiolated hydroxypropyl cellulose. *Polym Chem* 2: 672–8.

Tassa, C., Shaw, S.Y., and Weissleder, R. 2011. Dextran-coated iron oxide nanoparticles: A versatile platform for targeted molecular imaging, molecular diagnostics, and therapy. Acc. *Chem Res* 44: 842–52.

Vasile, C. and Nita, L.E. 2011. Novel multi-stimuli responsive sodium alginate-grafted-poly(N-Isopropylacrylamide) copolymers: II. Dilute solution properties. *Carbohydr Polym* 86: 77–84.

Wang, Y., Hosta-Rigau, L., Lomas, H., and Caruso, F. 2011. Nanostructured polymer assemblies formed at interfaces: Applications from immobilization and encapsulation to stimuli-responsive release. *Phys Chem* 13: 4782–801.

Wu, J. and Sailor, M.J. 2009. Chitosan hydrogel-capped porous SiO_2 as a pH responsive nano-valve for triggered release of insulin. *Adv Funct Mater* 19: 733–41.

Wu, W., Shen, J., Banerjee, P., and Zhou, S. 2010. Chitosan-based responsive hybrid nanogels for integration of optical pH-sensing, tumor cell imaging and controlled drug delivery. *Biomaterials* 31: 8371–81.

Yang, J.A., Kong, W.H., Sung, D.K., Kim, H., Kim, T.H., Lee, K.C., and Hahn, S.K. 2015. Hyaluronic acid – tumor necrosis factor-related apoptosis-inducing ligand conjugate for targeted treatment of liver fibrosis. *Acta Biomater* 12: 174–82.

Yang, X., Kim, E., Liu, Y., Shi, X.W., Rubloff, G.W., Ghodssi, R., Bentley, W.E., Pancer, Z., and Payne, G.F. 2010. In-film bioprocessing and immunoanalysis with electroaddressable stimuli-responsive polysaccharides. *Adv Funct Mater* 20 (10): 1645–52.

Yang, X.Y., Li, Y.X., Li, M., Zhang, L., Feng, L.X., and Zhang, N. 2013. Hyaluronic acid-coated nanostructured lipid carriers for targeting paclitaxel to cancer. *Cancer Lett* 334: 338–45.

Yin, S., Huai, J., Chen, X., Yang, Y., Zhang, X., and Gan, Y., et al. 2015. Intracellular delivery and antitumor effects of a redox-responsive polymeric paclitaxel conjugate based on hyaluronic acid. *Acta Biomater* 26: 274–85.

Zhang, J.L., Srivastava, R.S., and Misra, R.D. 2007. Core – shell magnetite nanoparticles surface encapsulated with smart stimuli-responsive polymer: Synthesis, characterization, and LCST of viable drug-targeting delivery system core – shell magnetite nanoparticles surface encapsulated with smart stimuli. *Langmuir* 23: 6342–51.

10 Advancement of Biodegradable Polysaccharide Nanocarriers for Delivery of Herbal Extracts and Bio-Actives

Pallavi Krishna Shetty and Chethan Gejjalagere Honnappa

CONTENTS

10.1 INTRODUCTION: BACKGROUND

Modern pharmaceutical technology has observed tremendous growth in an ever-growing field of research, and is still developing every day. In recent years, nanotechnology and novel drug delivery systems are the new face of technology in the biomedical drug development field. Owing to the poor absorbability of herbal extracts, bio-active constituents are attracting novel approaches to enhance sustained delivery at the site of action. The advancement in novel drug delivery systems assist in delivery of phytoconstituents to enhance patient compliance by increasing bioavailability and reducing repeated administration and toxicity. Nanotechnology is one of the thriving areas used for drug delivery. The phytochemical and phytopharmacological sciences have also received a considerable amount of attention due to the advancement in the elucidation of structural compositions and biological actions of several medicinal plants. Further, the active constituents present in medicinal plants are responsible for promising therapeutic activity. Therefore, herbal extracts and bio-active constituents such as flavonoids, tannins, and terpenoids occupy a major focus in the industry. Bio-active constituents themselves are less soluble, poorly permeable and bioavailable, and unstable in biological environment. Likewise, herbal bio-actives are unable to cross the lipid barrier of the cells because of their high molecular weight and hence are poorly absorbed, resulting in loss of bioavailability and efficacy, thus limiting their clinical use. Hence, these limitations can be overcome by encapsulating or attaching them with nanocarriers and novel drug delivery systems (Devi et al. 2010; Singh et al. 2016). Nanosized systems for herbal drugs enrich the use of many active constituents and help to overcome many of the problems associated with drug delivery. The biodegradable and biocompatible nature of polysaccharides makes them an ideal candidate for drug delivery (Puglia et al. 2017; Ansari and Farha Islam 2012). This chapter will highlight the use of biodegradable polysaccharides for delivery of herbal medicines for biomedical applications.

10.2 HERBAL EXTRACT AND BIO-ACTIVES

10.2.1 BRIEF OVERVIEW

Traditional medicines have been in use since ancient times and are broadly used around the world, particularly in developing countries where around 80% of people depend on traditional medicines (Kamboj 2000; Bonifacio et al. 2014; Bhattaram et al. 2002). Further, Indian systems of medicine mainly Siddha, Ayurveda & Unani encompass the use of herbal medicines.

Herbal medicines refer to use of various parts of the plant such as leaves, flowers, barks, fruits, seeds, and roots for their medicinal values, and also herbal preparations that are produced by extraction, fractionation, purification, concentration (e.g. herbal extracts and tincture), and finished products (Ekor 2014; Singh 2016).

Recently there has been a growing interest in use of the herbal medicines in the form of herbal extracts and/or the bio-actives of plants which demonstrate lesser side effects as compared to present medicines. The major classes of bio-active compounds are flavonoids, polyphenols, tannins, alkaloids, terpenoids, etc. Further, various active constituents including piperine, silibinin, catechin, quercetin, genistein, naringin, and curcumin have proven to be useful in various therapeutic actions of different classes of drugs, such as anti-hypertensive, anticancer, anti-viral, anti-tubercular, antifungal, etc. (Kesarwani and Gupta 2013; Kulkarni 2011).

10.2.2 LIMITATIONS OF HERBAL EXTRACTS

The main limitations of herbal medicines are solubility, permeability, stability, and inadequate potency. Despite the promising *in-vitro* findings, herbal medicines display less *in-vivo* effects due to their hydrophobic nature and hence have reduced absorption and bioavailability limiting their use. Also, oral administration or topical application of phytoconstituents is limited because of their poor absorption. Many of the herbal extracts or bio-actives (e.g. phenolics, glycosides, flavonoids, xanthan, etc.) are unstable at an extremely acidic pH, undergo first pass metabolism in the liver, and are water soluble molecules with poor lipid solubility and stability issues, which can result in reduced drug levels in the plasma with less therapeutic effect. Hence, researchers are giving importance to developing herbal drugs with various novel drug delivery systems to attain the required active constituent at the target site (Kalita et al. 2013; Kulkarni 2011; Puglia et al. 2017).

10.3   NOVEL DRUG DELIVERY SYSTEMS (NDDS) FOR THE DELIVERY OF HERBAL EXTRACTS AND BIO-ACTIVES

Advances in novel drug delivery systems have led to the improvement in effective delivery of herbal drugs. Several of the herbal actives, especially compounds containing phenolic, are water soluble and hence they are unable to cross lipid barriers and are less bioavailable. There is a need for development of novel drug delivery systems that deliver herbal components in a novel manner to reduce repeated administration and enhance patient compliance by reducing toxicity and improving bioavailability. Advanced novel drug delivery systems like phytosomes, liposomes, transfersomes, ethosomes, polymeric nanoparticles, micelles, nanoemulsions, niosomes, and solid-lipid nanocarriers can enhance their bioavailability and enable them to cross the lipid rich barriers. Incorporation of bio-actives in the delivery system helps to increase solubility, stability, protection from toxicity, enhanced pharmacological activity, improve tissue macrophage distribution, sustain delivery, and protect from physical and chemical degradation.

In brief, various NDDS used for herbal drug delivery may be classified as

- Vesicular type (e.g. liposomes, ethosomes, transferosomes, phytosomes)
- Particulate type (e.g. microspheres, nanoparticles)
- Biphasic systems (e.g. micro/nanoemulsions)

Many of these nanocarriers such as liposomes, nanoparticles, transferosomes, phytosomes, ethosomes, and lipid-based systems are developed for effective delivery of numerous herbal bio-actives and extracts.

Liposomes containing the essential oil of *Atractylodes macrocephala koidz* and its oxidative derivatives were prepared to enhance solubility and bioavailability with reduced side effects (Wen et al. 2010). Liposomes of the herbal extract *Tripterygium wilfordi* led to enhancement of stability with reduced side effects (Li et al. 2007). Formulated quercetin liposomes for oral and intranasal delivery showed anxiolytic and enhanced cognitive effects in rats. Intranasal liposomes have shown a decrease in dose and improved bioavailability compared to oral administration (Priprem et al. 2008). Silymarin-extract liposomes were prepared for management of liver disorders via the buccal route. The formulated liposomes showed enhancement in permeation with improved bioavailability. The interaction between the phospholipids of liposomes increased mucoadhesion and promoted better hepatoprotection (El-Samaligy et al. 2006). Liposomes containing *Artemisia arborescens L* showed enhancement in stability and anti-herpetic activity (Sinico et al. 2005). Capsaicin liposomes were prepared for transdermal application which showed enhanced permeation via the skin with a prolonged duration of action (Mahajan et al. 2010). Taxanes possess antitumor activity, their inclusion in liposomes reduced the tissue related toxicity of the bio-active with improved efficacy (Straubinger and Balasubramanian 2005). Despite the various advantages of liposomal formulations there have been few limitations such as reduced shelf life, degradation of the active moiety in liposome core, decreased bioavailability and limited loading potential, random clearance by reticule endothelial system (RES), and erratic drug release (Alexander et al. 2016). Some of the herbal actives involving phytosomes are briefly explained in this paragraph. Yanyu and his co-workers developed silybin phytosome and evaluated its pharmacokinetic effects in rats. The bioavailability of silybin was increased after oral administration of prepared silybin-phospholipid complex due to the improved lipophilic properties of silybin phytosomes (Yanyu et al. 2006). Maiti and his co-researches formulated a quercetin-phospholipid phytosome complex which exerted better therapeutic efficacy than the quercetin moiety in rat liver injury induced by carbon tetrachloride (Maiti et al. 2005). Further, from the same research group phytosomes of curcumin and naringenin were prepared and evaluated. The phytosome of curcumin was formulated to overcome the limitation of absorption and to investigate the protective effect of curcumin phospholipid complex on carbon tetrachloride-induced acute liver damage in rats. The complex showed enhanced aqueous or n-octanol solubility and significant improvements in the anti-oxidant activity of the complex compared to pure curcumin. The phytosome of naringenin produced better anti-oxidant activity and sustained duration of action than the free compound (Maiti et al. 2006; Maiti et al. 2007). Also, a novel hesperetin phytosome was prepared by complexing hesperetin with hydro-genated phospha-tidyl choline and evaluated for anti-oxidant activity. The results showed that the hesperetin phyto-some exhibited higher anti-oxidant activity and improved bioavailability than the pure molecule at the same dose. The phytosome formulation helps to enhance the absorption of active ingredients upon topical application and improves systemic bioavailability after oral administration (Venkatesh et al. 2008). Numerous phytosomal formulations have been evaluated for the delivery of poorly lipid soluble herbal drugs and extracts such as extracts of boswellia serrata, ginkgo biloba, hawthorn, green tea, and ginseng (Marena and Lampertico 1991).

10.4 NANOCARRIERS FOR DELIVERY OF HERBAL EXTRACTS AND BIO-ACTIVES

Nanoparticles are a novel approach for drug delivery to achieve better therapeutic action, bioavail-ability, and reduce toxicity. Formulation of nanoparticles for herbal extracts and bio-actives reduces degradation of actives in the gastrointestinal tract after oral administration and decreases first pass metabolism and distribution of actives in non-targeted sites. Hence nanoparticles for bio-actives improve therapeutic efficacy and patient compliance by reducing side effects (Kulkarni 2011; Kesarwani and Gupta 2013). Numerous bio-actives like flavonoids, terpenoids, and tannins show improved therapeutic effect at less or similar dose when combined into nanocarriers as compared to plain herbal extracts. Hence, there is a boundless possibility in formulation of nanoparticles for therapeutic effective herbal extracts and bio-actives as it provides therapeutically effective and cost effective delivery of the drug. Many bio-active formulations including glycyrrhizin, curcumin, morin, quercetin, naringin, silibinin, catechins, piperine, and genistein have proven their ability to increase bioavailability (Alexander et al. 2014; Ansari and Farha Islam 2012).

Nanotechnology helps in targeted and controlled drug delivery bio-actives for various chronic diseases. Nanocarriers provide a more efficient and appropriate route for administration, reduced toxicity, and health-care costs. Nanomaterials are colloidal particles with numerous physicochemi-cal properties such as small size, high solubility, large surface area, decreased immunogenicity, high reactivity, unique drug release patterns, and drug loading capacity. By varying formulation compositions, nanoparticles can be used for both hydrophilic and lipophilic drug candidates. Nano sized materials have unique properties such as solubility, drug release patterns, and immunogenic-ity. The recent past has resulted in the therapeutic advancement for the treatment of various ailments such as diabetes, asthma, infectious diseases, cancer, etc. (Keservani et al. 2017; Alexander et al. 2016; Wani et al. 2015; Ansari and Farha Islam 2012).

Nanocarriers for delivery of herbal active constituents carry numerous advantages correspond-ing to enhancement of their solubility, bioavailability and therapeutic effect, controlled release, and protection from degradation. Therefore, nanoparticles of herbal drugs carry potential advan-tages by overcoming the disadvantages related with plant medicines. In addition, they carry the drug to the action site by overcoming barriers such as the acidic pH of the stomach, the increasing metabolism in the liver, and the enhanced blood circulation due to their smaller size. Further, nanoparticles can be used to target specific tissues or selectively deliver drugs and also they have potential for extended circulation in human body. Hence, application of herbal drugs as remedies in the form of nanoparticles will enhance the development of herbal remedies to treat various dis-orders (Puglia et al. 2017).

The progress of advanced drug delivery systems for herbal medicines includes, nano dose, enhancing the solubility and bioavailability, protection from toxicity, sustained delivery, etc. Such novel drug delivery systems have site specific action and a predetermined rate. Nano drug delivery systems are very useful for optimal use and for improving the cost-effectiveness of the expensive phyto products. Nanocarriers can be targeted to particular tissues or organs enhancing their circulation time in the body. Hence, application of herbal drugs as remedies in the form of nanocarriers will enhance development of the use of herbal remedies to treat various disorders (Saraf 2010; Puglia et al. 2017).

10.5 POLYSACCHARIDE NANOCARRIER FOR DELIVERY OF HERBAL EXTRACT AND BIO-ACTIVES

Polysaccharides are the most commonly used materials for the preparation of nanocarriers, due to their structural flexibility, biocompatibility, and biodegradability. Polysaccharides are the most abundant macromolecules that exist in the biosphere. Polysaccharides are long chain monosaccharides and may have a linear or branched structure based upon the type of monosaccharide unit. Polysaccharides have a high number of functional groups, a wide range of molecular weights (100–1000 Da) with varying chemical and structural compositions, which contribute to their diversity in structure and in physical properties. Further, polysaccharides have different reactive groups such as hydroxyl, carboxyl, and amino groups which are available for chemical modification to enhance bioavailability. Polysaccharides are easily obtained from natural sources and are extracted from plants, bacteria, fungi, or algae. Polysaccharides have significant importance in the biomedical applications of drug carriers due to their favorable properties such as improved solubility and biocompatibility, enhanced release, reduced immunogenicity and toxicity, stealth nature, bioadhesion, easy to modify, etc., thus making them an ideal candidate for drug delivery (Nicolas et al. 2013).

Polysaccharides exhibit numerous advantages including enhanced solubility, potential for modification, biodegradability and biocompatibility, and innate bioactivity (Pushpamalar et al. 2016). Complex carbohydrates constituted of monosaccharides joined together by glycosidic bonds are often one of the main structural elements of plants and animals. Polysaccharides can be extracted from numerous sources of plants and animals. Polysaccharides from animal sources include mainly chitin and chondroitin; and polysaccharides from plant sources include cellulose, dextran, lectin, agarose, pectin, starch, hemicellulose, hyaluronate, alginate, guar gums, etc. As these biomaterials occur naturally, they are typically very stable, hydrophilic, non-toxic, and biodegradable.

Due to the presence of various derivable groups on the molecular chains, polysaccharides can be easily modified chemically and biochemically, resulting in different polysaccharide derivatives. Particularly, most of natural polysaccharides have hydrophilic groups such as hydroxyl, carboxyl, and amino groups, which could form non-covalent bonds with biological tissues (mainly epithelia and mucous membranes). Adding to this, polysaccharides can be modified easily as they exist in different positive, negative, or neutral charge states. Even some of these polysaccharides are bio-active and if used in developing nanocarriers can improve therapeutic effect and enhance the targeting efficiency of the system.

10.5.1 STARCH-BASED NANOCARRIERS FOR DELIVERY OF HERBAL EXTRACTS AND BIO-ACTIVES

Starch is made up of two types of polymers: amylose and amylopectin. Amylose is a linear homopolymer of α-1,4-linked glucose with a low level of branching and a α-1,6-linkage. Amylose makes up ~35% of starch and in solution amylose forms hydrogen bonds with other amylase molecules to yield rigid gels. Amylopectin is a highly branched form of amylose. Recently researchers have reported on nanoparticles with a shell of starch/cellulose and a core of alginate/the drug as nanocarriers for the treatment of osteoporosis. An extract of the herb *Amaranthus retroflexcus L* when encapsulated into nanoparticles performed more action compared to the industrial drug calcitonin (Esmaeili and Behzadi 2017).

10.5.2 Dextran-Based Nanocarriers for Delivery of Herbal Extracts and Bio-Actives

Dextran is a polysaccharide consisting of glucose molecules coupled into long branched chains, mainly through 1,6-glucosidic and some through 1,3-glucosidic linkages. Dextrans are colloidal, hydrophilic, and water-soluble substances, inert in biological systems. They are used medicinally as an anti-thrombotic (anti-platelet), to reduce blood viscosity, and as a volume expander in anemia.

Polyethylenimine-dextran sulfate nanoparticles were prepared via a complexation technique using polymers polyethylenimine (PEI) and dextran sulfate (DS) for *Punica granatum* peel extract. Mucoadhesive polyethylenimine-dextran sulfate nanoparticles were effective for local oral mucosa delivery to treat infections (Tiyaboonchai et al. 2015).

Doxorubicin used for the treatment of cancer has side effects such as cardiotoxicity. To reduce the side effects, doxorubicin was coupled with dextran and then formed into a conjugate encapsulated in biodegradable, biocompatible, long circulating hydrogel nanoparticles. The formulated nanoparticles were effective in the treatment of tumors with reduced side effects (Mitra et al. 2001). Chitosan-dextran sulfate nanoparticles were prepared to avoid the short residence time of topical drugs. Nanoparticles loaded with rhodamine B were produced via a polyelectrolyte complexation technique using cationic chitosan (CS), and anionic dextran sulfate (DS) for drug delivery to the ocular surface (Chaiyasan et al. 2013).

Further, formulated β-Lactoglobulin-dextran conjugate nanoparticles were prepared via a homogenization-evaporation method to load β-carotene. The results indicated that the prepared nanoparticles were more stable to aggregation under gastric pH conditions with good release and permeability properties (Yi et al. 2014).

Zheng Li and Liwei Gu reported on ovalbumin-dextran (O-D) conjugate nanoparticles loaded with EGCG. The Maillard reaction was employed for the conjugation of the ovalbumin with the dextran. The formulated O-D conjugate nanoparticle maintained a particle size in the range of 183–349 nm. The nanoparticle formulation significantly enhanced the apparent permeability coefficient and thus improved the absorption of EGCG (Li and Gu 2014).

10.5.3 Pullulan-Based Nanocarrier for Delivery of Herbal Extract and Bio-Actives

Pullulan is a polysaccharide polymer consisting of α-(1–6)-linked maltotriose units. Three glucose units in maltotriose are connected through an 1,4-glycosidic bond, whereas consecutive maltotriose units are connected to each other by an 1,6-glycosidic bond. Pullulan is produced from starch by the fungus *Aureobasidium pullulans*. Pullulan has film forming ability being non-hygroscopic in nature. It has ability to form films, nanoparticles, flexible coatings, and nanofibers.

Pullulan being biodegradable, undergoes degradation by hydrolysis of glycoside bonds and gets metabolized into glucose units (Teramoto and Shibata 2006).

10.5.4 Cyclodextrins-Based Nanocarriers for Delivery of Herbal Extracts and Bio-Actives

Cyclodextrins (CDs), are cyclic oligosaccharides which can be produced through the enzymatic degradation of starch derived from potatoes, corn, rice, or other sources. CDs, consists of a lipophilic cavity surrounded by hydrophilic surface. This lipophilic core present in cyclodextrin allows non-polar drugs to form inclusion complexes. Cyclodextrin form complexes via the van der Waals interaction, hydrophobic interaction or hydrogen bonds. The rate of complexation will be more when the drug and cyclodextrin share opposite charges and are at low temperatures (Ilarduya et al. 1998; Stella and He 2008).

Cyclodextrins are also helpful in altering the physicochemical properties (solubility/stability) of entrapped actives. Paclitaxel-loaded polycationic amphiphilic cyclodextrins nanoparticles were able to enhance anticancer activity, overcoming the problem of surfactant-induced toxicity.

Cationic cyclodextrin nanoparticles proved to be promising carriers for delivery of Paclitaxel (Varan et al. 2017). Olive leaf extract containing oleuropein and hydroxytyrosol was encapsulated in β-CD, increasing the water solubility and anti-oxidant capacity of the encapsulated polyphenols. Mohammadi and his co-researchers reported that water/oil/water emulsion with whey protein concentrate (WPC) and pectin complexes of olive leaf phenolic compounds resulted in a high stability and controlled release of the encapsulated compounds (Mohammadi et al. 2016).

Resveratrol is a naturally occurring polyphenol with anti-oxidant, anti-inflammatory, anticancer, and anti-aging properties with its main application in the treatment of obesity and diabetes. Resveratrol was complexed with cyclodextrin using a crosslinker such as carbonyldiimidazole to form cyclodextrin-based nanosponges. The particle sizes of the formulated nanosponges were in the range of 400–500 nm with increased solubility, stability, and permeation of resveratrol. The results of the resveratrol nanosponge formulation suggested that they can be used for buccal and topical delivery (Ansari et al. 2011).

Bis-demethoxy curcumin analog (BDMCA)-loaded chitosan-starch (CS) nanocomposite particles were developed using different ratios of chitosan and starch (3:1, 1:1, and 1:3) by an ionic gelation method. The entrapment efficiency and drug loading capacity were found to be high for the formulation with the ratio 3:1 of BDMCA:CS. The *in vitro* drug release profile of the BDMCA-CS nanocomposite particles showed a very slow and sustained diffusion-controlled release of the drug (Subramanian et al. 2014). Also, EGCG nanoparticles were encapsulated by crosslinking chitosan hydrochloride and sulfobutylether-β-cyclodextrin sodium, which can be used as a promising carrier for tea polyphenols (Liu et al. 2016).

10.5.5 Cellulose-Based Nanocarriers for Delivery of Herbal Extracts and Bio-Actives

Cellulose is an organic compound with the formula $(C_6H_{10}O_5)$ in a polysaccharide consisting of a linear chain of several hundred to over ten thousand 1,4-linked D-glucose units. Cellulose is the structural component of the primary cell wall of green plants, many forms of algae, and the oomycetes. Some species of bacteria secrete it to form biofilms. Cellulose is the most common organic compound on earth (Namazi et al. 2012).

10.5.6 Chitosan-Based Nanocarriers for Delivery of Herbal Extracts and Bio-Actives

Chitosan is a modified natural carbohydrate polymer prepared by the partial N-deacetylation of the crustacean-derived natural biopolymer chitin. Chitosan is a cationic polysaccharide with natural occurrence. It is extensively used in controlled delivery applications due to its cationic nature, biocompatibility, and mucoadhesive properties. Chitosan nanoparticles show site-specific delivery as they solubilize various lipophilic drug moieties, increase bioavailability, and have a long circulation in the blood. Coating of nanoparticles with cationic chitosan or ions protects them from endolysosomal degradation in enterocytes (Rejman et al. 2004). Due to different applications, chitosan has been formulated as powders, gels and films, sponges, intragastric floating tablets and especially spherical particles (micro and nanoparticles).

Researchers from the Key Laboratory of Forest and Plant Ecology, China, formulated carboxymethyl chitosan nanoparticles loaded with resveratrol. The formulated nanoparticles (155 nm in size; 44% encapsulation efficiency) showed improved solubility and anti-oxidant activity of resveratrol. Resveratrol-loaded carboxymethyl chitosan nanoparticles indicated a higher body localization of the drug in comparison to the active drug alone (Zu et al. 2016). Further, researchers from Monash University, Australia, encapsulated epigallocatechin- 3-gallate (EGCG) into chitosan to form nanoparticles. The formulated nanoparticles with a size of 165 nm and zeta potential of 33 mV were able to increase EGCG stability and bioavailability (Dube et al. 2010a). Also, catechin (C) and EGCG were loaded into chitosan which enhanced intestinal absorption and bioavailability due to the stabilization of these molecules after encapsulation (Dube et al. 2010b).

EGCG-loaded nanoparticles prepared from chitosan and polyaspartic acid (average size 102 nm) were evaluated against rabbit atherosclerosis. The effectiveness of EGCG against rabbit atherosclerosis was significantly improved by EGCG nanoformulations (Hong et al. 2014). EGCG was also encapsulated in novel nanocomplexes (size: 150.0 ± 4.3 nm and charge: 32.2 ± 3.3 mV) made up of bio-active peptides, caseinophosphopeptides, and chitosan. The intestinal permeability of EGCG was enhanced significantly by nanoparticles, which also indicated further improvement of EGCG bioavailability (Hu et al. 2012). Chitosan nanoparticles were formulated using carboxymethyl chitosan and chitosan hydrochloride as carriers by ionic gelation method for the delivery of tea polyphenols. The synthesized nanoparticles with an average size of 407 nm demonstrated sustained release of EGCG. Cytotoxicity studies of chitosan-coated tea polyphenols nanoparticles revealed significant antitumor activities (Liang et al. 2011).

Zhang and his co-workers prepared and evaluated the antibacterial activity of catechins and catechins-Zn complex-loaded β-chitosan nanoparticles (β-CS-NPs). The catechins-Zn complex-loaded β-CS NPs of smaller particle sizes showed higher antibacterial activity than that of larger particle sizes (Zhang et al. 2016). Hydroxytyrosol is a powerful anti-oxidant and anti-inflammatory agent present in olive oil. Anti-inflammatory effects are mediated by reducing the secretion of lipoxygenase-5, lipoxygenase-12, and various prostaglandins underlying inflammation cascades. Hydroxytyrosol was encapsulated into chitosan to form nanoparticles which provided beneficial effect in the treatment of atopic dermatitis (Katas et al. 2013). Siddique et al., reported hydrocortisone and hydroxytyrosol-loaded chitosan nanoparticles (235 nm in size with a zeta potential of +39.2 mV). The nanoencapsulation significantly reduced the toxic effects of hydrocortisone when incorporated into aqueous cream (Siddique et al. 2015).

Ellagic acid, which is present in pomegranate (*Punica granatum*), is used for its anticancer, antiviral, and anti-oxidant properties. Arulmozhi and his co-workers formulated ellagic acid containing chitosan nanoparticles (particle size of 176 nm; 94% drug encapsulation efficiency and loading efficiency of 33%) for oral cancer therapy (Arulmozhi et al. 2013). Das et al., formulated nanoparticles of curcumin with a tripolymeric composite (alginate-chitosan-pluronic) by ionotropic pre-gelation followed by polycationic crosslinking for treatment of cancer (Das et al. 2010). Alpha-tocopherol was encapsulated into chitosan nanoparticles coated with Zein. Hydrogen bonds and hydrophobic interactions between drugs and the Zein/chitosan complex resulted in formation of nanoparticles. The tocopherol nanoparticles (size ranging from 200–300 nm) protected degradation in the GI tract with controlled release (Luo et al. 2011).

Tang et al., encapsulated tea catechins in chitosan and an edible polypeptide, i.e. poly(γ-glutamic acid) for oral delivery. The results exhibited that chitosan and poly(γ-glutamic acid) nanoparticles can act as effective carrier (Tang et al. 2013). A group of researchers from Nanjing Agricultural University, China, formulated genipin-crosslinked caseinophosphopeptide (CPP)-chitosan (CS) nanoparticles loaded with polyphenol. The formulated nanoparticle (300 nm size) significantly improved stability and resistance in the gastrointestinal tract (Hu et al. 2014).

10.5.7 GLYCOSAMINOGLYCAN AS NANOCARRIER FOR DELIVERY OF HERBAL EXTRACT

Glycosaminoglycans (GAGs) are complex polysaccharides distributed in the animal kingdom and to a lesser extent produced by bacteria. They are broadly classified as sulfated and non-sulfated. Sulfated GAGS are further subclassified into hepain/heparin sulfate (HS), keratan sulfate (KS), dermatan sulfate (DS), and chondroitin sulfate (CS). Hyaluronan sulfate represents non-sufated GAGs. Amino sugar and hexuronic acid forms the basic skeleton of GAGs (Yamada et al. 2011). GAGs attached to a protein moiety are referred to as proteoglycans (PG). GAGs and PGs are highly negatively charged and are widely used as nanocarriers for the delivery of natural compounds (Misra et al. 2015).

GAGs are useful in improving the stability and therapeutic potential of flavonoids. One such flavanoid is anthocyanin. Anthocyanins are water-soluble pigments widely distributed in the plant kingdom. These flavonoids are primarily found in fruits although they are present in other plants parts as well. Historically, anthocyanins were used as coloring agents and are one of the 13 natural color pigments allowed by Europe (Bridle and Timberlake 1997). Anthocyanin, apart from coloring properties, have a plethora of health benefits including being anti-oxidative, anticancer, choleretic, and anti-inflammatory activity (Kowalczyk et al. 2003). However, its therapeutic benefit is not fully achieved due to low absorption and high excretion rate (Khoo et al. 2017). Previous studies have shown that cellular uptake and anti-oxidant properties of anthocyanin can be improved by using nanocarriers such as PLGA (Amin et al. 2017). However, polysaccharides could serve as an alternative natural nanocarrier system for delivery of anthocyanin.

Chondroitin sulfate (CS) consists of glucuronic acid and N-acteyl glucosamine. The number of disaccharides may vary from 40 units to more than 100 units. CS is useful as a nanocarrier for delivery of anthocynanin (anth). The anti-oxidant properties of anthocyanin are protected by preparing it in the form of a CS-anth nanocomplex. Ninety-nine percent of the anth is entrapped within the intermolecular stacking. Thus, CS provides a nanocarrier system with high entrapment efficiency. The size of these nanocomplexes was reported to be 300 nm. The stability of the complexed anth increased by eight times and the anti-oxidant and *in vitro* anticancer activity of the CS-anth nanocomplex was higher than the free anth (Sugahara et al. 2003; Jeong and Na 2012). Hyaluronic acid was used for formulating mucoadhesive lipidic nanoemulsion co-encapsulating two polyphenols (resveratrol and curcumin) for nose to brain delivery to treat neurodegenerative diseases (Nasr 2016). Even though considerable research has already initiated in polysaccharide-based drug delivery systems, innovative multifunctional systems are very much required owing to the complexity of diseases in the human body, and to overcome the limitations.

10.6 DELIVERY OF HERBAL EXTRACT AND BIO-ACTIVES USING POLYSACCHARIDE NANOCARRIERS

The principle advantage of polymeric nanocarriers is their robust structural characteristics imparting a very high stability within the gastrointestinal tract. Furthermore, the hydrophobicity and hydrophilicity within the polymeric system can be manipulated to accommodate a wide variety of drug molecules (Plapied et al. 2011). Literature review on some of the herbal extracts and their formulations are discussed in the following section.

10.6.1 Quercetin

Quercetin is a flavonoid widely distributed in nature with various pharmacological effects that include anti-oxidant, ant-allergic, anti-viral, anti-inflammatory, anti-artherogenic, and anti-cancinogenic properties. However, its usage is limited due to its disadvantages such as poor solubility, bioavailability, permeability, instability, and extensive first pass effect. Quercetins are rapidly hydrolyzed in the small intestine or in the colon by bacterial activity to generate the quercetin aglycones, which are further, metabolized into the glucuronidated or sulfated form of quercetin. This molecule is retained in the large intestine for approximately 6 h after oral administration. Various techniques have also been used to increase the solubility of quercetin including the complexation with cyclodextrin (Pralhad and Rajendrakumar 2004). Quercetin molecules have been successfully encapsulated into chitosan nanoparticles. Tan and his co-workers loaded quercetin in lecithin-chitosan nanoparticles (particle size 95.3 nm, entrapment efficiency 48.5%, and drug loading of 2.45%) using tocopheryl propylene glycol succinate for topical delivery. The lecithin-chitosan nanoparticles acted as a promising carrier for the topical delivery of quercetin (Tan et al. 2011). However, the detailed characterizations of the chitosan-nanoencapsulated quercetin molecules were not reported. To overcome the problems associated with the quercetin molecules they were entrapped/adsorbed into biodegradable polymeric nanoparticles.

In 2007, chitosan nanoparticles loaded with quercetin were prepared based on the ionic gelation of chitosan with tripolyphosphate (TPP) anions. TPP is a polyanion, which can interact with the cationic chitosan by electrostatic forces. The quercetin-loaded chitosan nanoparticles were helpful in improving the bioavailabilty of quercetin (Zhang et al. 2008).

10.6.2 CURCUMIN

Curcumin obtained from the rhizomes of turmeric (*Curcuma longa*) possess anti-oxidant, anti-inflammatory, and anticancer activity but its administration is limited due to its poor aqueous solubility and bioavailability. It has been widely studied for its anticancer properties (Panahi et al. 2015). PLGA nanoparticles loaded with curcumin and conjugated with anti-P-glycoprotein resulted in enhanced solubility of curcumin as well as cellular uptake with decreased cell viability. It also exhibited cytotoxic effects on human cervical carcinoma KB-V1 and KB-3-1 cells (Punfa et al. 2012). A thermoresponsive nanoformulation of a curcumin with chitosan-g-poly(N-isopropylacrylamide) copolymer was evaluated for anticancer effects in various cancer cell lines. The formulation yielded a better uptake of curcumin by cancerous cells, decreased cell viability, and augmented apoptosis in PC3 cells, as well as a diminished mitochondrial membrane potential in PC3 cells (Rejinold et al. 2011). Curcumin were loaded in ovalbumin-dextran nanogels prepared by the Maillard reaction to improve bioavailability (Feng et al. 2016).

10.6.3 SILIBININ

Silibinin (also known as silybin, a major active constituent of *Silybum marianum*), a natural polyphenol bio-active has been used traditionally to treat a range of acute and chronic liver disorders, hepatitis, cirrhosis, and inflammation of the bile duct. Silibinin primarily contains three flavonoids of the flavonol subclass (having a fully saturated c-ring). Silybin predominates, followed by silydianin and silychristin. The anti-oxidant capacity of silibinin substantially boosts the liver's resistance. Additionally, research endeavors are increasing to elucidate silibinin's potential against cancer and diabetes. However, very low solubility in water and poor bioavailability limit the therapeutic applications of Silibinin (Zhang et al. 2007; Iqbal et al. 2012; Kuen et al. 2017). In recent years, many authors have proposed a nanoparticle design for silibinin in biodegradable and biocompatible polymers to overcome the therapeutic inadequacy of silibinin.

10.6.4 EPIGALLOCATECHIN-3-GALLATE (EGCG)

The major catechin in tea is epigallocatechin-3-gallate (EGCG), which besides being a powerful anti-oxidant, has antitumor and anticancer activities. Epigallocatechin-3-gallate, the natural active ingredient of green tea, is the most widely used natural product and has shown excellent potential in several studies to treat and prevent many cancers including prostate cancer. But after oral administration it gets degraded in the gastrointestinal tract (acidic pH) by various enzymes and gastric juices. Thus, chitosan nanoparticle formulation of EGCG (Chit-nanoEGCG) is suitable for oral delivery. Formulated chitosan nanoparticles of EGCG are stable in acidic environments and prevent release of EGCG in the stomach. The nanoparticles carry a positive charge which enhances their adhesion time in the gastrointestinal tract. Thus, the nanoformulation of EGCG is able to enhance retention time, and has an ultrafine size and the ability to release the drug for a longer time, which makes them an ideal vehicle for oral delivery (Lin et al. 2014).

Alginate is used in encapsulation because of its low toxicity, low cost, biodegradability, and ability to form gels. It consists of linear chains of b-D-mannuronic acid and α-L-guluronic acid, and is widely used (Gazori et al. 2009). Alginate beads coated with chitosan improves stability, and encapsulation efficiency compared with that of alginate and chitosan beads alone (Singh et al. 2011). Rocha and co-workers formulated nanoparticles of EGCG by using gum arabic and maltodextrin. The formulated EGCG nanoparticles improved drug encapsulation efficiency (85%) and stability via reduced oxidation (Rocha et al. 2011).

10.6.5 PACLITAXEL

Paclitaxel, obtained from a natural source (pacific yew tree bark; *Taxus brevifolia*) is an effective chemotherapeutic agent used for treatment of a variety of tumors particularly brain, ovarian, and breast cancer. It is a white crystalline powder, which is highly lipophilic and hence has poor oral bioavailability limiting its clinical application (Fisusi et al. 2018; Ma and Mumper 2013). The biodegradable nanoparticle-based delivery system is the most common approach in improving pharmacokinetic profile and to demonstrate better patient compliance by reducing toxic effects with a controlled and sustained delivery (Trickler et al. 2008).

The US FDA approved paclitaxel albumin-bound nanoparticle formulation, (Abraxane®) for the treatment of metastatic breast cancer (MBC) in 2005, non-small-cell lung cancer (NSCLC) in 2012, and metastatic pancreatic cancer in 2013 (Surapaneni et al. 2012; Zhao et al. 2015; Kundranda and Niu 2015). Nanoparticle formulation of paclitaxel and doxorubicin was prepared by using a brij 78 surfactant which showed increased anticancer activity by inhibiting p-gp mediated drug resistance (Dong et al. 2009).

In addition, a number of novel paclitaxel nanoparticle formulations are currently undergoing clinical trials and may soon be available for medical practitioners. Further, readers can refer to the article by Kundranda and Niu for a comprehensive list of the various paclitaxel nanoparticle formulations which are under different stages (II/III/IV) of clinical trials for several types of cancers including MBC, NSLCC, and metastatic pancreatic cancer (Kundranda and Niu 2015).

10.6.6 TRIPTOLIDE

Triptolide (TP) is a diterpenoid tricpoxides isolated from the extract of the whole plant of the *Tripterygium wilfordii*. Triptolide is used for the immunosuppressive, anti-inflammatory, anti-fertility, and antitumor activities. It causes adverse reactions in the gastrointestinal tract when administered orally (Abirami et al. 2014). Triptolide-loaded nanoparticles were prepared using poly(D,L-lactic acid) for the beneficial effect on arthritis in rats. Also, to overcome the problems of the poor solubility and toxicity of triptolide, Liu and co-workers developed triptolide-loaded nanoparticles with biodegradable and biocompatible poly(D,L-lactic acid) (Liu et al. 2005).

10.7 FUTURE PROSPECTS AND OPPORTUNITIES

Herbal extracts and bio-actives have a lot of therapeutic potential. But problems like large molecular weight, lipid solubility, and degradation in the acidic stomach, limit their therapeutic activity. Novel drug delivery systems, like nanoparticles, help in developing drug delivery systems which progress the scope for the treatment and diagnosis of diseases. Formulation of nanocarriers for herbal extracts and bio-actives offer a valuable tool in developing future herbal medicine with increased permeability, solubility, reduced toxicity, and enhanced bioavailability. Nanotechnology is rapidly expanding with tremendous implications for many industries including medicine and cosmetics. Moreover, recent progress in polysaccharide chemistry and nanotechnologies allow for elaboration of new dedicated nanosystems.

Hence, there is a great potential for the development of novel drug delivery systems for herbal drugs as they provide efficient, safe, and economical drug delivery.

REFERENCES

Abirami, A., Halith, K., and Pillai, C.A. 2014. Herbal nanoparticle for anticancer potential - a review. *World J Pharm Sci* 3: 2123–32.

Alexander, A., Patel, R.J., Saraf, S., and Saraf, S. 2016. Recent expansion of pharmaceutical nanotechnologies and targeting strategies in the field of phytopharmaceuticals for the delivery of herbal extracts and bioactives. *J Control Release* 241: 110–24.

Alexander, A., Qureshi, A., Kumari, L., et al. 2014. Role of herbal bioactives as a potential bioavailability enhancer for active pharmaceutical ingredients. *Fitoterapia* 97: 1–14.

Amin, F.U., Shah, S.A., Badshah, H., Khan, M., and Kim, M.O. 2017. Anthocyanins encapsulated by PLGA@ PEG nanoparticles potentially improved its free radical scavenging capabilities via p38/JNK pathway against Aβ 1–42-induced oxidative stress. *J Nanobiotechnology* 15 (1): 12.

Ansari, K.A., Vavia, P.R., Trotta, F., and Cavalli, R. 2011. Cyclodextrin-based nanosponges for delivery of resveratrol: In vitro characterisation, stability, cytotoxicity and permeation study. *AAPS Pharm Sci Tech* 12 (1): 279–86.

Ansari, S. and Farha Islam, M. 2012. Influence of nanotechnology on herbal drugs: A Review. *J Adv Pharm Technol Res* 3 (3): 142.

Arulmozhi, V., Pandian, K., and Mirunalini, S. 2013. Ellagic acid encapsulated chitosan nanoparticles for drug delivery system in human oral cancer cell line (KB). *Colloids Surf B Biointerfaces* 110: 313–20.

Bhattaram, V.A., Graefe, U., Kohlert, C., Veit, M., and Derendorf, H. 2002. Pharmacokinetics and bioavailability of herbal medicinal products. *Phytomedicine* 9: 1–33.

Bonifacio, B.V., Da Silva, P.B., Dos Santos Ramos, M.A. et al. 2014. Nanotechnology-based drug delivery systems and herbal medicines: A review. *Int J Nanomedicine* 9: 1.

Bridle, P. and Timberlake, C. 1997. Anthocyanins as natural food colours—selected aspects. *Food Chem* 58 (1–2): 103–9.

Chaiyasan, W., Srinivas, S.P., and Tiyaboonchai, W. 2013. Mucoadhesive chitosan–dextran sulfate nanoparticles for sustained drug delivery to the ocular surface. *J Ocul Pharmacol Ther* 29 (2): 200–7.

Das, R.K., Kasoju, N., and Bora, U. 2010. Encapsulation of curcumin in alginate-chitosan-pluronic composite nanoparticles for delivery to cancer cells. *Nanomedicine* 6 (1): 153–60.

Devi, V.K., Jain, N., and Valli, K.S. 2010. Importance of novel drug delivery systems in herbal medicines. *Pharmacogn Rev* 4 (7): 27.

Dong, X., Mattingly, C.A., Tseng, M.T. et al. 2009. Doxorubicin and paclitaxel-loaded lipid-based nanoparticles overcome multidrug resistance by inhibiting P-glycoprotein and depleting ATP. *Cancer Res* 69 (9): 3918–26.

Dube, A., Ng, K., Nicolazzo, J.A., and Larson, I. 2010a. Effective use of reducing agents and nanoparticle encapsulation in stabilizing catechins in alkaline solution. *Food Chem* 122 (3): 662–7.

Dube, A., Nicolazzo, J.A., and Larson, I. 2010b. Chitosan nanoparticles enhance the intestinal absorption of the green tea catechins (+)-catechin and (–)-epigallocatechin gallate. *Eur J Pharm Sci* 41 (2): 219–25.

Ekor, M. 2014. The growing use of herbal medicines: Issues relating to adverse reactions and challenges in monitoring safety. *Front Pharmacol* 4: 177.

El-Samaligy, M.S., Afifi, N.N., and Mahmoud, E.A. 2006. Evaluation of hybrid liposomes-encapsulated silymarin regarding physical stability and in vivo performance. *Int J Pharm* 319 (1–2): 121–9.

Esmaeili, A. and Behzadi, S. 2017. Performance comparison of two herbal and industrial medicines using nanoparticles with a starch/cellulose shell and alginate core for drug delivery: In vitro studies. *Colloids Surf B Biointerfaces* 158: 556–61.

Feng, J., Wu, S., Wang, H., and Liu, S. 2016. Improved bioavailability of curcumin in ovalbumin-dextran nanogels prepared by Maillard reaction. *J Funct Foods* 27: 55–68.

Fisusi, F.A., Schätzlein, A.G., and Uchegbu, I.F. 2018. *Nanomedicines in the Treatment of Brain Tumors. Nanomedicine (Lond)* 13: 579–583.

Gazori, T., Khoshayand, M.R., Azizi, E. et al. 2009. Evaluation of alginate/chitosan nanoparticles as antisense delivery vector: Formulation, optimization and in vitro characterization. *Carbohydr Polym* 77 (3): 599–606.

Hong, Z., Xu, Y., Yin, J.-F. et al. 2014. Improving the effectiveness of (–)-epigallocatechin gallate (EGCG) against rabbit atherosclerosis by EGCG-loaded nanoparticles prepared from chitosan and polyaspartic acid. *J Agric Food Chem* 62 (52): 12603–9.

Hu, B., Ting, Y., Zeng, X., and Huang, Q. 2012. Cellular uptake and cytotoxicity of chitosan–caseinophosphopeptides nanocomplexes loaded with epigallocatechin gallate. *Carbohydr Polym* 89 (2): 362–70.

Hu, B., Xie, M., Zhang, C., and Zeng, X. 2014. Genipin-structured peptide–polysaccharide nanoparticles with significantly improved resistance to harsh gastrointestinal environments and their potential for oral delivery of polyphenols. *J Agric Food Chem* 62 (51): 12443–52.

Ilarduya, M.T.D., Martían, C., Goni, M., and Martinez-Oharriz, M. 1998. Solubilization and interaction of sulindac with β-cyclodextrin in the solid state and in aqueous solution. *Drug Dev Ind Pharm* 24 (3): 301–6.

Iqbal, M.A., Md, S., Sahni, J.K. et al. 2012. Nanostructured lipid carriers system: Recent advances in drug delivery. *J Drug Target* 20 (10): 813–30.

Jeong, D. and Na, K. 2012. Chondroitin sulfate based nanocomplex for enhancing the stability and activity of anthocyanin. *Carbohydr Polym* 90 (1): 507–15.

Kalita, B., Das, M., and Sharma, A. 2013. Novel phytosome formulations in making herbal extracts more effective. *Research Journal of Pharmacy and Technology* 6 (11): 1295–301.

Kamboj, V. 2000. Herbal medicine. *Curr Sci* 78 (1): 35–9.

Katas, H., Amin, M.C.I., Sahudin, S., Buang, F. 2013. Chitosan-based skin-targete d nanoparticle drug delivery system and method. Patent application WO2015072846A1.

Kesarwani, K. and Gupta, R. 2013. Bioavailability enhancers of herbal origin: An overview. *Asian Pac J Trop Biomed* 3 (4): 253–66.

Keservani, R.K., Sharma, A.K., and Kesharwani, R.K. 2017. *Drug Delivery Approaches and Nanosystems, Volume 1: Novel Drug Carriers.* CRC Press.

Khoo, H.E., Azlan, A., Tang, S.T., and Lim, S.M. 2017. Anthocyanidins and anthocyanins: Colored pigments as food, pharmaceutical ingredients, and the potential health benefits. *Food Nutr Res* 61 (1): 1361779.

Kowalczyk, E., Krzesiński, P., Kura, M., Szmigiel, B., and Blaszczyk, J. 2003. Anthocyanins in medicine. *Pol J Pharmacol* 55 (5): 699–702.

Kuen, C.Y., Fakurazi, S., Othman, S.S., and Masarudin, M.J. 2017. Increased loading, efficacy and sustained release of silibinin, a poorly soluble drug using hydrophobically-modified chitosan nanoparticles for enhanced delivery of anticancer drug delivery systems. *Nanomaterials* 7 (11): 379.

Kulkarni, G.T. 2011. Herbal drug delivery systems: An emerging area in herbal drug research. *J Chronotherapy Drug Deliv* 2 (3): 113–9.

Kundranda, M.N. and Niu, J. 2015. Albumin-bound paclitaxel in solid tumors: Clinical development and future directions. *Drug Des Devel Ther* 9: 3767.

Li, H., Li, S., and Duan, H. 2007. Preparation of liposomes containing extracts of Tripterygium wilfordii and evaluation of its stability. *China Journal of Chinese Materia Medica* 32 (20): 2128–31.

Li, Z. and Gu, L. 2014. Fabrication of self-assembled (–)-Epigallocatechin Gallate (EGCG) ovalbumin–dextran conjugate nanoparticles and their transport across monolayers of human intestinal epithelial Caco-2 cells. *J Agric Food Chem* 62 (6): 1301–9.

Liang, J., Li, F., Fang, Y. et al. 2011. Synthesis, characterization and cytotoxicity studies of chitosan-coated tea polyphenols nanoparticles. *Colloids Surf B Biointerfaces* 82 (2): 297–301.

Lin, Y. H., Feng, C.-L., Lai, C.-H., Lin, J.-H., and Chen, H.-Y. 2014. Preparation of epigallocatechin gallate-loaded nanoparticles and characterization of their inhibitory effects on Helicobacter pylori growth in vitro and in vivo. *Sci Technol Adv Mater* 15 (4): 045006.

Liu, F., Antoniou, J., Li, Y. et al. 2016. Chitosan/sulfobutylether-β-cyclodextrin nanoparticles as a potential approach for tea polyphenol encapsulation. *Food Hydrocoll* 57: 291–300.

Liu, M., Dong, J., Yang, Y., Yang, X., and Xu, H. 2005. Anti-inflammatory effects of triptolide loaded poly (D, L-lactic acid) nanoparticles on adjuvant-induced arthritis in rats. *J Ethnopharmacol* 97 (2): 219–25.

Luo, Y., Zhang, B., Whent, M., Yu, L.L., and Wang, Q. 2011. Preparation and characterization of zein/chitosan complex for encapsulation of α-tocopherol, and its in vitro controlled release study. *Colloids Surf B Biointerfaces* 85 (2): 145–52.

Ma, P. and Mumper, R.J. 2013. Paclitaxel nano-delivery systems: A comprehensive review. *Journal of Nanomedicine & Nanotechnology* 4 (2): 1000164.

Mahajan, A., Mangat, P., Bhatia, A., and Katare, O. 2010. A novel herbal capsaicin loaded liposomal formulation: Design, development and evaluation. *Pharmaceutical Sciences* (July): section 11.

Maiti, K., Mukherjee, K., Gantait, A., et al. 2005. Enhanced therapeutic benefit of quercetinphospholipid complex in carbon tetrachloride-induced acute liver injury in rats: A comparative study. *Iranian Journal of Pharmacology and Therapeutics* 4 (2): 84–90.

Maiti, K., Mukherjee, K., Gantait, A., Saha, B.P., and Mukherjee, P.K. 2006. Enhanced therapeutic potential of naringenin-phospholipid complex in rats. *J Pharm Pharmacol* 58 (9): 1227–33.

Maiti, K., Mukherjee, K., Gantait, A., Saha, B. P., and Mukherjee, P. K. 2007. Curcumin–phospholipid complex: Preparation, therapeutic evaluation and pharmacokinetic study in rats. *Int J Pharm* 330 (1–2): 155–63.

Marena, C. and Lampertico, M. 1991. Preliminary clinical development of silipide: A new complex of silybin in toxic liver disorders. *Planta Med* 57 (S2): A124–5.

Misra, S., Hascall, V.C., Atanelishvili, I. et al. 2015. Utilization of glycosaminoglycans/proteoglycans as carriers for targeted therapy delivery. *Int J Biochem Cell Biol* 2015.

Mitra, S., Gaur, U., Ghosh, P., and Maitra, A. 2001. Tumour targeted delivery of encapsulated dextran–doxorubicin conjugate using chitosan nanoparticles as carrier. *J Control Release* 74 (1–3): 317–23.

Mohammadi, A., Jafari, S.M., Assadpour, E., and Esfanjani, A.F. 2016. Nano-encapsulation of olive leaf phenolic compounds through WPC–pectin complexes and evaluating their release rate. *Int J Biol Macromol* 82: 816–22.

Namazi, H., Fathi, F., and Heydari, A. 2012. Nanoparticles based on modified polysaccharides. In: Hashim, A.A. (Ed.), *The Delivery of Nanoparticles*. InTechOpen.

Nasr, M. 2016. Development of an optimized hyaluronic acid-based lipidic nanoemulsion co-encapsulating two polyphenols for nose to brain delivery. *Drug Deliv* 23 (4): 1444–52.

Nicolas, J., Mura, S., Brambilla, D., Mackiewicz, N., and Couvreur, P. 2013. Design, functionalization strategies and biomedical applications of targeted biodegradable/biocompatible polymer-based nanocarriers for drug delivery. *Chem Soc Rev* 42 (3): 1147–235.

Panahi, Y., Badeli, R., Karami, G.R., and Sahebkar, A. 2015. Investigation of the efficacy of adjunctive therapy with bioavailability-boosted curcuminoids in major depressive disorder. *Phytother Res* 29 (1): 17–21.

Plapied, L., Duhem, N., Des Rieux, A., and Préat, V. 2011. Fate of polymeric nanocarriers for oral drug delivery. *Curr Opin Colloid Interface Sci* 16 (3): 228–37.

Pralhad, T. and Rajendrakumar, K. 2004. Study of freeze-dried quercetin–cyclodextrin binary systems by DSC, FT-IR, X-ray diffraction and SEM analysis. *J Pharm Biomed Anal* 34 (2): 333–9.

Priprem, A., Watanatorn, J., Sutthiparinyanont, S., Phachonpai, W., and Muchimapura, S. 2008. Anxiety and cognitive effects of quercetin liposomes in rats. *Nanomedicine* 4 (1): 70–8.

Puglia, C., Lauro, M.R., Tirendi, G.G. et al. 2017. Modern drug delivery strategies applied to natural active compounds. *Expert Opin Drug Deliv* 14 (6): 755–68.

Punfa, W., Yodkeeree, S., Pitchakarn, P., Ampasavate, C., and Limtrakul, P. 2012. Enhancement of cellular uptake and cytotoxicity of curcumin-loaded PLGA nanoparticles by conjugation with anti-P-glycoprotein in drug resistance cancer cells. *Acta Pharmacol Sin* 33 (6): 823.

Pushpamalar, J., Veeramachineni, A.K., Owh, C., and Loh, X.J. 2016. Biodegradable polysaccharides for controlled drug delivery. *Chempluschem* 81 (6): 504–14.

Rejinold, N.S., Sreerekha, P., Chennazhi, K., Nair, S., and Jayakumar, R. 2011. Biocompatible, biodegradable and thermo-sensitive chitosan-g-poly (N-isopropylacrylamide) nanocarrier for curcumin drug delivery. *Int J Biol Macromol* 49 (2): 161–72.

Rejman, J., Oberle, V., Zuhorn, I.S., and Hoekstra, D. 2004. Size-dependent internalization of particles via the pathways of clathrin-and caveolae-mediated endocytosis. *Biochem J* 377 (1): 159–69.

Rocha, S., Generalov, R., Pereira, M.D.C. et al. 2011. Epigallocatechin gallate-loaded polysaccharide nanoparticles for prostate cancer chemoprevention. *Nanomedicine* 6 (1): 79–87.

Saraf, S. 2010. Applications of novel drug delivery system for herbal formulations. *Fitoterapia* 81 (7): 680–9.

Siddique, M.I., Katas, H., Amin, M.C.I.M. et al. 2015. Minimization of local and systemic adverse effects of topical glucocorticoids by nanoencapsulation: In vivo safety of hydrocortisone–hydroxytyrosol loaded chitosan nanoparticles. *J Pharm Sci* 104 (12): 4276–86.

Singh, B.N., Shankar, S., and Srivastava, R.K. 2011. Green tea catechin, epigallocatechin-3-gallate (EGCG): Mechanisms, perspectives and clinical applications. *Biochem Pharmacol* 82 (12): 1807–21.

Singh, R., Kumari, P., and Kumar, S. 2016. Nanotechnology for enhanced bioactivity of bioactive phytomolecules. In: Grumezescu, A.M. (Ed.), *Nutrient Delivery*. Elsevier.

Sinico, C., De Logu, A., Lai, F. et al. 2005. Liposomal incorporation of Artemisia arborescens L. essential oil and in vitro antiviral activity. *Eur J Pharm Biopharm* 59 (1): 161–8.

Stella, V.J. and He, Q. 2008. Cyclodextrins. *Toxicol Pathol* 36 (1): 30–42.

Straubinger, R.M. and Balasubramanian, S.V. 2005. Preparation and characterization of taxane-containing liposomes. *Methods Enzymol* 391: 97–117.

Subramanian, S.B., Francis, A.P., and Devasena, T. 2014. Chitosan–starch nanocomposite particles as a drug carrier for the delivery of bis-desmethoxy curcumin analog. *Carbohydr Polym* 114: 170–8.

Sugahara, K., Mikami, T., Uyama, T. et al. 2003. Recent advances in the structural biology of chondroitin sulfate and dermatan sulfate. *Curr Opin Struct Biol* 13 (5): 612–20.

Surapaneni, M.S., Das, S.K., and Das, N.G. 2012. Designing paclitaxel drug delivery systems aimed at improved patient outcomes: Current status and challenges. *ISRN Pharmacol* 2012.

Tan, Q., Liu, W., Guo, C., and Zhai, G. 2011. Preparation and evaluation of quercetin-loaded lecithin-chitosan nanoparticles for topical delivery. *Int J Nanomedicine* 6: 1621.

Tang, D.-W., Yu, S.-H., Ho, Y.-C. et al. 2013. Characterization of tea catechins-loaded nanoparticles prepared from chitosan and an edible polypeptide. *Food Hydrocoll* 30 (1): 33–41.

Teramoto, N. and Shibata, M. 2006. Synthesis and properties of pullulan acetate. Thermal properties, biodegradability, and a semi-clear gel formation in organic solvents. *Carbohydr Polym* 63 (4): 476–81.

Tiyaboonchai, W., Rodleang, I., and Ounaroon, A. 2015. Mucoadhesive polyethylenimine–dextran sulfate nanoparticles containing Punica granatum peel extract as a novel sustained-release antimicrobial. *Pharm Dev Technol* 20 (4): 426–32.

Trickler, W., Nagvekar, A., and Dash, A. 2008. A novel nanoparticle formulation for sustained paclitaxel delivery. *AAPS PharmSciTech* 9 (2): 486.

Varan, G., Benito, J.M., Mellet, C.O., and Bilensoy, E. 2017. Development of polycationic amphiphilic cyclodextrin nanoparticles for anticancer drug delivery. *Beilstein J Nanotechnol* 8: 1457–68.

Venkatesh, M., Mukherjee, K., Maiti, K., and Mukherjee, P. 2008. Enhancement of bioavailability of phytomolecules with value added formulation. *Planta Med* 74 (09): PC11.

Wani, K., Tarawadi, K., and Kaul-Ghanekar, R. 2015. Nanocarriers for delivery of herbal based drugs in breast cancer - an overview. *J Nano R* 34: 29–40.

Wen, Z., Liu, B., Zheng, Z. et al. 2010. Preparation of liposomes entrapping essential oil from Atractylodes macrocephala Koidz by modified RESS technique. *Chem Eng Res Des* 88 (8): 1102–7.

Yamada, S., Sugahara, K., and Özbek, S. 2011. Evolution of glycosaminoglycans: Comparative biochemical study. *Commun Integr Biol* 4 (2): 150–8.

Yanyu, X., Yunmei, S., Zhipeng, C., and Qineng, P. 2006. The preparation of silybin–phospholipid complex and the study on its pharmacokinetics in rats. *Int J Pharm* 307 (1): 77–82.

Yi, J., Lam, T.I., Yokoyama, W., Cheng, L.W., and Zhong, F. 2014. Controlled release of β-carotene in β-lactoglobulin–dextran-conjugated nanoparticles' in vitro digestion and transport with Caco-2 monolayers. *J Agric Food Chem* 62 (35): 8900–7.

Zhang, H., Jung, J., and Zhao, Y. 2016. Preparation, characterization and evaluation of antibacterial activity of catechins and catechins–Zn complex loaded β-chitosan nanoparticles of different particle sizes. *Carbohydr Polym* 137: 82–91.

Zhang, J., Liu, J., Li, X., and Jasti, B. 2007. Preparation and characterization of solid lipid nanoparticles containing silibinin. *Drug Deliv* 14 (6): 381–7.

Zhang, Y., Yang, Y., Tang, K., Hu, X., and Zou, G. 2008. Physicochemical characterization and antioxidant activity of quercetin-loaded chitosan nanoparticles. *J Appl Polym Sci* 107 (2): 891–7.

Zhao, M., Lei, C., Yang, Y. et al. 2015. Abraxane, the nanoparticle formulation of paclitaxel can induce drug resistance by up-regulation of P-gp. *PloS one* 10 (7): e0131429.

Zu, Y., Zhang, Y., Wang, W. et al. 2016. Preparation and in vitro/in vivo evaluation of resveratrol-loaded carboxymethyl chitosan nanoparticles. *Drug Deliv* 23 (3): 971–81.

11 Use of Polysaccharide Nanocarrier Systems for the Delivery of Curcumin and Its Derivative

Narayanan Kasinathan and Kiran S. Avadhani

CONTENTS

11.1 INTRODUCTION

Curcumin is chemically known as bis-α,β-unsaturated β-diketone. It is a hydrophobic polyphenol, an active compound extracted from *Curcuma longa* (Anand et al. 2007). The U.S. FDA and the WHO Expert Committee on Food considers curcumin as safe (Lee 2015). Curcumin is a light sensitive molecule and due to its hydrophobic nature is poorly absorbed upon oral administration. In addition, it undergoes a rapid first pass metabolism and is quickly cleared from systemic circulation. This results in a short half-life causing low availability of active component at the target site (Mahmood et al. 2016; Bisht and Maitra 2009).

Curcumin as an active molecule is more than two centuries old and use of *Curcuma longa* as "curry powder" is known from time immemorial in certain parts of the world. Curcumin was first isolated in 1815 and pure crystalline was first obtained in 1870 (Bisht and Maitra 2009). From the time curcumin was isolated in pure form, research on its therapeutic efficacy has increased tremendously. Even a dose of curcumin as high as 12g/day is known to be safe (Anand et al. 2007). In spite of its lower plasma level, curcumin is effective against a myriad of diseases such as cancer, Crohn's disease, arthritis, and various neurological and inflammatory conditions. Even though the safety and efficacy of curcumin is documented, curcumin is not yet commercially available for treating any of the diseases against which it is proven to be effective (Anand et al. 2007). Therefore, curcumin has remained elusive for use in a clinical setting.

In an aqueous-based buffer system of pH 5, curcumin has a solubility of 11 ng/ml making curcumin unsuitable to be developed and administered in the form of tablets, capsules, or suspensions in absence of a carrier (Tønnesen and Loftsson 2002). Its lower oral bioavailability has led to an increase in research focusing on the topical application of curcumin and its analogues particularly for treating wounds. This is due to the ease of accessibility that curcumin has to the target site (Shoba et al. 1998).

As the research on understanding pharmacological activity of curcumin continues to increase, there are efforts to study the activity of curcumin metabolites. Curcumin along with its analogues demethoxycurcumin and bisdemethoxycurcumin exhibits various pharmacological activities. Studies show that analogues have more of a synergistic effect in enhancing the efficacy of curcumin (Sandur et al. 2007).

Curcumin undergoes degradation by both enzymatic and non-enzymatic pathways (Douglass and Clouatre 2015). Curcumin is degraded by either enzymatic dependent or enzyme independent pathways. Enzymatically, curcumin is degraded to an inactive metabolite by beta-glucuronidase and sulfatase. Oxidation and pH level leads to the degradation of curcumin *via* enzyme independent pathways (Douglass and Clouatre 2015). Within the liver, curcumin undergoes metabolism in two phases: phase 1 being reduction of the double bonds and phase 2 being conjugation (Hassaninasab et al. 2011). Even the microbiota found in the gastro intestinal (GI) system is known to degrade curcumin thereby further reducing the availability of curcumin for absorption (Hassaninasab et al. 2011). However, an interesting observation is that tetrahydrocurcumin, formed due to the action of microbes particularly *Escherichia coli,* is more potent than the curcumin itself (Hassaninasab et al. 2011).

A Number of approaches are continuously studied to improve the oral bioavailability of curcumin. Co-administering agents capable of blocking enzymes degrading curcumin in the liver, using lipid-based delivery systems, nanoparticulate delivery systems, dispersion/emulsion-based delivery systems, and various other approaches are being studied to improve the bioavailability of curcumin (Anand et al. 2007). Co-administration of piperine results in a higher plasma level of curcumin. Piperine is an inhibitor of glucuronidation which is involved in the degradation of curcumin. The effect is more prominent in humans (Shoba et al. 1998; Bisht and Maitra 2009).

11.2 NANOPARTICLE-BASED DELIVERY SYSTEMS

Due to their very small size, nanoparticles can enter smallest capillary pores. After entry into circulation, nanoparticles continue to remain for a long time as they escape capture and subsequent degradation by phagocytes. In addition, nanoparticles/nanocarriers can be designed as such that the "cargo" is released in a controlled manner only to the target site or in response to a stimuli guaranteeing a "tailored pharmacokinetics" (Liu et al. 2008; Liu et al. 2016). Higher intracellular penetration and enhanced permeability and retention property of these molecules is useful in specifically loading the "cargo" into the target site during conditions such as cancer (Zhang et al. 2017; Liu et al. 2016).

11.2.1 Lipid-Based Delivery Systems

Hydrophobic drugs have been historically delivered using liposome, micelles, and phospholipid complex-based delivery system. This is due to the ability of these delivery systems, particularly liposomes, to encapsulate and deliver both hydrophilic and hydrophobic drugs (Anand et al. 2007; Alkhader et al. 2017). Absorption of curcumin in the GI can also be improved by using micelles and phospholoipids (Anand et al. 2007). The level of cholesterol dictates absorption and subsequent bioavailability of curcumin. This is due to the enhanced stability of curcumin in the presence of a higher lipid at neutral pH (Chen et al. 2009; Bisht and Maitra 2009). However, instability of liposomes has always been a concern and this has led to research focusing on more stable carrier-based delivery system.

11.2.2 Polysaccharide-Based Nanocarrier Systems

Of late, research focuses more on the selection of appropriate carrier material, utilizing more than one carrier material and modifying the surface property of the carrier system. Biodegradability and biocompatibility are the most important characteristics that a carrier system should possess. Ease of availability and lower cost further makes polysaccharides one of the more preferred carrier materials (Liu et al. 2008; Zhang et al. 2017).

Polysaccharides, that consist of repeating units of monosaccharide, can be obtained from a wide variety of sources *viz.*, microbes, algae, plants, and animals (Liu et al. 2008; Sinha and Kumria 2001). Polysaccharides can be poly or non-polyelectrolyte. Polysaccharides are normally safe, stable, biodegradable, and can be customized, i.e., chemically and biochemically modified. Many of the polysaccharides have good adhesive properties that are utilized in preparing a prolonged release product. Recent development allows preparation of amphiphilic co-polymers by grafting hydrophilic chains with hydrophobic chains. These are particularly useful in delivery of hydrophobic molecules (Liu et al. 2008; Liu et al. 2016). Upon exposure to environments, these polymers form micelles spontaneously resulting in a thermodynamically stable particle with unique rheological properties and a smaller hydrodynamic radius (Letchford and Burt 2007). Polysaccharide-based nanocarrier systems including amphiphiles can be either prepared using a covalent or non-covalent method. While preparing covalent-based nanocarriers, care should be taken to ensure that the cross-linkers used for generating covalent linkages is non-toxic. In such situations, crosslinking *via* ionic interaction would be better although such interactions will be relatively weak. Electrostatic interaction, host-guest recognition, and π-π stacking constitute a non-covalent method (Liu et al. 2008; Liu et al. 2016).

11.3 POLYSACCHARIDE NANOCARRIER SYSTEMS FOR THE DELIVERY OF CURCUMIN AND ITS DERIVATIVE

Nanocarrier systems thus provide an alternative delivery system for the delivery of a wide variety of drugs that were considered challenging to be delivered into systemic circulation. With recent approval of nanoparticle-based delivery system by the U.S. FDA, there is an optimism that nanoparticle-based systems will help to achieve the higher and reproducible levels of curcumin in systemic circulation that has been evading humans for such a long period. Curcumin can be encapsulated within carrier systems and its size can be maintained in nanometer (Kasinathan et al. 2016). Proteins and polysaccharides are the most common carrier systems used for preparing nanoparticle-based delivery systems for hydrophobic drugs (Bai et al. 2017; Amirthalingam et al. 2017).

The following sections explain some of the polysaccharide-based nanocarrier systems used for the delivery of curcumin.

11.3.1 Carrageenan Nanocarrier Systems for the Delivery of Curcumin

Carrageenans are sulfated galactans. These were originally believed to be part of the extracts obtained from *Chondrus* and *Gigartina* species. However, many species belonging to the family *Rhodophycea* are found to produce carrageenan. The backbone of polysaccharide is produced by *Rhodophycea*, commonly known as red seaweed, β-d-galactose and 3,6-anhydro-α-d-galactose. Based on the predominant monosaccharide units, carrageenan is categorized into kappa, lambda, mu, and nu carrageenan (Whistler 2012). Readers can refer to "Industrial gums: Polysaccharides and their derivatives" for further details on the structural differences among various carrageenan (Whistler 2012).

Carrageenan-based carrier systems are effective in delivering curcumin. By combining with anionic, polysaccharides such as sodium alginate, carrageenan can be developed as hydrogels. The level of carrageenan determines the percentage of curcumin encapsulated (Guzman-Villanueva et al. 2013). These carrier systems can be further improved by preparing in the nanosized hydrogels. A complex coacervation technique is useful to fabricate carrageenan with proteins such as lysozyme. Curcumin encapsulated in such carrier systems has a higher stability against thermal and ultraviolet (UV) induced degradation (Xu et al. 2014). ι-Carrageenan stabilizes bovine serum albumin (BSA) through electrostatic interaction. This allows binding of curcumin to the hydrophobic regions of BSA. Curcumin bound to BSA-ι-carrageenan is reported to be more stable and possess higher radical scavenging activity (Yang et al. 2013).

Curcumin encapsulated within κ-carrageenan was effective at a concentration as low as 40 μg/ml. Curcumin-loaded κ-carrageenan was prepared using a solvent evaporation technique and was able to release a maximum amount of the drug at pH 5.0. Curcumin was stable at low acidic conditions indicating that κ-carrageenan can be useful in delivering curcumin into a tumor microenvironment. A tumor microenvironment is known to be acidic in nature (Sathuvan et al. 2017).

11.3.2 Chitosan Nanocarrier Systems for the Delivery of Curcumin

Chitosan (CS) is a naturally available carbohydrate-based biodegradable polymer. It is a chemically deacetylated derivative of chitin, composed of β-(1,4)-2-amino-2-deoxy-d-glucopyranose units and small amount of N-acetyl-d-glucosamine residues (Martins et al. 2013). Chitosan and its derivatives have potential roles in medical and pharmaceutical fields. Chitosan has excellent properties such as hydrophilicity, biocompatibility, low toxicity, and mucoadhesivity. Due to its cationic nature, CS offers multiple advantages for ionic interactions which can lead to chitosan nanoparticles as drug carriers by a simple ion gelation technique (Zheng et al. 2016). CS is also used as a biomaterial in targeted drug delivery systems (Facchi et al. 2016). Chitosan can be modified suitably for use as drug carriers (Martins et al. 2015).

Chitosan nanoparticles (CNP) can be prepared via an ion gelation technique using tripolyphosphate as crosslinking agents with suitable surfactants. CNP can be either prepared by using chitosan as the only carrier material or by conjugating chitosan with other polysaccharide-based polymers (Martins et al. 2013). CNP improves the water solubility and bioavailability of the drugs.

11.3.3 Chondroitin Sulfate Nanocarrier Systems for Delivery of Curcumin

Chondroitin sulfate (ChS) belongs to glycosoaminoglycans consisting of repeating units of N-acetyl galactosamine and D-glucuronic acid. Based on a sulfation pattern, i.e., number and position of sulfate group, ChS is classified into chondroitin-4-sulfate, chondroitin-6-sulfate, chondroitin-2,5-sulfate, and chondroitin-4,6-sulfate (Zhao et al. 2015; Kasinathan et al. 2016). ChS is a highly anionic mucopolysaccharide. Presence of a large number of functional groups allows for the ease of modifying ChS as a carrier for variety of molecules. Degradation of colonic micro flora makes ChS useful in targeting the colon. ChS is also useful to target sites, as it is capable of binding to CD 44. ChS can be used in preparing self-assembling nanovehicles (Zhao et al. 2015). Using an ionic gelation method, it is possible to prepare ChS-chitosan nanoparticles that can be used as a carrier for delivery of curcumin. The diameter of curcumin-loaded ChS-chitosan nanoparticles was in the range of 474–599 nm. Maximum encapsulation was around 68%. Curcumin releases from the carrier system by diffusion and was able to control proliferation of adenocarcinoma cells (Jardim et al. 2015).

11.3.4 Cyclodextrin Nanocarrier Systems for the Delivery of Curcumin

Cycoldextrin (CD) are cyclic oligosaccharides with a hydrophilic surface outside and lipophilic cavity inside (Rajesh et al. 2015). CDs are useful in developing supramolecular amphilic delivery systems (Liu et al. 2016). Through the van der Waals interaction, CD is able to form inclusion complexes with lipophilic drugs such as curcumin. While the benzene ring of curcumin remains within the CD cavity, OH groups of the enol interacts with the hydroxyl group of CD forming an OH-O bond (Mohan et al. 2012). For every two mole of CD, either one or two mole of curcumin is entrapped within the internal cavity (Tang et al. 2002; Mohan et al. 2012). Under suitable conditions, the CD-curcumin complex dissociates and curcumin is released into the target site (Pinho et al. 2014; Purpura et al. 2017). Based on a number of glucopyranose units, CD is categorized into α, β, and γ-CD containing six, seven, and eight units respectively. The glucopyranose units are linked by α-(1,4) linkage providing a truncated conical structure (Saha et al. 2016). Apart from these three types of CD, their derivatives are also commonly utilized in improving the solubility and stability of curcumin. However, the solubility and stability of curcumin varies depending the type of CD. While hydroxypropyl-β-CD provides a higher stability to curcumin in comparison to the 2-O-methyl-β-CD and hydroxypropyl-γ-CD (HP-γ-CD), HP-γ-CD provides a higher solubility (Tomren et al. 2007).

Cyclodextrins are useful in improving stability, dissolution rates, and bioavailability of poorly soluble drugs (Rajesh et al. 2015). Cyclodextrin forms an inclusion complex with lipophilic drugs thereby improving aqueous solubility, absorption, and bioavailability of hydrophobic drugs like curcumin (Purpura et al. 2017). Solubility of curcumin increases by 31-fold when complexed with β-CD. In addition, β-CD further provides photo stability by providing protection against sunlight (Mangolim et al. 2014).

The ability of curcumin to improve the dissociation of protein aggregates has been known for a long time. This anti-aggregating property of curcumin is useful in treating pathological conditions resulting from the mutation of P23H. P23H mutation causes misfolding of rhodopsin. Oral administration of curcumin in rats delayed and slowed retinitis pigmentosa (RP) caused due to mutation of P23H. Curcumin was administered by mixing it with hypoallergic milk powder (Vasireddy et al. 2011). Curcumin was effective even when administered orally. Milk (powder in this case) is a kind of emulsion consisting of a mixture of fats and proteins. Therefore, milk is known to be effective in improving the absorption of curcumin. However, a high dose of curcumin (100 mg/kg) was required to be administered to achieve clinical significance. As a result of the positive outcome of this study conducted by Vasireddy et al (Vasireddy et al. 2011), new studies were conducted focusing on developing curcumin into a suitable dosage form for treating retinal degenerations. Retinal degenerations affect millions of people around the globe, resulting in permanent blindness (Vasireddy et al. 2011). Curcumin complexed with CD can be directly administered on the eyes. β-CD-curcumin complexes are water-soluble and therefore can be given as eyedrops. This would be useful in treating ocular diseases such as retinitis pigmentosa (Maria et al. 2017). Such water soluble β-CD-curcumin complexes provide a sustained release of curcumin for more than 96 h. In addition, the amount of curcumin released was higher than the amount reported by Vasireddy et al. (Vasireddy et al. 2011; Maria et al. 2017).

β-CD-curcumin complexes are effective in treating melanoma when delivered in the form of transdermal formulations. Poloxamer molecules are useful in preparing in situ-forming hydrogel. These hydrogels are helpful in delivering β-CD-curcumin complexes as transdermal formulations. Complex released from the formulations had a higher solubility and permeability, and induced apoptosis in B16-F10 cells (Sun et al. 2014). Efficacy of CD-curcumin is further enhanced by encapsulating CD-curcumin complex within other nanocarrier system. HP-γ-CD-curcumin can be encapsulated within chitosan to prepare HP-γ-CD-curcumin-chitosan nanoconjuagate with an average size of 190 nm. A sustained release of curcumin from this complex was achieved for more than 72 h. The drug-loaded carrier was more effective against squamous cell carcinoma than the free drug (Popat et al. 2014). Administration of HP-γ-CD-curcumin entrapped into liposomes significantly reduces proliferation of osteosarcoma and breast cancer cell lines by inducing apoptosis in a caspase dependent pathway. The mean size of the HP-γ-CD-curcumin-liposomes nanoparticles was 98 nm. This complex was also effective in vivo in controlling progression of human osteosarcoma induced in nude mice (Dhule et al. 2012). Clinical studies conducted by Purpura et al. (Purpura et al. 2017) shows that effectiveness of CD-curcumin complexes observed in animals are reproducible in human also.

11.3.5 DEXTRAN NANOCARRIER SYSTEMS FOR THE DELIVERY OF CURCUMIN

Drugs can be conjugated to dextran either by direct esterification or conjugating through non-polar bonds that utilize the reaction between primary amino groups and iminocarbonate dextran (Molteni 1985). For the reactions involving the conjugation of dextran to the drug, it is important to inactivate unreacted epoxy radicals by treating them with an excess of a nucleophile such as glycine. This reduces the possibility of adverse reactions due to the epoxy radicals (Molteni 1985).

Dextran is known to protect even highly sensitive drugs such as proteins (Wu et al. 2013). The dextran confers a stability to the drugs from light, temperature, hydrolysis, and upon injections retard tubular filtration thereby increasing the circulation time (Molteni 1985).

Using succinic acid as a spacer, hemocompatible curcumin-dextran micelles can be prepared. Curcumin can therefore be conjugated to the hydrophilic backbone of dextran through this spacer. This conjugate self-assembles to form micelles. Using this technique, micelles with a maximum particle size of 200 nm and with a higher water solubility and longer stability at neutral pH in PBS can be easily achieved. In addition, conjugation helps in delivering curcumin into the glioma cells through macropinocytosis, thus increasing the efficacy of curcumin (Raveendran et al. 2016). Stability of casein micelles are improved by conjugating with dextran. Non-toxic amadori rearrangements of the Maillard reaction are utilized to conjugate protein to polysaccharide (Wu and Wang 2017). Conjugates are formed due to the covalent interaction between the amino group of protein and reducing group of carbohydrate (de Oliveira et al. 2016). The resulting self-assembling micelles consist of a core region made up of hydrodophobic protein and the shell made up of polysaccharide. Curcumin is entrapped due to a hydrophobic interaction with the core region of the micelles. The average diameter of curcumin-casein-dextran is 75 nm and it has a higher radical scavenging activity (Wu and Wang 2017).

Hepatacarcinoma can be specifically targeted by modifying the surface of dextran-based nanocarriers with glycyrrhetinic acid. By grafting polymers formed from 2-hydroxyethyl methacrylate on dextran, the biocompatibility and chemical stability of the nanocarrier system is further improved. While ceric ammonium nitrate acts as an initiator for this reaction, ethylene glycol dimethacrylate acts as crosslinker. By optimizing the pH and concentration of dextran-glycyyrhetinic acid grafted polymer, curcumin can be adsorbed onto the surface of this nanocarrier. This drug entrapped nanocarrier system is 40–50 nm in size and is highly effective against HepG2 cells (Anirudhan and Binusreejayan 2016).

11.3.6 Gum Arabic Nanocarrier Systems for the Delivery of Curcumin

Gum arabic (GA) which also called as gum acacia are acidic polysaccharides obtained from the stems of *Acacia senegal* and *Acacia seyal* which has been used in the pharmaceutical industry as stabilizers (Dauqan and Abdullah 2013; Bhardwaj et al. 2000). GA is a complex polysaccharide consisting of a mixture of polysaccharide and glycoprotein. The polysaccharide unit is composed of arabinose and rhamnose with (1,3) linked β-D-galactopyranosyl backbone (Benfattoum et al. 2017). Under the acidic conditions of the GI tract, GA protects the encapsulated drug by shrinking. The drug is released under an alkaline or neutral condition as GA swells. In addition, GA is completely degraded by large intestinal microbiota (Benfattoum et al. 2017; Dauqan and Abdullah 2013).

GA-based drug carrier systems have been effective in the delivery of drugs such as insulin and diclofenac (Benfattoum et al. 2017; Avadi et al. 2010). More than 90% of curcumin can be entrapped in GA-BSA coacervate using an emulsification-coacervation technique (Shahgholian and Rajabzadeh 2016). GA, due to an electrostatic interaction, can form complex coacervates with proteins. This interaction is dependent on the pH and ionic strength of the system (Weinbreck et al. 2003). These complex coacervates can be used in drug delivery. In the case of GA-BSA coacervate, the complex coacervate is stabilized by the hydrogen and hydrophobic bond in addition to the electrostatic interaction between the protein and polysaccharide (Shahgholian and Rajabzadeh 2016; Pathak et al. 2014). GA can be combined with chitosan and developed into a carrier system for the delivery of curcumin. The maximum size of the chitosan-GA carrier system was 245 nm (Avadi et al. 2010). GA is useful in increasing the solubility and degree of supersaturation (Patcharawalai et al. 2013). The selectivity of curcumin against hepatic carcinoma cells can be improved by conjugating curcumin to GA. This results in formation of drug-loaded micelles with a higher selectivity (Sarika et al. 2015a). Although there was no sufficient data on the size of such curcumin-loaded micelles, research focusing on achieving size in the range of nanometer could further improve the efficacy.

Binary systems utilize desirable characteristics of two materials to offer a single combined carrier system. For example, Sodium casein (SC) when combined with GA, offers the benefits of the biocompatibility and functionality of casein and the high pH stability and solubility of GA. By optimizing the level of tween-20, it is possible to prepare nanodispersion of SC-GA. Although the precise mechanism of the role of tween-20 is yet to be understood, it is believed that the surfactant affects the electrostatic interaction between the protein and polysaccharide. The reduction in the zeta potential of the SC-GA carrier system upon addition of tween-20 indicates the possibility of a steric barrier in the interaction between SC and GA. This nanodispersion is used as a carrier system in delivering curcumin. The mean particle size of curcumin-SC-GA was 72 nm (Sheikhzadeh et al. 2016).

Nanoemulsions are useful in improving stability and delivering hydrophobic drugs. However, emulsions as a system by themselves are sensitive to changes in temperature, pH, and salt concentration, particularly in systems that utilize proteins as emulsifier. These problems can be overcome by using polysaccharide such as GA as an emulsifying agent. Nanoemulsion containing curcumin as a drug and GA as an emulsifier is more stable than protein-based nanoemulsion. The mean particle size of GA-based nanoemulsion with curcumin was 600 nm. GA forms a thick layer at the interface providing stability against pH. Steric repulsion that plays a role in the formation of polysaccharide-based emulsions provides stability against higher ionic strengths and temperatures (Wu et al. 2017).

The anticancer property of curcumin is improved when encapsulated within GA aldehyde-gelatin nanogels (Sarika and Nirmala 2016). GA aldehyde-gelatin nanogels are prepared using an inverse mini-emulsion technique. These nanogels are non-toxic in nature (Sarika and James 2015). Curcumin-loaded GA aldehyde-gelatin nanogels are prepared by dissolving curcumin in acetone and then dispersing into the gels. As the organic solvent evaporates, curcumin dispersed in GA aldehyde-gelatin nanogels, are entrapped within the carrier. In addition, hydrogen bonding between the drug and the carrier further stabilize the interaction. The average size of the drug-loaded nanogels thus formed is 452 nm. These nanogels were hemocompatible and had a higher cytotoxic activity against MCF-7 cells possibly due to an enhanced permeation and retention (EPR) effect (Sarika and Nirmala 2016).

11.3.7 GUM TRAGACANTH NANOCARRIER SYSTEMS FOR THE DELIVERY OF CURCUMIN

Tragacanth gum (TG) is a gummy exudate obtained from various species of *Astragalus*. Depending on the species, the physical properties of gum will change. TG consists of a water-soluble portion called tragacanthin and a water-insoluble portion bassorin that swells in water. Tragacanthin is composed of acidic polysaccharides containing D-galactourinic acid. Bassorin is made up of methylated acid polysaccharides (Whistler 2012).

Among the natural plant-derived gum, TG is the most viscous. Among various applications as drug carriers, an important application of TG is in the preparation of hydrogels. Hydrogels are insoluble under aqueous conditions but have ability to swell (Hosseini, Hemmati, and Ghaemy 2016). Hydrogels have a large number of hydrophilic groups with a higher tissue permeability and drug residence time due to their mucoadhesive and bioadhesive properties. Partition co-efficient dictates drug release from hydrogel (Hemmati et al. 2015). TG is stable over a wide pH range. By suitable chemical modification, TG can be made pH dependent so that the drug release can be controlled. For example, TG nanohydrogels when modified chemically using glycidylmethacrylate and cross-linked through free radical polymerization result in the formation of nanohydrogels. The drug loading capacity can be controlled by controlling the crosslinker. This gel has a high swelling property at pH 7.0 in comparison to exposure to other pH levels, making them useful for delivery of drugs in a pH dependent way (Hemmati et al. 2015). TG can also be used in preparing nanohydrogels by using other crosslinkers such as glutaraldehyde, diglycidylether, and polyvinyl alcohol (Hemmati and Ghaemy 2016).

Comb-shaped amphiphilic polymers are useful in encapsulating hydrophobic drugs. In aqueous conditions, due to hydrophobic interactions, these comb-shaped amphiphilic polymers self-assemble. However, hydrophilic portions of the polymers still the maintain solubility of the polymer in aqueous solutions. Such polymers can be further made into a pH-temperature combo type by using ring-opening polymerization, atom transfer radical polymerization, and click reactions (Hemmati and Ghaemy 2016). TG is also useful in preparation of coacervate by complexing it with sodium alginate. The size of coacervate ranges in nanometer. These are formed due to electrostatic interaction. Size of coacervates are dependent on the pH (Gorji et al. 2014).

By blending GT with poly(vinyl alcohol) (PVA), a GT-PVA scaffold can be produced. By using an electrospinning technique, GT- PVA can be spun into nanofibers with curcumin entrapped within the fibers. Interestingly, the water-soluble portion of GT is found to be important in obtaining smooth and uniform nanofibers. GT extracted from *A. fluccosus* contains a higher portion of water-soluble components. Around 3% (w/v) of curcumin was reported to be entrapped. The maximum size of curcumin-fabricated nanofibers was 216 nm. This curcumin scaffold supported proliferation of fibroblast, which shows that it could be useful in the treatment of wounds and burns (Ranjbar-Mohammadi et al. 2017).

11.3.8 HYALURONIC ACID NANOCARRIER SYSTEMS FOR THE DELIVERY OF CURCUMIN

Hyaluronic acid (HA) is a naturally occurring linear polysaccharide (glycosaminoglycan). HA is composed of glucosamine and glucuronic acid. HA is a highly hydrated polyanionic macromolecule. It is present in human and animal connective tissues in the extracellular matrix (ECM) of cartilage tissues especially the skin (Burdick and Prestwich 2011). HA has been used alone as a drug carrier in various drug delivery systems such as topical, ophthalmic, parenteral, nasal, and pulmonary drug delivery systems (Eenschooten et al. 2012).

Hydrogels can be prepared by conjugating HA with polymers and other polysaccharides. These conjugated polymers are utilized as targeted drug delivery systems for delivering anticancer molecules (Chen et al. 2016).

Increase in uptake and cytotoxicity against human colon carcinoma cells is observed when curcumin conjugated to HA delivers using silica nanoparticles in comparison to curcumin delivered using silica nanoparticles without conjugating with chitosan (Singh et al. 2015b). Curcumin conjugated to hyaluronic acid has a higher aqueous solubility due to the formation of stable micelles (Manju and Sreenivasan 2011). A oligo-hyalurosomes nano delivery system containing hyaluronic acid as a key polymer is useful in delivering curcumin along with resveratrol. The drug-loaded conjugate system had higher stability, bioavailability, and anti-oxidant activity than the individual component (Guo et al. 2018).

Pulmonary cancer can be effectively treated by delivering curcumin using a HA-chitosan nanocarrier system. Due to the hydrophilicity, safe, non-toxic, mucoadhesive, and target specific properties of chitosan and hyaluronic acid, these biopolymers play an important role in cancer-targeted delivery systems.

11.3.9 PECTIN NANOCARRIER SYSTEMS FOR THE DELIVERY OF CURCUMIN

Pectin is a polysaccharide consisting of galacturonic acid residues and neutral sugar side chains. It is derived from plants, particularly from citrus and apple. It has a negative charge although the net negative charge and charge distribution changes based on the degree of esterification (Lee 2015).

The most common use of pectin in the pharmaceutical industry is as thickening agent. However, it is also a good carrier system for improving the bioavailability of curcumin. Pectin can be used either alone or in combination with other polysaccharides and protein (Ashford et al. 1993; Sriamornsak 2011; Pandey et al. 2013). Pectin has an important advantage, as while pectin is stable in the gut, it becomes unstable in the colon due to degradation by the microflora present in the colon. Therefore, the drug that is entrapped within the pectin will be released in the colon. This degradation of pectin in the colon has been adapted for delivering drugs specifically to the colon thereby it is useful in treating colon related diseases (Liu et al. 2003). The longer transit time and higher absorption capacity of the colon increases the possibility of drugs getting absorbed in a higher quantity. In addition, under alkaline conditions, pectin adheres to the mucosa of the colon. This further increases the residence time of drug-loaded pectin in colon (Lee 2015; Alkhader et al. 2017).

Microbeads prepared using a combination of pectin and alginate can entrap curcumin. Although the sizes of such particles are in microns, higher availability of curcumin in the colon is achieved (Sattarahmady et al. 2016). In another study, more than 99% of curcumin was encapsulated in pectin. The resulting pectin-curcumin hydrogel was effective in controlling adipogenesis (Lee 2015). This shows that an improvement in stability of curcumin could be achieved by entrapping curcumin in polysaccharides, and reducing the size, even at a micro scale.

Using an esterification reaction, pectin can be conjugated to curcumin. The maximum size of such pectin-curcumin conjugates is 190 nm. This conjugate increases the stability of curcumin in an aqueous environment retaining the anti-oxidant effect of curcumin. In addition, anticancer activity of curcumin is also enhanced. Synergistic interaction between the carrier and the entrapped molecule is believed to have contributed to this enhancement in anticancer activity (Bai et al. 2017).

Pectin can be used in conjunction with other polymers or as a coating polymer. The drawback of using pectin as a single carrier system is the burst release of the drug upon reaching the colon. This is due to swelling under alkaline pH. This can be overcome by using pectin in combination with other polysaccharides. For example, when pectin is used in combination with chitosan, chitosan-pectin-curcumin nanoparticles of sizes around 206 nm can be achieved. Curcumin nanoparticles have net positive charge. The chitosan-pectin, which is initially formed due to an electrostatic interaction, is stabilized due to crosslinking by sodium tripolyphosphate. The entrapped curcumin is stable under highly acidic conditions of pH <2 and is released when the composite is exposed to alkaline conditions (Alkhader et al. 2017). Pectin improves the functionality and stability of nanoparticles prepared using a protein-based nanocarrier (Chang et al. 2017b). Casein-zein-curcumin nanoparticles are more stable when linked to pectin (Chang et al. 2017a).

11.3.10 PULLULAN NANOCARRIER SYSTEMS FOR THE DELIVERY OF CURCUMIN

Pullulan is a neutral polysaccharide produced by black yeasts *Aureobasidium pullulans* and other species of *Aureobasidium* (Dionísio et al. 2013; Singh et al. 2015a). Pullulan has both hydrophilic and hydrophobic characteristics due to its unique structure, which consists of both α-(1,4) and α-(1,6) linkages. Depending upon the fungal species, there could be a small difference in the backbone of this glucan containing polysaccharide (Singh et al. 2015a). Presence of at least nine hydroxyl groups for each repeating units allows customization and preparation of various derivatives through the chemical modification of pullulan (Shingel 2004). For example, sulfation or amination allows pullulan to assemble into nanoparticles when complexed with other polysaccharides such as chitosan. The interaction between pullulan and other polysaccharides is reported to be a polyelectrolyte complexation (Dionísio et al. 2013).

Pullulan can be prepared into nanocarriers. They are known to undergo integrin-mediated adhesion resulting in internalization into the cell. This allows delivery of the drugs into the cells. Through active and passive targeting, pullulan can be customized to deliver its cargo only to the targeted site (Singh et al. 2015a; Shingel 2004). Upon intravenous injection, more than 80% of the high molecular weight pullulan tends to accumulate in liver. This is probably due to the presence of lectin-like receptors expressed in the liver (Yamaoka et al. 1993). This results in shorter half-life. However, this allows for targeting and specifically delivering drugs to the liver (Singh et al. 2015a). With a decrease in molecular weight, the extent of pullulan accumulated in the liver decreases, possibly due to a high vascular permeability (Yamaoka et al. 1993).

Galactosylated pullulan is useful in delivering curcumin specifically to the liver. Curcumin when encapsulated within chemically modified pullulan accumulates preferentially within HepG2 cells. This results in selective toxicity toward HepG2. Galactosylated pullulan was obtained by sequentially modifying the structure of pullulan. First pullulan was oxidized, followed by the grafting of aminated ligand. This was followed by the grafting of modified curcumin to the pullulan containing the ligand. The mean particle size of curcumin-loaded galactosylated pullulan was reported to be 355 nm (Sarika et al. 2015b; Yang et al. 2012).

11.3.11 STARCH NANOCARRIER SYSTEMS FOR THE DELIVERY OF CURCUMIN

Starch consists of amylase and amylopectin. Industrial application of starch is limited due to the insolubility of starch in cold water, its tendency to deteriorate, and the formation of high viscous solution upon gelatinization (Jivan et al. 2014). In plant, starch serves as the reserve source for its energy (Smith 2005). Starch consists of monosaccharides linked together with α-D-(1,4) and/or α-D-(1,6) linkage. Monosaccharides linked with only a α-D-(1,4) linkage are called amylose whereas amylopectin consists of a linear polymer linked by α-D-(1,4) branches crosslinked with each other via a α-D-(1,6) linkage (Rodrigues and Emeje 2012; Green et al. 1975).

In the past, soluble starch has been used extensively in the textile and food industry. Of late, soluble starch is being explored as a nanocarrier system for delivery of drugs (Hasanvand et al. 2015; Won et al. 1997; Liu et al. 2015; Yang et al. 2014). Depending on the method of preparation, it is possible to prepare starch-based nanocarriers with varying degree of physic-chemical properties (Rodrigues and Emeje 2012).

Hydrophobically modified starch (HMS) is an amphiphilic polymer that can be used for encapsulating and delivering curcumin. Curcumin can be entrapped using a polymeric micellar encapsulation technique without affecting the micellar structure of HMS. Entrapped curcumin exhibits 1640-fold increase in aqueous solubility and enhanced anticancer activity against HepG2 cell lines (Yu and Huang 2010). Hydrophobic starch acetate can be synthesized by acetylation. Such acetylated starch acts as a good nanocarrier. Curcumin can be entrapped in native and acetylated starch by a nanoprecipitation technique. More than 80% of curcumin was encapsulated and the resulting nanoparticles had a mean particle size of 135 and 192 nm for the native and acetylated starch respectively. The particles are ellipsoidal in morphology with zeta potential greater than −30 mV (Acevedo-Guevara et al. 2018). Desolvation is another technique that is utilized in encapsulating curcumin within starch to achieve a sustained release of curcumin for 96 h. Via this technique, 14.3% of curcumin is encapsulated. The mean particle size of curcumin-loaded starch is reported to be 61.1 nm with a zeta potential of −14.7 mV. The carrier system is effective against *Streptococcus mutans* (Maghsoudi et al. 2017).

By using a facile solution mixing method, curcumin can be entrapped within soluble starch. Depending on the percentage of curcumin loaded, the size of drug-loaded nanoparticles ranges from 182 to 255 nm. Efficiency was highest when 3% of the drug was entrapped and it showed potent anti-oxidant activity (Li et al. 2016). A loading efficiency of 78% is achieved when curcumin-starch nanoparticles are prepared using *in situ* nanoprecipitation and microemulsion techniques. A mean particle size of 87 nm is achieved by this technique. Loading efficiency was significantly dependent on the surfactant and hold time. Curcumin from this carrier system is released over ten days in a sustained manner (Chin et al. 2014).

Cassava starch with poly(vinyl alcohol) (PVA) nanocomposite represent a useful delivery system for controlled release of curcumin. Initially, starch nanoparticles are prepared followed by entrapment of curcumin within the nanoparticles. This is followed by incorporation of starch-curcumin nanoparticles (SCN) into starch-PVA nanocomposite. SCN was spherical and had maximum size of 200 nm. Curcumin release is dictated by diffusion and erosion. Anticancer activity of curcumin-loaded nanocomposite against skin carcinoma cells was significantly higher than free curcumin (Athira and Jyothi 2015).

11.4 CLINICAL STUDIES

Although research in the area of the therapeutic evaluation of curcumin and its delivery continue to increase, the outcome will not benefit human beings until benefits are successfully demonstrated through clinical trials. A number of clinical trials have been conducted using either curcumin extract or cucrumin as pure compound, which have demonstrated the safety and pharmacological benefits of curcumin. In addition, various clinical trials show that carrier systems are useful in enhancing bioavailability of curcumin.

Administration of oral curcuma extract in patients with colorectal cancer shows that curcumin extract is safe even at higher doses. Even though the patients did not respond to the treatment, non-toxicity to high doses suggest that an extensive clinical trial at higher doses could provide some lead in using curcumin for treating colorectal cancer (Sharma et al. 2001). A randomized, single-blind, crossover trial conducted with 23 volunteers showed higher oral bioavailability of curcumin when administered as a micellar formulation (Kocher et al. 2015). Phase I clinical trials were conducted in 25 patients with pre-malignant lesions to understand the biologically effective dose, pharmacokinetics, and toxicity of curcumin in humans. The median age of the selected subjects was 60 years. In this study, no toxicity was observed for a dose up to 8 g/day when given for three months. Curcumin was administered in tablet form. The maximum concentration in the serum was observed 1–2 h after oral administration. There was no multi-dose effect observed in selected patients. This study demonstrated the chemopreventive activity of curcumin against pre-malignant lesions. The study also shows that curcumin is poorly absorbed from the GI tract and its metabolic pathway may be more complicated than it was previously reported (Hsieh 2001). A separate set of studies conducted in human volunteers confirmed that upon oral administration, curcumin is primarily conjugated as curcumin glucuronide and to a smaller extent as curcumin sulfate. This proves that curcumin is transported to sites other than the intestinal tract (Vareed et al. 2008).

In phase II clinical studies, even with limited oral bioavailability, some patients with advanced pancreatic cancer responded to the treatment and no toxicity was reported in any of the volunteers (Dhillon et al. 2008).

A range of clinical studies has been conducted to understand the benefits of administering curcumin *via* carriers. These studies were undertaken for understanding the possibility of using a carrier system to achieve a higher bioavailability. Even the preclinical studies conducted in rats shows that nanocarrier systems such as nanoemulsions significantly improve oral bioavailability of curcumoids (Lu et al. 2018). In an attempt to understand the benefits of delivering liposomal curcumin, safety of the liposomal curcumin was assessed in a phase I clinical trial conducted in healthy volunteers. The tolerability and pharmacokinetics were also studied. Fifty subjects were part of this double-blind dose escalation study. The liposomal curcumin was administered as intravenous injections. The study shows that plasma concentration increases in a dose dependent manner and a dose of up to 120 mg/m^2 was safe (Storka et al. 2015).

In a randomized double-blind cross over study, 42 volunteers were administered with either curcumin micelles or a placebo. The study was conducted for six weeks and the subjects on micellar curcuminoids were given 294 mg. This was equivalent to 241 mg of pure curcumin. At the end of the study, no toxicity was observed. In addition, no effect on glucose and iron homoeostasis was also reported (Kocher et al. 2016). In another separate study, oral bioavailability and safety of micronized powder and liquid micelles of curcumin was compared to the native powder. Twenty-three healthy volunteers were subjected to this crossover study. While both micronization and micelles improved the oral bioavailability, C_{max} was particularly high in the case of micellar curcumin (Schiborr et al. 2014).

In a further development toward a novel delivery system utilizing polysaccharides as a nanocarrier system, a set of researchers from Tokyo developed a nanoparticle colloidal dispersion of curcumin by using gum ghatti. The efficacy of this formulation, which is called Theracurmin™, was first studied in rats. The study showed that there was a 40-fold increase in oral bioavailability in comparison to the free drug. Therefore, this polysaccharide-based nanocarrier system was further studied in 14 healthy volunteers. In humans, there was a 27-fold increase in the AUC in comparison to the free drug (Sasaki et al. 2011). In a double-blinded crossover clinical study conducted with 12 healthy volunteers, a significant increase in the absorption of curcumin was observed when curcumin was administered as γ-CD-curcumin complex in comparison to unformulated curcumin (Purpura et al. 2017).

11.5 COMMERCIALLY AVAILABLE CURCUMIN-BASED NEUTRACEUTICAL

There are only a few curcumin-based neutraceuticals that are marketed for treatment of various ailments. The following section describes some of these supplements available on market.

11.5.1 BioPerine®

BioPerine® is piperine extracted from *Piper nigrum* marketed by the Sabinsa Corporation. Absorption and hence bioavailability of curcumin is increased when co-administered with BioPerine®. There is at least a 20-fold increase in the bioavailability of curcumin.

11.5.2 Cavacurmin®

Cavacurmin® is another commercially available neutraceutcial manufactured by Wacker Chemie AG. It is an inclusion complex of 95% curcuminoids within gamma-cyclodextrin. Curcuminoids consists of 65%–80% curcumin, 15%–20% demethoxycurcumin and 2%–5%

bis-demethoxycurcumin. A 49-fold increase in bioavailability of curcumin is observed upon administration of Cavacurmin®.

11.5.3 InvigoFlex® CS

InvigoFlex® CS is a commercially available neutraceutical used as a supplement for strengthening articular surface and cartilage. It is manufactured and marketed by WynnPharm, USA. It is formulated and administered as capsules and consists of chondroitin sulfate and curcumin along with other excipients.

11.5.4 Longvida®

Longvida® contains curcumin prepared using solid lipid curcumin particle technology. Verdure Sciences® markets Longvida®. This lipophilic matrix-based preparation provides 24 hour circulating curcumin. In addition, curcumin has a higher permeability with the ability to cross the blood brain barrier.

11.5.5 Meriva-SF®

Meriva-SF® is a phytosome-based curcumin supplement developed and marketed by USA-based Throne Research. It has a higher absorption rate in comparison to free curcumin and it is marketed for the treatment of joint and muscle soreness.

11.5.6 Theracurmin® HP

Theracurmin® HP is manufactured as capsules and contains curcumin prepared using colloidal dispersion along with other excipients. It is developed and marketed by Integrative Therapeutics. Theracurmin increases the bioavailability of curcumin by 27 times.

Clinical trials conducted on curcumin provide evidence for the clinical efficacy of curcumin in spite of poor oral absorption. The study also confirms safety of curcumin even at a higher dose. Most research shows that the true therapeutic efficacy of curcumin can be realized if higher availability of curcumin is achieved at the target site. Although a dose, more than 8 g/day can be administered to achieve a higher bioavailability; it would be difficult for patients to ingest such a high quantity. The issues of reducing the degradation of curcumin in the GI tract, improving the stability, reducing the intake of high dose, increasing bioavailability, and increasing the half-life, can be achieved by utilizing the recent developments in drug delivering systems. Nanocarriers are one such promising delivery system wherein a high bioavailability is achieved even at low dose. By utilizing polysaccharides as nanocarriers, limitations observed with administration of free curcumin could be overcome. The few studies conducted using polysaccharide-based nanocarrier systems for delivery of curcumin prove that these carrier systems can be successfully used in humans. Already a few neutraceuticals are utilizing carrier-based delivery systems to achieve a higher bioavailability. Some of these marketed neutraceuticals are classic examples that demonstrate the progression of understanding derived from academic research for developing products on large scale. However, more research on polysaccharide nanocarrier systems for delivery of curcumin are required to translate this research into commercial products for the benefits of the normal population and people in "disease".

11.6 CONCLUSION

With recent progress in the field of nanotechnology and polysaccharides, it is possible to utilize polysaccharides as nanocarrier systems and utilize the benefit offered by both polysaccharides and nanotechnology in the field of drug delivery. The benefit of using polysaccharides as nanocarrier systems ranges from reduction in cost, non-toxicity, biodegradability, better efficiency, higher stability, and so on. This would facilitate the maximum therapeutic benefit being gained from curcumin, which has not been the case so far. This is due to the sensitive physico-chemical properties of curcumin. There is good progress in understanding the limitations and a number of researches have tried in circumventing these limitations through nanocarrier-based delivery systems. A number of clinical trials clearly show the therapeutic benefits of curcumin and the benefits of polysaccharides as nanocarriers. As the efforts are made to improve the bioavailability of curcumin, it is also important to undertake more research to improve the analytical techniques for assessing the bioavailability of curcumin. This has proved more challenging due to the lack of information on the pharmacological activity of curcumin analogues and their degradation products, and the conflicting information on the efficacy of curcumin analogues.

CONFLICTS OF INTEREST

The authors declare that there is no conflict of interest. The opinions expressed in this article are the author's own and do not reflect or represent the view of any organization.

REFERENCES

Acevedo-Guevara, L., Nieto-Suaza, L., Sanchez, L.T., Pinzon, M.I., and Villa, C.C. 2018. Development of native and modified banana starch nanoparticles as vehicles for curcumin. *Int J Biol Macromol* 111: 498–504.

Alkhader, E., Billa, N., and Roberts, C.J. 2017. Mucoadhesive chitosan-pectinate nanoparticles for the delivery of curcumin to the colon. *AAPS Pharm Sci Tech* 18: 1009–18.

Amirthalingam, M., Kasinathan, N., Amuthan, A., Mutalik, S., Sreenivasa Reddy, M., and Nayanabhirama, U. 2017. Bioactive PLGA-curcumin microparticle-embedded chitosan scaffold: In vitro and in vivo evaluation. *Artif Cells Nanomed Biotechnol* 45: 233–41.

Anand, P., Kunnumakkara, A.B., Newman, R.A., and Aggarwal, B.B. 2007. Bioavailability of curcumin: Problems and promises. *Mol Pharm* 4 (6): 807–18.

Anirudhan, T.S. and Binusreejayan. 2016. Dextran based nanosized carrier for the controlled and targeted delivery of curcumin to liver cancer cells. *Int J Biol Macromol* 88: 222–35.

Ashford, M., Fell, J., Attwood, D., Sharma, H., and Woodhead, P. 1993. An evaluation of pectin as a carrier for drug targeting to the colon. *J Control Release* 26 (3): 213–20.

Athira, G.K. and Jyothi, A.N. 2015. Cassava starch-poly(vinyl alcohol) nanocomposites for the controlled delivery of curcumin in cancer prevention and treatment. *Starke* 67 (5–6): 549–58.

Avadi, M.R., Sadeghi, A.M., Mohammadpour, N., Abedin, S., Atyabi, F., Dinarvand, R. et al. 2010. Preparation and characterization of insulin nanoparticles using chitosan and Arabic gum with ionic gelation method. *Nanomedicine* 6 (1): 58–63.

Bai, F., Diao, J., Wang, Y., Sun, S., Zhang, H., Liu, Y. et al. 2017. A new water-soluble nanomicelle formed through self-assembly of pectin-curcumin conjugates: Preparation, characterization, and anticancer activity evaluation. *J Agric Food Chem* 65 (32): 6840–7.

Benfattoum, K., Haddadine, N., Bouslah, N., Benaboura, A., Maincent, P., Barillé, R. et al. 2017. Formulation characterization and in vitro evaluation of acacia gum-calcium alginate beads for oral drug delivery systems. *Polym Adv Technol* 29: 884–895.

Bhardwaj, T.R., Kanwar, M., Lal, R., and Gupta, A. 2000. Natural gums and modified natural gums as sustained-release carriers. *Drug Dev Ind Pharm* 26 (10): 1025–38.

Bisht, S. and Maitra, A. 2009. Systemic delivery of curcumin: 21st century solutions for an ancient conundrum. *Curr Drug Discov Techno* 6 (3): 192–9.

Burdick, J.A. and Prestwich, G.D. 2011. Hyaluronic acid hydrogels for biomedical applications. *Adv Mater* 23: H41–56.

Chang, C., Wang, T., Hu, Q., Luo, Y. 2017a. Caseinate-zein-polysaccharide complex nanoparticles as potential oral delivery vehicles for curcumin: Effect of polysaccharide type and chemical cross-linking. *Food Hydrocoll* 72: 254–62.

Chang, C., Wang, T., Hu, Q., and Luo, Y. 2017b. Zein/caseinate/pectin complex nanoparticles: Formation and characterization. *Int J Biol Macromol* 104: 117–24.

Chen, C., Johnston, T.D., Jeon, H., Gedaly, R., McHugh, P.P., Burke, T.G. et al. 2009. An in vitro study of liposomal curcumin: Stability, toxicity and biological activity in human lymphocytes and Epstein-Barr virus-transformed human B-cells. *Int J Pharm* 366 (1–2): 133–9.

Chen, Y.N., Hsu, S.L., Liao, M.Y., Liu, Y.T., Lai, C.H., Chen, J.F. et al. 2016. Ameliorative effect of curcumin-encapsulated hyaluronic acid–PLA nanoparticles on thioacetamide-induced murine hepatic fibrosis. *Int J Environ Res Public Health* 14 (1): 11.

Cheng, A.L., Hsu, C.H., Lin, J.K., Hsu, M.M., Ho, Y.F., Shen, T.S. et. al. 2001. Phase I clinical trial of curcumin, a chemopreventive agent, in patients with high-risk or pre-malignant lesions. *Anticancer Res* 21: 2895–900.

Chin, S.F., Yazid, S.N.A.M., and Pang, S.C. 2014. Preparation and characterization of starch nanoparticles for controlled release of curcumin. *Int J Polym Sci* 2014: 1–8.

Dauqan, E. and Abdullah, A. 2013. Utilization of gum arabic for industries and human health. *Am J Appl Sci* 10 (10): 1270–9.

de Oliveira, F.C., Coimbra, J.S., de Oliveira, E.B., Zuñiga, A.D., and Rojas, E.E. 2016. Food protein-polysaccharide conjugates obtained via the Maillard reaction: A review. *Crit Rev Food Sci Nutr* 56 (7): 1108–25.

Dhillon, N., Aggarwal, B.B., Newman, R.A., Wolff, R.A., Kunnumakkara, A.B., Abbruzzese, J. et al. 2008. Phase II trial of curcumin in patients with advanced pancreatic cancer. *Clin Cancer Res* 14 (14): 4491–9.

Dhule, S.S., Penfornis, P., Frazier, T., Walker, R., Feldman, J., Tan, G. et al. 2012. Curcumin-loaded γ-cyclodextrin liposomal nanoparticles as delivery vehicles for osteosarcoma. *Nanomedicine* 8 (4): 440–51.

Dionísio, M., Cordeiro, C., Remuñán-López, C., Seijo, B., Rosa da Costa, A.M. et al. 2013. Pullulan-based nanoparticles as carriers for transmucosal protein delivery. *Eur J Pharm Sci* 50 (1): 102–13.

Douglass, B.J. and Clouatre, D.L. 2015. Beyond yellow curry: Assessing commercial curcumin absorption technologies. *J Am Coll Nutr* 34 (4): 347–58.

Eenschooten, C., Vaccaro, A., Delie, F., Guillaumie, F., Tømmeraas, K., and Kontogeorgis, G.M. et al. 2012. Novel self-associative and multiphasic nanostructured soft carriers based on amphiphilic hyaluronic acid derivatives. *Carbohydr Polym* 87 (1): 444–51.

Facchi, S.P., Scariot, D.B., Bueno, P.V., Souza, P.R., Figueiredo, L.C., Follmann, H. et al. 2016. Preparation and cytotoxicity of N-modified chitosan nanoparticles applied in curcumin delivery. *Int J Biol Macromol* 87: 237–45.

Gorji, S.G., Gorji, E.G. and Mohammadifar, M.A. 2014. Characterisation of gum tragacanth (Astragalus gossypinus)/sodium caseinate complex coacervation as a function of pH in an aqueous medium. *Food Hydrocoll* 34: 161–8.

Green, M.M., Blankenhorn, G., and Hart, H. 1975. Which starch fraction is water-soluble, amylose or amylopectin? *J Chem Educ* 52: 729.

Guo, C., Yin, J., and Chen, D. 2018. Co-encapsulation of curcumin and resveratrol into novel nutraceutical hyalurosomes nano-food delivery system based on oligo-hyaluronic acid-curcumin polymer. *Carbohydr Polym* 181: 1033–7.

Guzman-Villanueva, D., El-Sherbiny, I.M., Herrera-Ruiz, D., and Smyth, H.D. 2013. Design and in vitro evaluation of a new nano-microparticulate system for enhanced aqueous-phase solubility of curcumin. *Biomed Res Int* 2013.

Hasanvand, E., Fathi, M., Bassiri, A., Javanmard, M., and Abbaszadeh, R. 2015. Novel starch based nanocarrier for vitamin D fortification of milk: Production and characterization. *Food Bioprod Process* 96: 264–77.

Hassaninasab, A., Hashimoto, Y., Tomita-Yokotani, K., and Kobayashi, M. 2011. Discovery of the curcumin metabolic pathway involving a unique enzyme in an intestinal microorganism. *Proc Natl Acad Sci USA* 108 (16): 6615–20.

Hemmati, K. and Ghaemy, M. 2016. Synthesis of new thermo/pH sensitive drug delivery systems based on tragacanth gum polysaccharide. *Int J Biol Macromol* 87: 415–25.

Hemmati, K., Masoumi, A., and Ghaemy, M. 2015. Synthesis and characterization of pH-responsive nanohydrogels as biocompatible drug carriers based on chemically modified tragacanth gum polysaccharide. *RSC Adv* 5 (104): 85310–8.

Hosseini, M.S., Hemmati, K., and Ghaemy, M. 2016. Synthesis of nanohydrogels based on tragacanth gum biopolymer and investigation of swelling and drug delivery. *Int J Biol Macromol* 82: 806–15.

Jaisamut, P., Wiwattanawongsa K., and Wiwattanapatapee R. 2013. Influence of natural gum on curcumin supersaturation in gastrointestinal fluids. *Int Scholar Sci Res Innov* 7 (12): 570–3.

Jardim, K.V., Joanitti, G.A., Azevedo, R.B., and Parize, A.L. 2015. Physico-chemical characterization and cytotoxicity evaluation of curcumin loaded in chitosan/chondroitin sulfate nanoparticles. *Mater Sci Eng C Mater Biol Appl* 56: 294–304.

Jivan, M.J., Yarmand, M., and Madadlou, A. 2014. Preparation of cold water-soluble potato starch and its characterization. *J Food Sci Technol* 51 (3): 601–5.

Kasinathan, N., Amirthalingam, M., Reddy, N.D., Jagani, H.V., Volety, S.M., and Rao, J.V. 2016. In-situ implant containing PCL-curcumin nanoparticles developed using design of experiments. *Drug Deliv* 23 (3): 1007–15.

Kasinathan, N., Volety, S.M., and Josyula, V.R. 2016. Chondroitinase: A promising therapeutic enzyme. *Crit Rev Microbiol* 42 (3): 474–84.

Kocher, A., Bohnert, L., Schiborr, C., and Frank, J. 2016. Highly bioavailable micellar curcuminoids accumulate in blood, are safe and do not reduce blood lipids and inflammation markers in moderately hyperlipidemic individuals. *Mol Nutr Food Res* 60 (7): 1555–63.

Kocher, A., Schiborr, C., Behnam, D., and Frank, J. 2015. The oral bioavailability of curcuminoids in healthy humans is markedly enhanced by micellar solubilisation but not further improved by simultaneous ingestion of sesamin, ferulic acid, naringenin and xanthohumol. *J Funct Foods* 14: 183–91.

Lee, J.Y. 2015. Pectin hydrogels of curcumin and obesity applications. Master of Science, University of Georgia, Athens, Georgia.

Letchford, K. and Burt, H. 2007. A review of the formation and classification of amphiphilic block copolymer nanoparticulate structures: Micelles, nanospheres, nanocapsules and polymersomes. *Eur J Pharm Biopharm* 65 (3): 259–69.

Li, J., Shin, G.H., Lee, W., Chen, X., and Park, H.J. 2016. Soluble starch formulated nanocomposite increases water solubility and stability of curcumin. *Food Hydrocoll* 56: 41–9.

Liu, K., Jiang, X., and Hunziker, P. 2016. Carbohydrate-based amphiphilic nano delivery systems for cancer therapy. *Nanoscale* 8 (36): 16091–156.

Liu, K., Wang, Y., Li, H., and Duan, Y. 2015. A facile one-pot synthesis of starch functionalized graphene as nano-carrier for pH sensitive and starch-mediated drug delivery. *Colloids Surf B Biointerfaces* 128: 86–93.

LinShu, L. Fishman, M.L., Kost J. et al. 2003. Pectin-based systems for colon-specific drug delivery via oral route. Biomaterials 24 (19): 3333–43.

Liu, Z., Jiao, Y., Wang, Y., Zhou, C., and Zhang, Z. 2008. Polysaccharides-based nanoparticles as drug delivery systems. *Adv Drug Deliv Rev* 60 (15): 1650–62.

Lu, P.S., Inbaraj, B.S., and Chen, B.H. 2018. Determination of oral bioavailability of curcuminoid dispersions and nanoemulsions prepared from curcuma longa linnaeus. *J Sci Food Agric* 98 (1): 51–63.

Maghsoudi, A., Yazdian, F., Shahmoradi, S., Ghaderi, L., Hemati, M. and Amoabediny, G. 2017. Curcumin-loaded polysaccharide nanoparticles: Optimization and anticariogenic activity against Streptococcus mutans. *Mater Sci Eng C Mater Biol Appl* 75: 1259–67.

Mahmood, K., Zia, K.M., Zuber, M., Nazli, Z.H., Rehman, S., and Zia, F. 2016. Enhancement of bioactivity and bioavailability of curcumin with chitosan based materials. *Korean J Chem Eng* 33: 3316–29.

Mangolim, C.S., Moriwaki, C., Nogueira, A.C., Sato, F., Baesso, M.L., Neto, A.M. et al. 2014. Curcumin–β-cyclodextrin inclusion complex: Stability, solubility, characterisation by FT-IR, FT-Raman, X-ray diffraction and photoacoustic spectroscopy, and food application. *Food Chem* 153: 361–70.

Manju, S. and Sreenivasan, K. 2011. Conjugation of curcumin onto hyaluronic acid enhances its aqueous solubility and stability. *J Colloid Interface Sci* 359 (1): 318–25.

Martins, A.F., Bueno, P.V., Almeida, E.A., Rodrigues, F.H., Rubira, A.F., and Muniz, E.C. 2013. Characterization of N-trimethyl chitosan/alginate complexes and curcumin release. *Int J Biol Macromol* 57: 174–84.

Martins, A.F., Facchi, S.P., Monteiro, J.P., Nocchi, S.R., Silva, C.T., Nakamura, C.V. et al. 2015. Preparation and cytotoxicity of N, N, N-trimethyl chitosan/alginate beads containing gold nanoparticles. *Int J Biol Macromol* 72: 466–71.

Mohan, P.R.K, Sreelakshmi, G., Muraleedharan, C.V., and Joseph, R. 2012. Water soluble complexes of curcumin with cyclodextrins: Characterization by FT-Raman spectroscopy. *Vib Spectrosc* 62: 77–84.

Molteni, L. 1985. [22] Dextran and inulin conjugates as drug carriers. *Methods Enzymol* 112: 285–98.

Maria, D.N., Mishra, S.R., Wang, L., Abd-Elgawad, A.H., Soliman, O.A., El-Dahan, M.S. et al. 2017. Water-soluble complex of curcumin with cyclodextrins: Enhanced physical properties for ocular drug delivery. *Curr Drug Deliv* 14 (6): 875–86.

Pandey, S., Mishra, A., Raval, P., Patel, H., Gupta, A., and Shah, D. 2013. Chitosan–pectin polyelectrolyte complex as a carrier for colon targeted drug delivery. *J Young Pharm* 5 (4): 160–6.

Pathak, J., Rawat, K., and Bohidar, H.B. 2014. Surface patch binding and mesophase separation in biopolymeric polyelectrolyte-polyampholyte solutions. *Int J Biol Macromol* 63: 29–37.

Pinho, E., Grootveld, M., Soares, G., and Henriques, M. 2014. Cyclodextrins as encapsulation agents for plant bioactive compounds. *Carbohydr Polym* 101: 121–35.

Popat, A., Karmakar, S., Jambhrunkar, S., Xu, C., and Yu, C. 2014. Curcumin-cyclodextrin encapsulated chitosan nanoconjugates with enhanced solubility and cell cytotoxicity. *Colloids Surf B Biointerfaces* 117: 520–7.

Purpura, M., Lowery, R.P., Wilson, J.M., Mannan, H., Münch, G., and Razmovski-Naumovski, V. 2017. Analysis of different innovative formulations of curcumin for improved relative oral bioavailability in human subjects. *Eur J Nutr* 57(3): 929–38.

Rajesh, Y., Narayanan, K., Reddy, M.S., Bhaskar, V.K., Shenoy, G.G., Subrahmanyam, V.M. et al. 2015. Production of β-cyclodextrin from pH and thermo stable cyclodextrin glycosyl transferase, obtained from arthrobacter mysorens and its evaluation as a drug carrier for irbesartan. *Curr Drug Deliv* 12 (4): 444–53.

Ranjbar-Mohammadi, M., Kargozar, S. Bahrami, S.H., and Joghataei, M.T. 2017. Fabrication of curcumin-loaded gum tragacanth/poly (vinyl alcohol) nanofibers with optimized electrospinning parameters. *J Ind Text* 46 (5): 1170–92.

Raveendran, R., Bhuvaneshwar, G.S., and Sharma, C.P. 2016. Hemocompatible curcumin-dextran micelles as pH sensitive pro-drugs for enhanced therapeutic efficacy in cancer cells. *Carbohydr Polym* 137: 497–507.

Rodrigues, A. and Emeje, M. 2012. Recent applications of starch derivatives in nanodrug delivery. *Carbohydr Polym* 87 (2): 987–94.

Saha, S., Roy, A., Roy, K., and Roy, M.N. 2016. Study to explore the mechanism to form inclusion complexes of β-cyclodextrin with vitamin molecules. *Sci Rep* 6: 35764.

Sandur, S.K, Pandey, M.K., Sung, B., Ahn, K.S., Murakami, A., Sethi, G. et al. 2007. Curcumin, demethoxycurcumin, bisdemethoxycurcumin, tetrahydrocurcumin and turmerones differentially regulate anti-inflammatory and anti-proliferative responses through a ROS-independent mechanism. *Carcinogenesis* 28 (8): 1765–73.

Sarika, P.R. and James, N.R. 2015. Preparation and characterisation of gelatin-gum arabic aldehyde nanogels via inverse miniemulsion technique. *Int J Biol Macromol* 76: 181–7.

Sarika, P.R., James, N.R., Kumar, P.R., Raj, D.K., and Kumary, T.V. 2015a. Gum arabic-curcumin conjugate micelles with enhanced loading for curcumin delivery to hepatocarcinoma cells. *Carbohydr Polym* 134: 167–74.

Sarika, P.R., James, N.R., Nishna, N., Anil Kumar, P.R., and Raj, D.K. 2015b. Galactosylated pullulan-curcumin conjugate micelles for site specific anticancer activity to hepatocarcinoma cells. *Colloids Surf B Biointerfaces* 133: 347–55.

Sarika, P.R. and Nirmala, R.J. 2016. Curcumin loaded gum arabic aldehyde-gelatin nanogels for breast cancer therapy. *Mater Sci Eng C Mater Biol Appl* 65: 331–7.

Sasaki, H., Sunagawa, Y., Takahashi, K., Imaizumi, A., Fukuda, H., Hashimoto, T. et al. 2011. Innovative preparation of curcumin for improved oral bioavailability. *Biol Pharm Bull* 34 (5): 660–5.

Sathuvan, M., Thangam, R., Gajendiran, M., Vivek, R., Balasubramanian, S., Nagaraj, S. et al. 2017. κ-Carrageenan: An effective drug carrier to deliver curcumin in cancer cells and to induce apoptosis. *Carbohydr Polym* 160: 184–93.

Sattarahmady, N., Moosavi-Movahedi, A.A., Bazzi P., Heli, H., and Pourtakdoust, S. 2016. Improving pharmaceutical characteristics of curcumin by alginate/pectin microparticles. *Pharm Chem J* 50 (3): 131–6.

Schiborr, C., Kocher, A., Behnam, D., Jandasek, J., Toelstede, S., and Frank, J. 2014. The oral bioavailability of curcumin from micronized powder and liquid micelles is significantly increased in healthy humans and differs between sexes. *Mol Nutr Food Res* 58 (3): 516–27.

Shahgholian, N. and Rajabzadeh, G. 2016. Fabrication and characterization of curcumin-loaded albumin/gum arabic coacervate. *Food Hydrocoll* 59: 17–25.

Sharma, R.A., McLelland, H.R., Hill, K.A., Ireson, C.R., Euden, S.A., Manson, M.M. et al. 2001. Pharmacodynamic and pharmacokinetic study of oral curcuma extract in patients with colorectal cancer. *Clin Cancer Res* 7 (7): 1894–900.

Sheikhzadeh, S., Alizadeh, M., Rezazad, M., and Hamishehkar, H. 2016. Application of response surface methodology and spectroscopic approach for investigating of curcumin nanoencapsulation using natural biopolymers and nonionic surfactant. *J Food Sci Technol* 53 (11): 3904–15.

Shingel, K.I. 2004. Current knowledge on biosynthesis, biological activity, and chemical modification of the exopolysaccharide, pullulan. *Carbohydr Res* 339 (3): 447–60.

Shoba, G., Joy, D., Joseph, T., Majeed, M., Rajendran, R., and Srinivas, P.S. 1998. Influence of piperine on the pharmacokinetics of curcumin in animals and human volunteers. *Planta Med* 64 (04): 353–6.

Singh, R.S., Kaur, N., and Kennedy, J.F. 2015a. Pullulan and pullulan derivatives as promising biomolecules for drug and gene targeting. *Carbohydr Polym* 123: 190–207.

Singh, S.P., Sharma, M., and Gupta, P.K. 2015b. Cytotoxicity of curcumin silica nanoparticle complexes conjugated with hyaluronic acid on colon cancer cells. *Int J Biol Macromol* 74: 162–70.

Sinha, V.R. and Kumria, R. 2001. Polysaccharides in colon-specific drug delivery. *Int J Pharm* 224 (1–2): 19–38.

Smith, Ray. 2005. *Biodegradable Polymers for Industrial Applications*. CRC Press.

Sriamornsak, P. 2011. Application of pectin in oral drug delivery. *Expert Opin Drug Deliv* 8 (8): 1009–23.

Storka, A., Vcelar, B., Klickovic, U., Gouya, G., Weisshaar, S., and Aschauer, S. et al. 2015. Safety, tolerability and pharmacokinetics of liposomal curcumin (Lipocurc™) in healthy humans. *Int J Clin Pharmacol Ther* 53: 54–65.

Sun, Y., Du, L., Liu, Y., Li, X., Li, M., Jin, Y., and Qian, X. 2014. Transdermal delivery of the in situ hydrogels of curcumin and its inclusion complexes of hydroxypropyl-β-cyclodextrin for melanoma treatment. *Int J Pharm* 469 (1): 31–9.

Tang, B., Ma, L., Wang, H.Y., and Zhang, G.Y. 2002. Study on the supramolecular interaction of curcumin and β-cyclodextrin by spectrophotometry and its analytical application. *J Agric Food Chem* 50 (6): 1355–61.

Tomren, M.A., Másson, M., Loftsson, T., and Tønnesen, H.H. 2007. Studies on curcumin and curcuminoids: XXXI. Symmetric and asymmetric curcuminoids: Stability, activity and complexation with cyclodextrin. *Int J Pharm* 338 (1–2): 27–34.

Tønnesen, H.H., Másson, M., and Loftsson, T. 2002. Studies of curcumin and curcuminoids. XXVII. Cyclodextrin complexation: solubility, chemical and photochemical stability. *Int J Pharm* 244 (1): 127–35.

Vareed, S.K., Kakarala, M., Ruffin, M.T., Crowell, J.A., Normolle, D.P., Djuric, Z. et al. 2008. Pharmacokinetics of curcumin conjugate metabolites in healthy human subjects. *Cancer Epidemiol Biomarkers Prev* 17 (6): 1411–7.

Vasireddy, V., Chavali, V.R., Joseph, V.T., Kadam, R., Lin, J.H., Jamison, J.A. et al. 2011. Rescue of photoreceptor degeneration by curcumin in transgenic rats with P23H rhodopsin mutation. *PLoS One* 6 (6): e21193.

Weinbreck, F., de Vries, R., Schrooyen, P., and de Kruif, C.G. 2003. Complex coacervation of whey proteins and gum arabic. *Biomacromolecules* 4 (2): 293–303.

Whistler, Roy. 2012. *Industrial Gums: Polysaccharides and Their Derivatives*. Elsevier.

Won, C.Y., Chu, C.C., and Yu, T.J. 1997. Synthesis of starch-based drug carrier for the control/release of estrone hormone. *Carbohydr Polym* 32 (3–4): 239–44.

Wu, F., Zhou, Z., Su, J., Wei, L., Yuan, W., and Jin, T. 2013. Development of dextran nanoparticles for stabilizing delicate proteins. *Nanoscale Res Lett* 8 (1): 197.

Wu, M.H., Yan, H.H., Chen, Z.Q., and He, M. 2017. Effects of emulsifier type and environmental stress on the stability of curcumin emulsion. *J Dispers Sci Technol* 38 (10): 1375–80.

Wu, Y. and Wang. 2017. Binding, stability, and antioxidant activity of curcumin with self-assembled casein-dextran conjugate micelles. *Int J Food Prop* 20: 1–13.

Xu, W., Jin, W., Zhang, C., Li, Z., Lin, L., and Huang, Q. 2014. Curcumin loaded and protective system based on complex of κ-carrageenan and lysozyme. *Food Res Int* 59: 61–6.

Yamaoka, T., Tabata, Y., and Ikada, Y. 1993. Body distribution profile of polysaccharides after intravenous administration. *Drug Deliv* 1 (1): 75–82.

Yang, J., Huang, Y., Gao, C., Liu, M., and Zhang, X. 2014. Fabrication and evaluation of the novel reduction-sensitive starch nanoparticles for controlled drug release. *Colloids Surf B Biointerfaces* 115: 368–76.

Yang, M., Wu, Y., Li, J., Zhou, H., and Wang, X. 2013. Binding of curcumin with bovine serum albumin in the presence of ι-carrageenan and implications on the stability and antioxidant activity of curcumin. *J Agric Food Chem* 61 (29): 7150–5.

Yang, R., Zhang, S., Kong, D., Gao, X., Zhao, Y., and Wang, Z. 2012. Biodegradable polymer-curcumin conjugate micelles enhance the loading and delivery of low-potency curcumin. *Pharm Res* 29 (12): 3512–25.

Yu, H. and Huang, Q. 2010. Enhanced in vitro anti-cancer activity of curcumin encapsulated in hydrophobically modified starch. *Food Chem* 119 (2): 669–74.

Zhang, L., Pan, J., Dong, S., and Li, Z. 2017. The application of polysaccharide-based nanogels in peptides/proteins and anticancer drugs delivery. *J Drug Targe* 25 (8): 673–84.

Zhao, L., Liu, M., Wang, J., and Zhai, G. 2015. Chondroitin sulfate-based nanocarriers for drug/gene delivery. *Carbohydr Polym* 133: 391–9.

Zheng, Y., Chen, Y., Jin, L.W., Ye, H.Y., and Liu, G. 2016. Cytotoxicity and genotoxicity in human embryonic kidney cells exposed to surface modify chitosan nanoparticles loaded with curcumin. *AAPS PharmSciTech* 17 (6): 1347–52.

12 Polysaccharide-Based Nanocarriers for Drug Delivery into and through the Skin

Hemant Ramchandra Badwaik

CONTENTS

12.1 INTRODUCTION

The field of nanomedicine has emerged as a promising platform for the development of novel drug delivery systems that delivers the therapeutic molecules in a sustained and controlled manner at a targeted site (Giri et al. 2016; Giri et al. 2017). Nanotechnology has progressed in the pharmaceutical field owing to its capability to resolve solubility, stability, absorption, permeation, and toxicity related issues (Bawarski et al.2008; Bibi et al. 2017). Nanotechnology comprises of distinct materials of varying shapes and sizes. For the fabrication of drug delivery carriers, availability, safety, and toxicity issues must be considered seriously. The polysaccharides play a very significant role in overcoming these hurdles (Giri et el. 2015; Giri et el. 2013). Thus, the remarkable features of polysaccharides offer enormous potential for their applicability in the designing of drug delivery systems (Martínez et al. 2012). Recently, polysaccharide-based nanostructural systems have emerged as attractive vehicles for delivering the drug into the skin (local action) and through the skin (systemic action). This chapter explores the mechanism of the fabrication of polysaccharide-based nanocarriers and their application as potential drug delivery vehicles for local and systemic action.

12.2 HUMAN SKIN

In an adult human body, skin is considered to be the largest organ, constituting about 10% of total body weight, and extending approximately over a 2 m^2 surface area (Prausnitz et al. 2012; Prow et al. 2011). Among the numerous roles of human skin, its most crucial activity is to provide defensive protection against the invasive organisms from the environment. The skin has developed various defense systems which provides it with numerous barrier mechanisms such as physical, metabolic, immunological, and UV-protective barriers to permit inhibition against microbial attack, UV radiation, toxic and harmful chemicals, and particulate materials occurring in the environment (e.g. nanoparticles, etc.) (Roberts and Walters 2008). Apart from that, skin also acts as a port of entry for drugs, vaccines, and other therapeutic substances.

12.2.1 Structure of Human Skin

Skin comprises of two major layers, dermis and epidermis. The dermis layer of skin consists of numerous types of cells, blood vessels, nervous tissues, and lymphatic vessels embedded within its connective tissue network. The epidermal layer comprises mainly of stratified keratinocytes, in which the stratum corneum (SC) cells or corneocytes remains immersed in a proteinaceous covering, with an outer lipid covering, encompassed by an extracellular lipid matrix. Dermis and epidermis are separated by a layer called the basal membrane. The keratinocytes are interspersed with viable epidermis cells which play a role in the production of melanin (melanocytes), cells for sensory perception (Merkel cells), and immunological function cells (Langerhans cells and others). Varying appendages such as the pilosebaceous units (hair follicles and their associated sebaceous glands), apocrine, and eccrine sweat glands also form part of the epidermal layer of skin (Desmond 2006). An illustration of human skin comprising of the major structural parts with varying cell types is depicted in Figure 12.1.

12.2.2 The Barrier of the Stratum Corneum

The layer of SC forms the chief physical barricade of the skin which limits the permeation of a drug or any other foreign molecules across the skin (Desmond 2006). This layer also serves as a major barrier for water diffusion into the skin and vice versa (Elias and Friend 1975). The corneocytes of SC are flattened, anuclear, protein rich, and profoundly packed within the matrix of extracellular

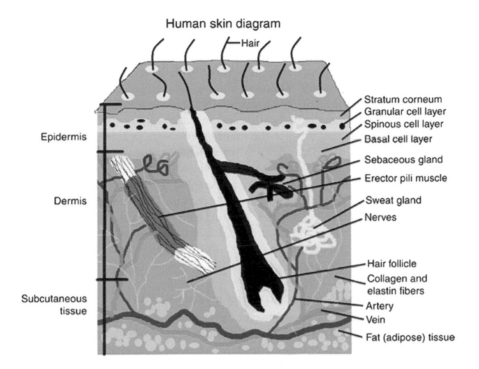

FIGURE 12.1 Anatomy of human skin comprising of three main layers: epidermis, dermis, and hypodermis. (Reprinted from Bibi, N., Ahmed, N., and Khan, G.M. *Nanostructure for drug delivery*, 639–68, Copyright 2017, with permission from Elsevier.)

lipid in a bilayer arrangement (Elias and Menon 1991). This arrangement is commonly known as a "bricks and mortar" arrangement (Michaels et al. 1975). The drug and other substances permeate the SC mainly via passive diffusion, and this is known to be carried out via three major routes, i.e. intercellular, transcellular, and appendageal routes.

12.2.2.1 Skin Turnover as a Moving Barrier

The stratum dysjunctum (the outermost layer of the SC), is prone to desquamation, which allows the SC to be turned over completely in approximately 14 days in human beings, governed by age and anatomical region (Reddy et al. 2000). Thus, Stratum dysjunctum cells can be observed as a dynamic and continually renewable barrier which provides an integral system that prevents any foreign molecules from skin penetration (Marks 2004). The constant migration of corneocytes followed by sloughing from the upper surface of the skin assists in the removal of pathogenic microorganisms, malignant cells, and any other particles from external environment.

12.2.2.2 Intercellular Spacing

The intercellular route is favored for most penetrants, while trying to move across the skin. Several small molecules are free to move about in the intercellular spaces while their diffusion rates are mainly dependent on their lipophilicity. The rate of the diffusion of drugs across the skin is governed by numerous physicochemical parameters including their solubility, molecular weight or volume, and their ability to form hydrogen bonding (Potts et al. 1995). The macromolecules or other larger particles, however, cannot move freely owing to the physical restriction provided by the lipid channels (Merwe et al. 2006; Baroli et al. 2007). Thus, it is suggested that the SC creates an additional barrier for such kind of molecules, but not for tiny particles.

12.2.2.3 Routes of Transportation for Exogenous Substances Across the Stratum Corneum

Initially, polar and non-polar solutes were assumed to be permeated via the SC through different routes – the polar solutes passes via transcellular route while lipophilic solutes travel through the intercellular lipids (Scheuplein 1965). However, continuous segregation between hydrophilic and lipophilic compartments in the SC is not always feasible, making this pathway almost implausible in several instances. The present theory is also encouraged by various theoretical and histochemical evidences which suggest that most of the solutes diffuse via intercellular lipids (Albery and Hadgraft 1979; Grice et al. 2010). Drug delivery through the appendageal route is considered to be more effective alternative to the SC route, regardless of the scarcity of these attributes on the surface of the skin (Roberts and Walters 1989). It is the tendency of the hair follicles to extend to deeper layers of the skin. There is a progressive decline in the thickness of the SC layer as it extends to the deeper layers. A network of blood capillaries is available to promote transportation of solutes that diffuses out of the follicle. The possibilities are that drug partitioning into sebum as well as targeted delivery to follicles with novel approaches including drug-loaded nanoparticles can prove to be quite effective routes of drug delivery (Lademann et al. 2007).

12.2.2.4 Acid Mantle Maintains the Stratum Corneum Barrier

The pH of the skin surface is acidic and ranges between 4.2 and 5.6 in human beings (Schmid-Wendtner and Korting 2006). This surface of the skin can be also referred to as the acid mantle. Various factors governing the pH of the skin surface include the anatomical site and sex, hydration, sweat, and sebum (Hanson et al. 2002; Krien and Kermici 2000). The pH gradient across the SC layer is quite sharp; while the upper viable layers of the stratum granulosum are of a neutral pH. By utilizing two-photon fluorescence lifetime imaging of a pH-sensitive fluorophore that was applied over the SC layer of hairless mice, acidic micro domains were detected in the extracellular matrix, which continued to become less persistent on moving from the surface toward the viable epidermis (Hanson et al. 2002). Texier et al. 1996 proposed that this results in the pH gradient, notwithstanding the fact that specific biochemical mechanisms have been suggested that lead to acidification, such as the production of transurocanic acid by histidase-catalyzed degradation of histidine. The acid mantle possesses numerous associated applications, including defense against microorganisms, the maintenance of optimal integrity, and cohesion of corneocyte, modulated by pH-sensitive proteolysis enzymes, the preservation of the permeability barrier by exerting effects on organization and processing of extracellular lipids and also restricts inflammatory response by the inhibition of pro-inflammatory cytokines release (Janssens et al. 1996; Genotelle et al. 2004; Li et al. 2005; Tereno et al. 2008).

A noticeable relevance is observed between the increased pH of the skin and diseases like atopic dermatitis, with remarkable pH differences between the skin of affected and unaffected patients (Seidenari and Giusti 1995). The acidic environment of the skin surface may also assist the skin's barricade against penetration of nanoparticles owing to the diminishing electrostatic forces at the lowered pH of the solution (Murphy et al. 2010). Aggregated particles are very unlikely to penetrate via the SC layer; while, the embedded particles would not be easily sloughed off during desquamation upon proper maintenance of the integrity and cohesive strength of the SC layer. Moreover, in the case of metal nanoparticles, such as zinc oxide nanoparticles, the acidic pH might influence the aggregation and dissolution kinetics of nanoparticles, thereby restricting their applicability on skin penetration experiments (Tso et al. 2010).

12.2.2.5 Viable Epidermis

12.2.2.5.1 Tight Junctions

The stratum granulosum shows the existence of functional tight junctions (Langbein et al. 2002). These tight junctions are considered to be vital elements of the epidermal barriers. The expression and localization of tight junction proteins are altered in diseased conditions leading to a damaged skin barrier, such as in case of psoriasis (Kirschner et al. 2009; Watson et al. 2007).

12.2.2.5.2 Skin Deactivation of Nanoparticles

Due to their versatile functions, the skin may also act as a chemical or metabolic barrier, where enzymes are present in the basal layer of the viable epidermis, the extracellular region of the SC layer, and also the appendages in the dermal layer (Guy et al. 1987; Oesch et al. 2007). The nanoparticles are biodegraded through various processes such as hydrolysis and enzymatic degradation, while physical forces cause the merging of liposomes with the intercellular lipids (Bouwstra and Honeywell-Nguyen 2002). Zinc oxide nanoparticles get hydrolyzed at a neutral pH and to a greater extent at an acidic pH, converting them to zinc ions, which get accelerated upon light exposure (Tso et al 2010; Domenech and Costa 1986). The process of hydrolysis, however, can be complex and governed by the variation in the local environment. Cross et al. 2007, demonstrated that any significant difference was not observed in the extent of zinc ions passing via human epidermal layer from zinc oxide nanoparticles in comparison to controls (Cross et al. 2007). As discussed above, the nanoparticles undergo a phenomenon equivalent to first pass metabolism, which results from the enzymatic as well as physical and chemical destruction of nanoparticles. In a similar manner the skin metabolism is utilized for the development of prodrug or soft-drug delivery strategies, the nanoparticles can also be employed in a novel drug delivery approach (Gysler et al. 1999).

12.2.3 SKIN PENETRATION OF NANOPARTICLES

Numerous researchers have elucidated the fact that skin penetration of drugs is governed by the physicochemical attributes of nanoparticles including particle size, solubility, surface area, surface charge, influence of solvents, chemical composition, and salt form of the drug (Liang et al. 2013; Labouta et al. 2011; Agharkar et al. 1976; Berge et al. 1977). Amongst these aspects, the most widely explored features are the size and charge of the nanoparticles.

Particle size is the most crucial factor which governs the penetration of molecules across the skin. Varying size nanoparticles comprising of divergent materials with different surface properties when analyzed exhibited that the smaller sized nanoparticles undergo skin penetration to a greater extent than compared to the larger ones. Additionally, hair follicles are regarded as a vital shunt route for the entry of nanoparticles. The nanoparticles of 300–600 nm size range display extensive penetration into hair follicles in which they are stored for a longer duration than in the SC layer (Patzelt 2011; Lademann et al 2011). The penetration of drug moieties across the skin is also affected by the surface charge of the nanoparticles. While several experiments demonstrate the elevated skin penetration ability of the positively charged nanoemulsions, other researches revealed that greater skin penetration is achieved by negatively charged nanoformulations. The positively charged nanoemulsions displayed greater potential in enhancing the bioavailability of drugs owing to the higher binding affinity of these tiny droplets to skin. The negative charge on the surface of the skin is attributable to the presence of epithelial cells on the surface of the skin and also due to the protein residues that resides on the outer cell membrane in the skin and other tissues (Rojanasakul et al. 1992; Piemi et al. 1999; Yilmaz et al. 2005). As indicated by Jung et al. (2006), cationic liposomes tend to penetrate into the hair follicles to a deeper extent as compared to the anionic liposomes. In contrast, Gillet et al. (2011) outlined an increased permeation of negatively charged liposomes of betamethasone and betamethasone dipropionate into the skin. The salt form of the drug plays a very crucial role in enhancing percutaneous absorption where the physicochemical parameters of the parent drug are inappropriate.

12.3 POLYSACCHARIDES

Polysaccharides are natural, hydrophilic, biodegradable polymers and they possess unique characteristics such as they are safe, highly stable, and non-toxic in nature (D'Ayala et al. 2008).

Polysaccharides are ubiquitous in nature; hence these are cheap and their processing is also cost effective (Badwaik et al. 2016a; Badwaik et al. 2013). Natural polysaccharides may be of plant (gum arabic and guar gum), animal (chondroitin and chitosan), microbial (dextran, gellan gum pullulan gum and xanthan gum), and algal (fucoidan and alginate) origin (Badwaik et al. 2017, Giri et al. 2012a, Giri et al. 2012b, Hovgaard et al. 1996). Polysaccharides are universally present in several plant parts such as the seeds, leaves and stems, animal body fluids, shells of various insects, and crustaceans (Singh et al. 2012). They are also extensively present in the extracellular fluids and cell walls of numerous microorganisms such as bacteria, yeast, and fungi, and thus act as renewable reservoirs for the synthesis of high yielded materials (Davidson 1980; Bemiller and Whistler 1992). The heterogeneity observed in the nature, chemical composition, and structural framework of polysaccharides might be attributable to the presence of various reactive functional groups on their backbone. The existence of numerous functional moieties on their molecular chain makes it possible for the easy modification of polysaccharides by various chemical and biochemical means (Prabaharan and Jayakumar 2009; Prabaharan 2008). Most of the polysaccharides possess characteristic bioadhesive features owing to the existence of hydrophilic functional moieties including amino, carboxyl, and hydroxyl groups. The bioadhesive nature of polysaccharides might be attributable to the non-covalent bond formation between the hydrophilic functional moieties of polysaccharides and epithelial and mucous membranes of various living tissues (Lee et al. 2000). Due to their ubiquitous nature, low price, wide regulatory acceptance, and the versatility in their modification ability of drug release profile, polysaccharides has gained increasing attention by researchers in designing controlled and sustained drug delivery systems (Prabaharan 2011; Rubinstein 2000; Badwaik et al 2014; Badwaik et al. 2016b; Vandamme et al. 2002; Lemarchand et al. 2014). Recently, several investigations were carried out to explore the application of polysaccharides and their modified derivatives for fabricating nanoparticulate drug formulations (Liu et al. 2008).

12.4 POLYSACCHARIDE-BASED NANOPARTICLES

In order to prepare polysaccharide-based nanoparticles, four different mechanisms are involved. In the year 2008, Liu et al. presented an outstanding review, which explored the techniques for the fabrication of polysaccharide-based nanoparticles and their utility in drug delivery. In this chapter we have categorized the method of preparation for polysaccharide nanoparticles on the basis of physical and chemical means. Various approaches for the preparation of polysaccharide nanoparticles are depicted in Figure 12.2.

12.4.1 CHEMICAL METHODS

In order to prepare polysaccharide nanoparticles with the desired and modified mechanical properties, the chemical crosslinking method is highly adaptable one. Owing to the existence of varying functional moieties (e.g. -OH, -NH$_2$, -COOH) in polysaccharides, it reacts with

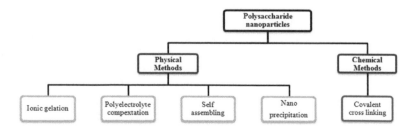

FIGURE 12.2   Synthetic approaches for the fabrication of polysaccharide-based nanoparticles.

the complementary groups of chemical crosslinking agent to form the chemical bond (Verma et al. 2017). Among several chemical crosslinking agents, glutaraldehyde is quite frequently employed for chemical crosslinking of polysaccharide nanoparticles (Sarmah et al. 2014; Liu et al. 2007). However, the toxic nature of glutaraldehyde restricts its widespread use; while promoting the utilization of alternative biocompatible covalent crosslinkers like succinic acid, citric acid, tartaric acid, and maleic acid in the formulation of polysaccharide nanoparticles (Bodnar et al. 2005a; Bodnar et al. 2005b). During the synthesis of nanoparticles by chemical means, the utilization of toxic crosslinkers or the presence of reactants as by-products in the finally yielded nanoparticles cannot be totally circumvented. From the biomedical point of view, the toxicity may render the nanoparticles non-biocompatible in case of short-term and long-term use. In order to outwit this inadequacy, physical crosslinking methods can be employed.

12.4.2 Physical Methods

The formulation of polysaccharide nanoparticles by physically crosslinked methods includes ionotropic gelation, self-assembling, polyelectrolyte complexation, and nanoprecipitation techniques.

12.4.2.1 Ionic Gelation

Ionic gelation, formerly designated as "ion-induced gelation", is employed for preparing nanoparticles by implementing chemical crosslinking of low-molecular-weight polyanionic polysaccharides with polycationic counterparts and vice versa. The most widely investigated anionic and cationic crosslinker for preparing polysaccharide nanoparticles is sodium tripolyphosphate (TPP) and calcium, respectively.

12.4.2.2 Polyelectrolyte Complexation

The basic mechanism for the preparation of polysaccharide-based nanoparticles by polyelectrolyte complexation involves intermolecular electrostatic interactions between two oppositely charged polyelectrolytes.

12.4.2.3 Self-Assembly

Self-assembly is a phenomenon where the molecules undergo disorder-to-order transition spontaneously with the aid of non-covalent interactions, including the hydrogen bonding, hydrophobic interactions and van der Waals forces (Myrick et al. 2014). Polysaccharide nanoparticles by self-assembly can be formulated via electrostatic interaction of oppositely charged ionic polysaccharides (Liu et al.2012). Ionic complexes present a very attractive strategy owing to their simplicity and due to the fact that their self-assembly is responsive to various stimuli including pH and ionic strength.

12.4.2.4 Nanoprecipitation

Another technique for fabricating polysaccharide-based nanoparticles is by employing the nanoprecipitation technique. Nanoparticles are fabricated by blending the polymer solution with an appropriate non-solvent system. The rapid diffusion of the polymer solution in the non-solvent system might result into the rapid generation of polysaccharide nanocarrier system (Martínez et al. 2012).

Apart from these techniques for fabricating polysaccharide-based nanoparticles, polysaccharides are also employed for preparing metal nanoparticles by green synthetic methods. On account of their low cost, extensive availability, negligible side effects, and enhanced efficiency, polysaccharides are nowadays preferred over chemical reducing agents for the synthesis of nanoparticles (Banerjee et al. 2017).

Various techniques for the fabrication of polysaccharide nanoparticles are depicted in Table 12.1.

TABLE 12.1

Various Techniques for the Synthesis of Polysaccharide-Based Nanoparticles

Sl. No.	Mechanism of NPs Formation	Polysaccharides	Size of NPs in nm	Reference
1	Ionic crosslinking	Alginate	236	Ahmed et al. 2016
2	Ionic crosslinking	Alginate	564	Reis et al. 2008
3	Ionic crosslinking	Alginate	80	You and Peng 2004
4	Ionic crosslinking	Alginate-chitosan	1280	Reis et al. 2007
5	Ionic crosslinking	Alginate-chitosan	196–430	Azizi et al. 2010
6	Ionic crosslinking	Alginate-dextran	267–2760	Reis et al. 2007
7	Ionic crosslinking	Chitosan	250–400	Pan et al. 2002
8	Ionic crosslinking	Chitosan	301–424	Cetin et al. 2007
9	Ionic crosslinking	Chitosan	75	Lu et al. 2006
10	Ionic crosslinking	Chitosan	200–700	Katas and Alpar 2006
11	Ionic crosslinking	Chitosan	30–150	Zhi et al. 2005
12	Ionic crosslinking	Chitosan	250–400	de la Fuente et al. 2010
13	Ionic crosslinking	N-(2-hydroxyl) propyl-3-trimethyl ammonium chitosan chloride	110–180	Xu et al. 2003
14	Ionic crosslinking	Deacetylated Chitosan	90–200	Zhang et al. 2004
15	Covalent crosslinking	Alginate-albumin	42–388	Martínez et al. 2011
16	Covalent crosslinking	Guar gum	200–300	Sarmah et al. 2014
17	Polyelectrolyte complexation	Alginate-poly-L-lysine	28–100	Gonzalez Ferreiro et al. 2002
18	Polyelectrolyte complexation	Chitosan-alginate	423–580	Sarmento et al. 2006
19	Polyelectrolyte complexation	Chitosan-alginate	323–1600	Douglas and Tabrizian 2005
20	Polyelectrolyte complexation	Chitosan-carboxymethyl gum kondagogu	285.9	Kumar, and Ahuja 2013
21	Polyelectrolyte complexation	Chitosan-dextran	423–580	Sarmento et al. 2006
22	Polyelectrolyte complexation	Chitosan-gum ghatti	126.6	Shelly et al. 2013
23	Polyelectrolyte complexation	Chitosan-dextran sulfate	600–800	Tiyaboonchai and Limpeanchob 2007
24	Polyelectrolyte complexation	Chitosan-glucomannan	200–700	Alonso-Sande et al. 2006
25	Self-assembling	β-cyclodextrin	50	Jones et al.2009
26	Self-assembling	Chitosan-cholesterol	417	Wang et al.2007
27	Self-assembling	Chitosan-PEG	262	Yang et al. 2008; Yoksan et al 2004
28	Self-assembling	Chitosan-stearic acid	28–175	Hu et al. 2006
29	Self-assembling	Pullulan-cholesterol	20–30	Akiyoshi et al. 1998
30	Nanoprecipitation	Guar gum	19–32	Soumya et al. 2010
31	Nanoprecipitation	Chitosan	700–1100	Berthold et al. 1996
32	Nanoprecipitation	β-cyclodextrin	90–150	Skiba et al. 1996
33	Nanoprecipitation	Acetylated cashew gum	179–302	Dias et al. 2016

12.5 APPLICATION OF POLYSACCHARIDE-BASED NANOCARRIERS FOR DELIVERING DRUGS INTO THE SKIN

Owing to its ease of accessibility, skin offers an excellent route for drug delivery in case of both local and systemic action (Williams 2003). Recently, the cosmetic industry is also focusing on the skin delivery of active compounds. However, the presence of barriers makes it quite difficult for the molecules to permeate across the skin. To overcome these hurdles, numerous nanocarriers are designed for modulating the barrier of skin and/or to provide a novel system for drug delivery. For optimizing the localized delivery of therapeutic moieties, topical administration of molecules has emerged as an interesting non-invasive technique, improving patient acceptability and pharmacokinetic profile of drugs which are easily prone to degradation, thereby minimizing several dose related side effects (De Louise 2012; Mathias and Hussain 2010; Bolzinger et al. 2012).

Over the past few years, polysaccharide-based nanocarriers have gained growing attention from the researchers of the skin administration of therapeutic compounds due to the sustained and controlled delivery of the active ingredients encapsulated within their polymeric matrix, which diffuses through them for permeation through the skin. The stable structures of these nanocarriers are attributable to their rigid matrix and the integrity of their structures is maintained over long periods of time upon topical administration (Lboutounne 2004).

12.5.1 CHITOSAN-BASED NANOCARRIERS FOR DRUG DELIVERY INTO THE SKIN

Among numerous natural polysaccharide nanoparticles, chitosan-based nanoparticles are most widely investigated for topical delivery to the skin. Chitosan, considered to be the N-deacetylated derivative of chitin, is a naturally abundant, biodegradable, polycationic linear polysaccharide which comprises mainly of glucosamine units (Giri et al. 2012a). It was been suggested that the anti-microbial, anti-inflammatory, and anti-oxidant properties of chitosan renders it a promising carrier for transporting therapeutic ingredients across the skin to treat dermatological disorders. In addition, the protonated amino groups of chitosan carry positive charges at physiological pH. The positive charge in solution promotes the crosslinking with poly anions to form nanoparticles, which encapsulates negatively charged drugs by electrostatic interaction, and also helps in the cellular internalization of drug-loaded chitosan nanoparticles. The biocompatible and low-toxic nature of this polymer accompanied by its excellent biopharmaceutical features makes it an interesting candidate for investigation by the researchers (Kim et al. 2006; Rangari and Ravikumar 2015). In an interesting research work, a nanoformulation of vitamin A derivative (i.e. retinol) was incorporated within chitosan-based nanoparticles. It is widely known that retinol and its other derivatives are widely employed in the pharmaceutical and cosmeceutical industry. The incorporation of retinol within chitosan nanoparticles reduces its irritability and toxic properties, and also enhances its solubility. These nanoparticles can be beneficially utilized for the treatment of acne and wrinkles (Kim et al. 2006). In another work by Şenyigit et al. (2010), chitosan-lecithin nanoparticles were incorporated within a chitosan gel formulation that delivered corticosteroid clobetasol-17-propionate to the epidermal and dermal layers of skin. Such formulations have potential for commercial purpose. Tan et al. (2011) reported the formulation of Quercetin incorporated lecithin-chitosan nanoparticles comprising of D-α-tocopheryl polyethylene glycol 1000 succinate (TPGS). The incorporation of TPGS within the nanocarrier system leads to an enhancement in the drug loading ability and entrapment efficiency of quercetin. It was observed that the quercetin-loaded nanoparticles lead to an elevation in the skin permeation of quercetin as compared to the quercetin propylene glycol solution, both in vitro and in vivo, and successfully helps in retaining quercetin in the epidermal region. The nanoparticle interaction with the surface of the skin alters the morphology of the SC layer and ruptures the firmly attached layers of corneocyte cells, resulting in the enhanced skin permeability of quercetin (Partha et al. 2010).The alteration in the surface of the skin with the aid of the nanoparticles might be due to their particular framework.

The presence of positively charged amino groups in chitosan warrant close association of nanoparticles with the skin. Chitosan hydrates the external environment of the skin, while the surface properties of TPGS also imparts outstanding wettability to the skin, thereby altering the barrier function of the skin and inhibiting its dehydration. Moreover, the permeation of the drug into the epidermis is facilitated with the increased hydration of the SC layer. Subsequent to the interaction of the nanoparticles with the skin, the lecithin present on the nanoparticle surface could integrate with the lipids present in the skin and disorganize the skin structure and lamellarity of the lipids in order to thicken the stratum corneum.

Partha et al. (2010) formulated and investigated ampicillin trihydrate-encapsulated chitosan nanoparticles via the modified ionotropic gelation technique. In the preparation of nanoparticles, chitosan was used as a polymer while sodium tripolyphosphate (TPP) acted as crosslinker. The formulated nanoparticles exhibited excellent stability and the drug was released in a sustained manner. Since chitosan itself acts as an antibacterial agent, the researcher reported the synergistic effect of ampicillin trihydrate in the chitosan nanoparticles. The encapsulation of amphotericin B (AmB) in the chitosan nanoparticles was reported by Sanchez et al. (2014). Chitosan nanoparticles can successfully deliver the incorporated drug moieties across the biological barriers of the skin. The investigators evaluated the potential of amphotericin B encapsulated in chitosan nanoparticles for cutaneous drug delivery in healing murine burn wound infection. The encapsulation of AmB within the nanoparticles can significantly reduce systemic side effects and promotes localized delivery of the drug. The efficacy of amphotericin B nanoparticles (AmB-np) was exhibited in vitro against yeast and fungal biofilm and moreover significantly minimized growth of fungus in vivo by the implication of a murine burn wound model. Polymeric nanoparticles were prepared by Hussain et al. (2013) for percutaneous delivery of hydrocortisone (HC)/hydroxytyrosol (HT) as depicted in Figure 12.3. The in vivo investigation revealed that co-loaded

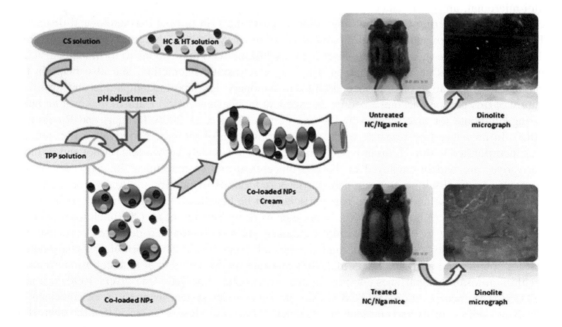

FIGURE 12.3 Schematic diagram illustrating the preparation and transdermal application of HC/HT co-loaded chitosan nanoparticles. (Reprinted from *Int J Pharm* 444, Hussain, Z., Katas, H., Amin, M., Kumolosasi, E., Buang, F., and Sahudin, S. Self-assembled polymeric nanoparticles for percutaneous co-delivery of hydrocortisone/hydroxytyrosol: An ex vivo and in vivo study using an NC/Nga mouse model, 109–19, Copyright 2013, with permission from Elsevier.)

chitosan NPs could effectively prevent transepidermal water loss, dermatitis index and intensity of erythema. This percutaneous co-delivery system has emerged as a favorable candidate for the transport of anti-oxidative and anti-inflammatory drugs for the therapeutic efficacy against atopic dermatitis (AD).

Shah et al. (2012) investigated bilayered nanoparticles by implementing poly-(lactide-co-glycolic acid) and chitosan for simultaneous administration of two anti-inflammatory drugs spantide II (SP) and ketoprofen (KP) by topical route. By altering the surface properties of the nanoparticles with oleic acid, skin penetration of nanoparticles encapsulated with fluorescent dye was enhanced by the translocation of nanoparticles deep into the skin with elevated intensities. From this research work, it was concluded that in vitro analysis of this nano gel system for human skin permeation showed efficient enhancement in permeation of ketoprofen and spantide II in both the epidermal and dermal region in comparison to the control groups (Shah et al. 2012). Such types of strategies could also be initiated for the treatment of several other skin infections such as bacterial, viral, fungal infections, and also skin carcinomas like melanoma.

12.5.2 ETHYL CELLULOSE-BASED NANOCARRIERS FOR DRUG DELIVERY INTO THE SKIN

Santhi et al. (2005) developed betamethasone-loaded nanospheres incorporated in a novel topical cream base. Ethyl cellulose was employed to formulate the nanospheres by a process of modified desolvation and crosslinking technique. Betamethasone nanosphere-loaded topical cream serves as a potential carrier for controlling and sustaining the release of the drug in cases of dermal delivery. Abdel-Mottaleb et al. (2012) formulated ethyl cellulose nanospheres by a modified desolvation technique followed by crosslinking. Betamethazone (a model drug) was encapsulated within nanospheres for targeted skin delivery of corticosteroids. The comparison of an in vitro diffusion study of formulated cream with that of the commercial cream exhibited significant decline in release rate of drug from nanospheres based cream. This formulation serves as an efficient delivery vehicle for controlling the release of the drugs in the case of dermal application. The authors came to the conclusion that the minute nanoparticles possessed three times deeper and stronger penetration ability, where drug is accumulated preferably in the inflamed hair follicles of the skin and sebaceous glands. The current strategy holds great promise for selectively delivering the drugs to the inflamed region of the skin by enhancing the availability in local intradermal region with reduced systemic adverse effects (Abdel-Mottaleb et al. 2012).

12.6 APPLICATION OF POLYSACCHARIDE-BASED NANOCARRIERS FOR DRUG DELIVERY THROUGH THE SKIN

Conventionally, the skin route was employed for local delivery of the drug, but since 1970 this route was widely explored for systemic drug delivery. Transdermal drug delivery systems (TDDS), also referred to as transdermal therapeutic systems are topical delivery carriers which provide systemic action of drugs via the skin (Paudel et al. 2010). Over several decades, TDDS has attracted researchers from the pharmaceutical field as one of the popular routes for systemic drug delivery (Zhao et al. 2014). TDDS is a non-invasive method of delivery of medications to bypass first pass metabolism where the plasma drug levels are maintained within the therapeutic window for a prolonged period of time (Yang et al. 2015). TDDSs represent an excellent alternative method when the oral route for drug administration is not practically possible or might lead to unpredictable bioavailability (Delgado-Charro and Guy 2014). By attaining these objectives, variability in drug responses could be lowered which may result in improved patient compliance (Wiedersberg and Guy 2014; Prausnitz et al. 2004). However, the impermeable layer of the skin comprising of epithelial tissue provides the main barricade for delivering drugs across the transdermal route. Chitosan is widely employed in transdermal systems owing to its appreciable features such as biodegradability, bioadhesion, permeability-increasing ability, and favorable physicochemical properties across the impermeable epithelial layer of the skin.

To attain therapeutic action of drugs via skin delivery, following consecutive steps are involved (Khalil et al. 2012):

1. Drug diffusion from its dosage form
2. Drug permeation across the barrier of skin
3. Exhibition of the desired pharmacological response

In TDDS, the therapeutic drugs must penetrate across the viable epidermal layer to enter into blood circulation via capillaries located in the dermal region of the skin (Prow et al. 2011). Numerous approaches are undertaken for improving drug delivery via the skin route. Among them, polysaccharide-based nanocarrier systems are one of the most interesting vehicles (Javadzadeh and Behri 2017) The transdermal polysaccharide-based nanocarriers that have gained more attention by the researchers are nanoparticles and nanofibers.

12.6.1 Nanoparticle-Based Carriers for Transdermal Applications

12.6.1.1 Chitosan-Based Nanoparticles

Chitosan is a natural polycationic polysaccharide, and is widely employed in transdermal systems owing to its appreciable features such as biodegradability, bioadhesion, permeability-increasing ability, and favorable physicochemical features (Mei et al. 2008: Uchechi et al 2014).

Cui and Mumper 2001 utilized two polysaccharides, chitosan and depolymerized oligomer of chitosan with carboxymethylcellulose to formulate cationic nanoparticles with a higher stability. They evaluated an efficient strategy to genetic immunization by the topical administration of plasmid DNA (pDNA) loaded chitosan-based nanoparticles.

Lee et al. (2008) demonstrated the preparation of chitosan (CS) and poly-γ-glutamic acid (γ-PGA) containing biodegradable polymeric nanoparticles by the ionotropic gelation technique for delivery of DNA via transdermal route. The formulated CS/γ-PGAs/DNA nanoparticles (as depicted in Figure 12.4) were reactive to stimuli, e.g. changes in pH and the internal structure of nanoparticles were more compact having higher density as compared to the conventional CS/DNA domain. In comparison with the CS/DNA domain, the CS/γ-PGA/DNA nanoparticles exhibited enhanced skin penetration of mice and increased gene expression, which might be a better alternative to gold nanoparticles for transdermal gene delivery (Lee et al. 2008).

Hasanovica et al. (2009) synthesized acyclovir-loaded chitosan-TPP nanoparticles and reported that the incorporation of acyclovir within the nanoparticles led to notably enhanced drug stability, decline in photo degradation, and increased penetration of the drug via porcine skin. Sadhasivam et al. (2015) developed and investigated insulin-encapsulated chitosan nanoparticles for transdermal delivery. The ionotropic gelation method was utilized to prepare nanoparticles where TPP was used as ionic crosslinking agent. For the study, it was suggested that the size of the NPs ranges were 465–661 nm and were incorporated in patches that significantly released insulin via the transdermal route. Al-Kassas et al. (2016) formulated propranolol-loaded chitosan nanoparticles by the ionotropic gelation technique by employing tripolyphosphate (TPP) as a crosslinking agent and incorporated in gel for transdermal delivery. The formulated nanogel showed thixotropic behavior and released the drug for a longer duration as illustrated by in vitro drug permeation studies performed on the ear skin of a pig. From the analysis, it was reported that the chitosan nanoparticles were permeated through the pig ear skin and acted as drug reservoir to release propranolol for a longer duration to reduce blood pressure. Hence, the nanoparticles incorporated in the gel base might be a novel approach for the transdermal application of propranolol.

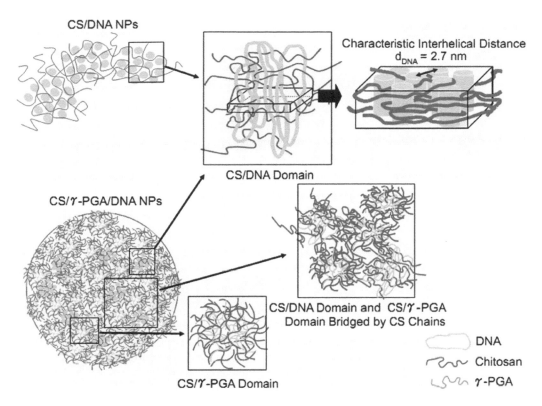

FIGURE 12.4 schematic representations of the internal structures of CS/DNA domain and CS/γ-PGA/ DNA. CS: chitosan; γ PGA: poly-γ-glutamic acid.(Reprinted from *Biomaterials* 29, Lee, P., Pen, S., Su, C., Mi, F., Chen, H., Wci, M., Lin, H., and Sung, H. The use of biodegradable polymeric nanoparticles in combination with a low pressure gene gun for transdermal DNA delivery, 742–51, Copyright 2013, with permission from Elsevier.)

12.6.1.2 Dextran and β-Cyclodextrin-Based Nanoparticles

Anirudhan et al. (2017) developed a novel solvent selective TDDS for simultaneously incorporating two drugs for the treatment of cancer as demonstrated in Figure 12.5. Dextran and β-cyclodextrin (β-CD) were implemented for preparing nanoparticles. The nanoparticles are loaded with two anti-cancer drugs, 5-flurouracil (5-FU) and curcumin (CUR), and the nanoparticle surfaces were coated with chitosan and alginate as illustrated in Figure 12.6. The surface charge on the nanoparticles assured satisfactory interaction among the NPs. The solvent selectivity of the drug carrier was exhibited by in vitro skin permeability studies on rat skin. By adjusting the copolymer composition, the sustainability of the drug release could be achieved. Moreover, biological evaluation performed on skin and melanoma cancer cell lines proposed the effectiveness of the formulated TDDS. It is also anticipated that this novel formulation can prove to be cost effective and patient compliant combination therapy for the targeting of CUR and 5-FU (Anirudhan et al. 2017).

12.6.1.3 Starch-Based Nanoparticles

Caffeine encapsulated nanoparticles prepared with starch derivatives were reported by Santander-Ortega et al. (2010). In vitro skin permeation studies performed by utilizing the skin of human beings showed that <0.2 mg/cm^2 of caffeine was permeated through the skin after 12 h in Franz diffusion cells. A novel polymer matrix nanocarrier system was synthesized by Saboktakin et al. (2014) containing carboxymethyl starch and 1,4-cis polybutadiene for transdermal delivery of clonidine.

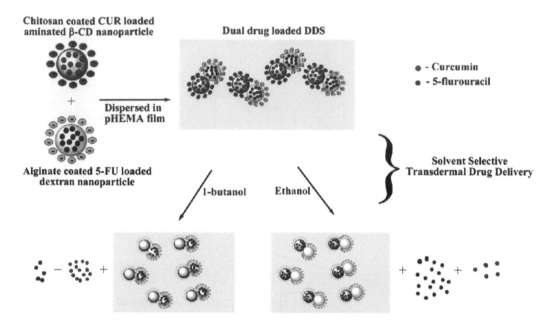

FIGURE 12.5 Schematic illustration of novel solvent selective TDDS formulation. (Reprinted from *Carbohydrate Polym* 173, Anirudhan, T.S., Nair, A.S., and Bino, S.J. Nanoparticle assisted solvent selective transdermal combination therapy of curcumin and 5-flurouracil for efficient cancer treatment, 131–42, Copyright 2017, with permission from Elsevier.)

12.6.1.4 Cashew Gum-Based Nanoparticles

Acetylated cashew gum nanoparticles were developed by Dias et al. (2016) by nanoprecipitation and dialysis techniques. Diclofenac diethyl amine was encapsulated as a model drug within the nanostructures and exhibited significant controlled drug delivery and promoted transdermal permeation in vitro. The excellent biocompatibility of NPs is indicated by the elevated cell viability rates, treated with blank and drug-loaded NPs. Therefore, it was noted that the acetylated cashew gum nanoparticles might prove to be quite effective drug delivery vehicle for anti-inflammatory drugs (Dias et al. 2016).

12.6.1.5 Hyaluronic Acid-Based Nanoparticles

A novel approach was initiated by Lim et al. (2012) for utilizing hydrogel nanoparticles for transdermal carriers. Figure 12.7 depicts a schematic illustration for this strategy based on hyaluronic acid (HA) for drug delivery by the transdermal route. Hyaluronic acid crosslinked with polyethylene glycol (PEG) was involved for the formulation of hydrogel nanoparticles of 37 nm size at dried condition. The investigators concluded that hydrogel nanoparticles based on HA might turn out to be a potential drug delivery carrier for transdermal delivery by carefully selecting the dispersing medium (Lim et al. 2012).

12.6.2 Nanofiber-Based Nanocarriers for Transdermal Applications

Electrospinning (ES) is a robust, unsophisticated, and effective technique for fabricating (bio) polymers constituting non-woven fibrillar structures and long-chain moieties which can be managed from micro to nanoscale size (Frenot and Chronakis 2003). Electrospinning allows the drugs to be directly encapsulated within the electrospun fibers (Zamani et al. 2013). Owing to the remarkable features of electrospun fibers such as high surface area, adjustable diameter, and surface properties, they are enormously explored in the arena of transdermal drug delivery (Kataria et al. 2014;

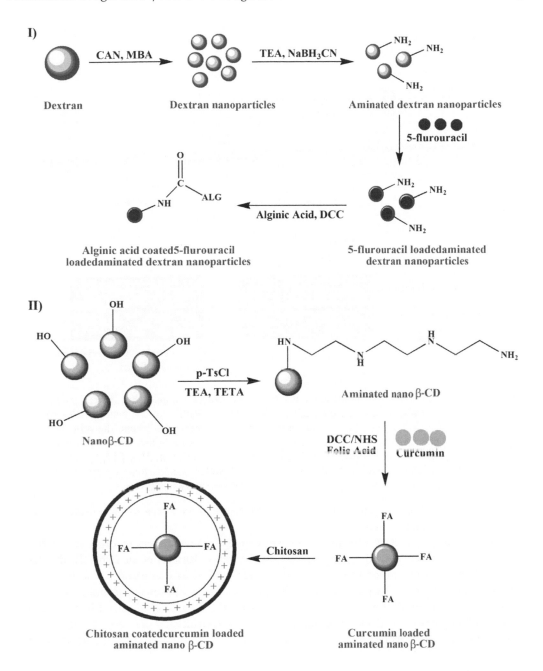

FIGURE 12.6 Schematic representation of formulation of dual drug-loaded nanoparticles.(Reprinted from *Carbohydrate Polym* 173, Anirudhan, T.S., Nair, A.S., and Bino, S.J. Nanoparticle assisted solvent selective transdermal combination therapy of curcumin and 5-flurouracil for efficient cancer treatment, 131–42, Copyright 2017, with permission from Elsevier.)

Madhaiyan et al. 2013; Rasekh et al. 2014; Taepaiboon et al. 2007). Ciprofloxacin-loaded electrospun nanofibers comprising of sodium alginate and poly(vinyl alcohol) were developed and evaluated as transdermal patches for the healing of wounds (Zamani et al. 2013). The time taken for wound healing by ciprofloxacin-loaded patches was comparatively less than the patches without drug. Indomethacin-loaded poly(vinylpyrolidone) electrospun nanofibers also finds potential application for adhesive patches and layering of the wound, without modifying their active mechanical

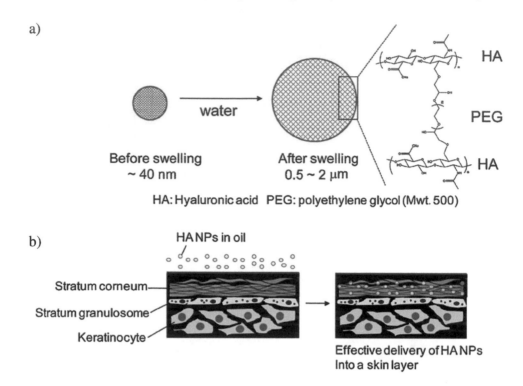

FIGURE 12.7 (a) A schematic demonstration of HA-based hydrogel nanoparticles. (b) For example, when the nanoparticles were dispersed in an oil medium, the reduced swelling of the nanoparticles from their dried state was expected, leading to an enhancement in their penetration ability into the skin. The viscosities of the medium and their chemical effects could also have an influence in the delivery efficiencies of the nanoparticles.(Reprinted from *Colloids Surf A Physicochem Eng Asp* 402, Lim, H.J., Cho, E.C., Lee, J.A., and Kim, J. A novel approach for the use of hyaluronic acid-based hydrogel nanoparticles as effective carriers for transdermal delivery systems, 80–7, Copyright 2012, With permission from Elsevier.)

features and controlling the rate of release of anti-inflammatory drugs to hasten the process of wound healing (Madhaiyan et al. 2013).

In another investigation, electrospun cellulose acetate (CA) nanofibers incorporated with vitamin A and E were synthesized for transdermal applications (Rasekh et al. 2014). In the case of CA nanofibers, controlled release of the vitamins was noticed as compared to the burst release shown in CA casted films. Taepaiboon et al. (2007) developed a vitamin-incorporated nanofibrous membrane for skin and the healing of wounds. Mendes et al. (2016) synthesized hybrid chitosan/phospholipid nanofibers by an electrospinning method for transdermal delivery of drugs. Because of the interacting reactions between the phospholipid layer and amino groups of chitosan in phosphate buffer saline (PBS) solution, chitosan/phospholipids hybrid nanofibers remained stable for up to seven days. Cellular investigations revealed that the nanofibers are of biocompatible nature. The release profiles of the incorporated drugs (curcumin, diclofenac, and vitamin B_{12}) from the chitosan/phospholipid hybrid nanofibers are controlled by their solubility behavior (Mendes et al. 2016). Liu et al. (2017) developed biobased fibrous membranes comprising of micro and nanofibers for the delivery of ibuprofen via the transdermal route. The novel dry-wet electrospinning technique was employed for the synthesis of cellulose micro/nanofiber matrices. In the process of electrospinning, the blunt metallic needle (24 G, 0.3 mm i.d.) of a syringe was rested in a vertical position above the collector. The tip of the needle was kept at 12 cm distance from the surface of the water bath. The heating cover was kept constant at a 103°C temperature, while the applied voltage was set to 10 kV. Subsequently after the electrospinning process, the prepared matrix was collected and placed in deionized water for 72 h at ambient room temperature before the ionic liquid is removed completely and dried for 24 h at room temperature (Liu et al. 2017). Because of their efficient biocompatible and ecofriendly nature, polysaccharide nanofibers possess tremendous features for industrial scale up as a drug delivery system via the transdermal route.

12.7 CONCLUSION

The versatile nature of polysaccharides is attributable to their complex structure and the presence of numerous reactive groups. Various chemical and biochemical derivatizations of polysaccharides are possible because of the existence of several functional moieties on their backbone. Therefore, during the last few decades, polysaccharides in their native as well as derived form are emerging as enormously investigated biomaterials in the field of nanoparticulate drug delivery. As reviewed above, several polysaccharides find potential application in developing nanoparticulate drug delivery systems. Polysaccharide-based nanocarrier systems are gaining an increasing importance for delivery to skin owing to the controlled release ability of its entrapped compounds, that diffuses through the polymeric matrices for permeating into the skin. These nanocarriers are rigid and possess stable structures and their structure is also retained for prolonged duration upon topical application.

Apart from exhibiting excellent potential for treating dermatological diseases, polysaccharide-based nanocarriers are efficiently utilized for transporting therapeutic agents across the skin. Their plethora of advantages such as nanoscale size, composition, stable structure, higher surface energy, and derivatization ability makes them potential candidate as transdermal delivery system.

In the present scenario, polysaccharide-based nanocarriers are not only potentially promising vehicles for the controlled delivery of anti-inflammatory, anticancer, anti-viral agents, etc., but also serve as an innovative strategy for genetic immunization. Topically administered polysaccharide-based nanocarrier formulations offer sophisticated and widespread applications in the pharmaceutical and cosmeceutical sector.

REFERENCES

Abdel-Mottaleb, M.M.A., Moulari, B., Beduneau, A., Pellequer, Y., and Lamprecht, A. 2012. Nanoparticles enhance therapeutic outcome in inflamed skin therapy. *Eur J Pharm Biopharm* 82: 151–7.

Agharkar, S., Lindenbaum, S., and Higuchi, T. 1976. Enhancement of solubility of drug salts by hydrophilic counterions: Properties of organic salts of an antimalarial drug. *J Pharm Sci* 65: 747–9.

Ahmed, T.A., El-Sa, K.M., Aljaeid, B.M., Fahmy, U.A., and Abd-Allah, F.I. 2016. Transdermal glimepiride delivery system based on optimized ethosomal nano-vesicles: Preparation, characterization, in vitro, ex vivo and clinical evaluation. *Int J Pharm* 500: 245–54.

Akiyoshi, K., Kobayashi, S., Shichibe, S. et al. 1998. Self-assembled hydrogel nanoparticle of cholesterol-bearing pullulan as a carrier of protein drugs: Complexation and stabilization of insulin. *J Control Release* 54: 313–20.

Albery, W. and Hadgraft, J. 1979. Percutaneous absorption: theoretical description. *J Pharm and Pharmacol* 31: 129–39.

Al-Kassas, R., Wen, J., Cheng, A.E., Kim, A.M., Liu, S.S.M., and Yu, J. 2016. Transdermal delivery of propranolol hydrochloride through chitosan nanoparticles dispersed in mucoadhesive gel. *Carbohydr Polym* 153: 176–86.

Alonso-Sande, M., Cuna, M., and Remunan-Lopez, C. 2006. Formation of new glucomannan-chitosan nanoparticles and study of their ability to associate and deliver proteins. *Macromolecules* 39: 4152–8.

Anirudhan, T.S., Nair, A.S., and Bino, S.J. 2017. Nanoparticle assisted solvent selective transdermal combination therapy of curcumin and 5-flurouracil for efficient cancer treatment. *Carbohydr Polym* 173: 131–42.

Azizi, E., Namazi, A., Haririan, I. et al. 2010. Release profile and stability evaluation of optimized chitosan/alginate nanoparticles as EGFR antisense vector. *Int J Nanomed* 5: 455–61.

Badwaik H.R., Giri, T.K., Nakhate, K.T., and Tripathi, D.K. 2013. Xanthan gum and its derivatives as a potential bio-polymeric carrier for drug delivery system. *Curr Drug Deliv* 10: 587–600.

Badwaik H.R., Sakure K., Alexander A., Ajazuddin., Dhongade, H., and Tripathi, D.K. 2016a. Synthesis and characterization of poly (acrylamide) grafted carboxymethyl xanthan gum copolymer. *Int J Biol Macromol* 85: 361–9.

Badwaik, H.R., Sakure, K., Nakhate, K.T., Dhongade, H., Kashayap, P., and Tripathi, D.K. 2016b. Microwave assisted eco-friendly synthesis, characterization and *in vitro* release behavior of carboxymethyl xanthan gum. *Curr Microwave Chem* 3: 203–11.

Badwaik, H.R., Sakure, K., Nakhate, K.T. et al. 2017. Effect of Ca^{2+} ion on the release of diltiazem hydrochloride from matrix tablets of carboxymethyl xanthan gum graft polyacrylamide. *Int J Biol Macromol* 94: 691–7.

Badwaik, H.R., Thakur, D., Sakure, K., Giri, T.K., Nakhate, K.T., and Tripathi, D.K. 2014. Microwave assisted synthesis of polyacrylamide grafted guar gum and its application as flocculent for waste water treatment. *Res J Pharm Tech* 7: 401–7.

Banerjee, A., Halder, U., and Bandopadhyay, R. 2017. Preparations and applications of polysaccharide based green synthesized metal nanoparticles: A state-of-the art. *J Clust Sci* 28: 1803–13.

Baroli, B., Ennas, M.G., Loffredo, F., Isola, M., Pinna, R., and Lopez-Quintela, M.A. 2007. Penetration of metallic nanoparticles in human full-thickness skin. *J Invest Dermatol* 127: 1701–12.

Bawarski, W.E., Childlowsky, E., Bharali, D.J., and Mousa, S.A. 2008. Emerging nanopharmaceuticals. *Nanomedicine* 4: 273–82.

Bemiller, J.N. and Whistler, R.L. 1992. *Industrial Gums: Polysaccharides and Their Derivative.* 3rd ed. New York: Academic Press.

Berge, S.M., Bighley, L.D., and Monkhouse, D.C. 1977. Pharmaceutical salts. *J Pharm Sci* 66: 1–19.

Berthold, A., Cremer, K., and Kreuter, J. 1996. Preparation and characterization of chitosan microspheres as drug carrier for prednisolone sodium phosphate as model for anti-inflammatory drugs. *J Control Release* 39: 17–25.

Bibi, N., Ahmed, N., and Khan, G.M., 2017. Nanostructures in transdermal drug delivery systems. In A. Ecaterina and G. Alexandru (Eds.), *Nanostructure for Drug Delivery*, 639–67. New York: Elsevier.

Bodnar, M., Hartmann, J.F., and Borbely, J. 2005b. Nanoparticles from chitosan. *Macromolecular Symposia* 227: 321–6.

Bodnar, M., Hartmann, J.F., and Borbely, J. 2005a. Preparation and characterization of chitosan-based nanoparticles. *Biomacromolecules* 6: 2521–7.

Bolzinger, M.A., Briançon, S., Pelletier, J., and Chevalier, Y. 2012. Penetration of drugs through skin, a complex rate-controlling membrane. *Curr Opin Colloid Interface Sci* 17: 156–65.

Bouwstra, J.A. and Honeywell-Nguyen, P.L. 2002. Skin structure and mode of action of vesicles. *Adv Drug Deliv Review* 54: S41–55.

Cetin, M., Aktas, Y., Vural, I. et al. 2007. Preparation and in vitro evaluation of bFGF-loaded chitosan nanoparticles. *Drug Deliv* 14: 525–9.

Cross, S.E., Innes, B., Roberts, M.S., Tsuzuki, T., Robertson, T.A., and McCormick, P. 2007. Human skin penetration of sunscreen nanoparticles: In-vitro assessment of a novel micronized zinc oxide formulation. *Skin Pharmacol Physiol* 20: 148–54.

Cui, Z. and Mumper, R.J. 2001. Chitosan-based nanoparticles for topical genetic immunization. *J Control Release* 75: 409–19.

D'Ayala, G.G., Malinconico, M., and Laurienzo, P. 2008. Marine derived polysaccharides for biomedical applications: Chemical modification approaches. *Molecules* 13: 2069–106.

Davidson, R.L. 1980. *Handbook of Water-Soluble Gums and Resins.* New York: McGraw-Hill.

de la Fuente, M., Ravina, M., Paolicelli, P., Sanchez, A., Seijo, B., and Alonso, M.J. 2010. Chitosan-based nanostructures: A delivery platform for ocular therapeutics. *Adv Drug Deliv Review* 62: 100–17.

De Louise, L.A. 2012. Applications of nanotechnology in dermatology. *J Invest Dermatol* 132: 964–75.

Delgado-Charro, M.B. and Guy, R.H. 2014. Effective use of transdermal drug delivery in children. *Adv Drug Deliv Review* 73: 63–82.

Desmond, J.T. 2006. Biochemistry of human skin - our brain on the outside. *Chem Soc Rev* 35: 52–67.

Dias, S.F.L., Nogueira, S.S., Dourado, F.F. et al. 2016. Acetylated cashew gum-based nanoparticles for transdermal delivery of diclofenac diethyl amine. *Carbohydr Polym* 143: 254–61.

Domenech, J. and Costa, J.M. 1986. Photoelectrochemical oxidation of oxalate ion in aqueous dispersions of zinc-oxide. *Photochem Photobiol* 44: 675–7.

Douglas, K.L. and Tabrizian, M. 2005. Effect of experimental parameters on the formation of alginate-chitosan nanoparticles and evaluation of their potential application as DNA carrier. *J Biomater Sci, Polym Ed* 16: 43–56.

Elias, P.M. and Friend, D.S. 1975. The permeability barrier in mammalian epidermis. *J Cell Biol* 65: 180–91.

Elias, P.M. and Menon, G.K. 1991. Structural and lipid biochemical correlates of the epidermal permeability barrier. *Adv Lipid Res* 24: 1–26.

Frenot, A. and Chronakis, I.S. 2003. Polymer nanofibers assembled by electrospinning. *Curr Opi Colloid Interface Sci* 8: 64–75.

Genotelle, N., Lherm, T., Gontier, O., Le Gall, C., and Caen, D. 2004. Right uncontrollable haemothorax revealing a liver injury with diaphragmatic rupture. *Ann Fr Anesth Rèanim* 23: 831–4.

Gillet, A., Compère, P., Lecomte, F. et al. 2011. Liposome surface charge influence on skin penetration behaviour. *Int J Pharm* 411: 223–31.

Giri, T.K., Mukherjee, P., Barman, T.K., and Maity, S. 2016. Nano-encapsulation of capsaicin on lipid vesicle and evaluation of their hepatocellular protective effect. Int J Biol Macromol 88: 236–243.

Giri, T.K., Pramanik, K., Barman, T.K., and Maity, S. 2017. Nano-encapsulation of dietary phytoconstituent capsaicin on emulsome: Evaluation of anticancer activity through the measurement of liver oxidative stress in rats. *Anticancer Agents Med Chem* 17: 1669–78.

Giri, T.K., Thakur, A., Alexander, A., Ajazuddin., Badwaik, H., and Tripathi, D.K. 2012a. Modified chitosan hydrogels as drug delivery and tissue engineering systems: Present status and applications. *Acta Pharm Scin B* 2: 439–49.

Giri, T.K., Thakur, D., Alexander, A., Ajazuddin., Badwaik, H., and Tripathi, D.K. 2012b. Alginate based hydrogel as a potential biopolymeric carrier for drug delivery and cell delivery system: Present status and applications. *Curr Drug Deliv* 9: 539–55.

Giri, T.K., Verma, S., Alexander, A., Ajazuddin., Badwaik, H., Tripathy, M., and Tripathi, D.K. 2013. Crosslinked biodegradable hydrogel floating beads for stomach site specific controlled delivery of metronidazole. *Farmacia* 61: 533–50.

Giri, T.K., Verma, P., and Tripathi, D.K. 2015. Grafting of vinyl monomer onto gellan gum using microwave: Synthesis and characterization of grafted copolymer. *Adv Compos Mater* 24: 531–43.

Gonzalez Ferreiro, M., Tillman, L., Hardee, G., and Bodmeier, R. 2002. Characterization of alginate/poly-L-lysine particles as antisense oligonucleotide carriers. *Int J Pharm* 239: 47–59.

Grice, J.E., Ciotti, S., Weiner, N., Lockwood, P., Cross, S.E., and Roberts, M.S. 2010. Relative uptake of minoxidil into appendages and stratum corneum and permeation through human skin in vitro. *J Pharm Sci* 99: 712–8.

Guy, R.H., Hadgraft, J., and Bucks, D.A. 1987. Transdermal drug delivery and cutaneous metabolism. *Xenobiotica* 17: 325–43.

Gysler, A., Kleuser, B., Sippl, W., Lange, K., Korting, H.C., and Holtje, H.D. 1999. Skin penetration and metabolism of topical glucocorticoids in reconstructed epidermis and in excised human skin. *Pharm Res* 16: 1386–91.

Hanson, K.M., Behne, M.J., Barry, N.P., Mauro, T.M., Gratton, E., and Clegg, R.M. 2002. Two photon fluorescence lifetime imaging of the skin stratum corneum pH gradient. *Biophys J* 83: 1682–90.

Hasanovica, A., Martin, Z., Gottfried, R., and Claudia, V. 2009. Chitosan-tripolyphosphate nanoparticles as a possible skin drug delivery system for aciclovir with enhanced stability. *J Pharm Pharmacol* 61: 1609–16.

Hovgaard, L. and Brondsted, H. 1996. Current applications of polysaccharides in colon targeting. *Crit Rev Ther Drug Carrier Syst* 13: 185–23.

Hu, F.Q., Ren, G.F., Yuan, H., Du, Y.Z., and Zeng, S. 2006. Shell cross-linked stearic acid grafted chitosan oligosaccharide self-aggregated micelles for controlled release of paclitaxel. *Colloids Surf B Biointerfaces* 50: 97–103.

Hussain, Z., Katas, H., Amin, M., Kumolosasi, E., Buang, F., and Sahudin, S. 2013. Self-assembled polymeric nanoparticles for percutaneous co-delivery of hydrocortisone/hydroxytyrosol: An ex vivo and in vivo study using an NC/Nga mouse model. *Int J Pharm* 444: 109–19.

Janssens, R., Communi, D., Pirotton, S., Samson, M., Parmentier, M., and Boeynaems, J.M. 1996. Cloning and tissue distribution of the human P2Y1 receptor. *Biochem Biophys Res Commun* 221: 588–93.

Javadzadeh, Y. and Bahari, L.A. 2017. Therapeutic nanostructures for dermal and transdermal drug delivery. In: A. Ecaterina and G. Alexandru (Eds.), *Nano- and Microscale Drug Delivery Systems Design and Fabrication*, 131–46. New York: Elsevier.

Jones, L.C., Lackowski, W.M., Vasilyeva, Y., Wilson, K., and Checkik, V. 2009. Self-assembly of cross- linked beta-cyclodextrin nanocapsules. 2009. *Chem Comun (Camb)* 21: 1377–9.

Jung, S., Otberg, N., Thiede, G. et al. 2006. Innovative liposomes as a transfollicular drug delivery system: Penetration into porcine hair follicles. *J Invest Dermatol* 126: 1728–32.

Kataria, K., Gupta, A., Rath, G., Mathur, R.B., and Dhakate, S.R. 2014. In vivo wound healing performance of drug loaded electrospun composite nanofibers transdermal patch. *Int J Pharm* 469: 102–10.

Katas, H. and Alpar, H.O. 2006. Development and characterisation of chitosan nanoparticles for siRNA delivery. *Journal Control Release* 115: 216–25.

Khalil, S.K.H., El-Feky, G.S., El-Banna, S.T., and Khalil, W.A. 2012. Preparation and evaluation of warfarin-b-cyclodextrin loaded chitosan nanoparticles for transdermal delivery. *Carbohydr Polym* 90: 1244–53.

Kim, D.G., Young, J., Changyong, C. et al. 2006. Retinol-encapsulated low molecular water-soluble chitosan nanoparticles. *Int J Pharm* 319: 130–38.

Kirschner, N., Poetzl, C., von den Driesch, P. et al. 2009. Alteration of tight junction proteins is an early event in psoriasis: Putative involvement of proinflammatory cytokines. *Am J Path* 175: 1095–106.

Krien, P.M. and Kermici, M. 2000. Evidence for the existence of a self-regulated enzymatic process within the human stratum corneum an unexpected role for urocanic acid. *J Invest Dermatol* 115: 414–20.

Kumar, A. and Ahuja M. 2013. Carboxymethyl gum kondagogu-chitosan polyelectrolyte complex nanoparticles: Preparation and characterization. Int J Biol Macromol 62: 80–4.

Labouta, H.I., El-Khordagui, L.K., Kraus, T., and Schneider, M. 2011. Mechanism and determinants of nanoparticle penetration through human skin. *Nanoscale* 3: 4989–99.

Lademann, J., Richter, H., Schanzer, S. et al. 2011. Penetration and storage of particles in human skin: Perspectives and safety aspects. *Eur J Pharm Biopharm* 77: 465–8.

Lademann, J., Richter, H., Teichmann, A. et al. 2007. Nanoparticles an efficient carrier for drug delivery into the hair follicles. *Eur J Pharm Biopharm* 66: 159–64.

Langbein, L., Grund, C., Kuhn, C. et al. 2002. Tight junctions and compositionally related junctional structures in mammalian stratified epithelia and cell cultures derived there from. *Eur J Cell Biol* 81: 419–35.

Lboutounne, H., Faivre, V., Falson, F., and Pirot, F. 2004. Characterization of transport of chlorhexidine-loaded nanocapsules through hairless and Wistar rat skin. *Skin Pharmacol Physiol* 17: 176–82.

Le Texier, L., Favre, E., Redeuilh, C. et al. 1996. Structure–activity relationships in platelet activating factor (PAF). 7. Tetrahydrofuran derivatives as dual PAF antagonists and acetylcholinesterase inhibitors. Synthesis and PAF-antagonistic activity. *J Lipid Mediators Cell Signalling* 13: 189–205.

Lee, J.W., Park, J.H., and Robinson, J.R. 2000. Bioadhesive-based dosage forms: The next generation. *J Pharm Sci* 89: 850–66.

Lee, P., Pen, S., Su, C. et al. 2008. The use of biodegradable polymeric nanoparticles in combination with a low-pressure gene gun for transdermal DNA delivery. *Biomaterials* 29: 742–51.

Lemarchand, C., Gref, R., and Couvreur, P. 2004. Polysaccharide-decorated nanoparticles. *Eur J Pharm Biopharm* 58: 327–41.

Li, G.L., de Vries, J.J., van Steeg, T.J. et al. 2005. Transdermal iontophoretic delivery of apomorphine in patients improved by surfactant formulation pretreatment. *J Controlle Release* 101: 199–208.

Liang, X.W., Xu, Z.P., Grice, J., Zvyagin, A.V., Roberts, M.S., and Liu, X. 2013. Penetration of nanoparticles into human skin. *Curr Pharm Design* 19: 6353–66.

Lim, H.J., Cho, E.C., Lee, J.A., and Kim. J. 2012. A novel approach for the use of hyaluronic acid-based hydrogel nanoparticles as effective carriers for transdermal delivery systems. *Colloids Surf A Physicochem Eng Asp* 402: 80–7.

Liu, H., Chen, B., Mao, Z.W., and Gao, C.Y. 2007. Chitosan nanoparticles for loading of toothpaste actives and adhesion on tooth analogs. *J Appl Polym Sci* 106: 4248–56.

Liu, Y., Nguyen, A., Allen, A., Zoldan, J., Huang, Y., and Chen, J.Y. 2017. Regenerated cellulose micro-nano fiber matrices for transdermal drug release. *Mater Sci Eng C* 74: 485–92.

Liu, Y., Yang, J., Zhao, Z., Li, J., Zhang, R., and Yao, F. 2012. Formation and characterization of natural polysaccharide hollow nanocapsules via template layer-by-layer self-assembly. *J Colloid Interface Sci* 379: 130–40.

Liu, Z., Jiao, Y., Wang, Y., Zhou, C., and Zhang, Z. 2008. Polysaccharide-based nanoparticles as drug delivery systems. Adv Drug Deliv Rev 60: 1650–62.

Lu, B., Xiong, S.B., Yang, H., Yin, X.D., and Zhao, R.B. 2006. Mitoxantrone-loaded BSA nanospheres and chitosan nanospheres for local injection against breast cancer and its lymph node metastases. I: Formulation and in vitro characterization. *Int J Pharm* 307: 168–74.

Madhaiyan, K., Sridhar, R., Sundarrajan, S., Venugopal, J.R., and Ramakrishna, S. 2013. Vitamin B_{12} loaded polycaprolactone nanofibers: A novel transdermal route for the water soluble energy supplement delivery. *Int J Pharm* 444: 70–6.

Marks, R. 2004. The stratum conium barrier: The final frontier. *J Nutr* 134: 2017S–1S.

Martínez, A., Fernández, A., Pérez, E., Benito, M., Teijón J.M., and Blanco, M.D. 2012. Polysaccharide based nanoparticles for controlled release formulations. In: A.A. Hashim (Ed.), *The Delivery of Nanoparticles*, 185–222. London: In Tech.

Martínez, A., Iglesias, I., Lozano, R., Teijón, J.M., and Blanco, M.D. 2011. Synthesis and characterization of thiolated alginate-albumin nanoparticles stabilized by disulfide bonds, evaluation as drug delivery systems. *Carbohydr Polym* 83: 1311–21.

Mathias, N.R. and Hussain, M.A. 2010. Non-invasive systemic drug delivery: Developability considerations for alternate routes of administration. *J Pharm Sci* 99: 1–20.

Mei, D., Mao, S., Sun, W., Wang, Y., and Kisse, T. 2008. Effect of chitosan structure properties and molecular weight on the intranasal absorption of tetramethylpyrazine phosphate in rats. *Eur J Pharm and Biopharm* 70: 874–81.

Mendes, A.C., Gorzelanny, C., Halter, N., Schneider, S.W., and Chronakis I.S. 2016. Hybrid electrospun chitosan-phospholipids nanofibers for transdermal drug delivery. *Int J Pharm* 510: 48–56.

Merwe, D., Brooks, J.D., Gehring, R., Baynes, R.E., Monteiro-Riviere, N.A., and Riviere, J.E. 2006. A physiologically based pharmacokinetic model of organophosphate dermal absorption. *Toxicol Sci* 89: 188–204.

Michaels, A.S., Chandrasekaran, S.K., and Shaw, J.E. 1975. Drug permeation through human skin: Theory and in vitro experimental measurement. *AlChE J* 21: 985–6.

Murphy, R.J., Pristinski, D., Migler, K., Douglas, J.F., and Prabhu, V.M. 2010. Dynamic light scattering investigations of nanoparticle aggregation following a light-induced pH jump. *J Chem Phys* 132: 194903.

Myrick, J.M., Vendra, K.V., and Krishnan, S. 2014. Self-assembled polysaccharide nanostructures for controlled-release applications. *Nanotechnol Rev* 3: 319–46.

Oesch, F., Fabian, E., Oesch-Bartlomowicz, B., Werner, C., and Landsiedel, R. 2007. Drug-metabolizing enzymes in the skin of man, rat, and pig. Drug Metab Rev 39: 659–98.

Pan, Y.; Li, Y. J.; Zhao, H. Y. et al. 2002. Bioadhesive polysaccharide in protein delivery system: Chitosan nanoparticles improve the intestinal absorption of insulin in vivo. *Int J Pharm* 249: 139–47.

Partha, S., Amit, K.G., and Rath, G. 2010. Formulation and evaluation of chitosan-based ampicillin trihydrate nanoparticles. *Trop J Pharm Res* 9: 483–8.

Patzelt, A., Richter, H., Knorr, F. et al. 2011. Selective follicular targeting by modification of the particle sizes. *J Controlle Release* 150: 45–8.

Paudel, K.S., Milewski, M., Swadley, C.L., Brogden, N.K., Ghosh, P., and Stinchcomb, A.L. 2010. Challenges and opportunities in dermal/transdermal delivery. *Ther Deliv* 1: 109–31.

Piemi, M.P.Y., Korner, D., Benita, S., and Marty, J.P. 1999. Positively and negatively charged submicron emulsion for enhanced topical delivery of antifungal drugs. *J Control Release* 58: 177–87.

Potts, R.O. and Guy, R.H. 1995. A predictive algorithm for skin permeability: The effects of molecular size and hydrogen bond activity. *Pharm Res* 12: 1628–33.

Prabaharan, M. 2008. Review paper: chitosan derivatives as promising materials for controlled drug delivery. *J Biomater Appl* 23: 5–36.

Prabaharan M. 2011. Prospectus of guar gum and its derivatives as controlled drug delivery systems. *Int J Biol Macromol* 49: 117–24.

Prabaharan, M and Jayakumar, R. 2009. Chitosan-graft-β-cyclodextrin scaffolds with controlled drug release capability for tissue engineering applications. *Int J Biol Macromol* 44: 320–5.

Prausnitz, M.R., Elias, P.M., Franz, T.J. et al. 2012. Skin barrier and transdermal drug delivery. *Dermatology* 20: 65–73.

Prausnitz, M.R., Mitragotri, S., and Langer, R. 2004. Current status and future potential of transdermal drug delivery. *Nat Rev Drug Discov* 3: 115–24.

Prow, T.W., Grice, J.E., Lin, L.L. et al. 2011. Nanoparticles and microparticles for skin drug delivery. *Adv Drug Deliv Rev* 63: 470–91.

Qi Tan, W.L., Chenyu, G., and Guangxi, Z. 2011. Preparation and evaluation of quercetin-loaded lecithin-chitosan nanoparticles for topical delivery. *Int J Nanomed* 6: 1621–30.

Rangari, A.T. and Ravikumar, P. 2015. Polymeric nanoparticles based topical drug delivery: An overview. *Asian J Biomed Pharm Sci* 47: 05–12.

Rasekh, M., Karavasili, C., Soong, Y.L. et al. 2014. Electrospun PVP-indomethacin constituents for transdermal dressings and drug delivery devices. *Int J Pharm* 473: 95–104.

Reddy, M.B., Guy, R.H., and Bunge, A.L. 2000. Does epidermal turnover reduce percutaneous penetration. *Pharm Res* 17: 1414–9.

Reis, C.P., Ribeiro, A.J., Houng, S., Veiga, F., and Neufeld, R.J. 2007. Nanoparticulate delivery system for insulin: Design, characterization and in vitro/in vivo bioactivity. *Eur J Pharm Sci* 30: 392–7.

Reis, C.P., Ribeiro, A.J., Veiga, F., Neufeld, R.J., and Damge, C. 2008. Polyelectrolyte biomaterial interactions provide nanoparticulate carrier for oral insulin delivery. *Drug Deliv* 15: 127–39.

Roberts, M.S. and Walters, K.A. 1998. *Dermal Absorption and Toxicity Assessment*. New York: Marcel Dekker.

Roberts, M.S. and Walters, K.A. 2008. Human skin morphology and dermal absorption. In: M.S. Roberts and K.A. Walter (Eds.), *Dermal absorption and toxicity assessment*, 1–15. New York: Informa Healthcare.

Rojanasakul, Y., Wang, L.Y., Bhat, M., Glover, D.D., Malanga, C.J., and Ma, J.K. 1992. The transport barrier of epithelia-a comparative study on membrane-permeability and charge selectivity in the rabbit. *Pharm Res* 9: 1029–34.

Rubinstein, A. 2000. Natural polysaccharides as targeting tools of drugs to the human colon. *Drug Dev Res* 50: 435–9.

Saboktakin, M.R., Akhyari, S., and Nasirov, F.A. 2014. Synthesis and characterization of modified starch/ polybutadiene as novel transdermal drug delivery system. *Int J Biol Macromol* 69: 442–6.

Sadhasivam, L., Dey, N., Francis, A.P., and Devasena, A.P. 2015. Transdermal patches of chitosan nanoparticles for insulin delivery. *Int J Pharm Sci* 5: 84–8.

Sanchez, D.A., David, S., Chaim, T.V. et al. 2014. Amphotericin B releasing nanoparticle topical treatment of Candida spp. in the setting of a burn wound. *Nanomedicine* 10: 269–77

Santander-Ortega, M.J., Stauner, T., Loretz, B. et al. 2010. Nanoparticles made from novel starch derivatives for transdermal drug delivery. *J Control Release* 141: 85–92.

Santhi, K., Venkatesh, D.N., Dhanaraj, S.A., Sangeetha, S., and Suresh, B. Development and in-vitro evaluation of a topical drug delivery system containing betamethazone loaded ethyl cellulose nanospheres. *Trop J Pharm Res* 4: 495–500.

Sarmah, J.K., Bhattacharjee, S.K., Roy, S., Mahanta, R., and Mahanta, R. 2014. Biodegradable guar gum nanoparticles as carrier for tamoxifen citrate in treatment of breast cancer. *J Biomater Nanobiotechnol* 5: 220–8.

Sarmento, B., Martins, S., Ribeiro, A., Veiga, F., Neufeld, R., and Ferreira, D. 2006. Development and comparison of different nanoparticulate polyelectrolyte complexes as insulin carriers. *Int J Pept Res Ther* 12: 131–8.

Scheuplein, R.J. 1965. Mechanism of percutaneous adsorption. I. Routes of penetration and the influence of solubility. *J Invest Dermatol* 45: 334–46.

Schmid-Wendtner, M.H., and Korting, H.C. 2006. The pH of the skin surface and its impact on the barrier function. *Skin Pharmacol Physiol* 19: 296–302.

Seidenari, S. and Giusti, G. 1995. Objective assessment of the skin of children affected by atopic dermatitis: A study of pH, capacitance and TEWL in eczematous and clinically uninvolved skin. *Acta Derm Venereol* 75: 429–33.

Senyiğit, T., Sonvico, F., Barbieri, S., Ozer, O., Santi, P., and Colombo, P. Lecithin/chitosan nanoparticles of clobetasol-17-propionate capable of accumulation in pig skin. *J Control Release* 142: 368–73.

Shah, P.P., Desai, P.R., and Singh, M. 2012. Effect of oleic acid modified polymeric bilayered nanoparticles on percutaneous delivery of spantide II and ketoprofen. *J Control Release* 158: 336–45.

Shelly., Ahuja, M., and Kumar A. 2013. Gum ghatti-chitosan polyelectrolyte nanoparticles: Preparation and characterization. *Int J Biol Macromol* 61: 411–5.

Singh, V., Kumar, P., and Sanghi R. 2012. Use of microwave irradiation in the grafting modification of the polysaccharides-A review. *Prog Polym Sci* 37: 340–64.

Skiba, M., Wouessidjewe, D., Puisieux, F., Duchène, D., and Gulik, A. 1996. Characterization of amphiphilic fl-cyclodextrin nanospheres. *Int J Pharm*142: 121–4.

Soumya, R.S., Ghosh, S., and Abraham, E.T. 2010. Preparation and characterization of guar gum nanoparticles. *Int J Biol Macromol* 46: 267–9.

Taepaiboon, P., Rungsardthong, U., and Supaphol, P. 2007. Vitamin-loaded electrospun cellulose acetate nanofiber mats as transdermal and dermal therapeutic agents of vitamin A acid and vitamin E. *Eur J Pharm Biopharm* 67: 387–97.

Terreno, E., Sanino, A., Carrera, C. et al. 2008. Determination of water permeability of paramagnetic liposomes of interest in MRI field. *J Inorg Biochem* 102: 1112–9.

Tiyaboonchai, W. and Limpeanchob, N. 2007. Formulation and characterization of amphotericin B-chitosan-dextran sulfate nanoparticles. *Int J Pharm* 329: 142–9.

Tso, C.P., Zhung, C.M., Shih, Y.H., Tseng, Y.M., Wu, S.C., and Doong, R.A. 2010. Stability of metal oxide nanoparticles in aqueous solutions. *Water Sci Technol* 61: 127–33.

Uchechi, O., Ogbonna, J.D., and Attama, A.A. 2014. Nanoparticles for dermal and transdermal drug delivery. In: A.D. Sezer (Ed.), *Application of nano-technology in drug delivery*, 193–235. InTech: Rijeka, Croatia.

Vandamme, T.F., Lenourry, A., Charrueau, C., and Chaumeil, J. 2002. The use of polysaccharides to target drugs to the colon. *Carbohydr Polym* 48: 219–31.

Verma, V.S., Sakure, V., and Badwaik, H.R. 2017. Xanthan gum a versatile biopolymer: Current status and future prospectus in hydro gel drug delivery. *Curr Chem Biol* 11: 10–20.

Wang, Y.S., Liu, L.R., Jiang, Q., and Zhang, Q.Q. 2007. Self-aggregated nanoparticles of cholesterol-modified chitosan conjugate as a novel carrier of epirubicin. *Eur Polym J* 43: 43–51.

Watson, R.E., Poddar, R., Walker, J.M. et al. 2007. Altered claudin expression is a feature of chronic plaque psoriasis. *J Pathol* 212: 450–58.

Wiedersberg, S. and Guy, R.H. 2014. Transdermal drug delivery: 30þ years of war and still fighting! *J Control Release* 190: 150–6.

Williams, A.C. 2003. Structure and function of human skin. In: *Transdermal and Topical Drug Delivery*, 1–25. London and Chicago: Pharmaceutical Press.

Xu, Y.M., Du, Y.M., Huang, R.H., and Gao, L.P. 2003. Preparation and modification of N-(2-hydroxyl) propyl-3-trimethyl ammonium chitosan chloride nanoparticle as a protein carrier. *Biomaterials* 24: 5015–22.

Yang, X., Zhang, Q., Wang, Y. et al. 2008. Self-aggregated nanoparticles from methoxy poly(ethylene glycol)-modified chitosan: Synthesis; characterization; aggregation and methotrexate release in vitro. *Colloids Surf B Biointerfaces* 61: 125–31.

Yang. Y., Manda, P., Pavurala, N., Khan, M.A., and Krishnaiah, Y.S.R. 2015. Development and validation of in vitro & in vivo correlation (IVIVC) for estradiol transdermal drug delivery systems. *J Control Release* 210: 58–66.

Yilmaz, E. and Borchert, H.H. 2005. Design of a phytosphingosine-containing, positively-charged nanoemulsion as a colloidal carrier system for dermal application of ceramides. *Eur J Pharm Biopharm* 60: 91–8.

Yoksan, R., Matsusaki, M., Akashi, M., and Chirachanchai, S. 2004. Controlled hydrophobic/hydrophilic chitosan: Colloidal phenomena and nanosphere formation. *Colloid Polym Sci* 282: 337–42.

You, J.O. and Peng, C.A. 2004. Calcium-alginate nanoparticles formed by reverse microemulsion as gene carriers. *Macromol Symp* 219: 147–53.

Zamani, M., Prabhakaran, M.P., and Ramakrishna, S. 2013. Advances in drug delivery via electrospun and electrosprayed nanomaterials. *Int J Nanomedicine* 8: 2997–3017.

Zhang, H., Oh, M., Allen, C., and Kumacheva, E. 2004. Monodisperse chitosan nanoparticles for mucosal drug delivery. *Biomacromolecules* 5: 2461–8.

Zhao, L., Wang, Y., Zhai, Y., Wang, Z., Liu, J., and Zhai, G. 2014. Ropivacaine loaded microemulsion and microemulsion-based gel for transdermal delivery: Preparation, optimization, and evaluation. *Int J Pharm* 477: 47–56.

Zhi, J., Wang, Y.J., and Luo, G.S. 2005. Adsorption of diuretic furosemide onto chitosan nanoparticles prepared with a water-in-oil nanoemulsion system. *React Funct Polym* 65: 249–57.

13 Polysaccharide Nanoparticle-Based Drug Delivery Approaches for Efficient Therapy of Diabetes

Vaswati Rita Das, Dibyendu Dutta, and Srijita Halder

CONTENTS

13.1   INTRODUCTION

Diabetes mellitus (DM) is a metabolic or endocrine disorder which is characterized by increased serum glucose level due to insufficiency of insulin hormone, resulting in hyperglycemia as well as the affected carbohydrate, protein, and fat metabolism. The incidence of diabetes is increasing all over the world. The number of diabetic patients has been increased from 30 million in 1985 to 171 million in 2000 and it is suspected to increase to 366 million by 2025.

Diabetes can be classified into two main types. It has been broadly categorized as type 1 DM (T1DM) and type 2 DM (T2DM). Type 1 DM is insulin-dependent or juvenile diabetes where insulin deficiency is due to the destruction of β-cells of pancreatic islets of Langerhans which produces the insulin. Type 1 DM can also be further classified as Type 1A (autoimmune destruction of the β-cells) and another one is Type 1B (idiopathic insulin deficiency). Type 2 DM which is known as non-insulin dependent DM, is mainly characterized by insulin resistance or diminished insulin sensitivity due to the defective responsiveness in insulin receptors of cell membranes toward insulin. Besides these, there is gestational diabetes which happens only during pregnancy where also the serum glucose level gets high due to the lack of ability to produce enough insulin, and the last one is congenital diabetes mellitus, which is known as LADA or latent autoimmune diabetes of adults. The reasons behind this are: extensive pancreatic damage, over secretion of the insulin antagonistic hormones, etc. So, the management of diabetes is highly needed to control the blood glucose level as well as to abate the diseases related to diabetes like cardiovascular disease, diabetic nephropathy, diabetic retinopathy, neuropathy, and many others. Treatment of diabetes includes the persistent monitoring of the blood glucose level, physical exercise, oral medications, and insulin (subcutaneous therapy), which is the primary target of treatment, mainly in type 1 DM, where it is a basic need to survive. However, the oral hypoglycemic agents are another mode of treatment to better control type 2 diabetes mellitus. Although, there is an abundant supply of medicines on the market for treating this disease, still the overall and successful cure remains unreachable due to several adverse effects like hypoglycemia, lipoatrophy, lipohyperatrophy, obesity, neuropathy, and many other side effects. The treatment of diabetes also has poor patient compliance due to multiple and frequent dosing, and a medical expert is needed for the subcutaneous administration of doses (like insulin). Therefore, researchers are more eager to overcome such problems by developing safe, efficacious, and alternative non-invasive routes of administration of drugs, with controlled or sustained release properties.

There are a lot of non-invasive routes for administration like oral, buccal, rectal, nasal, pulmonary, ocular, and transdermal routes. However, there are also several problems in the administration of conventional dosage forms of the anti-diabetic drugs or the free macromolecules like insulin by these routes. Owing to several factors, eventually the bioavailability of the drugs becomes limited, therefore conventional delivery through non-invasive routes becomes a challenge. Researchers have endeavored to overcome this challenge by inventing many new and promising approaches.

The novel strategies based on nanotechnologies are one of the promising approaches that offers many benefits in terms of increased bioavailability, decreased dosing frequency, prevention of the drugs from degradation in the abrasive environment of gastrointestinal tract, decreased side effects, and also site-specific activity.

Among the disparate materials which are being used to prepare the nanoparticle drug delivery systems, polysaccharides offer more advantages than others such as biodegradability, versatility, mucoadhesivity, biocompatibility, lesser toxicity, high therapeutic efficacy, etc. So, nanoparticles based on the polysaccharides are a promising approach for the treatment of diabetes mellitus. This chapter portrays various advancements related to the non-invasive delivery of the anti-diabetics via polysaccharide nanoparticle delivery systems.

13.2 BARRIERS OF INSULIN AND OTHER ANTI-DIABETIC DRUGS VIA THE CONVENTIONAL DOSAGE FORMS

Most of the oral anti-diabetic drugs are available in the form of tablets and capsules, and also some injectable drugs (like insulin) which are intended to be introduced non-invasively, these conventional dosage forms divulge higher systemic toxicity, rapid clearance, a multiple and frequent dosing schedule, narrow therapeutic window, hepatic first pass metabolism, enzymatic degradation of the drugs, and significantly limited accessibility to the desired site due to absorption barriers and therefore a very low bioavailability which eventually affects the absorption of drugs. There are three main absorption barriers: 1. the enzymatic barrier 2. the physiological barrier, and 3. the physicochemical properties of protein drugs.

13.2.1 ENZYMATIC BARRIER

There are various enzymatic barriers in the gastrointestinal tract for oral insulin and other anti-diabetic drugs. These can be denatured by the enzymes like, intracellular enzymes (e.g. cathepsins), many proteolytic enzymes of the stomach and the lumen of the intestines (like pepsin, tripsin), bacterial flora of the mucous layer and intestinal epithelial cells and the enzymes at the membrane of the brush border (endopeptidases). The efflux transporters like p-glycoprotein (P-gp) which are present on enterocytes, also renders low bioavailability and absorption.

13.2.2 PHYSIOLOGICAL BARRIER

The intestinal epithelial cells contain tight junctions (zona occludens), where the outer surface is covered by mucous and glycocalyx layers, which stymies the permeation of insulin and other oral anti-diabetic drugs and the subsequent absorption (Damgé et al. 2007). The absorption can be increased using many absorption enhancers like EDTA, bile salts, trisodium citrates, and polysaccharides (e.g. chitosan), that may help to broach the intestinal epithelial tight junctions (Herrero et al. 2012; Li and Deng 2004).

13.2.3 PHYSICOCHEMICAL PROPERTIES OF PROTEIN DRUGS

The radius of the pores in intestinal mucosa (7–15 Å) are an important barrier in protein drugs like insulin translocation. These molecules are always prone to aggregate at a concentration above 100 nm. The transformation of the monomeric protein drugs into hexameric conformation impairs the passage of protein drugs through intestinal epithelium (Damgé et al. 2008). Solvents, temperatures, and additives alter the amino acid (primary) sequence and the tertiary structure of the insulin. These alterations have an immense effect on the transportation of insulin. At physiological pH, amino acid and carboxylic acid groups of insulin get entirely ionized, and consequently form a zwitter ionic configuration. This will preclude the drug from transcellular diffusion, until and unless the charges get neutralized by the ion pairs (Damgé et al. 2008).

13.3 NANOCARRIERS IN THE ORAL DELIVERY OF INSULIN AND OTHER ANTI-DIABETIC DRUGS

To ensure successful delivery of insulin and other anti-diabetic drugs orally, the stability is exacted physiologically and biologically in the formulations and also in the gastrointestinal tract. Compared with the other delivery methods, nanoparticles have the ability to cellular uptake. Nanotechnology mainly deals with the manipulation of atoms and molecules, which in turn makes it efficient with new, advantageous properties. Nanoparticles are structures with sizes ranging from 1 to 100 nm (Suri et al. 2007). Nanoparticles are suitable for varied molecules like proteins, vaccines, etc. (des Rieux et al. 2006) In oral drug delivery, nanotechnologies are helpful in the transcytosis of drugs through the tight epithelial barrier, in the delivery of poorly hydrophilic drugs, in the targeted drug delivery to a desired site in the gastrointestinal tract and the transcellular and intracellular delivery of the drugs (Farokhzad and Langer 2009). Nanocarriers must be non-toxic, biodegradable, non-immuno-genic, non-inflammatory, non-thrombogenic, stable, and should be able to escape via the reticulo-endothelial system (Kumari et al. 2010; Chakraborty et al. 2013). So, they can also be successfully utilized as a carrier for the oral delivery of insulin and other anti-diabetic drugs. Nanocarriers are capable of being transported and internalized through the epithelial membrane of intestine, which affects the pharmacokinetic activity of insulin (Mukhopadhyay et al. 2013). Nanoparticles tender a huge range of advantages in oral drug delivery, i.e. they increases the tolerability, therapeutic index specificity, and efficacy of drugs (Hall et al. 2007). Also, to make the oral absorption of proteins as well as peptides drugs more feasible, nanocarriers are being modified by specific ligands and are targeted to the specific receptors of the epithelial cell membrane (Kavimandan et al. 2006; Roger et al. 2010; Vandamme et al. 2010; Lochner et al. 2003; Chalasani et al. 2007a). Nanoparticles can also protect the insulin and peptide drugs from hydrolysis and enzymatic degradation in the abrasive environment of the gastrointestinal tract (Jung et al. 2000; Galindo-Rodriguez et al. 2005; Damgé et al. 2008; Shaji and Patole 2008). The efficiency of nanoparticles for oral insulin and other oral anti-diabetic drug delivery is affected by various parameters like surface charge, particle size, properties of polymer, drug-polymer interaction, drug loading, release profile of drug, residence time at the desired site of absorption, and the rate of clearance from the body (Woitiski et al. 2011).

13.4 POLYSACCHARIDE NANOPARTICLES IN THE ORAL DELIVERY OF INSULIN AND OTHER ANTI-DIABETIC DRUGS

To achieve more advantages from the nanoparticular drug delivery system, polymeric nanopar-ticular formulation has been a great approach in the oral delivery of macromolecules, like insulin. Among other polymers, naturally occurring polysaccharides are preferable because of their bio-compatible, biodegradable, pH-sensitive, and bioadhesive properties, and they can also be used to prepare a unit molecule with insulin, proteins, and peptides. These biodegradable polymers act as better alternatives for oral insulin and other forms of anti-diabetic drug delivery. Moreover, the sta-bility and functional ability of these particles can be enriched by these excipients which are capable of maintaining pH-responsiveness and the P-gp effect. These are excellent polymers to block the efflux of P-gp. Being pH-sensitive, these nanocarriers can overcome the obstacles for the delivery of drugs orally and are observed to decrease the serum glucose level for a longer time. The bioadhesive properties of the nanoparticles tend to prolong the particle's residence time within the gastrointes-tinal tract and eventually enhance the total uptake of nanoparticles. Polysaccharide nanoparticles adhere with the biological tissues via strong adhesive interactions through different types of bonds (van der Waals, hydrogen bonds, etc.) to keep the nanoparticles in contact with the intestinal epithe-lium for a protracted period of time. They can also reach the targeted site via their mucoadhesive properties which can maintain the close contact of the nanoparticles with the mucosal tissues and thus hinder the pre-systemic metabolism. This provides increased bioavailability which protects the drugs from the gastrointestinal tract and can also provide a sustained release effect of the drugs that can be accommodative in the reduction of dosing frequency, which can ultimately increase the patient compliance. These systems can also decrease the rate of insulin clearance from the absorption site and consequently increase the available absorption time.

13.5 PHYSICOCHEMICAL PROPERTIES OF POLYSACCHARIDE NANOCARRIER

Nanoparticles like colloidal systems differ from macromolecular particles because of the presence of certain properties such as high energy, high surface area, and the high movement of particles, known as the Brownian motion. The physical properties of the drug substance (physical state, size, morphology) which have to be encapsulated play a vital role in the control of the release of the drug and degradation of the nanoparticles. The nanoparticle's surface charge is measured by zeta potential. Coating with polymers which have mucoadhesive properties like poly(acrylic acid), sodium alginate, chitosan, and poloxamers, helps to develop the bioavailability of the entrapped drug by enhancing the residence time of the nanoparticle at the mucosal site. This occurs because of the ionic interaction between amino groups (positively charged) of chitosan and the sialic acid residues (negatively charged) in mucus. A de-swelling process also occurs due to the alteration of pH value from acidic to basic value.

13.6 CHARACTERISTICS OF POLYSACCHARIDES

Polysaccharides are a diverse class of polymer materials derived from natural origin like animal, plant, and algae, which is formed by monosaccharides linked with glycosidic linkages (Shukla and Tiwari 2012). Polysaccharides can have a linear or branched architecture, depending on the monosaccharide unit's nature. In addition to structural diversity, polysaccharides possess a number of functional groups in its chemical structure such as hydroxyl, carboxylic acid, and amino groups, indicating the feasibility for chemical modification (Liu et al. 2008). Moreover, polysaccharide molecular weight can vary between hundreds to thousands of Daltons, showing further diversity (kumar et al. 2012). Herein, we will discuss the characteristics of polysaccharides, including solubility, biocompatibility, biodegradability, and the potentiality for modification of several polysaccharides, which makes them important for being used in drug delivery systems.

13.6.1 SOLUBILITY

The functional groups with polysaccharide backbones, specially hydroxyl, and also the amine groups but to a lesser extent, which are responsible for a high water solubility. Albeit, this solubility can be adjusted by modification of the monomer. For example, chitosan, which is composed of N-acetyl-D-glucosamine and D-glucosamine linked by β-(1–4), is prepared by chitin deacetylation. The solubility properties of the chitosan in the acidic medium can be tuned by varying the parent compound's degree of deacetylation or changing the ratio between the chitin and the alkali. More the degrees of deacetylation indicate a higher number of protonated and available free amino groups along the polysaccharide backbone and consequently enhance solubility (Morris et al. 2010).

13.6.2 BIODEGRADABILITY AND BIOCOMPATIBILITY

Polysaccharides possess low toxicity levels compared to many other synthetic polymers. For example, dextrans which are the biopolymers composed of glucose units, linked through α-1,6 linkages with feasible branching from α-1,2 to α-1,4 linkages, that elicit much less toxicity and higher biocompatibility. As a result, the dextrans have formed a basis of hydrogels which is biocompatible for a prolonged controlled release delivery system (Coviello et al. 2007). Moreover, dextrans have also exhibited biocompatibility in the microspheres formulation, and because of their native presence in the body, most of the polysaccharides experience enzymatic degradation. Polysaccharides can get broken down to monomer or oligomer blocks and then recycled for further use as storage, cell signaling applications, and structural support (Jain et al. 2007). For example, glycosidases have the ability of catalyzing the hydrolysis of different glycosidic linkages (Jain et al. 2007). In comparison to glycosidase, other enzymes are highly polysaccharide specific. Hyaluronidase degrades the hyaluronic acid (HA) polysaccharide cleaving the β-1,4 linkages between D-glucuronic acid and D-N-acetylglucosamine, specifically in high HA concentrated regions (Jain et al. 2007).

It is noticeable that few polysaccharides are particularly inclined to lysosomal enzymatic degradation, including esterases, proteases, and glycosidases pursuing endocytosis (Mehvar 2003). Thus, the enzymatic degradation allows the release of the drugs which is associated with a delivery system based on polysaccharides (Mehvar 2003).

13.6.3 EASE OF MODIFICATION

Polysaccharides are highly susceptible to modification. There are a lot of glucose-based polysaccharides, like amylopectin, amylose, cellulose, and glycogen, which tender a remarkable number of free hydroxyl groups. Polysaccharides, which have both hydroxyl as well as carboxylic acid groups, can be easily modified. The modification of chitosan has been reviewed extensively. Particularly, the quarterization of the amines (primary) with a varied alkyl groups is used for the enhancement of solubility and alteration of the bioactivity.

A lot of polysaccharides exhibit innate bioactivity, specifically mucoadhesive, anti-inflammatory, and anti-microbial properties. Mucoadhesion is the interaction of material with a mucosal layer of the gastrointestinal (GI) tract, airway or can be of the nasal pathway. Chitosan is the only positively charged, natural polysaccharide which has the capability of binding to the mucosal layers which are negatively charged. This binding of chitosan to mucosal layers occurs through an ionic interaction between them (Mourya and Inamdar 2009; Thanou et al. 2001a; Thanou et al. 2001b). Therefore, in oral drug delivery, chitosan has become a great interest for research by many investigators. For negatively charged or neutral polysaccharides like HA, the alternative mechanism for mucoadhesion is hydrogen bonding.

13.7 PREPARATION METHODS OF POLYSACCHARIDE-BASED NANOPARTICLES

There are several techniques widely used to prepare polysaccharide based nanoparticles, namely precipitation/coacervation, ionotropic gelation, emulsification-solvent diffusion, self-assembly, and polyelectrolyte complexation.

13.7.1 PRECIPITATION/COACERVATION

Precipitation/coacervation involves the use of aqueous solution and gentle processing conditions, thereby it is an ideal technique for the maintenance of the stability of proteins and peptides. The advantage of this technique is the use of the physicochemical properties of the polysaccharides. Chitosan is not soluble in alkaline pH but it tends to precipitate when it comes into contact with an alkaline medium. Nanoparticles are formed by blowing the chitosan into an alkali medium such as NaOH-methanol, ethanediamine, or sodium hydroxide using a compressed air nozzle to prepare the coacervate droplets then evaporation and ultimately purification of the particles which is achieved by the successive washing with the help of hot as well as cold water. The method is diagrammatically represented in Figure 13.1.

Chitosan nanoparticles preparation using a precipitation/coacervation technique can be achieved by dissolving the chitosan in acetic acid solution containing Tween 80. The nanoparticle is formed by the subsequent addition of sodium sulfate solution at a 1 mL/min rate to the solution of chitosan under continuous sonication and gentle agitation. The suspension is then centrifuged for 30 min and the supernatant is separated. Before being resuspended in the water and further centrifuged for 30

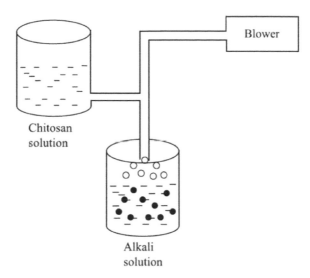

FIGURE 13.1 Chitosan nanoparticle preparation through coacervation/precipitation. (Reprinted from *J Controlled Release* 100, Agnihotri, S.A., Mallikarjuna, N.N., and Aminabhavi, T.M. Recent advances on chitosan-based micro- and nanoparticles in drug delivery, 5–28, Copyright 2004, with permission from Elsevier.)

min, and again the supernatant is discarded. The nanoparticles are kept overnight for being freeze dried and the particle size ranges from 100 to 1000 nm (Berthold et al. 1996). Chitosan/dextran sulfate nanoparticles were developed using this technique and the particles formed had a mean diameter of 223 nm, below optimal conditions, with a zeta potential of about -32.6 mV. The release and the physicochemical features of the nanoparticles could be modulated by changing the ratio of the two ionic polymers (Chen et al. 2003).

13.7.1.1 Modified Coacervation

The coacervation technique involves the separation of a polymer solution into two coexisting phases: one is a dense coacervate phase where the colloids are abundant and other is the supernatant where fewer amounts of colloids are present. In the modified coacervation method there is continuous liquid/liquid phase where separation occurs due to the electrostatic attraction resulting from the mixture of the two oppositely charged colloids (Kumar et al. 2012). In chitosan-alginate nanoparticle preparation, sodium alginate aqueous solution is sprayed into a solution of chitosan under magnetic stirring at a 1000 rpm rate for 30 min. Thus, the nanoparticles form because of the interaction between the chitosan's amino group which is positively charged and alginate's negative groups which are collected via the centrifugation technique (Calvo et al. 1997).

13.7.2 IONOTROPIC GELATION

The mechanism behind the chitosan nanoparticle formulation is based on the electrostatic interaction between the chitosan's amine groups and the polyanion groups like tripolyphosphate. In the ionic gelation method, to get the cation of the chitosan, the chitosan polysaccharide is dissolved in an aqueous acetic acid solution. This solution is then dropwise added to the poyanionic tripolyphosphate solution under a continuous stirring condition. Because of the complexation between the two species being oppositely charged, chitosan undergoes ionic gelation and precipitates spherical-shaped nanoparticles. The method is diagrammatically represented in Figure 13.2.

The surface charge as well as the size of the particles can both be modified through varying the chitosan and stabilizer ratio (Calvo et al. 1997). Ca-alginate nanoparticles were prepared by ion-inducing gelification. The drug encapsulation efficiency of the nanoparticles was found to be

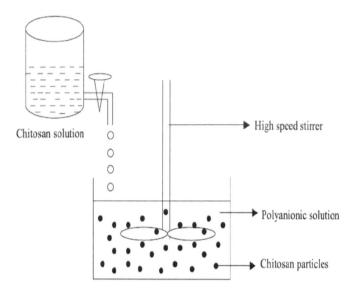

FIGURE 13.2 Chitosan nanoparticle preparation by ionic gelation.(Reprinted from *J Controlled Release* 100, Agnihotri, S.A., Mallikarjuna, N.N., and Aminabhavi, T.M. Recent advances on chitosan-based micro- and nanoparticles in drug delivery, 5–28, Copyright 2004, with permission from Elsevier.)

70%–90% for pyrazinamide and isoniazid, and for rifampicin, it was 80%–90%. The encapsulated drug had a higher relative bioavailability as compared to the free drug. Drugs were found higher than the MIC (minimum inhibitory concentration) in organs up to 15 days post administration (Ahmad et al. 2005).

13.7.3 Emulsification-Solvent Diffusion

This technique is based on the evaporation of the internal phase of emulsion through agitation, so it requires neither elevated temperatures nor the use of phase-separation agents. This method is based on the partial miscibility of an organic solvent with water. The steps of this method are summarized in Figure 13.3.

Under continuous mechanical stirring pursued by a high homogenization pressure, an o/w type emulsion was obtained through injecting the organic phase into a solution of chitosan with

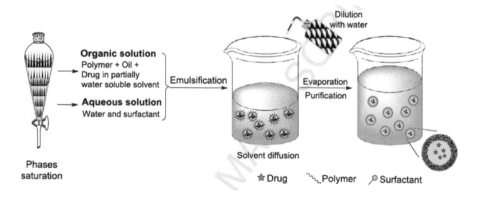

FIGURE 13.3 Polysaccharide nanoparticle preparation through solvent diffusion. (Reprinted from *Mater Sci Eng C*, Crucho, C.I.C. and Barros, M.T. Polymeric nanoparticles: A study on the preparation variables and characterization methods, 771–84, Copyright 2017, with permission from Elsevier.)

a stabilizing agent (poloxamer). Then, the emulsion was diluted by adding a plentiful amount of water and subsequently the precipitation of polymer took place as a result of the organic solvent's diffusion into water, which led to the nanoparticles formation. This method is suitable for hydrophobic drugs and exhibited a great drug entrapment percentage. The major drawbacks of this method includes abrasive processing conditions (organic solvent use) and high shear forces applied during the nanoparticle preparation (El-Shabouri 2002).

13.7.4 SPRAY DRYING

Spray drying is a very well-known technique for producing agglomerates, powders, and granules from the drugs and excipients mixed in solutions and suspensions. This method is basically based on the atomized droplets drying in the stream of hot air. Various process parameters should be controlled in order to achieve the required particle size. Particle size depends on the spray flow rate, size of the nozzle, atomization pressure, temperature of inlet air, and presence of crosslinking agent (Agnihotri et al. 2004). The technique is schematically represented in Figure 13.4. Spray drying is an advantageous technique of encapsulation in comparison to other nanoparticle formulation techniques, including ionotropic pre-gelation and nanoemulsion dispersion, because nanoparticles can be produced relatively quickly and the solution can be fed continuously. It takes only few hours to formulate nanoparticles using the spray drying technique where, as in the case of nanoemulsion dispersion technique, it can take up to a day. Insulin (100 IU/mL, 10 mL) was poured into a 1, 1.5, or 2% w/v alginate solution and gently mixed by using a magnetic stir bar at a speed of 250 rpm. The dispersion was then fed into a spray dryer at a 5 mL/min feed rate, at a 600 L/hour atomization air flow rate, at a 150^0C temperature of inlet and at a 38 m^3/hour aspirator rate. The formed dry particles were collected and stored at a temperature of 2°C–6°C. It was found that the resulting mean particle size was 1.83 ± 0.08 μm. The encapsulation efficiency (EE) using a 1, 1.5, and 2% alginate solution was found to be 16.5 ± 2, 25.9 ± 2, and 26.3 ± 4 respectively.

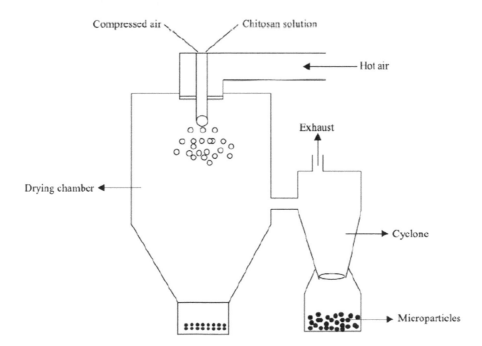

FIGURE 13.4 Preparation of nanoparticles by spray drying technique. (Reprinted from *J Controlled Release* 100, Agnihotri, S.A., Mallikarjuna, N.N., and Aminabhavi, T.M. Recent advances on chitosan-based micro- and nanoparticles in drug delivery, 5–28, Copyright 2004, with permission from Elsevier.)

13.7.5 POLYELECTROLYTE COMPLEXATION

Between the oppositely charged particles, polyelectrolyte complexes are being produced as association complexes. Due to the strong electrostatic interactions, the most remarkable and most extensively used factor in controlling the particle's strength is pH. There are two disparate approaches for preparing the nanoparticles by using two different types of glucomannan. These processes include the interaction between the chitosan and the glucomannan, in presence or absence of an ionic crosslinking agent (sodium tripolyphosphate). The nanoparticles thus formed having 200–700 nm size range as well as a -2–+39 mV zeta potential. Nanoparticles exhibited up to 89% encapsulation efficiency of the protein and peptide. Release of the peptide or protein can be altered by changing the ratio of the composition system (Alonso-Sande et al. 2006). Carboxymethyl konjac glucomannan and chitosan nanoparticles with bovine serum albumin was prepared through a polyelectrolyte complexation method (Du et al. 2005). The encapsulation efficiency and also in-vitro release of the drug was examined and it was found that the nanoparticles not only showed pH-responsive properties but also good ionic strength-sensitive features. Heparin/chitosan nanoparticles with proteins were prepared via a polyelectrolyte complexation method. The effects of the protein concentration on nanoparticle size, polymer molecular weight, protein entrapment efficiency and polymer concentration were studied in detail (Liu et al. 2007). Chitosan/glycyrrhetic acid nanocarriers were prepared through a polyelectrolyte complexation, encapsulation efficiency of the glycyrrhetic acid and also in-vitro drug release were studied in detail. Polyaspartic acid and chitosan nanocarriers with 5-flurouracil were prepared using a polyelectrolyte complexation method (Zheng et al. 2006).

13.7.6 SELF-ASSEMBLY OF HYDROPHOBICALLY MODIFIED POLYSACCHARIDES

Self-assembly is basically characterized by the diffusion pursued via molecular association through non-covalent interactions along with electrostatic or hydrophobic association. Grafting of hydrophilic polymers with hydrophobic chains results in amphiphilic copolymers. Polymeric amphiphiles instinctively form micelles which aggregate in the aqueous solution by inter or intra-molecular associations between the hydrophobic moieties, to reduce the interfacial free energy. The micelles exhibit a small hydrodynamic radius, unusual rheological properties depending upon the hydrophilic, and also hydrophobic moieties and thermodynamic stability. The hydrophilic outer shell that acts as a preservatory for the varied hydrophobic drugs encloses the hydrophobic domain of the micelle.

Chitosan as well as methoxy poly(ethylene glycol) conjugates were prepared by a grafting technique using the formaldehyde-linking method along with a 0.07 mg/mL critical aggregation concentration. The formed conjugates were spherical in shape and 261.9 nm in size.

13.8 MECHANISM OF POLYSACCHARIDIC NANOPARTICLES TRANSPORT

Intestinal epithelium is one of the cardinal absorption barriers in the macromolecular absorption from the lumen of the intestine into systemic circulation (Salama et al. 2006) after oral administration. The villi and micro-villi have a great role in the absorption of macromolecules (Figure 13.5). The epithelial cell layer of these villi and micro-villi is composed mainly of enterocytes, globlet cells, and M cells (Balcerzak et al. 1970; Cheng and Leblond 1974). The most plentiful intestinal epithelial cells are enterocytes which are mainly responsible for transporting the drugs through active transport and passive diffusion. The second most abundant cells are globlet cells, which secret mucus (Neutra et al. 1977; Neutra and Leblond 1966). Another one of the most specialized cells are M cells which reside in the Peyer's patches of ileum and can take up microorganisms and antigens from lumen (Kiyono and Fukuyama 2004). The mechanism for transportation of polysaccharidic nanoparticles in the intestinal epithelium involves either transcellular or paracellular transport. But as effective drug carrier and absorption enhancers (Lin et al. 2007), polysaccharide nanoparticles facilitates both the transcellular as well as the paracellular transport of macromolecules through the intestinal epithelium (Angelova and Hunkeler 2001).

13.8.1 Transcellular Pathway

The transcellular uptake of polysaccharidic nanoparticles takes place by the process of transcytosis through which these nanoparticles get taken up by the enterocytes/M cells, imitating the entry of pathogens, it is likely that chitosan-based nanocarriers are transported through this pathway. The effectiveness of this transcellular transport is enhanced through modifying the nanocarriers physicochemical properties like particle size, mucoadhesivity, etc. Polysaccharidic nanoparticles with a particle size under 100 nm are likely to get absorbed by the enterocytes. Whereas if they have a particle size of 500 nm they are taken up by the M cells of the Peyer's patches and thus overcome the pre-systemic metabolism to increase the drug bioavailability. The nanoparticles transport is achieved effectively by active transcellular transport (Shahbazi and Santos 2013). This transport involves macropinocytosis, phagocytosis, clathrin-mediated endocytosis and caveolin-mediated endocytosis (Chen et al. 2011). Many polysaccharidic nanoparticles (e.g. hyaluronic acid nanoparticles loaded with insulin) are transported through the caco-2 cell monolayer by this transcellular pathway and show a two-fold increase in the apparent permeability co-efficient from apical to basolateral side in comparison to the normal insulin solution (Han et al. 2012; Woitiski et al. 2011) (Figure 13.5).

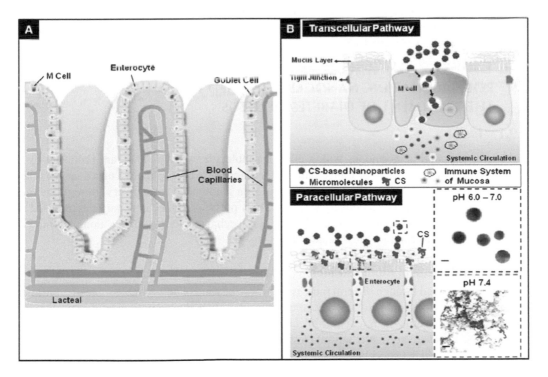

FIGURE 13.5 Mechanism of polysaccharidic nanoparticles transport. (Reprinted with permission from *Adv Drug Deliv Rev*, Chen, M.C., Mi, L.F., Liao, Z.X., Hsiao, C.W., Sonaje, K., Chung, M.F., Hsu, L.W., and Sung, H.W. Recent advances in chitosan-based nanoparticles for oral delivery of macromolecules, 865–9, Copyright 2012, with permission from Elsevier.)

13.8.2 PARACELLULAR PATHWAY

This pathway is the preferable pathway for transportation of hydrophilic drugs. This pathway stymies the entry of macromolecules and particles greater than 1 nm due to very small intercellular spaces as well as tight junctions between the intestinal epithelial cells of the intestine (diameter, 3–10.Å) (Chen et al. 2011). Hence, polysaccharide nanoparticles are not able to pass through the intestinal membrane via this paracellular pathway. In order to be able to transport trough this paracellular pathway, the tight junctions must be reversibly unsealed. This can be carried out by using permeation enhancers, like cationic enhancers (also chitosan and its derivatives) as well as anionic enhancers (also polyacrylic acid and derivatives). But these tight junctions are only opened by these enhancers to a width of <20 nm, which still enables the entry of nanoparticles of >20 nm into systemic circulation (Sonaje et al. 2009). As a denouement, the polysaccharidic nanoparticles should also be disintegrated as well as destabilized in the intercellular space when these nanoparticles approach the intestinal epithelial cells' tight junctions so that the entrapped drugs can be released and entered through the unsealed paracellular pathway. For example, chitosan or the poly(-glutamic acid) NPs (nanoparticles) loaded with insulin got disintegrated at a pH of 7.2–7.4 due to the deprotonization of chitosan and subsequent release of insulin and permeation through the tight junctions of the epithelial cells (Sonaje et al. 2009). Surface charge of the nanoparticles also has a great importance in the destabilization of the tight junctions. Indeed, the positively charged nanoparticles are prone to unseal these nanoparticles whereas the negatively charges nanoparticles do not have such effects. Chitosan works via an electrostatic interaction between the chitosan (positively charged) and cell membranes (negatively charged). Chitosan abates the transepithelial electrical resistance of the monolayers of caco-2 cells. Chitosan acts through the disruption of the tight junctions of the cell membranes, subsequently increasing the absorption of the insulin and eventually reducing the serum glucose level followed by the oral administration of anti-diabetic drug-loaded chitosan nanoparticles (Figure 13.5).

13.9 POLYSACCHARIDIC NANOCARRIERS USED FOR THE TREATMENT OF DIABETES MELLITUS

13.9.1 INSULIN

Insulin are polypeptidic hormones with a 6000 Da molecular weight. They are produced by the β-cells of the pancreatic islets of Langerhans of the intestines. Due to many consequences related to the subcutaneous administration of this drug, insulin is intended for delivery through the many non-invasive routes using novel delivery systems. Many polysaccharidic nanoparticles are used as a novel delivery system. Herein, the insulin-loaded polysaccharidic nanoparticles along with the different routes of administration are discussed below.

13.9.1.1 Oral Route of Administration

Insulin administrated through the oral route is the most convenient and suitable route of administration among the other available routes. The oral route can reduce the limitations of the subcutaneous administration of insulin such as pain, injection phobia, infection, and also the requirements of medical experts. There are many advantages to this route of administration such as there is very low permeability which takes place across the intestinal epithelium for two reasons, one is the high molecular weight of insulin and the other is the presence of the tight junctions of intestinal epithelial cells. Lastly, the cardinal problem associated with it is the low bioavailability of insulin due to the asperity of the gastric environment, which countenances the insulin getting degraded by the cytosolic enzymes of the stomach, like pepsin, trypsin, etc. To overcome such problems regarding the oral route of insulin administration, novel formulation is a remarkable invention. Nanotechnology applied for the loading of insulin is being focused on due its lower toxicity and scalable technologies using naturally occurring, biodegradable, and mucoadhesive polysaccharides such as alginate, chitosan, dextran, and many others.

13.9.1.1.1 Chitosan Nanocarriers

Chitosan is an innovative material which is extensively used as a polymer and copolymer because of its singular characteristics. It is a linear polysaccharide composed of D-glucosamine and N-acetyl-D-glucosamine linked with β-(1–4) (Sharma et al. 2015). This polysaccharide is extracted from the shells of crustaceans, such as shrimp, crabs, and other crustaceans. Chitosan is a naturally occurring polysaccharide, basic, cationic, biocompatible, and mucoadhesive polymer, which is approved by the U.S. FDA for drug delivery and tissue engineering. Chitosan is obtained from chitin. Chitin is abundantly found in natural sources and is bound to minerals and proteins, and must be removed before preparation of chitosan, through the acidification and alkalization processes. Then the purified chitin is N-deacetylated to the chitosan. The process is modified for controlling the properties of the end product (like molecular weight and pKa). Modification is achieved by controlling the degree of acetylation with some factors like reaction conditions (temperature, concentration, chitin to alkali ratio), the source of the chitin, and the extent of the reaction (Sorlier et al. 2001). Chitin is not soluble in water, alcohol, or dilute acids. A few properties, such as solubility in aqueous medium and its cationic character, has reportedly proven as the hallmark for extensive use of this polysaccharide. Among the investigated mucoadhesive polymers, chitosan has been given attention due to its biodegradability, biocompatibility, and its potency for performing the paracellular transport of drugs.

Chitosan acts as a permeation enhancer, by which the tight junctions between the intestinal epithelial cells get opened up by adhering to the mucous membrane and thereby it facilitates the hydrophilic drugs absorption to the blood stream. Chitosan interacts with mucous (negatively charged) forming a complex via hydrogen or ionic bonding and also through hydrophobic interactions. Depending upon the degree of N-deacetylation, the pKa of the chitosan's primary amine is ~6.5. This primary amine group makes a remarkable contribution to chitosan's solubility in acidic pH medium, and the partial neutralization of the primary amine group is responsible for the aggregation of chitosan in a neutral to high pH (Chen et al. 2013).

Graft copolymeric nanoparticles with novel characteristics consisting of chitosan and monomers of chitosan nanoparticles are prepared by ionotropic gelation. Their insulin association efficiency covers a broad range from 2% to 85%, depending on the process and formulation process, and they are highly sensitive to the pH of the formulation. Additionally, it has also been noticed that chitosan-insulin nanoparticles increase the insulin residence time in the small intestine and also enhance the paracellular absorption of insulin into the bloodstream (Sharma et al. 2015). The chitosan-insulin nanoparticle infiltrates into the mucosal layer and transiently opens up the tight junction between the epithelial cell, in turn the nanoparticle degrades because of the pH-sensitivity and thereby releases the insulin into the blood. The chitosan nanoparticle is modified to alter properties like mucoadhesion, stability, and solubility. Both the $-NH_2$ and OH groups are sites of modification.

13.9.1.1.2 Dextran Nanocarriers

Dextran is a naturally occurring polymer of glucose which is linked through α-1,6 glucopyranosidic linkages. It is produced from the sucrose of *Streptococcus mutans* as well as *Leuconostoc mesenteroides*. Dextran is soluble in water, di-methylsulfoxide, and formamide and insoluble in acetone and alcohol. Properties of this polysaccharide, such as it is hydrophilic, biocompatible, biodegradable and non-toxic, make it a potent drug delivery biopolymer (Seino et al. 2010). As insulin is marginally stable and can degrade during formulation (Sluzky et al. 1991), nanoparticular delivery systems encapsulating hydrophilic insulin have been developed in order to get the stable insulin formulation. The dextran-chitosan nanoparticle resulting from the electrostatic interaction between dextran and chitosan does not require any kind of stabilizing agents or external crosslinking agents, and the formulation exhibits excellent stability. Vitamin B12-dextran nanoparticle combinations act as an oral delivery system to protect the insulin against protease enzymes and also shows a faster insulin release profile (Chalasani et al. 2007b; Chalasani et al. 2007a). These conjugates are considered to be a viable carrier for oral insulin delivery for treating diabetes mellitus. A multilayered nanoparticle system containing mucoadhesive polymer, dextran sulfate, sodium alginate, and calcium has been developed to encapsulate insulin which consequently increases resident time at the absorption site. This formulation was further stabilized through chitosan-bound ploxamar 188, again coated with albumin A for giving protection to the insulin from cytosolic enzymatic degradation. This nanoparticular formulation of insulin exhibits an efficient and continual hypoglycemic effect on diabetic rats (Woitiski et al. 2010).

13.9.1.1.3 Polyalkylcyanoacrylated (PACA) Nanocarrier

Initially, PACA was being used as tissue glue (Woodward et al. 1965) due to its stability and biodegradable nature (Lenaerts et al. 1984). Recently, PACA has been used to transport insulin via an intestinal epithelial polymeric carrier via oral administration (Damgé et al. 1988). Insulin was kept unmodified during the covalent binding with the PACA nanoparticles (Kafka et al. 2010). Insulin entrapment in the PACA nanoparticles was achieved through microemulsions with different types of microstructures containing isopropyl myristate, polyglyceryl oleate, caprylocaproyl macrogolglycerides, and the PACA nanoparticle was then investigated for the in vitro release study as well as for bioactivity (Graf et al. 2009). It has been found that insulin-loaded polybutylcyanoacrylated nanoparticle exhibits a better hypoglycemic effect in diabetic rats. So, eventually, it can be concluded that insulin-loaded polyalkylcyanoacrylate nanoparticles have the ability to serve as a stable and trenchant delivery system for the oral administration of insulin (Hou et al. 2005).

13.9.1.1.4 Chitosan-Alginate Nanocarriers

Chitosan-alginate nanocarriers are prepared forming the alginate core's ionotropic pre-gelation that entraps the insulin, pursued by the polyelectrolyte complexation of chitosan, for the successful administration of insulin. Chitosan and alginate polysaccharides are extensively used in the research of drug delivery for giving a sustained release effect. Now we are all aware that chitosan is biocompatible, biodegradable, and effective in the delivery of insulin (Nagpal et al. 2010). Alginate is another linear, natural, and water soluble polysaccharide, which contains a variegated amount of and α-l-guluronic acid (G) as well as 1,4-linked β-d-mannuronic acid (M)) residues. It is a very PH-responsive polysaccharide owing to shrinkage at a lower pH (Dusseault et al. 2005). This enables the retention of the entrapped drug in the gastric environment while protecting it from cytosolic enzymatic degradation. Its biocompatible, biodegradable, mucoadhesive, and non-toxic nature (George and Abraham 2006; Esposito et al. 1996) renders it trenchant in the delivery of insulin orally. The biological efficiency of insulin is maintained by using a divalent ion and calcium in the crosslinking of the alginate (Lin et al. 2005). So, it can be concluded that the chitosan-alginate nanoparticles loaded with insulin provide a remarkable hypoglycemic effect, a sustained release effect, and a much better relative bioavailability.

13.9.1.2 Buccal Route of Administration

The buccal route is another advantageous non-invasive route for insulin delivery. The buccal mucosal layer has low enzymatic activity, excellent accessibility, a large absorptive area, along with an abundant supply of blood vessels and relatively immobile mucosa. This is an important feature for increased residence time, lower risk of trauma, good permeability, and perfusion. Insulin delivered via the buccal route is through aerosol spray into the oral cavity. There are several formulations that greatly influence the release of insulin through the buccal route. These formulations should have absorption enhancers such as bile salts, surfactants, sodium lauryl sulfate, etc., to increase membrane permeability. They should also have enzyme inhibitors to give protection from enzymatic degradation. For getting more advantage from the buccal delivery of insulin, the bioadhesive formulations are the best choice, for example, polysaccharidic nanoparticles like chitosan-reduced gold nanoparticles.

13.9.1.2.1   Chitosan-Reduced Gold Nanoparticles

One novel formulation for the buccal route of insulin delivery is chitosan polysaccharide-reduced gold nanoparticles. This novel formulation has the capability to increase the penetration of insulin through the buccal mucosal layer and remarkably reduce the serum blood glucose level (Bhumkar et al. 2007). Chitosan, which is the cationic natural polysaccharide obtained from chitin, has been mainly used for the synthesis of this novel formulation. Here the chitosan acts as a reducing agent and also as a penetration enhancer. The bovine insulin, chloroauric acid and alloxan are used in this formulation. Chitosan with concentration of 0.05, 0.01, 0.1, and 0.2 was used for the reduction of chloroauric acid for producing the gold nanoparticles. The evaluation parameters of gold nanoparticles are particle size analysis, transmission electron microscopy, viscosity measurements, zeta potential measurements, in-vitro dissolution studies, fluorescence spectroscopy measurements, and in vivo studies

13.9.1.3   Nasal Route of Administration

Nasal administration is another attractive approach for the delivery of insulin. The nasal cavities have a large surface area with a highly vascularized mucosal layer. This route of delivery mainly has two absorption barriers, proteolytic enzymes and mucociliary clearance (Owens et al. 2003). There are many factors that can influence the bioavailability of insulin through the nasal route such as, physicochemical properties, frequency and dosing of insulin administration, concentration of insulin, absorption enhancers, etc. Consequently, most of the nasal formulations have a bioavailability problem ranging between 8% and 15% (Cefalu 2004). To overcome such problems, novel formulation is one of the appropriate methods for the delivery of insulin through nasal route.

13.9.1.3.1   Chitosan Nanoformulation

Chitosan nanoparticles loaded with insulin is a novel formulation prepared by the ionic gelation technique using tripolyphosphate as a counterion. These nanoformulations have the ability to reduce the serum glucose level to 60% as compared to a chitosan-insulin formulation (85%). Other researchers have also focused on other formulations of chitosan delivery such as PEGlylated-trimethyl chitosan complexes loaded with insulin and thiolated-chitosan formulations (Mao et al. 2005) or even chitosan associated with other polysaccharides like alginate (Goycoolea et al. 2009). Chitosan-alginate nanoparticles exhibit the capability of enhancing systemic absorption, i.e. the bioavailability of insulin via the nasal route of administration. Chitosan is also associated with matellic nanoparticles (Bhumkar et al. 2007) like gold chitosan nanoparticles which can efficiently decrease blood glucose level up to 50%, 2 hours after the administration of insulin. This gold-level formulation has also demonstrated a remarkable improvement in chitosan-reduced gold particles uptake. In this formulation, chitosan has a dual activity, acting as a reducing agent in the production of gold nanoparticles and also promoting the penetration ability of insulin through the nasal mucosa.

13.9.1.3.2   Starch Nanoparticles

Other than the chitosan, many polysaccharides are effectively being used in the nasal delivery of insulin. Starch nanoparticles (Jain et al. 2008) loaded with insulin is one of them. These nanoparticles have a profound blood glucose level reduction ability at around 70% lasting for 6 hours.

13.9.1.4   Pulmonary Route of Administration

The lungs are another non-invasive route of drug delivery for getting a high systemic bioavailability. They can avoid the hepatic first pass metabolism, protect the drug from enzymatic degradation and also has a high bioavailability (Yang et al. 2008; Patton and Byron 2007). It is appropriate for the delivery of protein and peptide drugs like insulin. A lot of studies have been done using insulin as a protein drug to show its sustained release properties via the pulmonary route (Lim et al. 2009; Zhao et al. 2011; Xu et al. 2011). As insulin has a lot of problems with subcutaneous delivery as well as with the conventional dosage form, the invention of novel delivery formulations is desperately needed. Insulin-loaded gelatin polysaccharidic nanoparticles are effectively used for this purpose.

13.9.1.4.1 Gelatin Nanocarriers

As a natural polysaccharide, gelatin is highly biocompatible and cheap, and its degradation product is non-toxic and can be excreted from the body readily, which is its most remarkable feature. These properties enable it to be a significant ingredient in the formulation of gelatin-based nanoparticles, loaded with insulin and followed by pulmonary administration (Vandelli et al. 2001). As a soluble polymer, gelatin is not suitable for preparing the stable formulation, and it is too tough to control the rate of insulin release, so it needs modification to enable its use as a nanocarrier. D,L-glyceraldehyde is a non-toxic agent (Vandelli et al. 2001), which is utilized as a modifier for gelatin-based nanoparticles. Additionally, poloxamer 188 is also incorporated into the formulation to ameliorate the drug-holding capability as well as the penetration capability. The water-in-water (W/W) emulsion, this novel method of preparation was used for preparing nanoparticles, using mild conditions to assure the bioactivity of the insulin. The 1:1 ratio of the gelation to poloxamer 188 provided trenchant pulmonary insulin absorption and a high relative pharmacological bioavailability.

13.9.2 GLUCAGON-LIKE PEPTIDE 1(GLP)

Almost more than 20 peptide hormones get released by the gastrointestinal tract and glucagon-like peptide-1(GLP-1) is one of them. GLP-1 is a peptide of 30 amino acids which is secreted by the small intestinal L-cells (Herrmann et al. 1995). This hormone exhibits its effects through binding with GLP-1 receptors of the pancreatic β-cells, which is a G-protein coupled receptor. Only during hypoglycemia, the GLP-1 signaling pathway gets activated, which means that insulin secretion is restrained by GLP-1 in a glucose-dependent manner. GLP-1 also stymies the release of glucagon from the pancreas and the synthesis of glucose from the liver. Moreover, it occludes the B-cell apoptosis and delays gastric emptying. The beneficial effects depicted by GLP-1 intimated that it is a promising therapeutic substance for the management of type 2 diabetes mellitus.

However, GLP gets rapidly cleaved by dipeptidyl peptidase-IV (DPPIV). Even if, the GLP is able to escape the hepatic first pass metabolism, it gets exposed to degradation by the enzymes of the liver and eventually in blood circulation, leaving the peptide with a mere 2–3 min half-life. The problems regarding the oral administration of glucagon-like peptide 1 can be overcome through employing a novel delivery systems.

13.9.2.1 Chitosan Nanocarriers

Now we all are aware of the advantages of nanoparticle delivery systems over ordinary delivery. A oral nanoparticle formulation of GLP-1 needs to be protected from enzymatic degradation in the gastrointestinal tract to allow it to penetrate into the intestinal mucosal layer (Ensign et al. 2012). The latter is achieved through modifying the surface of the nanoparticles using bioadhesive polysaccharides such as chitosan (Araújo et al. 2014). In comparison to the non-coated poly(DL-lactic acid-co-glycolic acid) (PLGA) nanoparticles, the chitosan-coated porous silicon nanoparticles exhibited slower release of GLP-1 in the intestine. The amount of GLP-1 released from the silicon nanoparticles as well as from the chitosan-coated PGLA was 35% and 21% respectively. Although this release study was performed for only 6 hours, thereafter, the time taken for complete GLP-1 release from the nanoparticles and the release profile was not known. The researchers are now focused on addressing the stability of the porous silicon nanoparticles and chitosan-coated PLGA nanoparticulate systems that can withstand the abrasive environment of gastrointestinal tract. By applying the microfluidic technology (Araujo et al. 2015) as well as flow reactor technology (aerosol) (Shrestha et al. 2015), chitosan-coated nanoparticles loaded with GLP-1 were encapsulated into pH-responsive polymeric nanocarriers, which can also be loaded with the dipeptidyl peptidase-IV inhibitor (DPPIV inhibitor) forming a nano-in-nano delivery system. Consequently, GLP-1 released from the nanomatrix had much greater permeability through the intestinal cells as compared to the GLP-1, which was released from the chitosan-coated nanoparticles.

13.9.3 REPAGLINIDE

Repaglinide is another oral medication for treating diabetes mellitus. This drug mainly acts by sealing the potassium channels present in β-cells membrane which are ATP-dependent. Repaglinide is a fast acting meglitinide class medication with an extensively short biological half-life (1h) as well as a very low bioavailability (50%). To overcome such common problems related with conventional dosage forms, researchers' interests have inclined to the preparation of novel dosage formulations. Biodegradable nanoparticles are frequently used and preferable in the improvement of the therapeutic value of various water soluble and insoluble drugs because they can improve the bioavailability, solubility, and retention time of the drugs. Such nanoparticles also have the potential to provide a controlled and sustained release delivery of the drugs.

13.9.3.1 Chitosan Nanoparticles

Among all the various biodegradable polymers used for developing a sustained release drug delivery system, one of the most widely used polymers is chitosan and its derivatives. Repaglinide-loaded chitosan nanoparticles were successfully prepared by a solvent evaporation method. These repaglinide-loaded chitosan nanoparticles have a high loading and encapsulation efficiency as well as a small and narrow size distribution. In-vitro drug release studies have shown that these repaglinide-loaded nanoparticles are able to release the drug in a slow sustained manner. They can ameliorate the oral absorption of repaglinide owing to the high surface-to-volume ratio and higher biodistribution. Therefore, bioavailability can be improved and can also help to reduce the dose and frequency of the drug. So, ultimately it can be concluded that repaglinide-loaded chitosan nanoparticles are effective nanocarriers in the field of controlled release drug delivery of very poor water soluble drugs, like repaglinide.

13.9.4 GLIPIZIDE

Glipizide is a second generation sulfonyl urea, it helps to lower serum glucose levels in patients with type 2 diabetes mellitus by inducing the insulin from pancreatic β-cells. It has a several advantages, like low side effects, low cost, and it can also be administered to the renal failure patients. The only drawback is that the drug is very short acting in nature. It gets absorbed rapidly, reduces serum glucose level within 30 min, achieves peak concentration within 1–3 hours and then finally rapidly eliminates from the body owing to the very short half-life (2–4 hours). Therefore, the drug has to be given multiple times which results in patient noncompliance. To overcome these obstacles, researchers have endeavored to formulate novel formulations with a controlled release effect.

13.9.4.1 Alginate-Chitosan Nanoparticles

Alginate-chitosan nanoparticles are the more appropriate and convenient drug delivery approach for glipizide delivery. They have a lot of advantages such as a good release profile, good therapeutic efficacy, better maintenance on the plasma drug level, and many others, fewer side effects, and ultimately a controlled release profile. These formulations are biocompatible, non-toxic, stable, and have mucoadhesive property owing to the alginate-chitosan nanocarriers. These formulations have the ability to reduce the concentration fluctuation problem within the therapeutic window as well as the GIT side effects. Owing to the controlled release properties of the formulation, the plasma drug concentration maintained properly that enables lesser dosing frequency which in turn increases patient compliance. Also, due to the greater surface-volume ratio of this formulation, the concentration can readily achieve a therapeutic level. The water solubility properties can also resolve the low water solubility problem of glipizide. These alginate-chitosan-coated nanoparticles are prepared through an ionotropic controlled gelation method. The interaction between the alginate and the Ca^{+2} ion leads to the formation of a pre-gel state, which is also known as an egg- box structure, which avoids the gel point and produces the continuous phase. Subsequent administration of chitosan, as a poly cationic agent, results in the formation of poly electrolyte complex that can stabilize the pre-gel form of alginate into the nanoparticles. This method of preparation has many advantages, including absence of heat, share forces, and organic solvents.

13.9.5 Pioglitazone HCL

Chemically, pioglitazone HCL is a thiazolidinedione monohydrochloride which belongs in the class of thiazolidinedione. It is helpful in decreasing insulin resistance in the liver and in periphery and it is effectively used in the treatment of type 2 DM. It stimulates the peroxisome proliferator-activated receptor gamma (PPAR-ɣ). But very short half-life and low water-solubility restricts the feasible bioavailability. To evade this problem and provide a sustained release effect to this drug, novel delivery is approached.

13.9.5.1 Chitosan Nanoparticles

Chitosan nanoparticles are very efficient for the oral delivery of low solubility drugs like pioglitazon. They increase bioavailability through a particle uptake mechanism and also have very slow transit times which enhances the concentration gradient through the absorptive cells. These nanoparticles can be prepared through an ionic gelation method using mild conditions. The release pattern also shows a slow and controlled release effect of the drug.

13.10 FUTURE PROSPECTS AND CONCLUSION

Polysaccharidic nanoparticles are being used as a promising approach in the oral delivery of insulin and other anti-diabetic drugs. Many drawbacks can be overcome by this type of delivery, such as bioavailability, drugs protection from the abrasive gastrointestinal environment, stability, etc. This drug delivery system also provides protection of active ingredient from abrasive gastrointestinal environment and sustained/controlled released properties. Hence, a lot of investigation is ongoing in anticipation of the oral delivery of insulin and other anti-diabetic drugs through drug-loaded polysaccharide nanoparticular systems.

REFERENCES

Agnihotri, S.A., Mallikarjuna, N.N., and Aminabhavi, T.M. 2004. Recent advances on chitosan-based micro- and nanoparticles in drug delivery. *J Control Release* 100: 5–28.

Ahmad, Z., Zahoor, A., Sharma, S., and Khuller, G.K. 2005. Inhalable alginate nanoparticles as antitubercular drug carriers against experimental tuberculosis. *Int J Antimicrob Agents* 26: 298–303.

Alonso-Sande, M., Cuña, M., Remuñán-López, C., Teijeiro-Osorio, D., Alonso-Lebrero, J.L., and Alonso, M.J. 2006. Formation of new glucomannan–chitosan nanoparticles and study of their ability to associate and deliver proteins. *Macromolecules* 39: 4152–8.

Angelova, N. and Hunkeler, D. 2001. Effect of preparation conditions on properties and permeability of chitosan-sodium hexametaphosphate capsules. *J Biomater Sci Polym Ed* 12: 1317–37.

Araújo, F., Shrestha, N., Shahbazi, M.-A., Fonte, P., Mäkilä, E.M., Salonen, J.J., Hirvonen, J.T., Granja, P.L., Santos, H.A., and Sarmento, B. 2014. The impact of nanoparticles on the mucosal translocation and transport of GLP-1 across the intestinal epithelium. *Biomaterials* 35: 9199–207.

Balcerzak, S.P., Lane, W.C., and Bullard, J.W. 1970. Surface structure of intestinal epithelium. *Gastroenterology* 58: 49–55.

Berthold, A., Cremer, K., and Kreuter, J. 1996. Preparation and characterization of chitosan microspheres as drug carrier for prednisolone sodium phosphate as model for anti-inflammatory drugs. *J Control Release* 39: 17–25.

Bhumkar, D.R., Joshi, H.M., Sastry, M., and Pokharkar, V.B. 2007. Chitosan reduced gold nanoparticles as novel carriers for transmucosal delivery of insulin. *Pharm Res* 24: 1415–26.

Calvo, P., Remuñán-López, C., Vila-Jato, J.L., and Alonso, M.J. 1997. Novel hydrophilic chitosan-polyethylene oxide nanoparticles as protein carriers. *J Appl Polym Sci* 63: 125–32.

Cefalu, W.T. 2004. Concept, strategies, and feasibility of noninvasive insulin delivery. *Diabetes Care* 27: 239–46.

Chakraborty, C., Pal, S., Doss, G.P.C., Wen, Z.H., and Lin, C.-S. 2013. Nanoparticles as "smart" pharmaceutical delivery. *Front Biosci Landmark Ed* 18: 1030–50.

Chalasani, K.B., Russell-Jones, G.J., Jain, A.K., Diwan, P.V., and Jain, S.K. 2007a. Effective oral delivery of insulin in animal models using vitamin B12-coated dextran nanoparticles. *J Control Release* 122: 141–50.

Chalasani, K.B., Russell-Jones, G.J., Yandrapu, S.K., Diwan, P.V., and Jain, S.K. 2007b. A novel vitamin B12-nanosphere conjugate carrier system for peroral delivery of insulin. *J Control Release* 117: 421–9.

Chen, M.C., Sonaje, K., Chen, K.J., and Sung, H.W. 2011. A review of the prospects for polymeric nanoparticle platforms in oral insulin delivery. *Biomaterials* 32: 9826–38.

Chen, M.C., Mi, F.L., Liao, Z.X., Hsiao, C.W., Sonaje, K., Chung, M.F., Hsu, L.W., and Sung, H.W. 2013. Recent advances in chitosan-based nanoparticles for oral delivery of macromolecules. *Adv Drug Deliv Rev* 65: 865–79.

Chen, Y., Mohanraj, V.J., and Parkin, J.E. 2003. Chitosan-dextran sulfate nanoparticles for delivery of an anti-angiogenesis peptide. *Lett Pept Sci* 10: 621–9.

Cheng, H. and Leblond, C.P. 1974. Origin, differentiation and renewal of the four main epithelial cell types in the mouse small intestine. V. Unitarian theory of the origin of the four epithelial cell types. *Am J Anat* 141: 537–61.

Coviello, T., Matricardi, P., Marianecci, C., and Alhaique, F. 2007. Polysaccharide hydrogels for modified release formulations. *J Control Release* 119: 5–24.

Damgé, C., Michel, C., Aprahamian, M., and Couvreur, P. 1988. New approach for oral administration of insulin with polyalkylcyanoacrylate nanocapsules as drug carrier. *Diabetes* 37: 246–51.

Damgé, C., Maincent, P., and Ubrich, N. 2007. Oral delivery of insulin associated to polymeric nanoparticles in diabetic rats. *J Control Release* 117: 163–70.

Damgé, C., Reis, C.P., and Maincent, P. 2008. Nanoparticle strategies for the oral delivery of insulin. *Expert Opin Drug Deliv* 5: 45–68.

Du, J., Sun, R., Zhang, S., Zhang, L. F., Xiong, C.-D., and Peng, Y.-X. 2005. Novel polyelectrolyte carboxymethyl konjac glucomannan-chitosan nanoparticles for drug delivery. I. Physicochemical characterization of the carboxymethyl konjac glucomannan-chitosan nanoparticles. *Biopolymers* 78: 1–8.

Dusseault, J., Leblond, F.A., Robitaille, R., Jourdan, G., Tessier, J., Ménard, M., Henley, N., and Hallé, J.-P. 2005. Microencapsulation of living cells in semi-permeable membranes with covalently cross-linked layers. *Biomaterials* 26: 1515–22.

El-Shabouri, M.H. 2002. Positively charged nanoparticles for improving the oral bioavailability of cyclosporin-A. *Int J Pharm* 249: 101–8.

Ensign, L.M., Cone, R., and Hanes, J. 2012. Oral drug delivery with polymeric nanoparticles: The gastrointestinal mucus barriers. *Adv Drug Deliv Rev* 64: 557–70.

Esposito, E., Cortesi, R., and Nastruzzi, C. 1996. Gelatin microspheres: Influence of preparation parameters and thermal treatment on chemico-physical and biopharmaceutical properties. *Biomaterials* 17: 2009–20.

Farokhzad, O.C. and Langer, R. 2009. Impact of nanotechnology on drug delivery. *ACS Nano* 3: 16–20.

Galindo-Rodriguez, S.A., Allemann, E., Fessi, H., and Doelker, E. 2005. Polymeric nanoparticles for oral delivery of drugs and vaccines: A critical evaluation of in vivo studies. *Crit Rev Ther Drug Carrier Syst* 22: 419–64.

George, M. and Abraham, T.E. 2006. Polyionic hydrocolloids for the intestinal delivery of protein drugs: Alginate and chitosan—a review. *J Control Release* 114: 1–14.

Goycoolea, F.M., Lollo, G., Remuñán-López, C., Quaglia, F., and Alonso, M.J. 2009. Chitosan-alginate blended nanoparticles as carriers for the transmucosal delivery of macromolecules. *Biomacromolecules* 10: 1736–43.

Graf, A., Rades, T., and Hook, S.M. 2009. Oral insulin delivery using nanoparticles based on microemulsions with different structure-types: Optimisation and in vivo evaluation. *Eur J Pharm Sci* 37: 53–61.

Hall, J.B., Dobrovolskaia, M.A., Patri, A.K., and McNeil, S.E. 2007. Characterization of nanoparticles for therapeutics. *Nanomed* 2: 789–803.

Han, L., Zhao, Y., Yin, L., Li, R., Liang, Y., Huang, H., Pan, S., Wu, C., and Feng, M. 2012. Insulin-loaded pH-sensitive hyaluronic acid nanoparticles enhance transcellular delivery. *AAPS Pharm Sci Tech* 13: 836–45.

Herrero, E.P., Alonso, M.J., and Csaba, N. 2012. Polymer-based oral peptide nanomedicines. *Ther Deliv* 3: 657–68.

Herrmann, C., Göke, R., Richter, G., Fehmann, H.C., Arnold, R., and Göke, B. 1995. Glucagon-like peptide-1 and glucose-dependent insulin-releasing polypeptide plasma levels in response to nutrients. *Digestion* 56: 117–26.

Hou, Z., Zhang, Z., Xu, Z., Zhang, H., Tong, Z., and Leng, Y. 2005. The stability of insulin-loaded polybutylcyanoacrylate nanoparticles in an oily medium and the hypoglycemic effect in diabetic rats. *Yao Xue Bao* 40: 57–64.

Jain, A., Gupta, Y., and Jain, S.K. 2007. Perspectives of biodegradable natural polysaccharides for site-specific drug delivery to the colon. *J Pharm Sc* 10: 86–128.

Jung, T., Kamm, W., Breitenbach, A., Kaiserling, E., Xiao, J.X., and Kissel, T. 2000. Biodegradable nanoparticles for oral delivery of peptides: Is there a role for polymers to affect mucosal uptake? *Eur J Pharm Biopharm* 50: 147–60.

Kafka, A.P., Kleffmann, T., Rades, T., and McDowell, A. 2010. Characterization of peptide polymer interactions in poly(alkylcyanoacrylate) nanoparticles: A mass spectrometric approach. *Curr Drug Deliv* 7: 208–15.

Kavimandan, N.J., Losi, E., and Peppas, N.A. 2006. Novel delivery system based on complexation hydrogels as delivery vehicles for insulin-transferrin conjugates. *Biomaterials* 27: 3846–54.

Kiyono, H. and Fukuyama, S. 2004. NALT- versus Peyer's-patch-mediated mucosal immunity. *Nat Rev Immunol* 4: 699–710.

Kumar, S., Dilbaghi, N., Saharan, R., and Bhanjana, G. 2012. Nanotechnology as emerging tool for enhancing solubility of poorly water-soluble drugs. *Bio Nano Science* 4: 227–50.

Kumari, A., Yadav, S.K., and Yadav, S.C. 2010. Biodegradable polymeric nanoparticles based drug delivery systems. *Colloids Surf B Biointerfaces* 75: 1–18.

Lenaerts, V., Nagelkerke, J.F., Berkel, T.J.C.V., Couvreur, P., Grislain, L., Roland, M., and Speiser, P. 1984. In vivo uptake of polyisobutyl cyanoacrylate nanoparticles by rat liver kupffer, endothelial, and parenchymal cells. *J Pharm Sci* 73: 980–2.

Li, C.L. and Deng, Y.J. 2004. Oil-based formulations for oral delivery of insulin. *J Pharm Pharmacol* 56: 1101–7.

Lim, S.H., Park, H.W., Shin, C.H., Kwon, J.H., and Kim, C.W. 2009. Human insulin microcrystals with lactose carriers for pulmonary delivery. *Biosci Biotechnol Biochem* 73: 2576–82.

Lin, Y.H., Liang, H.F., Chung, C.K., Chen, M.C., and Sung, H.W. 2005. Physically crosslinked alginate/N,O-carboxymethyl chitosan hydrogels with calcium for oral delivery of protein drugs. *Biomaterials* 26: 2105–13.

Lin, Y.H., Mi, F.L., Chen, C.T., Chang, W.C., Peng, S.F., Liang, H.F., and Sung, H.W. 2007. Preparation and characterization of nanoparticles shelled with chitosan for oral insulin delivery. *Biomacromolecules* 8: 146–52.

Liu, Z., Jiao, Y., Liu, F., and Zhang, Z. 2007. Heparin/chitosan nanoparticle carriers prepared by polyelectrolyte complexation. *J Biomed Mater Res A* 83: 806–12.

Lochner, N., Pittner, F., Wirth, M., and Gabor, F. 2003. Wheat germ agglutinin binds to the epidermal growth factor receptor of artificial Caco-2 membranes as detected by silver nanoparticle enhanced fluorescence. *Pharm Res* 20: 833–9.

Mao, S., Germershaus, O., Fischer, D., Linn, T., Schnepf, R., and Kissel, T. 2005. Uptake and transport of PEG-graft-trimethyl-chitosan copolymer-insulin nanocomplexes by epithelial cells. *Pharm Res* 22: 2058–68.

Mehvar, R. 2003. Recent trends in the use of polysaccharides for improved delivery of therapeutic agents: Pharmacokinetic and pharmacodynamic perspectives. *Curr Pharm Biotechnol* 4: 283–302.

Morris, G., Kök, S., Harding, S., and Adams, G. 2010. Polysaccharide drug delivery systems based on pectin and chitosan. *Biotechnol Genet Eng Rev* 27: 257–84.

Mourya, V.K. and Inamdar, N.N. 2009. Trimethyl chitosan and its applications in drug delivery. *J Mater Sci Mater Med* 20: 1057–79.

Mukhopadhyay, P., Sarkar, K., Chakraborty, M., Bhattacharya, S., Mishra, R., and Kundu, P.P. 2013. Oral insulin delivery by self-assembled chitosan nanoparticles: In vitro and in vivo studies in diabetic animal model. *Mater Sci Eng C Mater Biol Appl* 33: 376–82.

Nagpal, K., Singh, S.K., and Mishra, D.N. 2010. Chitosan nanoparticles: A promising system in novel drug delivery. *Chem Pharm Bull (Tokyo)* 58: 1423–30.

Neutra, M. and Leblond, C.P. 1966. Synthesis of the carbohydrate of mucus in the golgi complex as shown by electron microscope radioautography of goblet cells from rats injected with glucose-H3. *J Cell Biol* 30: 119–36.

Neutra, M.R., Grand, R.J., and Trier, J.S. 1977. Glycoprotein synthesis, transport, and secretion by epithelial cells of human rectal mucosa: normal and cystic fibrosis. *Lab Investig J Tech Methods Pathol* 36: 535–46.

Owens, D.R., Zinman, B., and Bolli, G. 2003. Alternative routes of insulin delivery. *Diabet Med J Br Diabet Assoc* 20: 886–98.

des Rieux, A., Fievez, V., Garinot, M., Schneider, Y.J., and Préat, V. 2006. Nanoparticles as potential oral delivery systems of proteins and vaccines: A mechanistic approach. *J Control Release* 116: 1–27.

Roger, E., Lagarce, F., Garcion, E., and Benoit, J.P. 2010. Biopharmaceutical parameters to consider in order to alter the fate of nanocarriers after oral delivery. *Nanomed* 5: 287–306.

Salama, N.N., Eddington, N.D., and Fasano, A. 2006. Tight junction modulation and its relationship to drug delivery. *Adv Drug Deliv Rev* 58: 15–28.

Saravanakumar, G., Jo, D.-G., and Park, J.H. 2012. Polysaccharide-based nanoparticles: A versatile platform for drug delivery and biomedical imaging. *Curr Med Chem* 19: 3212–29.

Seino, Y., Nanjo, K., Tajima, N., Kadowaki, T., Kashiwagi, A., Araki, E., Ito, C., Inagaki, N., Iwamoto, Y., Kasuga, M. et al. 2010. Report of the committee on the classification and diagnostic criteria of diabetes mellitus. *J Diabetes Investig* 1: 212–28.

Shahbazi, M.A. and Santos, H.A. 2013. Improving oral absorption via drug-loaded nanocarriers: Absorption mechanisms, intestinal models and rational fabrication. *Curr Drug Metab* 14: 28–56.

Shaji, J. and Patole, V. 2008. Protein and peptide drug delivery: Oral approaches. *Indian J Pharm Sci* 70: 269–77.

Sharma, G., Sharma, A.R., Nam, J.S., Doss, G.P.C., Lee, S.-S., and Chakraborty, C. 2015. Nanoparticle based insulin delivery system: The next generation efficient therapy for Type 1 diabetes. *J Nanobiotechnology* 13.

Shrestha, N., Shahbazi, M.A., Araújo, F., Mäkilä, E., Raula, J., Kauppinen, E.I., Salonen, J., Sarmento, B., Hirvonen, J., and Santos, H.A. 2015. Multistage pH-responsive mucoadhesive nanocarriers prepared by aerosol flow reactor technology: A controlled dual protein-drug delivery system. *Biomaterials* 68: 9–20.

Shukla, R.K. and Tiwari, A. 2012. Carbohydrate polymers: Applications and recent advances in delivering drugs to the colon. *Carbohydr Polym* 88: 399–416.

Sluzky, V., Tamada, J.A., Klibanov, A.M., and Langer, R. 1991. Kinetics of insulin aggregation in aqueous solutions upon agitation in the presence of hydrophobic surfaces. *Proc Natl Acad Sci U S A* 88: 9377–81.

Sonaje, K., Lin, Y.H., Juang, J.H., Wey, S.P., Chen, C.T., and Sung, H.W. 2009. In vivo evaluation of safety and efficacy of self-assembled nanoparticles for oral insulin delivery. *Biomaterials* 30: 2329–39.

Sorlier, P., Denuzière, A., Viton, C., and Domard, A. 2001. Relation between the degree of acetylation and the electrostatic properties of chitin and chitosan. *Biomacromolecules* 2: 765–72.

Suri, S.S., Fenniri, H., and Singh, B. 2007. Nanotechnology-based drug delivery systems. *J Occup Med Toxicol Lond Engl* 2: 16.

Thanou, M., Verhoef, J.C., and Junginger, H.E. 2001a. Chitosan and its derivatives as intestinal absorption enhancers. *Adv Drug Deliv Rev* 50 Suppl 1: S91–101.

Thanou, M., Verhoef, J.C., and Junginger, H.E. 2001b. Oral drug absorption enhancement by chitosan and its derivatives. *Adv Drug Deliv Rev* 52: 117–26.

Vandamme, K., Melkebeek, V., Cox, E., Deforce, D., Lenoir, J., Adriaens, E., Vervaet, C., and Remon, J.P. 2010. Influence of reaction medium during synthesis of Gantrez AN 119 nanoparticles for oral vaccination. *Eur J Pharm Biopharm* 74: 202–8.

Vandelli, M.A., Rivasi, F., Guerra, P., Forni, F., and Arletti, R. 2001. Gelatin microspheres crosslinked with D,L-glyceraldehyde as a potential drug delivery system: Preparation, characterisation, in vitro and in vivo studies. *Int J Pharm* 215: 175–84.

Woitiski, C.B., Neufeld, R.J., Veiga, F., Carvalho, R.A., and Figueiredo, I.V. 2010. Pharmacological effect of orally delivered insulin facilitated by multilayered stable nanoparticles. *Eur J Pharm Sci* 41: 556–63.

Woitiski, C.B., Sarmento, B., Carvalho, R.A., Neufeld, R.J., and Veiga, F. 2011. Facilitated nanoscale delivery of insulin across intestinal membrane models. *Int J Pharm* 412: 123–31.

Woodward, S.C., Herrmann, J.B., Cameron, J.L., Brandes, G., Pulaski, E.J., and Leonard, F. 1965. Histotoxicity of Cyanoacrylate Tissue Adhesive in the Rat. *Ann Surg* 162: 113–22.

Xu, Y.Y., Lu, C.T., Fu, H.X., Zhao, Y.Z., Yang, W., Li, X., Zhang, L., Li, X.K., and Zhang, M. 2011. Comparing the enhancement efficiency between liposomes and microbubbles for insulin pulmonary absorption. *Diabetes Technol Ther* 13: 759–65.

Yang, X.D., Zhang, Q.Q., Wang, Y.S., Chen, H., Zhang, H.Z., Gao, F.P., and Liu, L.R. 2008. Self-aggregated nanoparticles from methoxy poly(ethylene glycol)-modified chitosan: synthesis; characterization; aggregation and methotrexate release in vitro. *Colloids Surf* B 61, 125–131.

Zhao, Y.Z., Xu, Y.-Y., Li, X., Lu, C.T., Zhang, L., Dai, D.-D., Sun, C.Z., Lv, H.F., Li, X.K., and Yang, W. 2011. An in vivo experiment to improve pulmonary absorption of insulin using microbubbles. *Diabetes Technol Ther* 13: 1013–21.

Zheng, Y., Wu, Y., Yang, W., Wang, C., Fu, S., and Shen, X. 2006. Preparation, characterization, and drug release in vitro of chitosan-glycyrrhetic acid nanoparticles. *J Pharm Sci* 95: 181–91.

14 Chitosan-Based Nanoparticulate System for Pulmonary Drug Delivery

Tapan Kumar Giri, Bijaya Ghosh, and Falguni Patra

CONTENTS

14.1 INTRODUCTION

The respiratory tract is an attractive target for delivery of drugs for both local and systemic effect. It is the target organ for treatment of respiratory diseases, as its high vascularity and wide surface area offer adequate scope for systemic absorption (Azarmi et al. 2008; Sung et al. 2007; Jaafar-Maalej et al. 2012). Compared to the oral route, this route also has the added advantage: the avoidance of the first pass effect (Sung et al. 2007) which allows for drug targetability and diminishes the side effects (Beck-Broichsitter et al. 2009; Beck-Broichsitter et al. 2012). Administration of drugs through the pulmonary route is not a new concept. Liquid nebulizers were developed at the start of 19th century and a number of drugs such as procaine insulin, adrenaline, steroids, and penicillin were available as inhalation therapy. But the introduction of a metered dose inhaler by the pharmaceutical aerosol industry in 1956 completely revolutionized the treatment of many difficult to treat respiratory diseases. The management of asthma and chronic obstructive pulmonary diseases became far more effective (McAllen et al. 1974).

With advances in science and technology, many more drugs have been successfully developed for inhalation therapy (O'Riordan 2000). Presently this route is being used for treatment of bacterial infections (Muttil et al. 2009; Geller et al 2011), fungal infections (Mohammad and Klein 2006), chronic obstructive pulmonary disease (Jones et al. 2011), cancer (Huland et al. 2003; Videira et al. 2012), influenza virus infection (Bernstein et al. 1988), diabetes (de Galan et al. 2006), and cystic fibrosis (Aitken et al. 1992). Additionally, it is being investigated for the non-invasive delivery routes for vaccines (Hokey and Misra 2011; Lu et al. 2010).

However, the majority of inhalable dosage forms suffer from the restrictions of low bioavailability because of normal mucociliary clearance. This results in a short half-life which necessitates repeated dosing. Hence, there is a need to discover strategies for overcoming these limitations and develop efficient inhalation therapies which would be able to deliver drugs for prolonged periods with a controlled therapeutic effect. Delivering drugs in nanoparticulate dosage forms is an important option when answering this need.

A significant branch of pharmaceutical research is devoted to the development of nanodosage forms as potential alternatives to conventional inhaled formulations. The objective of this type of research is to develop formulations with enhanced biopharmaceutical features (Roy and Vij 2010; Mansour et al. 2009 Bailey and Berkland 2009; Smola et al. 2008)

14.2 ANATOMY AND PHYSIOLOGY OF THE LUNG

The human respiratory system can be broadly divided into two sections; lower respiratory tract and the upper respiratory tract. The lower section consists of the lungs, larynx, bronchi, trachea, and alveoli, whereas the upper section comprises of the nose, nasal cavity, and pharynx. The two lungs of the human body are entrusted with the job of the supply of oxygen and gas exchange. The core of the lungs is full of tiny blood vessels, lymph tissue, bronchi, fine air passages, and more than 300 million alveoli (Paranjpe and Muller-Goymann 2014). Each alveolus is lined with a huge number of capillaries and provides a huge surface area for the blood gas barrier (El-Sherbiny et al. 2015). The alveoli are coated with mucus and alveolar fluids containing surface proteins and phospholipids which reduce surface tension and facilitate gas exchange. The layer is bounded with numerous cells, nerve endings, macrophages, fibroblasts, and lymph vessels making it a perfect location for drug administration for pulmonary and lymphatic diseases (Paranjpe and Muller-Goymann 2014). Endowed with a high vascularity and a large absorptive surface area, the respiratory tract is an exceedingly attractive target for non-invasive administration of drugs for systemic effect too.

For therapeutic effectiveness, inhaled drugs should proficiently deposit in the airways for local action and pass through the air-blood barrier for systemic action. Numerous conditions, such as anatomical, organic, and pathological factors, play an important role in controlling deposition and absorption of drugs administered through the pulmonary route.

One vital parameter that determines drug deposition in the respiratory tract is airway geometry. The airways of the lung are exceedingly branched and with each division the pathway gets narrower (Figure 14.1). Accordingly, the air velocity varies in different respiratory zones (De Marzo et al. 1989). Hence the likelihood of particle deposition in a specific lung area increases as airways decrease in radius. The size and distribution patterns of aerosolized droplets maybe different in lungs areas of different moisture content (Phipps et al. 1994). The high humidity of the lung also influences the particle deposition profile.

Particles having sizes in the range of 0.5–1 μm are mainly trapped in the alveolai; particles <0.5 μm are mostly exhaled (Yang et al. 2008). Usually nanoparticles released from an atomizer device aggregate to form bigger particles of micrometer sizes. The aggregates with an adequate mass form sediments in the respiratory tract and reside longer time to produce the desired effect in the bronchiolar region. Moreover, particle properties, their size, shape, and surface characteristics play a vital role in particle deposition. Air velocity, tidal volume, holding of breath, and breathing frequency are also important factors influencing the particle deposition pattern (Yang et al. 2008).

While passing through the respiratory tree most of the particles get impacted by the natural barriers of the system. The impaction can be diminished by slow inhalation of dosage form which also increases penetration of large particles into the lungs. However, very small particles are largely unaffected by slow or fast inhalation (Usmani et al. 2005). Particles <100 nm are deposited efficiently by random Brownian motion (Heyder et al. 1986). Particle shape can also influence the

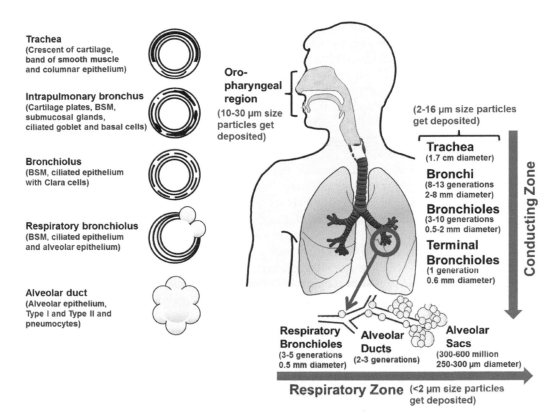

FIGURE 14.1 The number and dimensions of the airways of the adult lung and structure of the airway wall with generations as explained by Weibel's tracheo-bronchial tree. (Reprinted from *Eur J Pharm Sci* 49, Nahar, K., Gupta, N., Gauvin, R., Absar, S., Patel a, Gupta, V. et al, In vitro, in vivo, and ex vivo models for studying particle deposition and drug absorption of inhaled pharmaceuticals, 805–18, Copyright 2013, with permission from Elsevier.)

targetability at various regions in the lung and fibrous particles show deep lung deposition (Crowder et al. 2002). Higher toxicity of the lungs has been reported for particles with elongated shape in comparison to particles with spherical shape (Watanabe et al. 2002). In general, charged particles show faster deposition compared to neutral particles (Cohen et al.1998). Size of the particles usually increase through absorption of moisture during passage which enhances pulmonary deposition (Labiris and Dolovich 2003).

14.3 BARRIERS FOR PULMONARY DRUG DELIVERY

At present inhalation therapy is associated with a number of problems. Low therapeutic efficacy, short residence time in the lung and fast clearance are some of the problems that cause poor bioavailability at the target site. The low drug bioavailability and short half-life of inhaled drugs at the target site are caused by rapid systemic absorption, enzymatic degradation, clearance by alveolar macrophages, and mucociliary mechanism (Patton et al. 2010). Entry of foreign particles into the respiratory system is naturally prevented to keep it sterile and healthy through these defense mechanisms. When drug particles enter into the respiratory system, the system recognizes them as foreign bodies and eliminates them accordingly. Often the drug particles don't get enough time to interact with the target cells resulting in unsuccessful therapy. Macrophages clear the particles mainly from the alveoli while the ones trapped in the upper and lower part of the tracheobronchial tree are cleared by mucociliary mechanism (El-Sherbiny et al. 2015; Todoroff and Vanbever 2011; Beck-Broichsitter et a. 2012).

The mucociliary escalator of the upper airways consist of mucus producing (goblet) cells and ciliated cells. This system clears the particles by balancing the functions of mucus producing cells and ciliated cells. Larger sized inhaled particles are entrapped in the mucociliary escalator and get eliminated from the system by the process of swallowing or coughing (Patton et al. 2010; Hogg 1985). However, during lung inflammation or infection, the balance of the mucociliary escalator is disturbed. Usually the clearance of inhaled drug is accelerated which results in reduction of retention time and efficacy (El-Sherbiny et al. 2015).

However, smaller particles can escape the mucociliary escalator and travel through the entire length of the tracheobronchial tree and get deposited in the alveolar part. Mucociliary clearance velocities decrease with the decrease in diameter of the respiratory airways (Hofmann and Asgharian 2003). The mucus velocity measured in the bronchi is approximately 44% of that in trachea (2.4 and 5.5 mm/min respectively) (Foster et al. 1980). The higher the mucus velocity, the greater is the mucocillary clearance. Moller et al. (2008) had attempted to quantify this parameter with work on nanoparticles. Nanoparticles (100 nm size) were targeted to the lungs of the healthy volunteers using a bolus inhalation technique. Retention was noted after 24 h. It was observed that the percentage retention had been much higher in the peripheral branches of the lung (96%) compared to that of the airways (75%). Higher mucociliary clearance was suggested to be the cause of the diminished retention in the airways following administration of nanoparticles.

Another powerful clearance mechanism is operated by the phagocytic alveolar macrophages present in the lungs. This factor limits the residence time of drug in the alveoli, causing the doses to be repeated at frequent intervals. However, engulfment by the macrophages are usually size selective. It is reported that rather than nanoparticles, these macrophages have a preference for slightly bigger particles (1.5–3 µm) (El-Sherbiny et al. 2015). Hence designing particulate dosage forms for pulmonary administration is a tightrope walk. The particle size should be such that they can escape both alveolar macrophages as well as the mucociliary mechanism. Semmler-Behnke et al. investigated the effect of macrophage engulfment on particle size. They administered (inhalation) both micro and nanosized particles to rats and studied their uptake over 3 weeks by alveolar macrophages. As per their study, the microparticles were mainly retained (80% of the recovered microparticles) inside the alveolar macrophages. Only 20% of the recovered radioactivity was connected with alveolar macrophages indicating a significantly lesser retention of the nanosized particles (Semmler-Behnke et al. 2007). Geiser et al. also studied the role of macrophages in the clearance of inhaled nanoparticles (20 nm) from rat lungs. The uptake of the inhaled dose by lung macrophages was about 0.1% over 24 h (Geiser et al. 2008).

Inhaled drugs are usually subjected to enzymatic degradation resulting in decreased therapeutic activity. The enzymes of cytochrome P450 families are present in lungs which afford a defense against the inhaled xenobiotics. Numerous inhaled drugs such as theophylline, budesonide, salmeterol, and ciclesonide are degraded in the lungs through an enzymatic degradation process. Additionally, proteins and peptide drugs are vulnerable to proteases and peptidases present in lungs.

One more important challenge to inhalation therapy is the quick systemic absorption of the drugs from the lung area. This is due to the lungs' high vascularity, good epithelial permeability, and large surface area. The inhalable aerosols are designed for local action. To get a perfect local effect, an inhaled drug has to be absorbed in the lung tissue and retained there for an adequate period of time; systemic absorption results in a quick removal of the drug which produces adverse side effects. Hydrophobic and un-ionized drugs can cross the respiratory epithelia and enter into the systemic circulation faster in comparison to hydrophilic compounds. Small hydrophilic compounds have a greater mean absorption half-life (about 1 h), compared to small lipophilic molecules (about 1 min) (Patton et al. 2004). Moreover, the rate of transport of macromolecules from the airway lumen is inversely correlated to molecular weight. Following inhalation macromolecules (>40 kDa) need more time to be absorbed (several hours), contrary to smaller proteins or peptides which reach the bloodstream in a few minutes (Patton and Byron 2007). Absorption of hydrophilic drugs occur by diffusion through tight junctions whereas lipophilic drugs get absorbed by passive diffusion. Some compounds can only be absorbed by the active transport using drug transporters expressed in the lungs (Bosquillon 2010). Ipratropium bromide is actively transported within the tracheal tissue by using transporter Octn2 (Nakanishi et al. 2013). An in vivo study carried out in an isolated perfused rat lung model showed that pulmonary absorption of loperamide is actively prevented by P-glycoprotein-mediated efflux and rhodamine 123 from the lung airways to the perfusate (Al-Jayyoussi et al. 2013). Macromolecules can be transported into systemic circulation by receptor-mediated transcytosis (Matsukawa et al. 1997). Absorption of the drug from the lungs into the systemic circulation is higher from the lung periphery compared to the central region (Sangwan et al. 2001).

14.4 ABSORPTION OF THE DRUG THROUGH PULMONARY ADMINISTRATION

Drugs absorption profiles (local and systemic acting drugs) administered through the lungs are evaluated. Absorption profiles of locally acting drugs are determined to evaluate the amount of drug that reaches into systemic circulation. Absorption profiles of drugs into the lung also give information about the amount of drug that would be accessible locally to produce therapeutic activity in the lungs and the drug's overall systemic exposure. On the other hand, absorption of systemically acting drugs administered through pulmonary route are performed to establish bioavailability and biodistribution. In vitro cell culture studies have been used comprehensively for lungs drugs uptake, transport, and metabolism (Figure 14.2). In vitro cell culture studies have received suitability as a substitute to in vivo models since they have a reduced cost in comparison to animals and fast throughput.

An isolated perfused rat lung model was used for an absorption and deposition study of inhaled dosage form. Subsequent surgery, drugs, or formulations can be administered either directly into the lungs or in perfusate without the influence of the whole body to evaluate various pharmacokinetic parameters. Various perfusate media such as physiological salt solution-ficoll and albumin containing Krebs-Henseleit solution with or without hematocrit have been used in isolated perfused rat lung models. Usually, before performing surgery, perfusion medium is recirculated in the isolated perfused rat lung model instrument. A variety of drug delivery systems such as nebulizers, inhalable dry powders, dust gun aerosols, and metered dose propellant-based intratracheal dosing cartridges have been investigated for drug administration into the isolated lungs (Nahar et al. 2013).

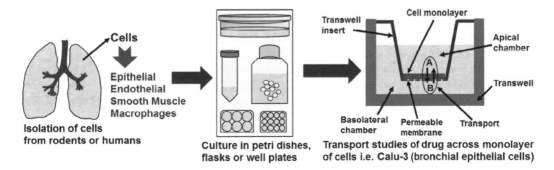

FIGURE 14.2 In vitro cell culture model to study drug uptake, absorption, and metabolism across the pulmonary epithelium. (Reprinted from *Eur J Pharm Sci* 49, Nahar, K., Gupta, N., Gauvin, R., Absar, S., Patel a, Gupta, V. et al. In vitro, in vivo, and ex vivo models for studying particle deposition and drug absorption of inhaled pharmaceuticals, 805–18, Copyright 2013, with permission from Elsevier.)

14.5   NANOTECHNOLOGY AND PULMONARY DELIVERY

The field of nanomedicines is huge. Depending upon structure, the nano drug delivery systems can be divided into two broad categories, particles and vesicles. Composition-wise the same can be divided into some more categories such as solid lipid nanoparticles, polymeric nanoparticles, liposomes, micelles, drug-polymer conjugates, and dendrimers. The size of the nanosystems also varies from a few nm to 1 μm (Roy and Vij 2010) As the sizes of the nanoparticles are similar to biological entities, nanoparticles can interact with biomolecules at the cell surface as well as structures within the cell (Todoroff and Vanbever 2011).

As a delivery route, the respiratory tract allows dual advantages. For respiratory diseases, drugs can be directly administered into the lungs, whereas wide surface and high blood supply allows adequate absorption for treatment of systemic diseases too. The introductions of nanodosage forms have augmented the efficacy of both the approaches.

As the particles of nano size range can escape the uptake by macrophages, they offer the option of a prolonged local delivery too (Todoroff and Vanbever 2011). Compared to other routes, delivery of nanomedicine to the pulmonary region is relatively easy. It can be carried out via several ways such as nebulizers, aerosols, dry powder, and metered dose inhalers which contain drug-loaded nanocarriers. Colloidal suspensions of drug-loaded nanoparticles can be easily incorporated in nebulizers (Dailey et al. 2003). Drug-loaded nanoparticles can also be incorporated in micro and porous dry powders for lung delivery (Tsapis et al. 2002). After deposition in the lungs, the microparticles release to generate the nanoparticles that act on the lung tissue. Preliminary results obtained with this system demonstrate potential benefits over the existing systems and promise further clinical exploitation in the near future (Videira et al. 2012; Bailey and Berkland 2009; Andrade et al. 2011). The therapeutic effectiveness of anti-infective drugs can be particularly enhanced by development of nanoparticles. Nanonization allows for enhancement of drug solubility as well as pulmonary accumulation which increases the local drug concentration leading to a decrease in the dosing frequency and side effects (Pandey and Khuller 2005; Garcia-Contreras et al. 2007).

14.6   PULMONARY DELIVERY OF CHITOSAN NANOCARRIER FOR LOCAL AND SYSTEMIC ACTION

The inner surface of the respiratory tract and lungs are in contact with the outer environment and are a site for exchange of gases. It is exposed to inorganic, organic, and biological components that can cause a variety of diseases. A host of viral, bacterial, parasitic, and fungal entities can affect lungs and progress to cause systemic infections like influenza, aspergillosis, pneumonia, and tuberculosis. The infection of the lower respiratory tract ranks among the three major causes of death and causes morbidity to about 3.5 million people annually (WHO). Another deadly disease of the lung is lung cancer and each year huge numbers of new patients are diagnosed with it. As nanomedicines bring the promise of enhanced retention as well as prolonged drug release in the lungs, they are particularly amenable for the treatment of such diseases (Azarmi et al. 2008).

Chitosan (Figure 14.3) is a natural cationic polysaccharide prepared by the partial deacetylation of chitin (Chandy and Sharma 1990; Venkatesan and Kim 2010). It has been broadly used as a carrier for controlled drug delivery, owing to its considerable chemical and biological properties such as bioactivity, biocompatibility, and biodegradability (Kumar et al. 2004).

Numerous polymeric nanoparticulate systems have been prepared using both natural and synthetic polymers, each with their own advantages and limitations. Natural polymers are mainly polysaccharides so they are biocompatible and devoid of any side effects (Giri et al. 13; Giri et al. 15; Giri et al. 17). Among the natural polymers, chitosan has been studied expansively for nanoparticle preparation. Nanoparticles prepared from chitosan have been reported with diverse characteristics with respect to drug delivery. Chitosan has also been extensively used to prepare pH-sensitive nanoparticles. Amino groups in chitosan are protonated at acidic conditions and chitosan can be

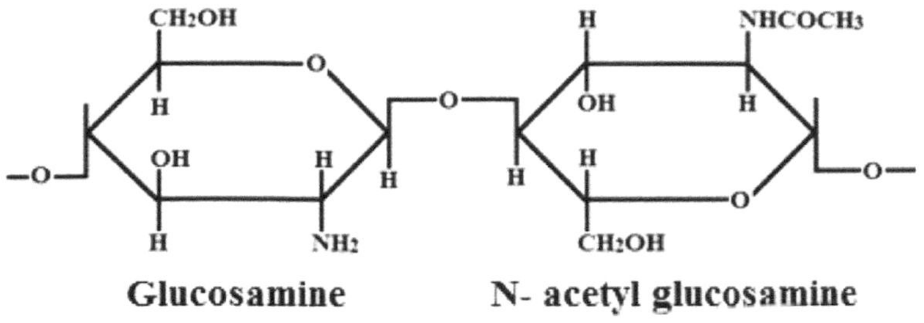

CH₂OH — Glucosamine / N- acetyl glucosamine

FIGURE 14.3 Chemical structure of chitosan.

responsive to external pH stimulation (Figure 14.4). Moreover, chitosan does not produce considerable toxicity to lung cells and tissue (de Jesús Valle et al. 2008; Grenha et al. 2007). Therefore, chitosan nanocarriers are an attractive drug delivery vehicle for treatment of both local and systemic lung diseases.

14.6.1 Pulmonary Delivery of Chitosan Nanoparticles for the Treatment of Pneumonia

Pneumonia is an infectious disease of the lung caused by viruses, fungi, and bacteria. The causative agents usually involved with this disease are *Acinetobacter baumannii, Haemophilus influenzae* type b, *Streptococcus pneumonia*, human respiratory syncytial virus, *Moraxella catarrhalis, Klebsiella pneumonia, Mycoplasma pneumoniae, Pneumocystis jiroveci, Chlamydophila pneumoniae*, Human parainfluenza virus, and *Legionella pneumophila*. In children under five years of age, the disease often turns fatal and is one of the foremost cause of death (Zumla 2012), with an annual death toll of approximately 1.8 million. Moreover, ventilated patients often suffer from nosocomial pneumonia (Rello and Diaz 2003) and development of resistant strains is a matter of great concern amongst health professionals.

Currently the disease is treated by an aminoglycoside antibiotic called gentamicin. But, the use of gentamicin in conventional dosage form is restricted by severe side effects as well as low bioavailability. To circumvent this problem, Huang et al. (2016) developed gentamicin-loaded chitosan nanoparticles for pulmonary delivery and tested them with an in vitro drug release. The formulation

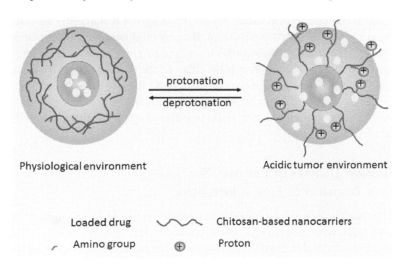

Physiological environment   Acidic tumor environment

protonation / deprotonation

Loaded drug   ⌒⌒ Chitosan-based nanocarriers
Amino group   ⊕ Proton

FIGURE 14.4 The pH-sensitive mechanism of chitosan-based nanoparticles. (Reprinted from *Colloids Surf B Biointerfaces* 148, Zhang, X., Yang, X., Ji, J., Liu, A., and Zhai, G. Tumor targeting strategies for chitosan-based nanoparticles, 460–73, Copyright 2016, with permission from Elsevier.)

could sustain drug release for 72 h with zero-order release for the first 10 h. On intra-tracheal administration too, the gentamicin nanoparticles exhibited a higher bioavailability and minimum inhibitory concentration ratio compared to intravenous administration. These translate to a significant reduction of systemic toxicity and an improvement in antimicrobial efficacy. Nosocomial infections in the human body are usually caused by the organism *Klebsiella pneumonia* and are difficult to treat because of antibiotic resistance. Chitosan nanoparticles loaded with antigen were evaluated by in vivo studies in rats (Menon 2015). The prepared nanoparticles showed a greater protection effect in comparison to the injectable vaccine.

14.6.2 Pulmonary Delivery of Chitosan Nanoparticles for the Treatment of Tuberculosis

Tuberculosis caused by *Mycobacterium tuberculosis* is an infectious disease that affects the lungs and until the late 20th century, it was one of the leading causes of death. As per WHO, worldwide approximately 8.7 million cases were diagnosed with tuberculosis in 2011. Around 0.43 million people suffered from HIV-allied tuberculosis and approximately 1 million morbidity was reported from HIV-negative people. Streptomycin, pyrazinamide, ethambutol, isoniazid, and rifampicin are the first-line drugs used to treat tuberculosis (Rastogi et al. 2006; Pinheiro et al. 2011). The current treatment option is a prolonged oral therapy with a combination of these antitubercular drugs. However, development of multidrug-resistant strains is a serious constraint to the approach. Traditional delivery has severe restrictions for drug infiltration and cytosolic availability to infected phagocytic cells. In infected hosts, *Mycobacterium tuberculosis* resides in alveolar macrophages inside the granulomatous fibrocystic layers. When systemically administered, some anti-tubercular drugs fail to infiltrate into this space causing a treatment failure. This constraint has been an impetus for development of nanocarrier drug delivery systems for these difficult to treat respiratory diseases. To circumvent the difficulties of multiple drug administration, all the drugs (pyrazinamide, rifampicin, and isoniazid) were simultaneously loaded into alginate-chitosan nanoparticles (Ahmad et al. 2005). Clinical trials for new anti-tubercular dosage forms are continuing with the hope for treatment of such resistant strains (Sosnik et al. 2010; Pandey and Khuller 2005)

Rifampicin-loaded liposomal dry powder formulations were developed and assessed for pulmonary delivery (Changsan et al. 2009). The prepared liposomal suspension was freeze dried using cryoprotectant which influenced the aerosolization properties. The chitosan-based coating of the liposomes enhanced the entrapment efficiency of the drug but it markedly affected the formulations nebulization properties (Zaru et al. 2009). But, on modification of the coating composition, mucoadhesiveness of liposome increased which resulted in greater accumulation of the rifampicin in the lung tissue and increased the therapeutic effect (Zaru et al. 2009). In vivo studies in guinea pigs showed that the drugs were present in plasma for more than 10 days. Moreover, the drugs were detected in the spleen, liver, and lungs above the minimum inhibitory concentration up to 15 days. Various chitosan nanocarrier-loaded with antitubercular drugs for pulmonary delivery are represented in Table 14.1.

14.6.3 Pulmonary Delivery of Chitosan Nanoparticles for the Treatment of Fungal Infections

Recently there has been a surge of lung fungal infections due to the increasing number of immune-compromised patients allied with cancer, organ transplantations, HIV, and hematologic disorders (Limper et al. 2011). Fungal infections that can often cause severe lung injury include: sporotrichosis (*Sporothrix schenkii*), histoplasmosis (*Histoplasma capsulatum*), coccidioidomycosis (*Coccidioides spp.*), blastomycosis (*Blastomyces dermatitidis*), cryptococcosis (*Cryptococcus spp.*), aspergillosis (*Aspergillus spp.*), paracoccidioidomycosis (*Paracoccidioides brasiliensis*), and candidiasis (*Candida spp.*) (Limper et al. 2011). A variety of antifungal drugs including itraconazole, caspofungin, amphotericin

TABLE 14.1

Chitosan Nanocarrier of Antitubercular Drug for Pulmonary Delivery

Drug	Composition	Research Finding	Reference
Isoniazid, rifampicin and pyrazinamide	Alginate/chitosan nanoparticles	Lower toxicity against A549 epithelial cells compared to free drug	Zaru et al. 2009
Rifampicin	Chitosan nanoparticles	Initial burst release followed by slow sustained drug release	Patel et al. 2013
Rifampicin	Chitosan nanoparticles	Almost complete drug release (81% in 10 h at pH 4.5)	Amirah et al. 2014
Rifampicin	Chitosan nanoparticles (freeze dried powder)	Longer residence and slow clearance of drug from the lungs	Rawal et al. 2017
Isoniazid	Chitosan-montmorillonite nanoparticles	Controlled release of isoniazid	Banik et al. 2012
Isoniazid	Chitosan nanoparticles	Sustained drug release (87% in 24 h)	Prashansa et al. 2014
Isoniazid	Fe_3O_4– containing chitosan nanoparticles (magnetic properties)	Initial burst release (10 h) followed by slow sustained release up to 48 h	Qin et al. 2015
Streptomycin, gentamicin and tobramycin	Chitosan nanoparticles	Successful growth inhibition of *Mycobacterium tuberculosis* in mouse model	Lu et al. 2009
Streptomycin	Chitosan nanoparticles with magnetic properties	Inhibition of *Mycobacterium* growth	El Zowalaty et al. 2015
Streptomycin	Chitosan nanoparticles with magnetic properties	Improved efficacy against methicillin-resistant *Staphylococcus aureus*	Hussein-Al-Ali et al. 2014

B deoxycholate, and voriconazole are available on the market for intravenous or oral administration (Limper et al. 2011). Amphotericin B deoxycholate is considered as the gold standard of antifungal drugs and is usually used to treat life-threatening cases. However, cardiotoxicity and nephrotoxicity is the main clinical drawback leading to the discontinuation of treatment (Laniado-Laborín and Cabrales-Vargas 2009). Recently, interest has been generated to formulate amphotericin B deoxycholate in different nano drug delivery systems (Vyas et al. 2005; Agrawal et al. 2002).

Chitosan oligosaccharide micelles (a nanostructure) grafted with stearic acid have been loaded with amphotericin B deoxycholate for the delivery of the drug to the lung (Gilani et al. 2011). The micelles showed the same antifungal efficacy as the market product Fungioze® with lower toxicity. The micelles formulations were proficiently nebulized and presenting up to 52% of fine particle fraction (Gilani et al. 2011).

Oral administration of itraconazole, an antifungal drug suffers from a low bioavailability because of low solubility. For effective treatment of lung infections, the pulmonary route is used for this drug. Aerosolized antifungal agents offer a greater benefit as they can offer high concentration of drug at the action site. Chitosan-based aerosolized nanoparticles of itraconazole, administered through the pulmonary route demonstrated greater efficacy by virtue of their greater pulmonary deposition.

Moazeni et al. also evaluated stearic acid grafted chitosan-based micelles as a nanocarrier for pulmonary delivery of itraconazole through inhalation (Moazeni et al. 2012). Entrapment of itraconazole in the prepared micelles was 43.2 µg per milliliter and the mean diameter of the particles were between 120 and 200 nm. The in vitro pulmonary profile of the prepared micelles was performed by using an air-jet nebulizer. Fine particle fraction was varied between 38% and 47% with maximum nebulization efficiency of 89%. Stability of the drug in the micelles was enough during nebulization process.

14.6.4 Pulmonary Delivery of Chitosan Nanoparticles for the Treatment of Viral Infections

Respiratory infections caused by viruses are a common phenomenon worldwide. Mainly viruses accountable for these infections include rhinovirus, influenza virus, echovirus, coxsackie virus, adenovirus, respiratory syncytial virus, corona virus, parainfluenza virus, torque tenovirus, human metapneumovirus, human bocavirus, polyomaviruses, polyomavirus, and avian influenza virus H5N1 (Jartti et al. 2012; Beckham et al. 2005; Rosenthal et al. 2010). However, worldwide the influenza virus is the foremost cause of pulmonary viral infections. Moreover, the viruses responsible for lower respiratory tract infection in children are the parainfluenza virus and the syncytial virus. At present, a small number of drugs like oseltamivir, rimantadine, and amantadine are available for treating such disorders which are administered through the oral route. Recently, a dry powder inhaler containing zanamivir was approved for the treatment of influenza.

14.6.5 Pulmonary Delivery of Chitosan Nanoparticles for the Treatment of Lung Cancer

Cancer of the lung is a deadly disease and is widely prevalent in both men and women (Goel et al. 2013). At present survival rate through conventional treatments such as chemotherapy, radiation, and surgical is quite poor (Roa et al. 2011). Systemic delivery of the chemotherapeutic drug has limited success because only a minimal fraction of the total dose reaches the tumor tissue in the lung. Greater fractions of the administered doses act on normal cells and inhibit the normal cell growth resulting in the death of the patient (Tseng et al. 2008). Improved delivery of the drug to the lung tumor region can be a useful weapon in the fight against cancer and can minimize systemic drug exposure to the normal tissue.

Gemcitabine is a deoxycytidine analog used to treat various types of cancer including lung cancer. However, this drug has the drawback of a short half-life and requires frequent administration to maintain the minimum effective concentration level. This results in high exposure to the normal tissue resulting in a higher toxicity. Surface-modified polymeric nanoparticles of chitosan and polyethylene glycol loaded with gemcitabine could preferentially target the cancer tissue and deliver the drug at a higher concentration compared to that in normal tissue (Garg et al. 2012).

14.7 STRATEGIES FOR TARGETING THE NANOPARTICLES TO PULMONARY TISSUE

Various strategies have been applied for targeting nanoparticles to tumor tissue. Nanoparticles have been attempted for delivery of the anticancer drug docetaxel too. PEGylated chitosan nanocapsules conjugated with the monoclonal antibody anti-TMEFF-2 were developed using the avidin-biotin approach (Figure 14.5). The effectiveness of these nanocapsules were demonstrated in lung carcinoma xenograft (non-small cell type) compared with free docetaxel. The developed nanocapsules exhibited a delayed and prolonged effect on tumor volume reduction with insignificant side effects while free docetaxel showed a fast and short action.

Work was carried on the anticancer drug lomustine. Mehrotra et al. (2011) prepared lomustine-loaded chitosan nanoparticles for the treatment of lung cancer. The prepared nanoparticles showed improved cytotoxicity in the L132 lung cancer cell line in comparison to the free drug. Recently, PLGA or PLA in combination with chitosan was used for the preparation of nanoparticles. The surface of these gene/drug-loaded nanoparticles were modified with chitosan to improve cellular uptake and cytotoxicity in lung cancer cells (Yang et al. 2009; Tahara et al. 2010). Chitosan-modified PLGA nanoparticles containing paclitaxel (size 200–300 nm) improved tumor uptake and cytotoxicity in A549 lung cancer cells. Moreover, the modified nanoparticle showed an increased biodistribution in the lung in a lung metastatic mouse model.

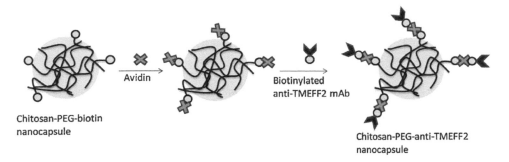

FIGURE 14.5 Schematic illustration for the preparation of PEGylated chitosan NPs conjugated to anti-TMEFF-2. (Reprinted from *Int J Biol Macromol* 72, Prabaharan, M. Chitosan-based nanoparticles for tumor-targeted drug delivery, 1313–22, Copyright 2015, with permission from Elsevier.)

To improve the targetability and retention in the lung tissue, nanoparticles are usually surface modified.

Nanoparticles were surface-coated with anisamide to improve lung targetability. For the preparation of anisamide-modified nanoparticles, tripolyphosphate was used as a crosslinking agent (Figure 14.6).

It was observed that the surface modified nanoparticles with anisamide accumulated in the tumor with a higher concentration compared to nanoparticles without surface modification. Surface modified nanoparticles exhibited outstanding cytotoxicity toward A549 cells and efficiently slow down A549 cell-bearing tumor growth in mice. The prepared nanoparticles showed nominal toxicity indicating that surface modification facilitates drug delivery to the targeted tumor sites, with minimum entrée to non-tumor tissues.

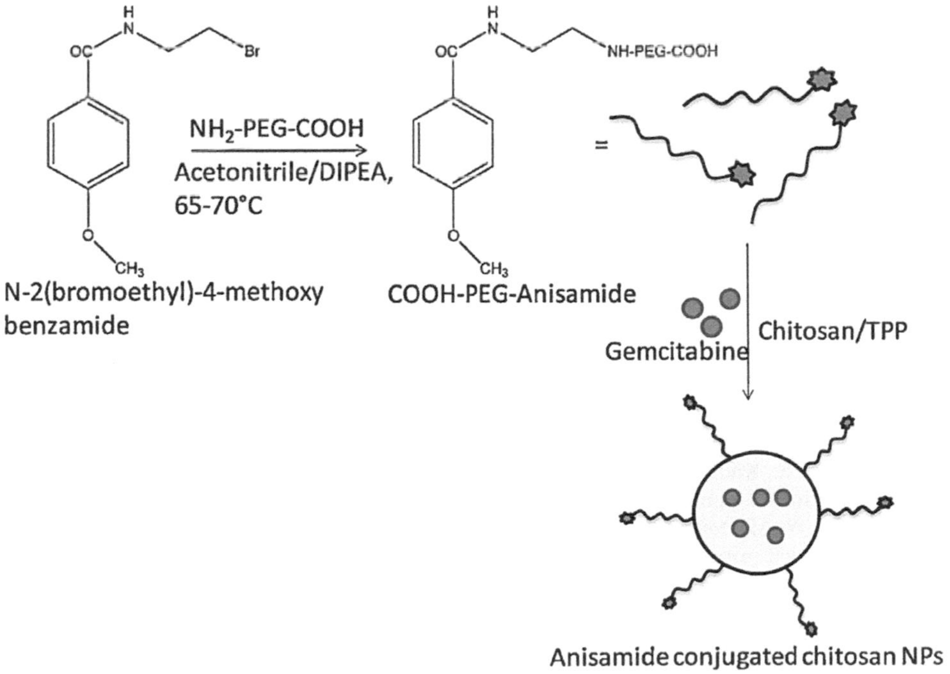

FIGURE 14.6 Schematic illustration of the preparation of anisamide-conjugated chitosan NPs. (Reprinted from *Int J Biol Macromol* 72, Prabaharan, M. Chitosan-based nanoparticles for tumor-targeted drug delivery, 1313–22, Copyright 2015, with permission from Elsevier.)

Antigen was extracted by a hot phenol extraction technique from *Klebsiella pneumonia*. The entrapment efficiency and size of the nanoparticles were 87.9% and 470 nm, respectively. In order to obtain an inhalable formulation, the prepared nanoparticles were spray dried using lactose as a carrier. In vivo studies were carried out by administering the prepared nanoparticles in rats through the mucosal route (pulmonary and intranasal). The antibody titres (IgA and IgG) were measured by ELISA followed by a bactericidal assay. Results of antibody titres and the bactericidal assay have shown a greater protecting effect in comparison to the injectable vaccine. Vllasaliu et al. (2010) established through MTS assays that chitosan nanoparticles were less toxic toward human airway epithelial cells (calu-3 cell lines) in comparison to chitosan solution with the same chitosan concentration. Similarly, chitosan nanoparticles showed an absence of toxicity in lung epithelial cells for up to 48 h using MTT assays (Grenha et al. 2007).

Chitosan nanoparticles loaded with isoniazid were prepared by an iontropic gelation method for controlled delivery of the drug to the pulmonary region (Pourshahab et al. 2011). Prepared nanoparticles were spray dried using excipients such as maltodextrin, mannitol, and lactose only or with leucine to prepare inhalable microparticles. An in vitro deposition study showed that the prepared spray dried particles with lactose and leucine resulted in inhalable powders with a 45% fine particle fraction (highest). It was observed that the release of drug from nanoparticles diminished with increasing chitosan concentration.

Jafarinejad et al. (2012) had prepared inhalable microparticles of itraconazole in a two-step process. Nanoparticles made by ionic gelation technique were incorporated into a suitable vehicle, and the combination was spray dried to obtain free-flowing microparticles suitable for pulmonary delivery (Jafarinejad et al. 2012). The highest encapsulation efficiency of 55% was obtained from nanoparticles prepared with chitosan and tripolyphosphate with a ratio of 1:3. Emitted dose percentage and fine particle fraction were measured by using a twin stage impinger. In vitro deposition data showed that the processing of nanoparticles with leucin and mannitol significantly improved the drug aerosolization properties.

14.8 CONCLUSION

Delivery of the drug to the pulmonary region is rapidly growing and the lungs offer a diversity of advantages compared to oral drug delivery. The absorption of the drugs in the pulmonary region is faster due to a large surface area and the elimination of the first pass effect. Biodegradable polymeric nanoparticles especially chitosan nanoparticles may exhibit a sustained release effect. Pulmonary research has vast opportunities for the success of chitosan nanoparticulate systems, which still needs thorough physicochemical and nanotoxicological analysis for possible human application.

REFERENCES

Agrawal, A.K., Agrawal, A., Pal, A., Guru, P.Y., and Gupta, C.M. 2002. Superior chemotherapeutic efficacy of amphotericin B in tuftsin-bearing liposomes against Leishmania donovani infection in hamsters. *J Drug Target* 10: 41–5.

Ahmad, Z., Sharma, S., Khuller, G.K. 2005. Inhalable alginate nanoparticles as antitubercular drug carriers against experimental tuberculosis. *Int J Antimicrob Agents* 26: 298–303.

Aitken, M., Burke, W., McDonald, G., Shak, S., Montgomery, A., and Smith, A. 1992. Recombinant human DNase inhalation in normal subjects and patients with cystic fibrosis. A phase 1 study. *JAMA* 267: 1947–51.

Al-Jayyoussi, G., Price, D.F., Francombe, D., Taylor, G., Smith, M.W., Morris, C., Edwards, C.D., Eddershaw, P., and Gumbleton, M. 2013. Selectivity in the impact of P-glycoprotein upon pulmonary absorption of airway-dosed substrates: A study in ex vivo lung models using chemical inhibition and genetic knockout. *J Pharm Sci* 102: 3382–94.

Amirah, M.G., Amirul A.A., and Habibah, A.W. 2014. Formulation and characterization of rifampicin-loaded p (3hb-co-4hb) nanoparticles. *Int J Pharm Sci* 6: 140–6.

Andrade, F., Videira, M., Ferreira, D., and Sarmento, B. 2011. Nanocarriers for pulmonary administration of peptides and therapeutic proteins. *Nanomedicine (Lond.)* 6: 123–41.

Azarmi, S., Roa, W.H., and Lobenberg, R. 2008.Targeted delivery of nanoparticles for the treatment of lung diseases. *Adv Drug Deliv Rev* 60: 863–75.

Bailey, M. and Berkland, C. 2009. Nanoparticle formulations in pulmonary drug delivery. *Med Res Rev* 29: 196–212.

Banik, N., Hussain, A., Ramteke, A., Sharma, H.K., and Maji, T.K. 2012. Preparation and evaluation of the effect of particle size on the properties of chitosan-montmorillonite nanoparticles loaded with isoniazid. *RSC Adv* 2: 10519–28.

Beck-Broichsitter, M., Gauss, J., Packhaeuser, C.B., Lahnstein, K., Schmehl, T., Seeger, W., Kissel, T., and Gessler, T. 2009. Pulmonary drug delivery with aerosolizable nanoparticles in an ex vivo lung model. *Int J Pharm* 367: 169–78.

Beck-Broichsitter, M., Kleimann, P., Gessler, T., Seeger, W., Kissel, T., and Schmehl, T. 2012. Nebulization performance of biodegradable sildenafil-loaded nanoparticles using the Aeroneb® Pro: Formulation aspects and nanoparticle stability to nebulization. *Int J Pharm* 422: 398–408.

Beck-Broichsitter, M., Merkel, O.M., and Kissel, T. 2012. Controlled pulmonary drug and gene delivery using polymeric nano-carriers. *J Control Release* 161: 214–24.

Beckham, J.D., Cadena, A., Lin, J., Piedra, P.A., Glezen, W.P., Greenberg, S.B., and Atmar, R.L. 2005. Respiratory viral infections in patients with chronic, obstructive pulmonary disease. *J Infect* 50: 322–30.

Bernstein, D.I., Reuman, P.D., Sherwood, J.R., Young, E.C., and Schiff, G.M. 1988. Ribavirin small-particle-aerosol treatment of influenza B virus infection. *Antimicrob Agents Chemother* 32: 761–4.

Bosquillon, C. 2010. Drug transporters in the lung—do they play a role in the biopharmaceutics of inhaled drugs? *J Pharm Sci* 99: 2240–55.

Chandy, T. and Sharma, C.P. 1990. Chitosan - as a biomaterial. Biomater. *Artif Cells Artif Organ* 18: 1–24.

Changsan, N., Chan, H.K., Separovic, F., and Srichana, T. 2009. Physicochemical characterization and stability of rifampicin liposome dry powder formulations for inhalation. *J Pharm Sci* 98: 628–39.

Cohen, B.S., Xiong, J.Q., Fang, C.P., and Li, W. 1998. Deposition of charged particles on lung airways. *Health Phys* 74: 554–60.

Crowder, T.M., Rosati, J.A., Schroeter, J.D., Hickey, A.J., and Martonen, T.B. 2002. Fundamental effects of particle morphology on lung delivery: Predictions of Stokes' law and the particular relevance to dry powder inhaler formulation and development. *Pharm Res* 19: 239–45.

Dailey, L.A., Schmehl, T., Gessler, T., Wittmar, M., Grimminger, F., Seeger, W., and Kissel, T. 2003. Nebulization of biodegradable nanoparticles: Impact of nebulizer technology and nanoparticle characteristics on aerosol features. *J Control Release* 86: 131–44.

de Galan, B., Simsek, S., Tack, C., and Heine, R. 2006. Efficacy and safety of inhaled insulin in the treatment of diabetes mellitus. *Neth J Med* 64: 319–25.

de Jesús Valle, M.J., Dinis-Oliveira, R.J., Carvalho, F., Bastos, M.L., and Sanchez Navarro, A. 2008. Toxicological evaluation of lactose and chitosan delivered by inhalation. *J Biomater Sci Polym Ed* 19: 387–97.

De Marzo, N., Di Blasi, P., Boschetto, P., Mapp, C.E., Sartore, S., Picotti, G., and Fabbri, L.M. 1989. Airway smooth muscle biochemistry and asthma. *Eur Respir J Suppl* 6: 473s–476s.

El Zowalaty, M.E., Hussein Al Ali, S.H., Husseiny, M.I., Geilich, B.M., Webster, T.J., and Hussein, M.Z. 2015. The ability of streptomycin-loaded chitosan-coated magnetic nanocomposites to possess antimicrobial and antituberculosis activities. *Int J Nanomedicine* 10: 3269–74.

El-Sherbiny, IM., El-Baz, N.M., and Yacoub, M.H. 2015. Inhaled nano- and microparticles for drug delivery. *Glob Cardiol Sci Pract* 2015: 1–14.

Foster, W.M., Langenback, E., and Bergofsky, E.H. 1980. Measurement of tracheal and bronchial mucus velocities in man: Relation to lung clearance. *J Appl Physiol Respir Environ Exerc Physiol* 48: 965–71.

Garcia-Contreras, L., Fiegel, J., Telko, M.J., Elbert, K., Hawi, A., Thomas, M., VerBerkmoes, J., Germishuizen, W.A., Fourie, P.B., Hickey, A.J., and Edwards, D. 2007. Inhaled large porous particles of capreomycin for treatment of tuberculosis in a guinea pig model, Antimicrob. *Agents Chemother* 51: 2830–6.

Garg, N.K., Dwivedi, P., Campbell, C., and Tyagi, R.K. 2012. Site specific/targeted delivery of gemcitabine through anisamide anchored chitosan/poly ethylene glycol nanoparticles: An improved understanding of lung cancer therapeutic intervention. *Eur J Pharm Sci* 47: 1006–14.

Geiser, M., Casaulta, M., Kupferschmid, B., Schulz, H., Semmler-Behnke, M., and Kreyling, W. 2008. The role of macrophages in the clearance of inhaled ultrafine titanium dioxide particles. *Am J Respir Cell Mol. Biol* 38: 371–6.

Geller, D.E., Flume, P.A., Staab, D., Fischer, R., Loutit, J.S., and Conrad, D.J. 2011. Levofloxacin inhalation solution (MP-376) in patients with cystic fibrosis with Pseudomonas aeruginosa. *Am J Respir Crit Care Med* 183: 1510–6.

Gilani, K., Moazeni, E., Ramezanli, T., Amini, M., Fazeli, M.R., and Jamalifar, H. 2011. Development of respirable nanomicelle carriers for delivery of amphotericin B by jet nebulization. *J Pharm Sci* 100: 252–9.

Gilani, K., Moazeni, E., Ramezanli, T., Amini, M., Fazeli, M.R., and Jamalifar, H. 2011. Development of respirable nanomicelle carriers for delivery of amphotericin B by jet nebulization. *J Pharm Sci* 100: 252–9.

Giri, T.K., Choudhary, C., Alexander, A., Ajazuddin., Badwaik, H., Tripathy, M., and Tripathi, D.K. 2013. Sustained release of diltiazem hydrochloride from cross-linked biodegradable IPN hydrogel beads based on pectin and modified xanthan gum. *Ind J Pharm Sci* 75: 619–27.

Giri, T.K., Pure, S., and Tripathi, D.K. 2015. Synthesis of graft copolymers of acrylamide for locust bean gum using microwave energy: Swelling behavior, flocculation characteristics and acute toxicity study. *Polimeros* 25: 168–74.

Giri, T.K., Verma, D., and Badwaik, H.R. 2017. Effect of aluminium chloride concentration on diltiazem hydrochloride release from pH-sensitive hydrogel beads composed of hydrolyzed grafted k-carrageenan and sodium alginate. *Curr Chem Biol* 11: 44–9.

Goel, A., Baboota, S., Sahni, J.K., and Ali, J. 2013. Exploring targeted pulmonary delivery for treatment of lung cancer. *Int J Pharm Investig* 3: 8–14.

Grenha, A., Grainger, C.I., Dailey, L.A., Seijo, B., Martin, G.P., Remuˉnán- López, C. et al. 2007. Chitosan nanoparticles are compatible with respiratory epithelial cells in vitro. *Eur J Pharm Sci* 31: 73–84.

Heyder, J., Gebhart, J., Rudolf, G., Schiller, C.F., and Stahlhofen, W. 1986. Deposition of particles in the human respiratory tract in the size range 0.005–15 µm, *J Aerosol Sci* 17: 811–25.

Hofmann, W. and Asgharian, B. 2003. The effect of lung structure on mucociliary clearance and particle retention in human and rat lungs. *Toxicol Sci* 73: 448–56.

Hogg, J.1985. Response of the lung to inhaled particles. *Med J Aust* 142: 675–8.

Hokey, D.A. and Misra, A. 2011. Aerosol vaccines for tuberculosis: A fine line between protection and pathology. *Tuberculosis (Edinb.)* 91: 82–5.

Huang, Y.C., Li, R.Y., Chen, J.Y., and Chen, J.K. 2016. Biphasic release of gentamicin from chitosan/fucoidan nanoparticles for pulmonary delivery. *Carbohydr Polym* 138: 114–22.

Huland, E., Burger, A., Fleischer, J., Fornara, P., Hatzmann, E., Heidenreich, A. et al. 2003. Efficacy and safety of inhaled recombinant interleukin-2 in high-risk renal cell cancer patients compared with systemic interleukin-2: An outcome study. *Folia Biol* 49: 183–90.

Hussein-Al-Ali, S.H., El Zowalaty, M.E., Hussein, M.Z., Ismail, M., and Webster, T.J. 2014. Synthesis, characterization, controlled release, and antibacterial studies of a novel streptomycin chitosan magnetic nanoantibiotic. *Int J Nanomedicine* 9: 549–57.

Jaafar-Maalej, C., Elaissari, A., and Fessi, H. 2012. Lipid-based carriers: Manufacturing and applications for pulmonary route. *Expert Opin Drug Deliv* 9: 1111–27.

Jafarinejad, S., Gilani, K., Moazeni, E., Ghazi-Khansari, M., Najafabadi, A.R., and Mohajel, N. 2012. Development of chitosan-based nanoparticles for pulmonary delivery of itraconazole as dry powder formulation. *Powder Technol* 222: 65–70.

Jartti, T., Jartti, L., Ruuskanen, O., and Söderlund-Venermo, M. 2012. New respiratory viral infections. *Curr Opin Pulm Med* 18: 271–8.

Jones, L.H., Baldock, H., Bunnage, M.E., Burrows, J., Clarke, N., Coghlan, M. et al. 2011.Price, Inhalation by design: Dual pharmacology β-2 agonists/M3 antagonists for the treatment of COPD. *Bioorg Med Chem Lett* 21: 2759–63.

Kumar, M.N., Muzzarelli, R.A., Muzzarelli, C., Sashiwa, H., and Domb, A.J. 2004. Chitosan chemistry and pharmaceutical perspectives. *Chem Rev* 104: 6017–84.

Labiris, N.R. and Dolovich, M.B. 2003. Pulmonary drug delivery. Part I: Physiological factors affecting therapeutic effectiveness of aerosolized medications. *Br J Clin Pharmacol* 56: 588–99.

Laniado-Laborín, R. and Cabrales-Vargas, M.N. 2009.Amphotericin B: Side effects and toxicity. *Rev Iberoam Micol* 26: 223–7.

Limper, A.H., Knox, K.S., Sarosi, G.A., Ampel, N.M., Bennett, J.E., Catanzaro, A. et al. 2011. An official American Thoracic Society statement: Treatment of fungal infections in adult pulmonary and critical care patients. *Am J Respir Crit Care Med* 183: 96–128.

Lu E, Franzblau S, Onyuksel H, and Popescu C. 2009. Preparation of aminoglycoside-loaded chitosan nanoparticles using dextran sulphate as a counterion. *J Microencapsul* 26: 346–54.

Lu, D., Garcia-Contreras, L., Muttil, P., Padilla, D., Xu, D., Liu, J., Braunstein, M., McMurray, D.N., and Hickey, A.J. 2010. Pulmonary immunization using antigen 85-B polymeric microparticles to boost tuberculosis immunity. *AAPS J* 12: 338–47.

Mansour, H.M., Rhee, Y.S., and Wu, X. 2009. Nanomedicine in pulmonary delivery. Int J *Nanomedicine* 4: 299–319.

Matsukawa, Y., Lee, V.H., Crandall, E.D., and Kim, K.J. 1997. Size-dependent dextran transport across rat alveolar epithelial cell monolayers. *J Pharm Sci* 86: 305–9.

McAllen, M.K., Kochanowski, S.J., and Shaw, K.M. 1974. Steroid aerosols in asthma: An assessment of betamethasone valerate and a 12-month study of patients on maintenance treatment. *Br Med J* 1: 171–5.

Mehrotra, A., Nagarwal, R.C., and Pandit, J.K. 2011. Lomustine loaded chitosan nanoparticles: Characterization and in-vitro cytotoxicity on human lung cancer cell line L132. *Chem Pharm Bull* 59: 315–20.

Menon, M.D. 2015. Capsular polysaccharide loaded chitosan nanoparticles for mucosal immunization via respiratory tract against Klebsiella pneumonia. 5th Asia Pacific Global Summit and Expo on Vaccines & Vaccination, Brisbane, Australia.

Moazeni, E., Gilani, K., Najafabadi, A.R., Reza Rouini, M., Mohajel, N., Amini, M., and Barghi, M.A. 2012. Preparation and evaluation of inhalable itraconazole chitosan based polymeric micelles. *DARU J Pharm Sci* 20: 85.

Mohammad, R.A. and Klein, K.C. 2006. Inhaled amphotericin B for prophylaxis against invasive aspergillus infections. *Ann Pharmacother* 40: 2148–54.

Moller, W., Felten, K., Sommerer, K., Scheuch, G., Meyer, G., Meyer, P., Haussinger, K., and Kreyling, W.G. 2008. Deposition, retention, and translocation of ultrafine particles from the central airways and lung periphery. *Am J Respir Crit Care Med* 177: 426–32.

Muttil, P., Wang, C., and Hickey, A.J. 2009. Inhaled drug delivery for tuberculosis therapy. *Pharm Res* 26: 2401–16.

Nahar, K., Gupta, N., Gauvin, R., Absar, S., Patel a, Gupta, V. et al. 2013. In vitro, in vivo and ex vivo models for studying particle deposition and drug absorption of inhaled pharmaceuticals. *Eur J Pharm Sci* 49: 805–18.

Nakanishi, T., Hasegawa, Y., Haruta, T., Wakayama, T., and Tamai, I. 2013. In vivo evidence of organic cation transporter-mediated tracheal accumulation of the anticholinergic agent ipratropium in mice. *J Pharm Sci* 102: 3373–81.

O'Riordan, T. 2000. Inhaled antimicrobial therapy: From cystic fibrosis to the flu. *Respir Care* 45: 836–45.

Pandey, R. and Khuller, G.K. 2005. Antitubercular inhaled therapy: Opportunities, progress and challenges. *J Antimicrob Chemother* 55: 430–5.

Paranjpe, M. and Muller-Goymann, C.C. 2014. Nanoparticle-mediated pulmonary drug delivery: A review. *Int J Mol Sci* 15: 5852–73.

Patel, B.K., Parikh, R.H., and Aboti, P.S. 2013. Development of oral sustained release rifampicin loaded chitosan nanoparticles by design of experiment. *J Drug Deliv* 2013: 1–10.

Patton, J.S. and Byron, P.R. 2007. Inhaling medicines: Delivering drugs to the body through the lungs. *Nat Rev Drug Discov* 6: 67–74.

Patton, J.S., Brain, J.D., Davies, L.A., Fiegel, J., Gumbleton, M., Kim, K.J., Sakagami, M., Vanbever, R., and Ehrhardt, C. 2010. The particle has landed-characterizing the fate of inhaled pharmaceuticals. *J Aerosol Med Pulm Drug Deliv* 23: (S2): S-71–S-87.

Patton, J.S., Fishburn, C.S., and Weers, J.G. 2004. The lungs as a portal of entry for systemic drug delivery. *Proc Am Thorac Soc* 1: 338–44.

Phipps, P.R., Gonda, I., Anderson, S.D., Bailey, D., and Bautovich, G. 1994. Regional deposition of saline aerosols of different tonicities in normal and asthmatic subjects. *Eur Respir J* 7: 1474–82.

Pinheiro, M., Lúcio, M., Lima, J.L., and Reis, S. 2011. Liposomes as drug delivery systems for the treatment of TB. *Nanomedicine (Lond.)* 6: 1413–28.

Pourshahab, P.S., Gilani, K., Moazeni, E., Eslahi, H., Fazeli, M.R., and Jamalifar, H. 2011. Preparation and characterization of spray dried inhalable powders containing chitosan nanoparticles for pulmonary delivery of isoniazid. *J Microencapsul* 28: 605–13.

Prashansa, S., Kumar, S.P., Bhushan, M.V., and Bhandari A. 2014. Preparation and characterization of isoniazid chitosan loaded nanoparticles. *J Drug Deliver Therapeutics* 4: 158–66.

Qin, H., Wang, C.M., Dong, Q.Q., Zhang, L., Zhang, X., Ma, Z.Y., and Han, Q.R. 2015.Preparation and characterization of magnetic Fe_3O_4–chitosan nanoparticles loaded with isoniazid. *J Magn Mater* 381: 120–6.

Rastogi, R., Sultana, Y., Ali, A., and Aqil, M. 2006. Particulate and vesicular drug carriers in the management of tuberculosis. *Curr Drug Deliv* 3: 121–8.

Rawal, T., Parmar, R., Tyagi, R.K., and Butani, S. 2017. Rifampicin loaded chitosan nanoparticle dry powder presents an improved therapeutic approach for alveolar tuberculosis. *Colloids Surf B Biointerfaces* 154: 321–330.

Rello, J. and Diaz, E. 2003. Pneumonia in the intensive care unit. Crit Care Med 31: 2544–51.

Roa, W.H., Azarmi, S., Al-Hallak, M.H., Finlay, W.H., Magliocco, A.M., Lobenberg, R. et al. 2011. Inhalable nanoparticles, a non-invasive approach to treat lung cancer in a mouse model. *J Control Release* 150: 49–55.

Rosenthal, L.A., Avila, P.C., Heymann, P.W., Martin, R.J., Miller, E.K., Papadopoulos, N.G., Peebles, R.S., and Gern, J.E. 2010. Infections and asthma committee, American academy of allergy, asthma & immunology, viral respiratory tract infections and asthma: The course ahead. J Allergy Clin Immunol 125: 1212–7.

Roy, I. and Vij, N. 2010. Nanodelivery in airway diseases: Challenges and therapeutic applications. *Nanomedicine* 6: 237–44.

Sangwan, S., Agosti, J.M., Bauer, L.A., Otulana, B.A., Morishige, R.J., Cipolla, D.C., Blanchard, J.D., and Smaldone, G.C. 2001. Aerosolized protein delivery in asthma: Gamma camera analysis of regional deposition and perfusion. *J Aerosol Med Pulm Drug Deliv* 14: 185–95.

Semmler-Behnke, M., Takenaka, S., Fertsch, S., Wenk, A., Seitz, J., Mayer, P., Oberdorster, G., and Kreyling, W.G. 2007. Efficient elimination of inhaled nanoparticles from the alveolar region: Evidence for interstitial uptake and subsequent re-entrainment onto airways epithelium. *Environ Health Perspect* 115: 728–33.

Smola, M., Vandamme, T., and Sokolowski, A. 2008. Nanocarriers as pulmonary drug delivery systems to treat and to diagnose respiratory and non respiratory diseases. *Int J Nanomedicine* 3: 1–19.

Sosnik, A., Carcaboso, A.M., Glisoni, R.J., Moretton, M.A., and Chiappetta, D.A. 2010. New old challenges in tuberculosis: Potentially effective nanotechnologies in drug delivery. *Adv Drug Deliv Rev* 62: 547–59.

Sung, J.C., Pulliam, B.L., and Edwards, D.A. 2007. Nanoparticles for drug delivery to the lungs. *Trends Biotechnol* 25: 563–70.

Tahara, K., Yamamoto, H., Hirashima, N., and Kawashima, Y. 2010. Chitosan-modified poly(d,l-lactide-co-glycolide) nanospheres for improving siRNA delivery and gene-silencing effects. *Eur J Pharm Biopharm* 74: 421–6.

Todoroff, J. and Vanbever, R. 2011. Fate of nanomedicines in the lungs. *Curr Opin Colloid Interface Sci*16: 246–54.

Torrecilla, D., Lozano, M.V., Lallana, E., Neissa, J.I., Novoa-Carballal, R., Vidal, A., Fernandez-Megia, E., Torres, D., Riguera, R., Alonso, M.J., and Dominguez, F. 2013. Anti-tumor efficacy of chitosangpoly(ethylene glycol) nanocapsules containing docetaxel: Anti-TMEFF-2 functionalized nanocapsules vs non-functionalized nanocapsules. *Eur J Pharm Biopharm* 83: 330–7.

Tsapis, N., Bennett, D., Jackson, B., Weitz, D.A., and Edwards, D.A. 2002. Trojan particles: Large porous carriers of nanoparticles for drug delivery. *Proc Natl Acad Sci U S A* 99: 12001–5.

Tseng, C.L., Wu, S.Y., Wang, W.H., Peng, C.L., Lin, F.H., Lin, C.C. et al. 2008. Targeting efficiency and biodistribution of biotinylated-EGF-conjugated gelatin nanoparticles administered via aerosol delivery in nude mice with lung cancer. *Biomaterials* 29: 3014–22.

Usmani, O.S., Biddiscombe, M.F., and Barnes, P.J. 2005. Regional lung deposition and bronchodilator response as a function of beta2-agonist particle size. *Am J Respir Crit Care Med* 172: 1497–504.

Venkatesan, J. and Kim, S.K. 2010. Chitosan composites for bone tissue engineering—An overview. *Mar Drugs* 8: 2252–66.

Videira, M., Almeida, A.J., and Fabra, A. 2012. Preclinical evaluation of a pulmonary delivered paclitaxel-loaded lipid nanocarrier antitumor effect. *Nanomedicine* 8: 1208–15.

Vllasaliu, D., Exposito-Harris, R., Heras, A., Casettari, L., Garnett, M., Illum, L. et al. 2010. Tight junction modulation by chitosan nanoparticles: Comparison with chitosan solution. *Int J Pharm* 400: 183–93.

Vyas, S.P., Quraishi, S., Gupta, S., and Jaganathan, K.S. 2005. Aerosolized liposome-based delivery of amphotericin B to alveolar macrophages. *Int J Pharm* 296: 12–25.

Watanabe, M., Okada, M., Kudo, Y., Tonori, Y., Niitsuya, M., Sato, T., Aizawa, Y., and Kotani, M. 2002. Differences in the effects of fibrous and particulate titanium dioxide on alveolar macrophages of Fischer 344 rats. *J Toxicol Environ Health A* 65: 1047–60.

Yang, R., Yang, S.G., Shim, W.S. et al. 2009. Lung-specific delivery of paclitaxel by chitosan-modified PLGA nanoparticles via transient formation of microaggregates. *J Pharm Sci* 98: 970–84.

Yang, W., Peters, J.I., and Williams, R.O. 2008. Inhaled nanoparticles-a current review. *Int J Pharm* 356: 239–47.

Zaru, M., Manca, M.L., Fadda, A.M., and Antimisiaris, S.G. 2009. Chitosan-coated liposomes for delivery to lungs by nebulisation. *Colloids Surf B Biointerfaces* 71: 88–95.

Zumla, A. 2012. Killer respiratory tract infections: Time to turn the tide. *Curr Opin Pulm Med* 18: 173–4.

15 Polysaccharide-Based Nanoparticles for Colon-Specific Drug Delivery

Moumita Das, Arindam Maity,
Debanjana Chakraborty, and Lakshmi Kanta Ghosh

CONTENTS

15.1 INTRODUCTION

The colon-targeting of biologically active molecules for treatment and management of colonic diseases is an area of research that has attracted a huge number of scientists over the last few decades. Drugs are targeted to the colon for both local action on diseases affecting the colon like inflammatory bowel diseases, colon cancer, etc., or for systemic absorption and action. Overall, colon-targeted formulations offer several advantages over conventional drug delivery systems. However, there are certain limitations due to which such formulations may not be as effective as desired. Nanoparticulate formulations would help to solve the limitations of colon-targeted drug delivery systems due to the several advantages of nanosize formulations which can penetrate the mucous layer and epithelial membrane effectively due to their smaller size and ensure better tissue penetration of the affected areas of the colon. Further, several types of polymers have been used in the preparation of such formulations. However, natural polysaccharides offer a distinct advantage over others as they are selectively metabolized in the colon due to the action of the huge bacterial population.

Therefore, in this chapter polysaccharide-based nanoparticulate formulations targeted for colonic delivery will be discussed, which will help us to understand the recent developments and technologies being utilized to target the colon for drug delivery in a much better and efficient manner.

15.2 PHYSIOLOGY AND CHARACTERISTIC FEATURES OF THE COLON

In this section we will discuss the physiology of the large intestine and colon highlighting its gross anatomy, microscopic anatomy, blood supply, and functions.

The human body has two types of intestines; one is the small intestine and the other is the large intestine (also called the colon). The large intestine is part of the final stages of digestion. The function of the small intestine is to handle the middle part of the digestion process.

The colon is a dynamic organ and plays a major role in maintaining human health, involved in various functions including absorption of electrolytes and water, the salvage of unabsorbed nutrients, and the transport of luminal contents as feces (Romanes 1986).

15.2.1 Gross Anatomy

The colon in present at the lower part of gastrointestinal tract, inverted, 5–6 ft long, and U-shaped (Figure 15.1). The cecum (and appendix) and ano-rectum are not included in the colon, but they are the parts of the large intestine.

The gut is divided into foregut, midgut, and hindgut. The first part of the colon from the ascending colon to the proximal transverse colon develops from the midgut, while the terminal part of the colon from the distal transverse colon to sigmoid colon develops from the hindgut. The colon is filled with air and fecal material as observed from abdominal radiographs. Another characteristic feature of the colon is the "haustra" which are small pouches in the colonic mucosa which develop due to sac formation or sacculation. They give the colon its segmented appearance.

15.2.1.1 Ascending Colon

The ascending colon is an important part of the four major regions of the colon situated in between the cecum and the transverse colon. It mainly occupies the right iliac fossa, right lumbar region, and right hypochondrium. The cecum is present at the proximal end (pouch) of the ascending colon. The ascending colon becomes the transverse colon when taking a right-angled turn just below the liver. The transverse colon is situated as a horizontal route from right to left occupying the right hypochondrium, epigastrium, and left hypochondrium. The ascending colon absorbs nutrients, water, and vitamins from the feces and deposits them into the blood stream. The vitamins are released by digestion of the transitory fecal matter with the help of bacteria.

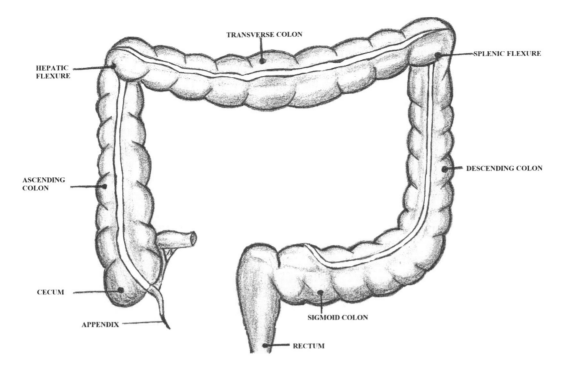

FIGURE 15.1 Anatomical features of the colon.

15.2.1.2 Transverse Colon

In between the ascending and descending colon lies the long transverse colon. It is the longest part of the colon and crosses the abdomen transversely from a right to left direction below the stomach. The ascending colon takes a right turn at the right colic flexure or hepatic flexure (as it is close to liver) to form the transverse colon. The transverse colon then takes a turn at the left colic flexure or splenic flexure (as it is close to the spleen) to descend down into the descending colon. A major amount of absorption takes place in the transverse colon forming a major bulk of feces. Therefore, it is a very important part of the gastrointestinal tract. Then the feces are transferred from the descending colon into the rectum and exit out of the body through the anus as stool. Like other parts of the large intestine, the transverse colon is susceptible to tumors and the onset of colon cancer (Grant et al. 1989).

15.2.1.3 Paracolic Gutters

The paracolic gutters are the spaces between the outer wall of the colon and back side of the abdominal wall. It is also named paracolic sulci or paracolic recesses. It is divided between the left and right lateral paracolic gutters. They both lie on the lateral side of the posterior abdominal wall alongside the ascending and descending colon. The right one is much larger than the left one and thus allows fluid/pus in the upper abdomen to trickle down into the pelvic cavity. The ascending and descending colon is related to the ureter, kidney, and gonadal vessels of the corresponding side that lie behind them in the retroperitoneum. The ascending colon is also related to the C loop (second part) of the duodenum.

15.2.1.4 Transverse Colon and Sigmoid Colon

The transverse colon is long and is located in between the ascending and descending colon and the sigmoid colon and is the part of the large intestine and near to the rectum and anus. The sigmoid colon is also called the pelvic colon. Both the colons have a mesentery that is the transverse mesocolon and sigmoid mesocolon, respectively. But the ascending and descending colon are retroperitoneal. The core of the transverse mesocolon is situated parallel over the duodenum and pancreas. The greater omentum has different parts like the 2-layered gastrocolic ligament attached to the transverse colon and the greater curvature of the stomach and the 4-layered omental apron sling of the transverse colon. Three perpendicular teniae coli are also present in the cecum, ascending colon, descending colon, transverse colon, and sigmoid colon but not present in the rectum. The teniae coli is also present anteriorly on the posterolateral and posteromedial aspects in both ascending and descending colon where they are appendages of fat, contain small blood vessels (called omental appendages or appendices epiploicae) and are also attached to the colon (Gray and Lewis 2000; Sinnatamby 1999).

15.2.2 Blood Supply

Both the superior mesenteric artery and the inferior mesenteric artery supply blood to the colon through their right and middle colic branches and through the left colic and sigmoid branches, respectively. The terminal branches of these arteries which enter in to the colonic mucosal wall are termed vasa recta. Further, there is also a series of anastomoses between the distal branch of the proximal artery and proximal branch of the distal artery which is termed the marginal artery of Drummond, which is present close to the inner lining of the colon. Anastomoses are connections between the branches of arteries or blood vessels. This artery can be useful for mobilization of a large part of the colon, like in the replacement of esophagus in the chest after an esophagectomy.

The lymphatic system supplying the colon consists of epicolic, paracolic, intermediate, and main lymph nodes. Epicolic lymph nodes are present on the surface of the colon, paracolic nodes are present next to the colon, intermediate lymph nodes are present in the mesocolon, and the main lymph nodes at the root of the mesocolon. The lymph flows through the lymph nodes as follows:

$$\text{epicolic} \rightarrow \text{paracolic} \rightarrow \text{intermediate} \rightarrow \text{main lymph node}$$

The mesocolon is the fold of the peritoneum (thin, transparent lining of the abdominal and pelvic cavity) which is present on one or more parts of the colon and connects it to the wall of the abdomen.

15.2.3 Microscopic Anatomy

There are four layers in the colon:

1. The mucosa: It contains columnar epithelium with goblet cells secreting mucosa, lamina propria and muscularis mucosa. Villi is absent.
2. The sub-mucosa: It contains Meissner nerve plexus and blood vessels.
3. Muscularis propria: It contains the myenteric nerve plexus, circular muscles in the inner layer and longitudinal muscles in the outer layer (contains three straps called teniae coli).
4. Serosa: It contains the visceral peritoneum.

The large intestine is much wider than the small intestine and has four main parts, namely, the cecum, the colon, the rectum, and the anal canal. The large intestine meets the terminal end of the small intestine in the pelvis at the right iliac region, then moves upward in the abdominal region and then moves downward and continues till the anal canal. The three straps of teniae coli, 1/5 in. wide, start from below the appendix and continue from the cecum to the rectum. Epiploic appendages run along the teniae coli and contain fat filled peritoneum tags. The lining of the large intestine contains columnar epithelium with intestinal glands and goblet cells secreting mucin which forms mucus in water.

The Crypt of Lieberkühn is an intestinal crypt that is found in both the small and large intestines. The crypts are covered by the epithelial cell layer which contains the goblet cells (secreting mucus) and the enterocytes (secreting electrolytes). It also contains stem cells at the basal layer.

Digestive enzymes (peptidases, sucrase, maltase, lactase, and intestinal lipase) are produced from the enterocytes which digest food when the food gets absorbed through the intestinal cells. As, the epithelial layer is worn out by the passing food, it is reformed at regular intervals. One of the causes of colorectal cancer is thought to be the loss of control over proliferation in crypts.

The transverse colon forms a bridge from the left to the right side and is the top arm. The descending colon forms the left arm from which the sigmoid hangs creating an s-shape and is called the "broken" part of the rectangle emptying into the rectum (Romanes 1986).

15.2.4 FUNCTIONS OF THE COLON

- The large intestine or the colon is the last part of the gastrointestinal tract. Its main functions are to store the undigested food passed from small intestine (such as fiber), absorb any remaining water, nutrients (like vitamins and minerals), and electrolytes from the food and to eradicate the waste matter from the body through the anus.
- The colon also helps to maintain the fluid balance in the body by absorbing water and electrolytes.
- Feces are formed in the colon from fiber, vitamins, and water along with mucus and bacteria found in the colon.
- Huge populations of bacteria in the colon (like *Bacillus coli* and *acidophillus*) helps:
  - To maintain pH balance
  - In the formation of nutrients (like folic acid, vitamin K, or some groups of vitamin B)
  - In digestion
  - In the prevention of the growth of harmful bacteria in the colon.
    Fiber acts as food for the bacteria in the colon which they convert into nutrients beneficial for the colonic tissues. Therefore, presence of fiber in food matter is very important for colonic health.
- Peristaltic movement in the rectum, the terminal part of the large intestine helps in the easy removal of waste matter through the anus (Romanes 1986).

15.2.5 COLONIC DISEASES AND CONDITIONS

- Colitis: The colon mucosa is inflamed which may be due to infection in the colon or inflammatory bowel diseases like Crohn's disease or ulcerative colitis.
- Diverticulosis: Small pouches, called diverticuli are formed in the weak areas of the colonic mucosa which crosses the cell lining of the colon.
- Diverticulitis: Infection or inflammation of the diverticuli with symptoms like fever, constipation or abdominal pain.
- Colonic hemorrhage or bleeding: Bleeding of the colon may occur in different types of colonic diseases, which may be seen in the stool.
- Inflammatory bowel disease (IBD): In this condition, the inflammation of the colon takes place like Crohn's disease or ulcerative colitis.
  - Crohn's disease: Inflammation of the colon and intestines with symptoms like abdominal pain and diarrhoea and bloody stools.
  - Ulcerative colitis: In this case, inflammation occurs in the colon and rectum and bloody stools are passed.
- Diarrhoea: Under this condition, the patient passes frequent, watery stools which is mostly due to infection in the intestines.
- Salmonellosis: Occurs due to infection caused by the bacteria *Salmonella*, usually in the small intestine with symptoms like diarrhoea and cramps in the stomach.
- Shigellosis: Occurs due to infection caused by the bacteria Shigella, usually in the colon with symptoms like diarrhoea and cramps in the stomach, fever, or bloody stools.

- Travelers' diarrhoea: Occurs due to contamination of food and water by bacteria; causes diarrhoea, fever, and nausea or vomiting.
- Colon polyps: Small outgrowths from the colonic mucosa which may develop into colon cancer in the long run. Therefore, preventive measures may be taken by removing them.
- Colon cancer: Cancerous growth in the colon which affects millions of people worldwide and can be prevented if proper screening is done at regular intervals.

15.3   ADVANTAGES OF A COLON-TARGETED DRUG DELIVERY SYSTEM (CDDS) OVER AN ORAL CONVENTIONAL DRUG DELIVERY SYSTEM

Conventional oral dosage forms, if targeted to treat and manage colonic diseases, like inflammatory bowel diseases or colon cancer, etc., would rarely produce desired results. As such, conventional systems release a major amount of the drug before reaching the colon in the upper gastrointestinal tract (GIT), the acidic stomach, or the alkaline small intestine. Therefore, the primary objective of the drug is treatment of colonic diseases; the dosage form must be targeted to the colon. Some of the advantages of colon-targeted drug delivery systems are highlighted as below:

1. Direct action at the disease site
   The CDDS which delivers the drug in high concentrations at the colonic site affected by a particular disease would definitely achieve better therapeutic effect for management of the disease. So colon-specific delivery has already been investigated for inflammatory bowel diseases of the colon; ulcerative colitis, Crohn's disease, and colon cancer, etc. These diseases can be treated well by the local action of the drugs (Maity and Sen 2017).
2. Reduction of dose
   Drugs administered by intravenous infusions or conventional oral delivery systems may reach the colonic site at much lower concentrations through the systemic circulation and thus a much higher dose of the drug may be required. CDDS releasing the drug near colonic mucosa would release the drug in high concentrations and then get absorbed through the colonic mucosa cells into blood circulation. Thus, the diseased site gets exposed to high concentration of the drug and a lower dose may be sufficient to achieve the required therapeutic effect.
3. Minimization of side effects
   One of the important advantages of local delivery is that a major amount of the drug acts locally and then a minimal amount enters into blood circulation. This restricts the systemic side effects of drugs. All drugs, especially anticancer or steroidal drugs, can have serious long-term adverse effects when they enter the systemic circulation in high amounts. CDDS can provide a distinct advantage in reducing such side or adverse effects.
4. Delivery of proteins and peptide molecules
   Certain biopharmaceutical drugs including proteins, peptides, DNA conjugates, etc., do not survive the acidic environment of the stomach or the alkaline intestinal fluid due to pH conditions, susceptibility to physical, chemical, and enzymatic degradation. The colon is relatively devoid of digestive enzymes and the pH conditions are neither highly acidic nor highly alkaline. Therefore, colonic delivery of protein and peptide molecules is being studied (Maity and Sen 2017; Walle 2011).
5. Prolonged drug delivery
   Dosage forms remain longer in the colon as compared to the stomach or the small intestine due to much higher transit times in the colon (approximately 35–36 h). Due to this factor prolonged drug delivery can be achieved when drug release is targeted in the colon with the help of suitable polymers (Friend 1992). Further, bioavailability of the poorly absorbed drugs can improve when the dosage form is retained for prolonged periods of time (Maity and Sen 2017).

15.4 VARIOUS APPROACHES FOR COLON TARGETED DRUG DELIVERY

The colon-targeting of drugs can be a challenging task and different approaches have been laid down for ensuring site-specific delivery of the drugs. Some of them are discussed briefly.

1. pH dependent systems

   It is already pointed out that within the GIT, the pH conditions vary from highly acidic to neutral to highly alkaline. The stomach pH is highly acidic and ranges from 1 to 3. In the small intestine, the pH rises gradually to reach 5–6 (duodenum), 6–7 (jejunum), and 6.5–7.5 (ileum). Interestingly in the colon, the pH drops and remains within 5–7 (Narang and Boddu 2015). The pH dependent systems for colon targeting are designed in such a way that the delivery system bypasses the stomach and major parts of the small intestine and maximum amount of drug release occurs in the colon. Core tablets with entrapped drugs are coated with pH-sensitive polymers like cellulose acetate phthalate, shellac, or eudragits which dissolve only at higher pHs, limiting the drug release in the stomach or small intestine considerably.

2. Time dependent systems

   Drug release from time dependent systems rely on the transit times of the dosage forms in the gastrointestinal tract. The average residence time of a dosage form in the upper GIT is around 5–6 h. However, this is around 24–36 h in the colon, due to which the drug may be targeted to release in larger amounts in the colon. However, during the 5–6 h of transit of the dosage form through the upper GIT, the release cannot be altogether avoided. Because of favorable environment for drug absorption, small amounts that may be released can be absorbed and metabolized to create potential side effects. To safeguard against this possibility, enteric coating is often applied over the pH dependent dosage form. Further, the transit times may vary from individual to individual and in certain conditions like IBD, carcinoid syndrome, diarrhoea, and ulcerative colitis, accelerated transit may occur. This causes speedy removal of the dosage form through defecation before releasing the drug in a sufficient amount for a proper therapeutic effect (Das and Ghosh 2013, Philip and Philip 2010).

3. Microbial-triggered systems

   The colonic fluid is a good reservoir of bacteria (1011–1012 CFU/mL) containing about 400 different species. It mainly consists of anaerobic bacteria like *Bacteroides*, *Bifidobacteria*, *Ruminococci*, *Eubacteria*, *Clostridia*, etc., which secrete a multitude of enzymes like glucoronidase, xylosidase, arabinosidase, galactosidase, nitroreductase, azareducatase, etc. Carbohydrates such as non-starch polysaccharides cannot be digested in the upper GIT. In contrast colonic bacteria can survive on them. Therefore, when a particular dosage form is developed with one such non-starch polysaccharide as the main excipient, the dosage form becomes colonic fluid selective or colon-targeted. The polysaccharide remains unaffected in the upper GIT and upon reaching the colon is acted upon by the enzymes produced by the bacterial population, and releases the drug slowly. Many polysaccharides like chitosan, amylose, pectin, guar gum, dextran, cyclodextrin, etc., have been studied for targeting drugs to the colon (Das and Ghosh 2013; Philip and Philip 2010).

4. Pressure controlled systems

   The viscosity of the colonic contents is high and the fluid volume in the colonic lumen is low. Therefore, the luminal pressure in the colon is higher than the pressure exerted in the upper GIT. Some novel delivery systems for colon delivery have been devised based on this difference in pressure in the upper GIT and the colon. The thickness of the membrane enclosing the formulation is devised in such a way that the device is able to withstand the pressure while passing the stomach and small intestine but opens up in the colon when it faces larger luminal pressure (Philip and Philip 2010).

5. Osmotically controlled systems

Such systems utilize osmotic pressure for controlled drug delivery. They are independent on the physiological conditions of the GIT and therefore have a distinct advantage compared to other approaches. The construction of these systems is simple. They usually contain a drug core with or without an osmogen, a semipermeable membrane that surrounds the core, a drilled orifice, through which the drug is released in a controlled manner. Drug solubility plays an important role in the design of such systems. Only one osmotic unit may be sufficient for drugs of moderate solubility, while 2–5 push pull units in a single capsule may be needed for poorly soluble drugs (Das and Ghosh 2013; Philip and Philip 2010).

6. Multiparticulate drug delivery systems

Single-unit dosage form always has the risk of failing as *in-vivo* conditions may defy our predictions and change due to intra-subject variability, food, or disease, etc.

Failure of a single unit containing a large amount of drug has a much higher potential for damage than multiparticulate systems where units contain smaller amounts of drugs. Hence, pellets, granules, microspheres, nanoparticles, liposomes, etc., can be enteric-coated and compressed into tablets or filled into capsules. When the tablet or capsule disintegrates in the GIT, constituent particles come in direct contact with luminal fluid and each act as an individual drug reservoir (Figure 15.2). The units spread over a large area and avoid dose dumping at the delivery site, reducing the risk of failure and increasing the therapeutic efficacy manifolds (Das and Ghosh 2013).

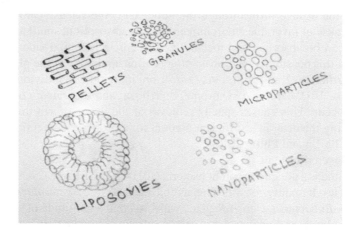

FIGURE 15.2   Different types of multiparticulate dosage forms.

15.5   ADVANTAGES OF POLYSACCHARIDE-BASED COLONIC DOSAGE FORMS

Polysaccharides have been used in colon delivery for various purposes. Synthetic polysaccharides like eudragits, cellulose derivatives, etc., have been mainly used as film formers for the coating of the colon-targeted systems. Natural polysaccharides are biodegradable and have several advantages which would be discussed below.

1. Enzyme and pH independence of gastric and small intestinal fluid

Natural polysaccharide-based systems are not degraded by the enzymes in the stomach or small intestine. The colon having high population of anaerobic bacteria secretes enzymes in the colonic fluid which degrades such polysaccharides. They are also not affected by the pH of the stomach or small intestine (Qiu et al. 2017; Valentine 2011).

2. Independence of gastric and small intestinal emptying time and target specificity

The intra-subject variability of emptying time in the stomach or small intestine does not affect the formulations prepared with natural polysaccharides as they are not degraded in the environment of the upper GIT. They start to degrade only when the formulation reaches the colonic environment with high counts of bacteria (Qiu et al. 2017). Hence, such formulations are highly target-specific.

3. Fasted and fed states have no impact on microflora induced drug release for polysaccharide-based colon-targeted systems.

   The constitution of colonic content does not undergo significant changes and the microflora in the colonic fluid remains more or less the same during the fasted or fed state. Therefore, the drug release from polysaccharide- based formulations would also be not affected by fasted or fed state, which ensures insignificant intra-subject variability (Alonso and Csaba 2012).

4. Ingested food has a temporary reservoir in the stomach from where it is released at a controlled rate to the small intestine.

5. Reduction of inter-subject variation of drug release

   It is reported that the microflora level remains constant over a diverse human population. Polysaccharide-based systems may reduce inter-subject variation of therapeutic efficacy among the patients. The release from polysaccharide-based systems is highly microflora dependent, therefore, a consistency in the microflora level may significantly reduce the variation of drug release and thereby ensure uniform therapeutic efficacy.

6. Biocompatible and non-toxic degradation products

   Natural polysaccharides are very safe and non-toxic. Even the degradation products are non-toxic. Therefore, they are much safer to use rather than the synthetic polymers which are not biocompatible (Rajpurohit et al. 2010).

7. They are inexpensive and freely available

   Natural polysaccharides are available freely and are economic to use as compared to synthetic polymer or polymeric derivatives (Rajpurohit et al. 2010).

8. Capable of chemical modification

   Polysaccharides have a variety of structures and can be modified or crosslinked easily to produce tailor-made dosage forms (Valentine 2011).

9. Stability and compatibility with other excipients in the formulation

   The natural polysaccharides are relatively stable polymers that can be combined with other excipients used in formulations (Rajpurohit et al. 2010).

15.6 SIGNIFICANCE OF NANOPARTICLES FOR DISEASE MANAGEMENT IN THE COLON

The local therapeutic effect of a particular drug in the colonic tissues can only be realised when the concerned drug is present in sufficient concentration at the site of action. This may be possible when the biological barriers separating the cells at the site of action are traversed by the formulation or drug particles successfully, allowing the drug to act and get retained at the affected cells without significant systemic absorption and side effects thereafter (Viscido et al. 2014). Such action can be achieved by nanoparticle formulations (NPs) of drugs. Nanoparticle formulations can be of various types and structures like nanospheres, nanocapsules, liposomes, or micelles as described in Figure 15.3 (Xu et al. 2013). Their physicochemical properties are discussed below:

1. NPs are retained in the colon luminal fluid for prolonged periods as they are unaffected by the flow of intestinal luminal fluid due to their small size (less than 100 nm) (Viscido et al. 2014; Murthy 2007). NPs in the luminal fluid undergo Brownian movement, which improves the probability of the particles hitting and adhering to the colonic mucosa (Viscido et al. 2014). The more the adherence of the NPs to the mucosa, more the probability of the drug getting absorbed in the mucosal cells.

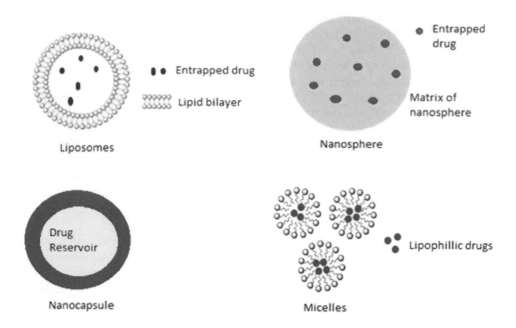

FIGURE 15.3 Different types of nanoparticle formulation.

2. The healthy intestinal mucosa consists of an inner and an outer mucous gel layer which act as barriers to the underlying selectively permeable epithelial layer which allows only absorption of nutrients (Figure 15.4). However, microfold cells (M cells) are present in certain parts of the mucosa which have reduced or no barrier layers. The inflamed colonic mucosa in the case of inflammatory bowel diseases or cancers, etc., loses its physical integrity and holes appear in the epithelial barrier layer of the cells which can be easily traversed by the NPs or smaller microparticles for entry into the mucosa. This process of entry of the NPs into the mucosa through such holes is called persorption. M cells of the epithelium affected by IBD take in the NPs through transcytosis. Further, inflamed areas of the mucosa become permeable to bacteria and therefore immune cells are generated in the mucosal tissues, which can take in the NPs preferentially (Viscido et al. 2014; Hua et al. 2015). Due to all these factors, selective absorption of NPs into the inflamed mucosa may take place.

3. Preferential uptake of the NPs by the mucosal cells helps to avoid their removal due to diarrhoeal conditions in the colonic lumen. Formulations may be thrown out of the colonic lumen under such conditions.

4. Once into the mucosa, bioadhesion of the small-sized NPs increase their residence time in the mucosal cells. They can also enter into the phagocytic cells present in the inflamed colonic mucosa which may further increase their distribution as well as retention time in the mucosal tissues (Viscido et al. 2014; Hua et al. 2015). Phagocytic cells are an important part of the immune system which helps to eradicate foreign particles or pathogens.

5. NPs, due to their small size, can penetrate deeper layers of the colonic mucosa while larger sized particles or microparticles are concentrated in the upper layers of the mucosa (Viscido et al. 2014). The deeper the NPs penetrate the more action they produce for deep rooted inflammation in the colonic mucosa, which spread to deeper layers of the tissue.

6. Finally, as multiple unit delivery system, the chance of failure of the delivery system is much less as compared to single-unit dosage forms. Nanoparticle-based systems consist of several single-unit delivery systems in a single formulation which spread in the lumen widely.

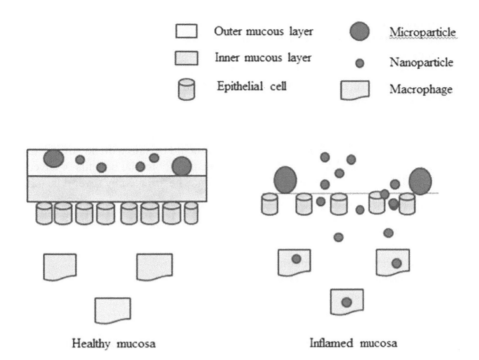

FIGURE 15.4 Selective uptake of nanoparticles from inflamed mucosa.

Hence, the NP formulations may provide a favorable option to treat and manage the diseases of the colon specifically the inflammatory diseases as they spread throughout the lumen, are taken up by the inflamed mucosa preferentially, passes through the epithelial cells and can penetrate deeper layers of the mucosa.

15.7 VARIOUS POLYSACCHARIDES: THEIR SPECIFIC CHARACTERISTICS, THEIR USE FOR COLON DELIVERY, SPECIFIC RESEARCH STUDIES FOR NANOPARTICLES OF EACH POLYSACCHARIDE

Polymers are large chain macromolecules made up with repetitive units of low or high molecular weight monomers containing different functional groups. They play a major role in the advancement of drug delivery. A selective consideration of polymers through their surface and bulk properties will lead to the development of newer novel drug delivery systems including colon-specific drug delivery (Pillai and Panchagnula 2001).

Colon-targeted drug delivery can be achieved by developing various mechanistic pathways (discussed in section 3). In colon targeted polysaccharide-based drug delivery systems, polysaccharide (present in the matrix or in the coating) starts to dissolve when it enters into the colon. The natural polysaccharides which remain undigested in the upper GIT get degraded enzymatically into organic derivatives like acetate, propionate, or butyrate derivatives due to the action of the huge pool of bacteria in the colon. The process of bacterial degradation of the polysaccharides is called fermentation. The fermentation products are beneficial for the mucosal cells of the colon. Once the polysaccharide is dissolved the formulation releases the entrapped drug easily (Joshi 2007).

The process of biodegradation is a natural activity where organic compounds are transformed to simple compounds and then redistributed in the environment. So, the biopolymers have been widely used in biomedical applications due to their well-known biocompatibility and biodegradability (Vert 1989). Further, polymers within this group maintain their properties for a limited period of time and then gradually degrade into soluble molecules and get excreted from the body (Vainionpaa 1989).

Due to the elimination of the depleted device by a surgical removal process, biodegradable polymers are mostly preferred for drug delivery applications. There are lots of biodegradable polymers present in nature, but only a few numbers of polymers are suitable for drug delivery applications. Suitable candidates should be properly biodegradable and biocompatible, should be able to go through processing, be sterilizable and be stable under various storage conditions. Only then can it be used for biomedical applications. (Kronenthal 1975).

A significant advantage of biodegradable polymers is that they are broken down or metabolized into substrates which are then removed from the body by normal metabolic pathways. However, the by-products produced through such metabolic pathways should be safe with no adverse reactions in the body. Such by-products should be tested to determine their potential benefits or adverse effects. Further, the degradation of the biodegradable materials may be affected by several factors, some of which are listed below:

- Chemical structure.
- Chemical composition.
- Distribution of repeat units in multimers.
- Presence of unexpected units or chain defects.
- Presence of ionic groups.
- Molecular weight.
- Molecular-weight distribution.
- Morphology (amorphous/semicrystalline, microstructures, residual stresses).
- Presence of low-molecular-weight compounds.
- Processing conditions.
- Annealing.
- Sterilization process.
- Storage history.
- Shape.
- Site of implantation.
- Adsorbed and absorbed compounds (water, lipids, ions, etc.).
- Physicochemical factors (ion exchange, ionic strength, and pH).
- Physical factors (shape and size changes, variations of diffusion coefficients, mechanical stresses, stress- and solvent-induced cracking, etc.).
- Mechanism of hydrolysis (enzymes versus water).
- Biodegradable polymers mainly investigated for drug delivery applications are of either natural or synthetic origin.

15.7.1 Natural Polymers in Colon-Targeting

Polysaccharides obtained from nature are one of the major sources extensively used for solid oral dosage forms of colonic drug delivery (Jain and Jain 2006). They are generally hydrophilic in nature and have a limited swelling property in acidic pH. The colon contains a number of bacteria which secretes many enzymes and cause hydrolytic cleavage of glycosidic bonds, e.g. β-D-galactosidase, β-D-glucosidase, α-D-xylosidase, amylase, pectinase, and dextranase. Guar gum, pectin, dextran, alginate, and chitosan are some of the few polysaccharides available in a variety of structures and commonly used in various colonic dosage forms (structures given in Figure 15.5 and Figure 15.6). These polysaccharides are intact in the stomach and small intestine but degrade in the human colon due to the action of bacteria which makes them useful for colon-targeting (Shirwaikar 2008).

The following are some of the natural polymers used in colon-targeted drug delivery systems:

1. Guar gum
2. Pectin

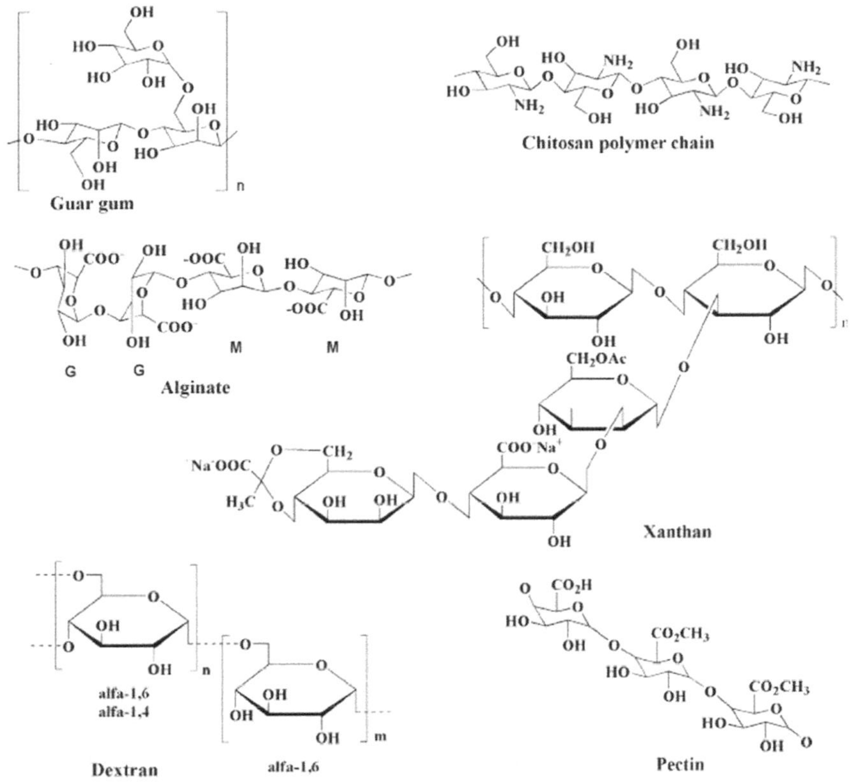

FIGURE 15.5 Structure of polysaccharides (guar gum, chitosan, alginate, xanthan, dextran, and pectin).

3. Xanthan Gum
4. Shellac
5. Chitosan
6. Dextran
7. Cyclodextrin
8. Chondroitin sulfate
9. Alginates
10. Inulin

15.7.1.1 Guar Gum

The gum is obtained by extraction from the seeds of the plant *Cyamopsis tetragonoloba*. It is a galactomannan consisting of galactose and mannose sugar moieties in the ratio of 1:2. The structure of guar gum includes a linear chain of β-1,4-linked mannose residues attached to 1,6-linked galactose residues at every second mannose, forming short side-branches (Figure 15.5) (Hartemink et al. 1999).

The polysaccharide remains unaffected in the upper GIT. Fermentation takes place in the colon by the action of certain strains of bacteria including *Bacteroides ovatus, Bifidobacterium dentium, Ruminococcus albus*, etc., to produce short chain fatty acids and gases as by-products. Thus, formulations containing guar gum release the entrapped drug only when they reach the colon and are colon-specific. Further, the gum can only form gels in aqueous environments which helps it to retard and sustain drug release. Guar gum containing colon-targeted systems include microspheres, matrix, and compression-coated tablets, as well as nanoparticle formulations (Al-Saidan et al. 2005; Krishnaiah et al. 2003).

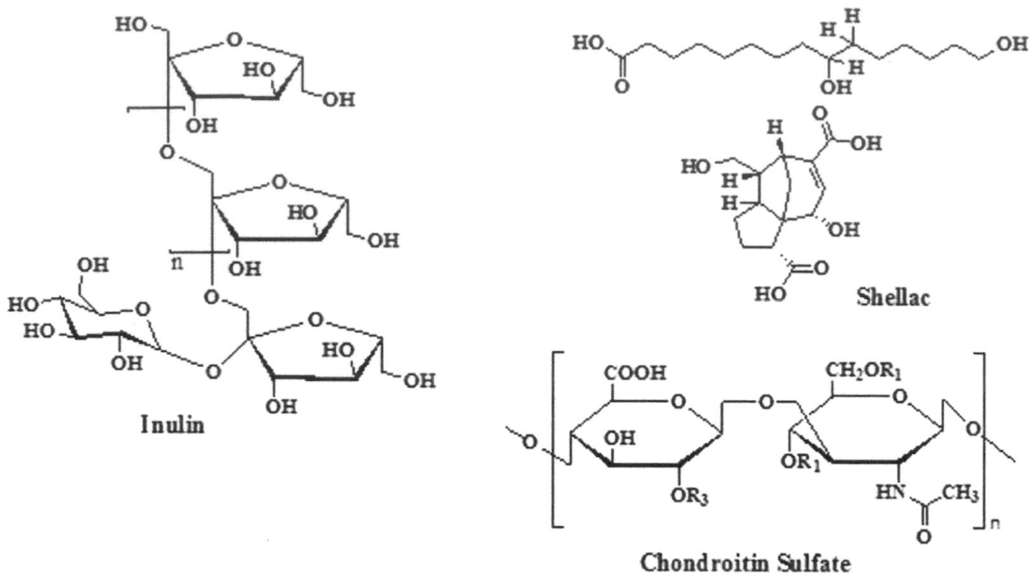

FIGURE 15.6 Structure of polysaccharides (inulin, shellac, and chondroitin sulfate).

Treatment and management of colonic diseases require colon-targeted drug delivery, may it be in the case of inflammatory bowel diseases like colitis, diarrhoea, or colon cancer. In the present study, Kumar et al. developed a formulation for targeting colon cancer cells. They prepared mesoporous silica nanoparticles covered with a guar gum layer. Mesoporous particles have a pore size in the range of 2–50 nm which help to entrap the drug within the mesoporous channels of the nanoparticles. The guar gum layer protected the drug in the upper GIT and released a major amount of the drug in the colonic environment which contained enzymes to degrade the gum. Further, significant anticancer activity was observed in *in-vitro* studies, conducted on cancer cell lines with the nanoparticle formulation. Therefore, the formulation developed by the researchers was fit to achieve colon-targeted release of the anticancer drug (Kumar et al. 2017).

Colon cancer affects huge numbers of people worldwide and novel strategies are constantly being developed to target the cancer cells at the molecular level and ensure better therapeutic efficacy of the administered drugs. Folate receptors are found on the cancerous cells in the colon in larger amounts than the normal cells and these receptors were studied by Sharma et al. to target drugs to colon cancer cells using the emulsion crosslinking method. Thus, nanoparticles were developed with guar gum and the surface of the nanoparticles was modified with folic acid by emulsion crosslinking. In an emulsion crosslinking method, the crosslinking agent is incorporated into the emulsion containing the polymer to form a complex with chemical groups on the monomer chain. Methotrexate was chosen as the anticancer drug and was loaded into the nanoparticles. Thus, the strategy was to avoid drug release in the upper parts of the GIT with the help of guar gum and once the guar gum is degraded by the colonic enzymes, the folic acid groups on the nanoparticles would selectively bind to the folate receptors on the cancer cells, increasing the specificity of the formulation for the diseased tissues and the retention of the nanoparticles in them. The nanoparticles would then release the drug within the cancer cells and produce a much better therapeutic efficacy with reduced side effects. *In-vitro* drug release and *in-vivo* studies with caco-2 cancer cells (epithelial cells collected from human colon carcinoma tissues) were performed for both surface modified and unmodified particles. The nanoparticles could successfully avoid drug release in the upper parts of GIT due to presence of guar gum and showed major amount of drug release in the simulated colonic fluid of pH 6.8. The modified nanoparticles showed better inhibition of caco 2 cells than the unmodified nanoparticles. It was claimed that the novel strategy can be useful to achieve site specific drug release and action for management of colon cancer (Sharma et al. 2013).

Anticancer drugs like 5-fluorouracil have several side effects like diarrhoea, mucositis, etc., and may cause substantial damage to the microflora in the colonic fluid. The bacterial population in the colon performs many important functions and plays a substantial role in metabolism. They are also important for the metabolism of the polysaccharides and release of the entrapped drugs in the colon. Therefore, reduction in the bacterial population in the colon may cause potential side effects in the body. Taking this into consideration, Singh et al. developed nanoparticles containing anticancer drug 5-fluorouracil coated with prebiotics like guar gum and xanthan gum and probiotic like *Bifidobacterium bifidum*. The prebiotic coating ensured the delivery of the drug in the colon avoiding the upper GIT, while the probiotic helped to maintain the bacterial population in the colon resulting in fewer side effects and metabolized the gums. *In-vitro* dissolution studies were performed in simulated fluids of the stomach, small intestine, and colon. The formulation released about 93% of the drug in simulated colonic fluid containing rat cecal contents. *In-vivo* tests were performed in rats with the formulation and with free drug powder and drug nanoparticles. The probiotic containing the formulation did not cause any diarrhoea, ulceration, or histopathological changes and normal cecum conditions were observed when compared with the drug powder and drug nanoparticles. Therefore, the developed formulation with the unique strategy can definitely be helpful for benefiting patients with safety and efficacy of treatment (Singh et al. 2015).

Guar gum is a natural polysaccharide which releases entrapped drug in the large intestine due to the action of bacterial enzymes. But in this particular study, Varma et al. modified the gum by grafting it with polyacrylamide to make the gum pH-sensitive. Grafting is a process by which new functional groups are introduced within a polymer chain under controlled conditions, by means like radiation or chemical hydrolysis, to alter its physicochemical properties. Esomeprazole magnesium (a proton pump inhibitor used to treat ulcers) was used as the model drug. The modified gum was used to prepare drug-loaded nanoparticles which released the drug at a higher pH and could delay drug release (Varma et al. 2016).

Guar gum was also used by Baboo et al. to apply a protective inner coating for granules containing raupya bhasma, guar gum, and xanthan gum which helped to avoid release in the small intestine (pH >7) and release the drug in the colon. The gums also helped to sustain drug release. The granules were further coated with eudragit FS30D for protection in the upper GIT. Raupya bhasma is an ayurvedic medicine used to treat memory loss, dizziness, excessive thirst, diabetes, etc. (Baboo et al. 2013).

15.7.1.2 Pectin

This polysaccharide can be found in the cell wall of plants. The structure of pectin is heterogeneous in nature and consists of poly(D-galacturonic acid) linked with (1→4) glycosidic linkage and 1,2 D-rhamnose with side chains of D-galactose and D-arabinose (Figure 15.5). It has an average molecular weight of between 50,000 and about 180,000 Da (Sinha and Kumria 2001). It is not affected by the fluids in the upper GIT but gets degraded by the pectinases produced by the colonic bacteria like *Bacteroides thetaiotaomicron* in the colonic fluid to produce soluble oligalactorunates and short chain fatty acids (Englyst 1987; Roy and James 1973; Dongowski et al. 2000).

It is soluble and swells in water. The entrapped drug within the pectin matrix is released through diffusion.

Modifications of polymers by suitable agents by grafting or crosslinking have been performed by researchers to alter the physicochemical properties of polymers for the benefits of drug delivery. In one study, Chang et al. complexed pectin with glutaraldehyde to impart pH-sensitivity to the polymer and developed a novel nanogel formulation containing nanosized spherical particles. The drug release from the nanogel was fast in alkaline pH which may be due to the pH-sensitive modified polymer. The release increased further in the presence of pectinolytic enzymes. The modified polymer had the dual advantage of selective hydrolysis in the colon as well as pH-sensitivity making the formulation more colon specific (Chang et al. 2007).

Though colon-targeted delivery systems using natural polysaccharides release drug selectively in the colon they suffer from the disadvantage of affecting both normal and cancer cells, causing damage to both and producing serious side effects. The problem can be minimized through selective drug binding by targeting receptors present specifically in the cancerous cells. Thus Subudhi et al. used a novel approach to target galectin-3 receptors in colon cancer cells. They developed citrus pectin nanoparticles containing the anticancer drug 5-fluorouracil. Citrus pectin can bind to galectin-3 receptors and thus attacked the cancerous cells selectively. The nanoparticles were coated with eudragit S100 to avoid release in the upper GIT. The eudragit S100 coating dissolved in the distal small intestine, releasing the nanoparticles (drug entrapped in citrus pectin) which selectively bound to the cancer cells present in the colon. *In-vitro* drug release studies with the nanoparticles showed 70% selective drug release after 24 h in the colonic region. Further, the efficacy of the nanoparticles was evaluated on HT-29 cancer cells along with free drug solution. The nanoparticles were 1.5-times more cytotoxic than the corresponding 5-FU solution. The pectin layer protected the nanoparticles in the small intestine which was acted upon by bacteria in the colon to release the drug. The drug then acted on the cancer cells and thus this resulted in better efficacy and lesser side effects (Subudhi et al. 2015).

Yet in another study by Tsai et al, hyaluronan receptors were identified in cancer cells and therefore, nanoparticles were prepared using hyaluronan to target those receptor-bearing cells. Cisplatin was the chosen anticancer drug. Nanoparticles bearing hyaluronan-cisplatin conjugate were prepared by stirring hyaluronan and cisplatin for 3 days in the absence of light. It was reported that the platinum atoms of the drug complexed with the carboxyl groups of hyaluronic acid to form conjugates on the nanoscale. The prepared nanoparticles were then entrapped within microbeads prepared with pectin and alginate by an electrospray method. In this process, the nanoparticles were added to the polymer solution (kept in a syringe) and connected to a positive electrode. The negative electrode was connected to the solution containing the complexing agent (calcium chloride). On applying voltage, the nanoparticles entrapped within microbeads of alginate/chitosan were produced. The microbeads were finally coated with eudragit S100 to protect them from gastric and intestinal fluids. Release studies using pH dependent process showed minimal release in simulated stomach and intestinal fluids and peak release (75.6%) at pH 7.4 which was due to the protective eudragit coating. The nanoparticles with the drug conjugate showed reduced nephrotoxicity compared to free drug solution when evaluated by an *in-vivo* nephrotoxicity study in Wistar rat model (Tsai et al. 2013).

Pectin is widely used in colon-targeted delivery due to its selective hydrolysis in the colonic medium. Cheng et al. prepared calcium pectinate nanoparticles containing insulin. Insulin is an important peptide drug which gets hydrolyzed by enzymes in the stomach or small intestine and thus colon targeted delivery may prove useful for its absorption through the colonic mucosa. Pectin with different molecular weights were taken and milled to smaller size particles. Nanoparticles were prepared using both milled and unmilled pectins which had similar particle size and insulin association. However, the insulin association was significantly affected by the pH of the formulation. When, the pH was increased from 2 to 3, the insulin association efficiency was increased by 3-times due to a higher charge density on the polymer. Charge density is a measure of the charge on a molecule. The nanoparticles were produced by ionic crosslinking using calcium chloride as the crosslinking agent. In the process of ionic crosslinking, interaction takes place between the oppositely charged ions (anion and cation) in the polymer and crosslinking agent resulting in the synthesis of crosslinked polymer and salts in solution. The variation in mean diameter was lesser in case of high molecular weight pectin. Further, change in formulation pH also affected the stability of the nanoparticles. Insulin release from the particles was dependent on the extent of dilution of nanoparticles in the dissolution medium as well as pH of the medium (Cheng and Lim 2004).

Approaches to drug delivery are continuously evolving in the field of colon cancer treatment as it is the third most common cancer in the world. A novel platinum complex (bipyridine ethyl dithiocarbamate Pt (II) nitrate) was thus, targeted to the colon by Izadi et al. using a novel nanoparticle comprising of pectin and β-lactoglobulin (a whey protein). β-lactoglobulin has the unique properties of not being affected by stomach pH as well as proteases in gastric fluid. Further, it can bind to hydrophobic ligands (molecules with functional groups that can bind to central metal atom of another molecule to form a complex). The stability of the carrier system was found to be concentration dependent and a certain combination 0.5 mg/ml of β-lactoglobulin and pectin concentration 0.025–0.05 wt% had the best particle size and stability. The formulation was stable at a low pH and released the drug in alkaline pH and therefore, was colon-specific (Izadi et al. 2016).

Dicer-substrate small interfering RNA (DsiRNA) has excellent anticancer efficacy but could not be used in drug delivery because it is not stable, easily degraded in gastrointestinal fluids, and its uptake in the cells is low. Dicer is an enzyme which reduces double stranded RNA into short fragments of 20–25 nucleotides called small interfering RNA. Dicer activates RNA induced silencing complex in cells which causes RNA interference and gene silencing which is helpful to combat cancer and other infections. Therefore, water soluble chitosan was used by Hussain et al. to form a complex with DsiRNA to make it pharmaceutically compatible. Nanoparticles were prepared from the developed complex and coated with pectin to lower cumulative release in the stomach (<15%) and small intestine (<30%) and achieve maximum release in the colon (>90%). Therefore, the DsiRNA was protected from the gastrointestinal fluids and made stable. Further, the efficacy of the formulation was tested on colorectal adenocarcinoma cells. It was found that inhibition of the cells was increased when amounts of chitosan-DsiRNA complex was increased during incubation of 24 to 48 h. Therefore, the uptake of the DsiRNA into the cells also improved (Hussain et al. 2017).

15.7.1.3 Xanthan Gum

Xanthan gum is produced from the fermentation of the gram negative bacterium *Xanthomonas campestris*. It has a cellulose backbone consisting of β-D-glucose residues and a side chain consisting of β-D-mannose, β-D-glucuronic acid and α-D-mannose. The mannose residues contain pyruvate and acetyl groups. Glucuronic acid and pyruvate groups render an anionic nature to the gum (Maity and Sen 2017).

The gum has a high molecular weight. It is available as a free flowing powder which is soluble in both hot and cold water and gives viscous solutions which are very effective as thickeners and stabilizers even in low amounts. The gum is stable under varying pH conditions (Mutalik et al. 2016).

The gum has been used for preparation of nanoparticles under various conditions. In a study by Xu et al., nanoparticles were prepared with the polymer and lysozyme having like charges and the interactions between them produced stable and spherical nanoparticles (Xu et al. 2015).

The gum has been used along with guar gum in coating of granules to make them colon specific and also as a prebiotic as described by Singh et al, earlier.

Inflammatory bowel disease or colitis is a painful condition of the colon with chronic inflammation, edema, or blood loss. However, in animal models, curcumin have been shown to be helpful in treating the symptoms of inflammatory bowel disease. Thus, Mutalik et al. prepared curcumin-loaded nanoparticles. They used xanthan gum which was grafted with polyacrylamide to make it more pH-sensitive and used it to develop the nanoparticles. The nanoparticles did not release curcumin in the upper GIT, but released the drug in simulated colonic fluid with rat cecal contents. Further, when tested on a colitis-induced rat model, myeloperoxidase and nitrite levels (markers for inflammation) were decreased and inflammation was curbed. Myeloperoxidase and nitrite levels are found to be much higher in patients with colitis. Therefore, the formulation was effective in delivering curcumin to the colon, which had promising effects to treat colitis (Mutalik et al. 2016).

Curcumin is considered to be a promising molecule endowed with anti-inflammatory, anticancer, and antioxidant properties. Jha et al. prepared curcumin-loaded xanthan gum nanoparticles for colonic delivery and made them pH-sensitive by coating with eudragit S100. The drug-loaded nanoparticles could release a major amount of the drug in the colon in a sustained manner. As curcumin is thought to be beneficial for colonic diseases like colitis or colon cancer, the successful colonic delivery opens the vista for delivering curcumin to affected sites to treat the diseases with improved efficacy (Jha et al. 2017).

15.7.1.4   Shellac

Shellac is a resin produced by the lady lac bug found in trees in the forests of India and Thailand. It is available as dry flakes which dissolve in ethanol.

Wang et al. used an electrospinning method to produce nanofibers of polymer solutions. In this method, electric force is applied to produce nanofibers from polymer solutions which would be devoid of the solvents used. Ferulic acid was mixed with shellac solution (polymer) in such a way that it stays dispersed within the shellac nanofibers. The release of the fibers was minimum at pH 2 while a sustained release was obtained at higher pH. When the fibers came into contact with the dissolution medium, the nanofibers were converted into nanoparticles with the release of ferulic acid which dissolved slowly (Wang et al. 2015).

Nanoparticles were prepared with shellac and a freeze dried probiotic "*Bifidobacterium*" for colonic delivery. The samples degraded by only 5% at pH 1.2 and 6.8 whereas degradation was complete within 10–11 h at pH 7.4 (Noel et al. 2017).

15.7.1.5   Chitosan

Biodegradable and biocompatible polymers like chitosan can be useful in colonic delivery as they have desirable properties for scaling up formulations from the laboratory level to commercial manufacturing for both oral and parenteral dosage forms (Tran et al. 2016). Chitosan is polycationic in nature with high molecular weight. It is obtained from chitin by alkali-based deacetylation method. Chitosan consists of repeated units of (2-amino-2-deoxy-D-gluco-pyranose) joined by (1–4) β-bonds (Wilson et al. 2008; Jain et al. 2007).

The colonic bacterial enzymes (glycosidases) are responsible for the hydrolysis of chitosan. The polymer is also degraded by anaerobic bacteria (*Bacteroides* and *Bifidobacteria*) in the human colon to form glucosamine and *N*-acetylglucosamine (Brondsted and Hovgaard 1996; Salyer 1979; Hawksworth et al. 1971).

Chitosan is a non-toxic and biodegradable polymer. It is also known to be biocompatible and bioactive. Chitosan has been used in controlled drug delivery systems. It has also been used to improve the bioavailability of proteins or to promote the uptake of water soluble materials across the epithelial tissues (Madziva et al. 2005).

Shimono et al. developed a drug delivery system for colon delivery which was claimed to be time dependent as well as site specific. The inner core of the formulation consisted of drug capsules which were coated with a layer consisting of chitosan and eudragit RS. Chitosan is a polysaccharide which is selectively degraded in the colon and therefore can ensure site-specific drug release. However, it is soluble in the acid medium of the stomach, therefore, it was dispersed in eudragit RS. Eudragit RS is a hydrophobic polymer which helps to sustain drug release. Further, a secondary enteric coat was given to protect the delivery system from gastric fluid (the chitosan is highly soluble in acid medium) to neutralise the possibility of premature release. The formulation was tested in beagle dogs. It was found that it reached the colon within 3 h and the drug was released in the colon. Once the enteric coat dissolves in the small intestine, the hydrophobic layer containing chitosan can protect the formulation. But when it reached the colon, chitosan was acted upon by enzymes and degraded creating channels within the hydrophobic layer through which drug got released from the inner core. The hydrophobic layer dissolved slowly, ensuring the sustained release of the drug from the capsules (Shimono et al. 2002).

Elzatahry and Eldin developed colon-targeted nanoparticles containing metronidazole. The nanoparticles were prepared by an ionotropic gelation method, the process already described earlier. The resulting nanoparticles were mucoadhesive indicating that they would adhere to the mucous layer in the colon for a prolonged period, facilitating drug release within the mucosal tissues. The mucoadhesive properties of the nanoparticles decreased with increasing drug concentration (in the particles) and was dependent on the size of the particles. Nanoparticles in the range of 200–300 nm had very good mucoadhesive properties. The formulation could sustain drug release in the colon for more than 12 h. Thus, chitosan attributed two important properties to the formulation; colon-specificity as well as mucoadhesiveness (Elzatahry and Eldin 2008).

Hyaluronan receptors present in the colon cancer cells have been utilized to target anticancer drugs to the cancerous cells (a study has been described for pectin). In this particular study, Jain et al. prepared a complex of hyaluronic acid with chitosan and developed nanoparticles of anticancer drug 5-fluorouracil using the complex as matrix. Drug release from the nanoparticles in simulated fluids of the stomach and intestine showed colon-specific release as chitosan got selectively hydrolyzed in the colon. Drug-loaded hyaluronan complexed chitosan nanoparticles, chitosan nanoparticles, and drug solution were compared for drug uptake in HT-29 colon cancer cells. The uptake for the hyaluronan complexed chitosan nanoparticles was 7.9 times and 2.6 times greater than that of chitosan nanoparticles and drug solution, respectively. The results show the promise of using chitosan-hyluronan complex to target the hyaluronan receptors of colon cancer cells for effective delivery of anticancer drugs (Jain and Jain 2008).

Immune cells, especially macrophage and dendritic cells, in the colonic mucosa help to identify the harmful and the helpful bacteria and protect the underlying cells from infection. However, dysregulation of these cells may cause infection and inflammation of the colon. Therefore, if the immune cells can be targeted through specific strategy, then the root cause of the inflammation may be prevented (Steinbach and Plevy 2014). Coco et al., in this study, developed a strategy for targeting the macrophages by introducing mannose in the polymer chain and a specific peptide for the inflamed mucosa. In colitis affected patients, macrophages carrying mannose receptors are increased and they are called wound healing macrophages (Kuhl et al. 2015). Three different polymers like polyethylene glycol (PEG), poly-lactic-co-glycolic acid (PLGA), and poly(ε-caprolactone) (PCL) were mixed to produce different formulations containing PLGA, PEG-PLGA, and PEG-PCL. The polymers could impart sustained release properties to the formulation. Mannose and peptide residues were introduced within the polymer chain via grafting for targeting the macrophages and inflamed colon, respectively. Nanoparticles were prepared with the grafted polymers along with ovalbumin as the active ingredient. Trimethylchitosan was used to impart mucoadhesive properties to the nanoparticles. Finally, they were coated with eudragit S100 to protect them from upper GIT conditions. To study the effect on the epithelial cells of the colon, caco-2 cells were used. The particles were tested on both normal cells and inflamed cells. Mucoadhesive nanoparticles had the highest drug permeability within the normal cells. However, all the formulations had similar permeability in case of inflamed tissues. The formulations were also tested in inflamed rat colonic mucosa. The nanoparticles which had mannose residues on the polymer chain produced the highest drug permeability, indicating that the mannose residues were selectively bonded to the mannose receptors of the inflamed tissues resulting in high drug release and greater penetration of the cells (Coco et al. 2013).

Ac-poly(amidoamine) is an active agent with efficacy on cancer cells. However, it is cytotoxic in nature due to its surface charges. Here chitosan was used to form a hydrophilic nanogel and loaded with 5-aminosalicylic acid. The formulation was pH-sensitive and degraded selectively in the colon. Drug release was tested through gel electrophoresis which separated the macromolecules under the influence of an electric field through a gel medium. Results indicated that the formulation is favorable for colonic delivery (Saboktakin et al. 2010). Both chitosan and oxidized sodium alginate are biocompatible and Chen et al. used the polymer duo to prepare a hydrogel by water-in-oil emulsification for delivering 5-aminosalicylic acid for intestinal inflammation. The formulation could protect the drug in simulated gastric conditions and release occurred only above pH 7.4 (Chen et al. 2013).

Nanoparticles prepared from hyaluronic acid-coupled chitosan have been previously discussed. In this particular study, Jain et al. loaded 5-fluorouracil into the nanoparticles and encapsulated them within pellets, given an enteric coating for colonic delivery and possible treatment of colon cancer. The formulation could deliver the nanoparticles in the colon due to the enteric coat. Further, *in-vivo* studies showed that the strategy for targeting hyaluronic receptors on the cancer cells with hyaluronic acid in the formulation was responsible for the retention and prolonged release of the drug from the nanoparticles (Jain and Jain 2016).

Nuclear factor kappa B is a transcription factor which has been observed to become activated in inflammatory diseases and a relationship between its activation and cancer cells generation has been predicted. Decoy oligonucleotides (short fragments of double stranded DNA) can inhibit the nuclear factor kappa B during the process of transcription or translation to control the growth of tumor. The oligonucleotide was encapsulated within chitosan-modified poly(D,L-lactide-co-glycolide) (PLGA) nanospheres using the force of electrostatic attraction. The PLGA has negative charged carboxyl groups on its surface while chitosan is cationic and hence reaction can yield surface-modified (with chitosan) PLGA nanoparticles. The nanospheres with modified PLGA (bearing positive charges) and unmodified PLGA (bearing negative charges) were tested on caco-2 cells. The uptake of the nanospheres with modified PLGA was much greater than the unmodified one. The formulations had better stability in gastric conditions. Daily oral administration of modified nanospheres in a rat model significantly improved symptoms of induced diarrhoea, bloody feces shortening of colon length, and myeloperoxidase activity. Furthermore, nanoparticles were observed to be deposited and adsorbed on the inflamed mucosal tissue of the colitis affected rat. These results suggested that the formulation provided an effective means of colon-specific delivery of the oligonucleotides in colitis (Tahara et al. 2011).

Insulin is indicated in diabetes mellitus which is the most common lifestyle disease affecting a huge number of people. However orally administered, insulin showed poor bioavailability due to the action of proteases in the GIT and low permeability through epithelial layer. Interestingly, in the colon, the quantity of protease is low and pH is neutral, offering a scope of colon-specific delivery. It is suggested that the long residence time in the colon can improve the chance of the permeation of insulin and other peptide drugs, but the adherence on the mucosal tissues and permeability through the colonic epithelium is a challenging proposition. To address this issue, Guo et al. developed nanoparticles using chitosan derivatives and cell-penetrating peptides for delivery of insulin to the colon. Chitosan was included to impart mucoadhesive properties to the formulation and cell-penetrating peptides (short chain peptides) to enhance the permeability into the epithelial tissues. Nanoparticles evaluated on caco-2 cells showed that the formulation with chitosan derivatives had a much higher cellular uptake and penetration than that of the chitosan nanoparticles. The efficacy of the formulation was further evaluated in diabetic rat models and it was observed that the hypoglycaemic effect of developed formulation was 1.79 times higher than corresponding chitosan nanoparticles. In *in-vivo* tests in mini-pigs, the formulations could reach the colon and produced the desired pharmacological effect. The researchers claimed that, the formulation could effectively improve the bioavailability of insulin through colonic absorption (Guo et al. 2016).

Efforts have been made to use the cytoskeleton network (filaments and tubules present in cytoplasm of cells to maintain its shape and structure) for targeted delivery of anticancer agents. Taranejoo et al. developed a formulation containing chitosan and albendazole which targeted the actin microfilament and microtubules in the cancer cells, respectively. The formulation was then evaluated to study the effect on the viscoelasticity of colonic adenocarcinoma cells, SW48. Significant changes in the elastic constants (K_1 and K_2) and the coefficient of viscosity (μ) of the cells were observed after 48 h of onset of study. Chitosan had pronounced effects on actin microfilament whereas albendazole affected the microtubules in the cells. The formulation selectively affected the cancer cells rather than the normal cells. The dual action of the drug and carrier (chitosan) led to better therapeutic efficacy (Taranejoo et al. 2016).

6-shoagol is an active ingredient extracted from ginger which exhibits anticancer activity. Zhang et al. loaded the drug in nanoparticles prepared with various polymers like poly(lactic-co-glycolic acid)/polylactic acid-polyethylene glycol-folate and tested the same on colon 26 and Raw 264.7 macrophage cells. Polyethylene glycol-folate nanoparticles showed promising results with respect to receptor mediated uptake in the cells. As previously described, folate receptors are over-expressed in cancer cells. Therefore, the nanoparticles bearing folate groups could be selectively bonded and taken up by the cancer cells. Further, the nanoparticles were encapsulated within chitosan/alginate hydrogels and tested *in-vivo* (oral administration). Significant improvement in colitis symptoms and inflammation were observed due to inhibition of inflammatory factors (Zhang et al. 2017).

15.7.1.6 Dextran

Dextran consists of α-1,6 D-glucose linkages in straight chain and branches of α-1,3 D-glucose units with chains of varying lengths (from 3 to 2000 kDa). Dental plaque is rich in dextran (Staat et al. 1973). This characteristic branching distinguishes a dextran from a dextrin, which is a straight chain glucose polymer bonded by α-1,4 or α-1,6 linkages.

Dextran was discovered by Louis Pasteur from wine as a microbial product (Pasteur 1861). However, it was produced in bulk by Allene Jeanes using lactic acid bacteria (*Leuconostoc mesenteroides* and *Streptococcus mutans*) from sucrose.

A soluble enzyme system, capable of hydrolyzing dextrans to dextrose as the sole or major product, has been obtained from an intestinal bacterium of the *Bacteroides* genus. This system evidently contains two different dextranases, since it can either "liquify" or "saccharify" (Theodore and Edward 1955).

The polysaccharide is readily soluble in water to form clear, stable solutions. The polymer is degraded by dextranase produced by bacteria in the colon (Quan 2013).

Dextran is a biodegradable and biocompatible polymer, used in the sustained release delivery systems consisting of various drugs, protein molecules, or vaccines.

Use of glucocorticoids like methylprednisolone and dexamethasone in colon inflammation has been limited due to their side effects. Thus, McLeod et al. prepared a prodrug formulation such that the systemic absorption of the steroids may be avoided by targeting them to the colon. Dextran was covalently linked with methylprednisolone and dexamethasone with succinic acid. Dexamethasone was also linked with glutaric acid chain to dextran molecule. The glucocorticoid esters and dextran-glucocorticoid conjugates were tested for their degradation in rat GIT. Most of the esters were degraded in the small intestine because the enzyme for their hydrolysis is present in a high concentration in the small intestine. In contrast, the prepared dextran conjugates were not degraded in the upper GIT, including the stomach and small intestine, but hydrolyzed in the colon due to the action of the bacterial enzymes (endodextranases) on dextran. Thus the conjugate showed the promise of colon targeted delivery for the glucocorticoids with better efficacy and lesser side effects (McLeod et al. 2006).

DNA molecules from all organisms bear the same structure, differing only in the nucleotide sequence. They have been used to identify the genes involved in inflammatory bowel diseases, or applied as anti-interferons in management of Crohn's disease. Interferons are produced by immune cells in response to bacterial or viral infections or tumor cells. Recombinant DNA products synthesized in the laboratory have been identified as producing beneficial effects in the large intestine. Therefore, Liptay et al. attempted to transfer recombinant DNA molecules within the colon epithelial cells using cationic liposomes and cationic dextran derivative. They prepared liposomes containing recombinant DNA (with acetyl transferase) and distributed it within a dextran matrix. The system could enable the uptake of DNA into the colonic epithelial cell layer *in-vivo*. Both liposomes and cationic diethylaminoethyl dextran have been reported to help in the transfer of negatively charged DNA molecules into the cells. The surface cationic charge of the system helped to adhere to the mucosal tissues and transfer the molecules within the cell membrane of the epithelial tissues.

This finding was supported by another study using "chloramphenicol acetyl transferase reporter plasmid", a bacterial enzyme synthesized from *Escherichia coli*. The plasmid was complexed with liposomes, mixed with diethylaminoethyl dextran and inserted into the colon of anaesthetized rats with the help of a catheter. Plasmid DNA molecules precipitated with calcium phosphate and naked DNA molecules were also given. The uptake of DNA in the liposomes and dextran derivatives was much higher than precipitated molecules. Naked DNA molecules were not taken up by the epithelial cells. The study suggests diethylaminoethyl dextran together with liposomes can be used effectively for the management of colonic diseases with gene therapy (Liptay et al. 1998).

Drug delivery systems prepared for ulcerative colitis suffer from certain challenges. The colon-targeted formulation acts on the entire colon affecting the normal cells resulting in increased drug absorption, metabolism, wastage, and side effects. Therefore, Vong et al. developed redox nanoparticles which would attack the reactive oxygen species (ROS) selectively in the inflamed tissues of the colon. To evaluate the efficacy of the formulation both *in-vitro* and *in-vivo* studies were performed. In *in-vitro* studies, uptake of the nanoparticles was much higher in ROS treated cells than in normal epithelial cells of the colon. In *in-vivo* studies, the nanoparticles were not taken up by the normal cells of colon but taken up by inflamed colonic tissues resulting in decreased inflammation and beneficial pharmacologic activity, compared to the free drug mesalamine. Dextran was used to induce colitis in an animal model for the test (Vong et al. 2015).

Fluorescein isothiocyanate dextran (FITC dextran) is a dextran derivative having fluorescent properties, used to trace the transfer of molecules into the cells by fluorescence microscopy. This can be of immense help when the permeability of tissues in disease and normal conditions needs to be studied. The quantity or concentration of molecules in tissue fluids can also be measured with its help. β-sitosterol β-D-glucoside (sit G) has been reported to be active on colon cancer cells *in-vitro*. In this study, Nakamura et al. developed a formulation containing nanoparticles prepared with FITC dextran (molecular weight 4400) and sit G and studied the effect of incorporation of sit G on the permeability of FITC dextran across the colonic tissues. It was observed that the absorption of FITC dextran improved significantly which may be due to the presence of glucose residues in the sit G molecule (Nakamura et al. 2003).

15.7.1.7 Cyclodextrin

This polysaccharide is a cyclic oligosaccharide which consists of 6–8 D-glucose units linked with α-(1→4) glucosidic bonds. D-glucose is the D-isomer of glucose also known as dextrose. The cyclodextrins with six, seven, and eight D-glucose units are known as α-, β-, and γ-cyclodextrins, respectively. The molecules have ring like structures which have an inner lipophilic layer and outer hydrophilic layer which increases water solubility. Like other polysaccharides, cyclodextrin is not degraded in the upper GIT but hydrolyzed in the colonic environment (Gerloczy et al. 1985; Flourie et al. 1993).

α-, β-, or γ-cyclodextrins can be modified to produce amphiphilic cyclodextrins which form nanoassemblies in contact with aqueous fluids like nanospheres, nanorods, vesicles, etc. Such nanorange systems may be used to encapsulate hydrophobic drugs in their lipophilic cavities and improve their solubility, bioavailability, and stability or in gene delivery or anticancer phototherapy (Zerkoune et al. 2014).

They get degraded by bacteroides via enzymes in the colon to form glucose, malto-oligosaccharides which are readily fermentable by colon anaerobes to form fatty acids and gases (Antenucci and Palmer 1984).

Biphenylacetic acid is a drug with an anti-inflammatory activity. The ester and amide groups of the drug were complexed with the -OH groups of α-, β-, and γ cyclodextrins to produce prodrugs. They were then tested *in-vivo* in rat GIT. The prodrugs were stable in the stomach and small intestine. However, after they reached the colon, biphenylacetic acid in blood samples was detected indicating that the drug absorption occurred only in the colon where the prodrug released the active drug by the action of colonic enzymes (Minami et al. 1998).

Gavini et al. prepared solid lipid nanoparticles of diclofenac sodium using hydroxypropyl β-cyclodextrin and eudragit L100 to produce a pH-sensitive formulation for systemic effect. The drug uptake was studied on caco-2 cells, pig mucosa and synthetic membrane. It was observed that cyclodextrin improved the drug uptake through pig mucosa (Gavini et al. 2011).

Carboxymethyl-β-cyclodextrin and glycol chitosan were used by Wang et al. to produce drug-loaded nanoparticles. Glycol chitosan has mucoadhesive properties, degrades in the colon selectively as well as being used to improve cell membrane permeability. Carboxymethyl-β-cyclodextrin is a derivative of β-cyclodextrin which can bind to hydrophobic drugs and help to transfer nucleic acids within cells. Drug-loaded (doxorubicin hydrochloride) nanoparticles were prepared with carboxymethyl-β-cyclodextrin and modified glycol chitosan and tested on human colon cancer cells. The nanoparticles inhibited the growth of the cancer cells compared to the free drug and sustained the drug release. The carboxymethyl-β-cyclodextrin and glycol chitosan therefore, proved to be helpful in the improved uptake of drug into the cells (Wang et al. 2015).

Diclofenac sodium-loaded solid lipid nanoparticles were prepared using compritol ATO888 and hydroxypropyl-β-cyclodextrin and evaluated by both *in-vitro* and *ex-vivo* studies.

Compritol ATO888 was used as a lipid excipient to sustain drug release. From the results, it was concluded that the formulations were safe and effective for colon-targeted delivery (Spada et al. 2012).

Small interfering RNA (siRNA) consists of short fragments of 20–25 nucleotides. They are useful in anticancer therapy for their gene-silencing effect. However, their uptake into the cancer cells is a challenging task. In one study, Arima et al. used polyamidoamine conjugated α-cyclodextrin to transfer the siRNA into the cells. Due to negative charges on the plasma membrane of cells, the entry of nucleic acids (negative charge) into cells becomes limited. Polyamidoamine dendrimers are branched molecules with amide and amine units bearing positive charges. Polyamidoamine dendrimers can form complex with the nucleic acids (due to opposite charges) and help in their transfer within cells. α-cyclodextrin can protect the entrapped molecules from degrading enzymes. The complex was tested on colon-26-luc cells and NIH3T3-luc cells and compared with siRNA delivery systems with other transfection agents. The polyamidoamine dendrimers had much better inhibition of the expression of proteins like lamin A/C and Fas (first apoptosis signal receptor) within the cells, and thus produced low toxicity. Lamins and Fas are expressed in malignant tumors (Arima et al. 2011).

Platinum nanoparticles have been reported previously to break DNA strands. Gehrke et al. had attempted to develop platinum nanoparticles distributed within the matrix of β-cyclodextrin and tested its efficacy on human colon cancer cells. The nanoparticles were taken up by the cells. Platinum ions were produced from the platinum nanoparticles within the cells, their amount increasing with time and concentration of the nanoparticles (Gehrke et al. 2011).

β-cyclodextrin nanoparticles were attempted for effective delivery of camptothecin too, another drug used for colon cancer with bioavailability and stability issues. Krishnan et al. prepared camptothecin-loaded nanoparticles using a combination of iron oxide and ethylenediaminetetra acetic acid (EDTA) crosslinked with β-cyclodextrin which improved both drug stability and solubility. EDTA crosslinked with β-cyclodextrin helped to improve the solubility while iron oxide helped to produce a magnetic nanocarrier which gave targeted release under the influence of an external magnetic field. The drug-loaded nanocarrier could achieve apoptosis or programmed cell death in colon cancer cells when administered in larger doses (Krishnan et al. 2017).

15.7.1.8 Chondroitin Sulfate

Chondroitin sulfate is manufactured from animal sources, such as shark and cow cartilage. It is a mucopolysaccharide which is soluble in water. It is degraded in the colon by *B. Thetaiotaomicron* and *B. Ovatus*. Due to its high solubility in water, formulation for targeting the colon may be difficult (Rubinstein et al. 1992). However, the same has been used to develop photosensitive cum stimuli activated nanoparticles of doxorubicin for targeted delivery to the cancer cells. Studies on colon cancer cells showed that LASER irradiation and tumor hypoxia resulted in inhibition of the cells.

Light triggered drug delivery systems can prove useful to target drug release in specific areas with photo-sensitive drugs or carriers using a high energy UV/visible light. However cellular damage and tissue penetration of light limits the use of such systems. In this study, Park et al. utilized a drug carrier which was stimulated by both light as well as by tumor hypoxia. Tumor hypoxia is a condition of low concentration of oxygen in tumor cells. As tumors grow rapidly, the supply of oxygen falls scarce, compared to normal tissues. Doxorubicin was loaded into the carrier along with chondroitin sulfate and a photosensitizer. In hypoxic conditions, a reactive oxygen species was released from the sulfate groups of chondroitin sulfate, which caused drug release. Further, the delivery system was found to be selectively accumulated in tumor tissues which proved that the system was able to achieve site-specific delivery (Park et al. 2016).

Hyaluronic acid and chondroitin sulfate are known to bind with CD44 receptors in cells. It was also reported that targeting of CD44 receptors on malignant cells resulted in their significant inhibition. Therefore, Oommen et al. prepared doxorubicin-loaded nanoparticles with hyaluronic acid and chondroitin sulfate and tested them on human colon cancer cell lines. They were taken up by the cells depending on the concentration of CD44 receptors and dose of nanoparticles (Oommen et al. 2016).

Studies have been done with ketoprofen too. Chondroitin sulfate is highly water soluble. Therefore, the polysaccharide was crosslinked with polyacrylic acid using diethylene glycol diacrylate to produce a polymer network for encapsulation of ketoprofen. The polymer network could hold the drug in the upper GIT releasing only 30 wt % of the drug at pH 1.2 and up to 80 wt % of the drug at pH 7.4. Thus, the drug-loaded polymer network developed in the study was effective in colonic delivery (Wang et al. 2002).

15.7.1.9 Alginates

With respect to formulation development alginates and its derivatives have favorable physicochemical properties. Structurally it is a heteropolysaccharide made of (1–4) linked β-D-mannuronic acid and L-guluronic acid. They are water soluble and can form gels and viscous solutions in water. They are biodegradable, biocompatible, non-immunogenic, and stable polymers which are relatively inexpensive (Keller and Modler 1989).

Alginates are widely available in the cell walls of brown algae (*Phaeophyceae*) including *Laminariahyperborea*, *Laminariadigitata*, *Laminariajaponica*, *Ascophyllumnodos,* and *Macrocystispyrifera* and extracted by treatment with aqueous alkali solutions, like NaOH (Smidsrod and Skjak-Bræk 1990; Clark and Green 1936). Bacterial alginate is also produced from *Azotobacter* and *pseudomonas*. It is a major component of the biofilms produced by *Pseudomonas aeruginosa*. As an anionic polysaccharide, it produces a viscous gum by binding with water. Its color ranges from white to yellowish-brown. It is sold in filamentous, granular, or powdered forms.

Alginates have been used in various types of drug delivery systems. In colon-targeted drug delivery, it has been used in both matrices as well as reservoir systems (coating). As it selectively dissolves in the colonic fluid it helps to release the drug in a sustained manner.

Numbers of studies have used alginate in combination with hyaluronic acid. Colon-specific delivery of cisplatin nanoparticles using hyaluronic acid along with alginate and pectin has already been discussed under the "pectin" section (15.7.1.2) (Tsai et al. 2013).

Ma et al. developed drug-loaded nanoparticles within alginate matrix for targeted drug release to the colon. In an experiment, eudragit RS (hydrophobic polymer) nanoparticles were distributed within alginate microcapsules. The release was negligible in simulated gastric and intestinal fluids. Yet in another experiment, indomethacin was encapsulated within eudragit S100 nanoparticles and further they were entrapped within alginate pellets. Eudragit S100 is a pH-sensitive enteric polymer which is soluble above pH 7. The nanoparticles released about 90% drug in upper GI fluids and only 10% reached the colon. Whereas, the nanoparticles trapped within alginate pellets released 60% of the drug in the colon, suggesting encapsulating drug-loaded nanodevices within alginate matrix can protect the formulation and achieve colon-specific delivery (Ma and Coombes 2014).

Paclitaxel is a reported anticancer drug, and iron-saturated bovine lactoferrin (protein in nature) is in the limelight as a promising candidate for a safe anticancer agent. The drugs were separately deposited on nanocores and encapsulated within an alginate and chitosan matrix by ionic gelation and nanoprecipitation by Kanwar et al. The formulation containing lactoferrin was tested *in-vitro* on caco-2 cells as well as fed to mice to test the prevention and treatment of cancer. When the formulation was injected into the mice a week before caco-2 cells were injected, no tumor growth was noticed, whereas the mice on a normal diet developed tumors when caco-2 cells were injected. The nanoparticles of both lactoferrin and paclitaxel given orally significantly inhibited tumor growth in a mice model. The lactoferrin nanoparticles were observed to be deposited on tumor cells (Kanwar et al. 2012).

The same research group also conjugated iron-saturated bovine lactoferrin nanoparticles with chitosan and coated the same with alginate to prepare a colon-specific sustained release formulation which induced apoptosis by the inhibition of survivin and cancer stem cells. Survivin is a protein which inhibits apoptosis. The formulation inhibited caco-2 cells, reducing levels of survivin and CD-44 cancer stem cells. The formulation given to mice inhibited tumor growth even after tumor cells were grafted into their tissues (Kanwar et al. 2015).

In another study by Roy et al., iron-saturated bovine lactoferrin was encapsulated in calcium phosphate nanoparticles, surrounded by an alginate layer and coated with chitosan along with locked nucleic acid-modified (nucleic acids with closed ribose rings) aptamers (short single strands of DNA/RNA) to produce a targeted nanoformulation and to study the effect on the epithelial cell adhesion molecule (EpCAM) and nucleolin markers. EpCAM and nucleolin markers are receptor molecules expressed in the cancer cells. The nanoformulation was fed orally to mice previously injected with EpCAM, CD133, and CD44 colon cancer stem cells. The complete inhibition of the tumor was found in 70% of mice, which relapsed in 30% of cases for non-targeted formulation and 10% in the cases of targeted formulation, thus improving the survival rate of the animals (Roy et al. 2015).

Lys-pro-val is a tripeptide that is used to reduce inflammation of the small intestine and colon. Laroui et al. prepared nanoparticles loaded with this peptide and dispersed them in a hydrogel consisting of alginate and chitosan to make the nanoparticles colon-specific. The formulation was evaluated *in-vitro* on caco-2 cells as well as *in-vivo* in a colitis-induced mouse model. The formulation was found to release the drug-loaded nanoparticles within the colon which released the peptide within the colonocytes. Reduced inflammation in caco-2 cells and in animal models confirmed the efficacy of the formulation. The formulation was able to achieve the desired anti-inflammatory activity in much low concentrations (12,000 times lower) when compared to a free peptide solution (Laroui et al. 2010).

Prednisolone and inulin-loaded nanocomposites were prepared with chitosan and alginate for colon-targeted delivery by a spray freeze drying method. In spray freeze drying, a liquid dispersion containing drugs and polymers is sprayed into a cryogenic liquid (a liquid which retains its liquid form at very low temperatures) to freeze the sample which is then heated slowly to remove water and solvents to precipitate the nanoparticles within excipient matrix. The nanoparticles had good yields. The drug release was tested in phosphate and Kreb's buffers along with lysozyme, bacteria, and faecal slurry. Alginate nanoparticles were better in terms of formulation parameters as well as degradation by bacteria, when compared to that of chitosan (Gamboa et al. 2015).

Pressure controlled systems are utilized for colon-targeted delivery as the luminal fluid pressure in the colon is higher than in the upper GIT. Hosseinifar et al. prepared pressure sensitive hydrogels by crosslinking alginate with β-cyclodextrin; nanoparticles were prepared by an emulsion method and 5-fluorouracil was encapsulated within the nanoparticles in aqueous solution. 5-fluorouracil is an anticancer drug which faces challenges in uptake by cells. The nanogel formulation could selectively release drug in *in-vitro* controlled conditions mimicking the colonic luminal pressure. The nanogels had a good drug encapsulation efficiency (>80%) and were rapidly taken up by colon cells, when tested on a HT-29 cell line. Further, the drug accumulation within the colonic cells was much greater than the free drug, resulting in apoptosis and cell death (Hosseinifar et al. 2017).

Metallic nanoparticles such as nanoparticulate platinum are well-known potent anticancer agents. In one study, El-Batal et al. prepared zinc nanoparticles and showed their anticancer activity on human colon cancer cells. The nanoparticles were prepared with polysaccharides, like chitosan, alginate, and citrus pectin, along with fermented fenugreek powder by γ-radiation. The polysaccharides got attached to the metal ions and stabilized the nanoparticles. γ-radiation produces electrons that reduces metal ions (in aqueous solutions) which later aggregate to form nanoparticles. Fermented fenugreek powder has been reported to produce gold nanoparticles by γ-radiation (El-Batal et al. 2017).

Folate receptors present on the cells can be used for drug targeting. Wang et al. prepared alginate nanoparticles with loaded paclitaxel and introduced chitosan and folate-chitosan in the alginate matrix by ionic crosslinking. Alginate and chitosan bear opposite charges which play a role in their crosslinking. It was observed that the folate containing nanoparticles were taken up by a colon cancer cell line in greater extent than the other nanoparticles. It was shown that the folate groups selectively bind to the folate receptors on the cells, improving cell adhesion and drug delivery (Wang et al. 2016).

Few other natural polysaccharides like locust bean gum or amylose have also been evaluated in colon-targeted systems by researchers. However, nanoparticulate formulations have not yet been developed.

15.7.1.10 Inulin

Inulin is a glucofructan which is found in nature. It consists of β-2,1-linked D-fructose molecule having a glycosul unit at the reducing end. Naturally it is present in different foods such as asparagus, leek, onions, banana, wheat, and garlic. It is also obtained in high concentrations in herbs like dandelion root, chicory root, and elecampane root. It can resist the hydrolysis and digestion in the upper GIT. Inulin is not hydrolyzed by the endogenous secretions of the human digestive tract (Dysseler and Hoffen 1995). However, *Bifido* bacteria present in the human colon can ferment inulin.

Vervoort et al. prepared inulin hydrogels for colon-targeted delivery and studied the swelling of the hydrogels *in-vitro* (Vervoort and Kinget 1996). They also studied the degradation of inulin by the inulinase enzyme synthesized from *Aspergillus niger* which showed that the enzymes could degrade inulin within the hydrogels (Vervoort et al. 1998).

Transport of drugs into the target cells is a challenging task as it requires penetration of the tight junctions of the epithelial cells which often cause potential side effects. Schoener and Peppas prepared a pH-dependent hydrogel with poly(methacrylic acid-grafted-ethylene glycol) dispersed within poly methyl methacrylate) and further, nanoparticles were prepared from the hydrogel. Inulin, carboxylated and conjugated with the drug doxorubicin, was loaded onto these nanoparticles. *In-vitro* dissolution of the loaded nanoparticles (pH 2 and pH 7.4) indicated the pH-sensitivity of the drug release. Nanoparticles released the drug predominantly at an alkaline pH (>90%). Further, they were also tested on cultured cells like caco-2 and electrical resistance of the cells was measured. Polarity is developed between the layers of epithelial cells which can be monitored by measuring the electrical resistance. The electrical resistance of cell layers was found to decrease with increased concentration of the nanoparticles. It was suggested that chelation of calcium ions in the cell layer by poly(methacrylic acid-grafted-ethylene glycol) resulted in the opening of the tight junctions of the cells and assisted in drug uptake (Schoener and Peppas 2013).

Inulin is an ampiphilic polysaccharide carrying both hydrophilic and hydrophobic parts in its structure. Sun et al. used this property of inulin to develop a complex with 4-aminothiophenol. They conjugated 4-aminothiophenol with carboxymethyl inulin and prepared nanoparticles with the polymer conjugate. Budesonide (indicated for colitis) was also loaded onto it. Drug release was studied in a media containing glutathione (a tripeptide, over-expressed in tumor tissues). Nanoparticles showed a low release in glutathione free media but release was much higher (>80%) in a glutathione media. Further, the nanoparticles were observed as being deposited on inflamed cells in colitis-induced mice and demonstrated significant anti-inflammatory activity when compared to the administered drug suspension. Thus, the developed formulation showed great promise for the treatment of inflammatory bowel diseases compared to the conventional formulations (Sun et al. 2017).

15.8 CONCLUSION: FUTURE PROSPECTS OF RESEARCH IN THIS AREA

Polysaccharide-based nanoparticles have immense possibilities for future research and development and for providing the best possible management of the colonic diseases whose treatment remains questionable. However, further research studies could be focused on proper clinical and *in-vivo* studies, which are very few in number and which may establish their efficacy strongly. Proper toxicological studies may be undertaken to establish the safety of the nanoparticulate formulations as they enter into deeper layers within the colonic mucosa. Such studies would definitely help to recognize the possible toxic effects, if any of such formulations. "Natural polysaccharides" are also an area of research that is constantly evolving and newer, safer natural polysaccharides are constantly being discovered. Hence, nanoparticles developed with newer polysaccharides, for colonic delivery, are always keeping the researchers busy. Lastly, understanding the mechanisms of nanoparticle up take and selective drug absorption in the colonic mucosa may be further studied as there are many questions which need more elaborate explanations based on robust experiments. Overall, nano delivery systems for the colon open an interesting area of research which needs to be explored more and more for production of better formulations targeted specifically to diseased sites, thus ensuring better efficacy and lower toxicity of the active ingredients given through the delivery systems. It would definitely be beneficial for the end users which is our "ultimate goal".

REFERENCES

Agur, A.M.R., Lee, M.J., and Grant, J.C.B. 1999. *Grant's Atlas of Anatomy*. London: Lippincott Williams and Wilkins.

Alonso, M.J. and Csaba, N.S. 2012. *Nanostructured Biomaterials for Overcoming Biological Barriers*. Cambridge: RSC Publishing.

Al-Saidan, S. M., Krishnaiah, Y. S., Satyanarayana, V., and Rao, G. S. 2005. In vitro and in vivo evaluation of guar gum-based matrix tablets of rofecoxib for colonic drug delivery. *Curr Drug Deliv* 2: 155–63.

Antenucci, R.N. and Palmer, J.K. 1984. Enzymic degradation of α- and β-cyclodextrins by Bacteroides of the human colon. *J Agric Food Chem* 32: 1316–21.

Arima, H., Tsutsumi, T., Yoshimatsu, A. et al. 2011. Inhibitory effect of siRNA complexes with polyamidoamine dendrimer/α-cyclodextrinconjugate (generation 3, G3) on endogenous gene expression. *Eur J Pharm Sci* 44: 375–84.

Baboo, S., Yashwant, P., and Aeri, V. 2013. Formulation and evaluation of dosage form of raupya (Silver) bhasma for colon targeted drug delivery. *Am J Pharm Tech Res* 3: 318–26.

Brondsted, H. and Hovgaard, L. 1996. Polysaccharide gels for colon targeting. *Macromol Symp* 109: 77–87.

Chang, C., Wang, Z.C., Quan, C.Y. et al. 2007. Fabrication of a novel pH-sensitive glutaraldehyde cross-linked pectin nanogel for drug delivery. *J Biomater Sci Polym* 18: 1591–9.

Chen, C., Gao, C., Liu, M. et al. 2013. Preparation and characterization of OSA/CS core-shell microgel: In vitro drug release and degradation properties. *J Biomater Sci Polym* 24: 1127–39.

Cheng, K. and Lim, L.Y. 2004. Insulin-loaded calcium pectinate nanoparticles: effects of pectin molecular weight and formulation pH. *Drug Deliv Ind. Pharm* 30: 359–67.

Clark, D.E. and Green, H.C. 1936. Alginic acid and process of making same. 2036922US Patent.

Coco, R., Plapied, L., Pourcelle, V. et al. 2013. Drug delivery to inflamed colon by nanoparticles: Comparison of different strategies. *Int J Pharm* 440: 3–12.

Das, M. and Ghosh, L.K. 2013. Colon targeting of drugs: The factors, targeting approaches and evaluation strategies. *Int J Pharm Tech Res* 5: 1416–25.

Dongowski, G., Lorenz, A., and Anger, H. 2000. Degradation of pectins with different degrees of esterification by *Bacteroides the taiotaomicron* isolated from human gut flora. *Appl Environ Microbiol* 66: 1321–7.

Dysseler, B.S. and Hoffen, M.J. 1995. Inulin. An alternative dietary fiber: Properties and quantitative analysis. *Eur J Clin Nutr* 49: S145–52.

El-Batal, A.I., Mosalam, F.M., Ghorab, M.M., Hanora, A., and Elbarbary, A.M. 2017. Antimicrobial, antioxidant and anticancer activities of zinc nanoparticles prepared by natural polysaccharides and gamma radiation. *Int J Biol Macromol* S0141–8130: 33196–3.

Elzatahry, A.A. and Eldin, M.S.M. 2008. Preparation and characterization of metronidazole loaded chitosan nanoparticles for drug delivery application. *Polym. Adv. Techno* 19: 1787–91.

Englyst, H. N. 1987. Digestion of the polysaccharides of potato in the small intestine of man. *Am J Clin Nutr* 45: 423–31.

Flourie, B., Molis, C., Achour, L., Dupas, H., Hatat, C., and Rambaud, J. C. 1993. Fate of Â-cyclodextrin in the human intestine. *J Nutr* 123: 676–80.

Friend, D.R. 1992. *Oral colon specific drug delivery*. Boca Raton, FL: CRC Press.

Gamboa, A., Araujo, V., Caro, N., Gotteland, M, Abugoch, L., and Tapia, C. 2015. Spray freeze-drying as an alternative to the ionic gelation method to produce chitosan and alginate nano-particles targeted to the colon. *J Pharm Sci* 104: 4373–85.

Gavini, E., Spada, G., Rassu, G. et al. 2011. Development of solid nanoparticles based on hydroxypropyl-β-cyclodextrin aimed for the colonic transmucosal delivery of diclofenac sodium. *J Pharm Pharmacol* 63: 472–82.

Gehrke, H., Pelka, J., Hartinger, C.G. et al. 2011. Platinum nanoparticles and their cellular uptake and DNA platination at non-cytotoxic concentrations. *Arch Toxicol* 85: 799–812.

Gerloczy, A., Fonagy, A., Keresztes, P., Perlaky, L., and Szejtli, J. 1985. Absorption, distribution, excretion and metabolism of orally administered 14 C- Â -cyclodextrin in rat. *Arzneim Forsch/Drug Res* 35: 1042–7.

Grant, J.C.B., Basmajian, J.V., and Slonecker, C.E. 1989. *Grant's Method of Anatomy: A Clinical Problem-Solving Approach*. London: Williams and Wilkins.

Gray, H. and Lewis, W.H. 2000. *Gray's Anatomy of the Human Body*. New York: Bartleby.

Guo, F., Zhang, M., Gao, Y. et al. 2016. Modified nanoparticles with cell-penetrating peptide and amphipathic chitosan derivative for enhanced oral colon absorption of insulin: preparation and evaluation. *Drug Deliv* 23: 2003–14.

Hartemink, R., Schoustra, S.E., and Rombouts, F.M. 1999. Degradation of guar gum by intestinal bacteria. *Biosci Microflora* 18: 17–25.

Hawksworth, G., Drasar, B.S., and Hill, M.J. 1971. Intestinal bacteria and hydrolysis of glycosidic bonds. *J Med Microbiol* 4: 451–9.

Hosseinifar, T., Sheybani, S., Abdouss, M., Hassani, N.S.A., and Shafiee, A.M. 2017. Pressure responsive nanogel based on alginate-cyclodextrin with enhanced apoptosis mechanism for colon cancer delivery. *J Biomed Mater Res A* (Epub ahead of print)

Hua, S., Marks, E., Schneider, J. J., and Keely, S. 2015. Advances in oral nano-delivery systems for colon targeted drug delivery in inflammatory bowel disease: Selective targeting to diseased versus healthy tissue. *Nanomed Nanotechnol* 11: 1117–32.

Hussain, Z., Katas, H., Yan, S. L., and Jamaludin, D. 2017. Efficient colonic delivery of DsiRNA by pectin-coated polyelectrolyte complex nanoparticles: Preparation, characterization and improved gastric survivability. *Current Drug Delivery* 14: 1016–27.

Izadi, Z., Adeleh, D., Saboury, A. A., and Sawyer, L. 2016. β-lactoglobulin-pectin-nanoparticle based oral drug delivery system for potential treatment of colon cancer. *Chem Biol Drug Des* 8: 209–16.

Jain, A., Gupta, Y., and Jain, S.K. 2007. Perspectives of biodegradable natural polysaccharides for site specific delivery to the colon. *J Pharm Sci* 10: 86–128.

Jain, A. and Jain, S.K. 2008. In vitro and cell uptake studies for targeting of ligand anchored nanoparticles for colon tumors. *Eur J Pharm Sci* 35: 404–16.

Jain, A. and Jain, S.K. 2016. Optimization of chitosan nanoparticles for colon tumors using experimental design methodology. *Artif Cells Nanomed Biotechnol.* 44: 1917–26.

Jain, S. and Jain, N.K. 2006. *Pharmaceutical Product Development*. New Delhi: CBS Publisher and Distributor.

Jha, G., Garud, A., Tailang, M., and Garud, N. 2017. Preparation and evaluation of pH dependent curcumin nanoparticles for colon drug delivery. *Research Pharmaceutica* 1: 11–6.

Joshi, S.R. 2007. *Microbes: Redefined Personality*. New Delhi: APH Publishing Corporation.

Kanwar, J.R., Mahidhara, G., and Kanwar, R.K. 2012. Novel alginate-enclosed chitosan-calcium phosphate-loaded iron-saturated bovine lactoferrin nanocarriers for oral delivery in colon cancer therapy. *Nanomedicine* 7: 1521–50.

Kanwar, J.R., Mahidhara, G., and Roy, K. 2015. Fe-bLf nanoformulation targets surviving to kill colon cancer stem cells and maintains absorption of iron, calcium and zinc." *Nanomedicine* 10: 35–55.

Keller, C. and Modler, R.C. 1989. Metabolism of fructooligosaccharides by Biffidobacterium spp. *Appl Microbiol Biotechnol* 31: 537–41.

Krishnaiah, Y. S. R., Satyanarayana, V., Kumar, D. B., Karthikeyan, R. S., and Bhaskar, P. 2003. In Vivo pharmacokinetics in human volunteers: Oral administered guar gum-based colon-targeted 5 fluorouracil tablets. *Eur J Pharm Sci* 19: 355–62.

Krishnan, P., Rajan, M., Kumari, S. et al. 2017. Efficiency of newly formulated camptothecin with β-cyclodextrin-EDTA-Fe3O4 nanoparticle-conjugated nanocarriers as an anti-colon cancer (HT29) drug. *Sci Rep* 7: 10962.

Kronenthal, R.L. 1975. *Biodegradable polymers in medicine and surgery.* New York: Plenum Press.

Kuhl, A.A., Erben, U., Kredel, L.L., and Siegmund, B. 2015. Diversity of intestinal macrophages in inflammatory bowel diseases. *Front Immunol* 6: 613.

Kumar, B., Kulanthaivel, S., Mondal, A. et al. 2017. Mesoporous silica nanoparticle based enzyme responsive system for colon specific drug delivery through guar gum capping. *Colloids Surf B Biointerfaces* 150: 352–61.

Laroui, H., Dalmasso, G., Nguyen, H.T., Yan, Y., Sitaraman, S.V., and Merlin, D. 2010. Drug-loaded nanoparticles targeted to the colon with polysaccharide hydrogel reduce colitis in a mouse model. *Gastroenterology* 138: 843–53.

Liptay, S, Weidenbach, H., Adler, G., and Schmid, R.M. 1998. Colon epithelium can be transiently transfected with liposomes, calcium phosphate precipitation and DEAE dextran in vivo. *Digestion* 59: 142–7.

Ma, Y. and Coombes, A.G. 2014. Designing colon-specific delivery systems for anticancer drug-loaded nanoparticles: An evaluation of alginate carriers. *J Biomed Mater Res A.* 102: 3167–76.

Madziva, H., Kailasapathy, K., and Phillips, M. 2005. Alginate-pectin microcapsules as a potential for folic acid delivery in foods. *J Microencap* 22: 343–51.

Maity, S. and Sen, K.K. 2017. *Bio-targets and Drug Delivery Approaches.* Boca Raton, FL: CRC Press.

McLeod, A.D, Friend, D.R., and Tozer, T.N. 2006. Glucocorticoid-dextran conjugates as potential prodrugs for colon-specific delivery: Hydrolysis in rat gastrointestinal tract contents. *J Pharm Sci* 83: 1284–8.

Minami, K., Hirayama, F., and Uekama, K. 1998. Colon specific drug delivery based on a cyclodextrin prodrug: Release behavior of biphenylylacetic acid from its cyclodextrin conjugates in rat intestinal tracts after oral administration. *J Pharm Sci* 87: 715–20.

Murthy, S. K. 2007. Nanoparticles in modern medicine: State of the art and future challenges. *Int J Nanomedicine* 2: 129–41.

Mutalik, S., Suthar, N.A., Managuli, R. S. et al. 2016. Development and performance evaluation of novel nanoparticles of a grafted copolymer loaded with curcumin. *Int J Biol Macromol* 86: 709–20.

Nakamura, K., Takayama, K., Nagai, T., and Maitani, Y. 2003. Regional intestinal absorption of FITC-dextran4,400 with nanoparticles based on beta-sitosterol beta-D-glucoside in rats. *J Pharm Sci* 92: 311–8.

Narang, A.S. and Boddu, S.H.S. 2015. *Excipient Application in Formulation Design and Drug Delivery.* Switzerland: Springer.

Noel, M., Gately, D., and Kennedy, J.E. 2017. The development of a melt-extruded shellac carrier for the targeted delivery of probiotics to the colon. *Pharmaceutics* 9: 38.

Philip, A.K. and Philip, B. 2010. Colon targeted drug delivery systems. *Oman Med J* 25: 79–87.

Oommen, P.O., Duehrkop, C., Nilsson, B., Hilborn, J., and Varghese, P.O. 2016. Multifunctional hyaluronic acid and chondroitin sulfate nanoparticles: Impact of glycosaminoglycan presentation on receptor mediated cellular uptake and immune activation. *ACS Appl Mater Interfaces* 8: 20614–24.

Park, W., Bae, B. C., and Na, K. 2016. A highly tumor-specific light-triggerable drug carrier responds to hypoxic tumor conditions for effective tumor treatment. *Biomaterials* 77: 227–34.

Pasteur, L. 1861. On the viscous fermentation and the butyrous fermentation. *Bull Soc Chim* 11: 30–1.

Pillai, O. and Panchagnula, R. 2001. Polymers in drug delivery. *Curr Opin Chem Biol* 5: 447–51.

Quan, Li. 2013. *Intelligent Stimuli-Responsive Materials: From Well-Defined Nanostructures to Applications.* New Jersey: John Wiley and Sons.

Rajpurohit, H., Sharma, P., Sharma, S. and Bhandari, A. 2010. Polymers for colon targeted drug delivery. *Indian J Pharm Sci* 72: 689–96.

Romanes, G.J. 1986. *Thorax and Abdomen: Cunningham's Manual of Practical Anatomy.* New York: Medical Publications, Oxford University Press.

Roy, L.W. and James N.B.M. 1973. *"Pectin" in Industrial Gums and Their Derivatives.* New York: Academic Press.

Roy, K., Kanwar, R.K., and Kanwar, J.R. 2015. LNA aptamer based multi-modal, Fe3O4-saturated lactoferrin (Fe3O4-bLf) nanocarriers for triple positive (EpCAM, CD133, CD44)colon tumor targeting and NIR, MRI and CT imaging. *Biomaterials* 71: 84–99.

Rubinstein, A., Nakar, D., and Sintov, A. 1992. Colonic drug delivery: Enhanced release of indomethacin from cross linked chondroitin matrix in rat cecal content. *Pharm Res* 9: 276–8.

Saboktakin, M.R., Tabatabaie, R.M., Maharramov, A., and Ramazanov, M.A. 2010. Synthesis and characterization of chitosan hydrogels containing 5-aminosalicylic acid nano pendents for colon: specific drug delivery. *J Pharm Sci* 99: 4955–61.

Salyer, A.A. 1979. Energy sources of major intestinal fermentative anaerobes. *Am J Clin Nutr* 32: 158–63.

Schoener, C.A. and Peppas, N.A. 2013. pH-responsive hydrogels containing PMMA nanoparticles: An analysis of controlled release of a chemotherapeutic conjugate and transport properties. *J Biomater Sci Polym* 24: 1027–40.

Sharma, M., Malik, R., and Verma, A. 2013. Folic acid conjugated guar gum nanoparticles for targeting methotrexate to colon cancer. *J Biomed Nanotechnol.* 9: 96–106.

Shimono, N., Takatori, T., Ueda, M., Mori, M., Higashi, Y., and Nakamura, Y. 2002. Chitosan dispersed system for colon-specific drug delivery. *Int J Pharm* 245: 45–54.

Shirwaikar, A., Shirwaikar, A.N., Prabu, S. L., and Kumar, G. A. 2008. Herbal excipients in novel drug delivery systems. *Indian J Pharm Sci* 70: 415–22.

Singh, S., Kotla, N. G., Tomar, S. et al. 2015. A nanomedicine-promising approach to provide an appropriate colon-targeted drug delivery system for 5-fluorouracil. *Int J Nanomed* 10: 7175–82.

Sinha, V.R. and Kumria, R. 2001. Polysaccharides in colon-specific drug delivery. *Int J Pharm.* 224: 19–38.

Sinnatamby, C.S. 1999. *Last's Anatomy: Regional and Applied.* Edinburgh: Churchill Livingstone.

Smidsrod, O. and Skjak-Bræk, G. 1990. Alginate as immobilization matrix for cells. *Trend Biotechnol* 8: 71–8.

Spada, G., Gavini, E., Cossu, M., Rassu, G., and Giunchedi, P.2012. Solid lipid nanoparticles with and without hydroxypropyl-β-cyclodextrin: A comparative study of nanoparticles designed for colonic drug delivery. *Nanotechnology* 23: 095101.

Staat, R.H., Gawronski, T.H., and Schachtele, C.F. 1973. Detection and preliminary studies on dextranase-producing microorganisms from human dental plaque. *Infect Immun* 8: 1009–16.

Steinbach, E.C. and Plevy, S.E. 2014. The role of macrophages and dendritic cells in the initiation of inflammation in IBD. *Inflamm Bowel Dis* 20: 166–75.

Subudhi, M.B., Jain, A., Jain, A. et al. 2015. Eudragit S100 coated citrus pectin nanoparticles for colon targeting of 5-fluorouracil. *Materials* 8: 832–49.

Sun, Q., Luan, L., Arif, M. et al. 2017. Redox-sensitive nanoparticles based on 4-aminothiophenol-carboxymethyl inulin conjugate for budesonide delivery in inflammatory bowel diseases. *Carbohydr Polym* 189: 352–359.

Tahara, K., Samura, S., Tsuji, K. et al. 2011. Oral nuclear factor-κB decoy oligonucleotides delivery system with chitosan modified poly(D,L-lactide-co-glycolide) nanospheres for inflammatory bowel disease. *Biomaterials* 32: 870–8.

Taranejoo, S., Janmaleki, M., Pachenari, M. et al. 2016. Dual effect of F-actin targeted carrier combined with antimitotic drug on aggressive colorectal cancer cytoskeleton: Allying dissimilar cell cytoskeleton disrupting mechanisms. *Int J Pharm* 513: 464–72.

Theodore, W.S. and Edward, J.H. 1955. *Degradation of Dextrans by Enzymes of Intestinal Bacteria.* New York: Department of Microbiology and Immunology, Cornell University Medical College.

Tran, T.T., Tran, P.H., Wang, Y., Li, P., and Kong, L. 2016. Nanoparticulate drug delivery to colorectal cancer: Formulation strategies and surface engineering. *Curr Pharm Des* 22: 2904–12.

Tsai, S.W., Yu, D.S., Tsao, S.W., and Hsu, F.Y. 2013. Hyaluronan-cisplatin conjugate nanoparticles embedded in Eudragit S100-coatedpectin/alginate microbeads for colon drug delivery. *Int J Nanomedicine.*8: 2399–407.

Vainionpaa, S., Rokkanen, P., and Tormala, P. 1989. Surgical applications of biodegradable polymers in human tissues. *Prog Polym Sci* 14: 679.

Valentine, P. 2011. *Polysaccharides in medicinal and pharmaceutical applications.* Shropshire: iSmithers.

Varma, V. N., Shivakumar, H.G., Balamuralidhara, V., Navya, M., and Hani, U. 2016. Development of pH sensitive nanoparticles for intestinal drug delivery using chemically modified guar gum co-polymer. *Iran J Pharm Res* 15: 83–94.

Vert, M. 1989. Bioresorbable polymers for temporary therapeutic applications. *Angew Makromol Chem* 166: 155–8.

Vervoort, L. and Kinget, R. 1996. In vitro degradation by colonic bacteria of inulin HP incorporated in Eudragit films. *Int J Pharm* 129: 185–90.

Vervoort, L., Rombaut, P., Mooter, G.V., Augustijns, P., and Kinget, R. 1998. Inulin hydrogels. II. In vitro degradation study. *Int J Pharm* 172: 137–45.

Viscido, A., Capannolo, A., Latella, G., Caprilli, R., and Frieri, G. 2014. Nanotechnology in the treatment of inflammatory bowel diseases. *J. Crohn's Colitis* 8: 903–18.

Vong, L.B., Mo, J., Abrahamsson, B., and Nagasaki, Y. 2015. Specific accumulation of orally administered redox nano therapeutics in the inflamed colon reducing inflammation with dose-response efficacy. *J Control Release* 210: 19–25.

Walle, C.V.D. 2011. *Peptide and protein delivery*. London: Academic Press, Elsevier.

Wang, F., Wang, J.M., and Chiang, Y.L. 2002. Insolubilization of sodium chondroitin sulfate by forming a semi-interpenetrating polymer network with acrylic acid: A potential carrier for colon-specific drug delivery. *J Appl Polym Sci* 85: 114–22.

Wang, F., Yang, S., Yuan, J., Gao, Q., and Huang, C. 2016. Effective method of chitosan-coated alginate nanoparticles for target drug delivery applications. *J Biomater Appl* 31: 3–12.

Wang, X., Yu, D.G., Li, X.Y., Bligh, S.W., and Williams, G.R. 2015. Electrospun medicated shellac nano fibers for colon-targeted drug delivery. *Int J Pharm* 490: 384–90.

Wang, Y., Qin, F., Tan, H. et al. 2015. pH-responsive glycol chitosan-cross-linked carboxymethyl-β-cyclodextrin nanoparticles for controlled release of anticancer drugs. *Int J Nanomedicine* 10: 7359–69.

Wilson, C.G., Mukherji, G., and Sha, H.K. 2008. *Biopolymers and Colonic Delivery*. New York: Informa Healthcare.

Xu, Q., Kambhampati, S.P., and Kannan, R. K. 2013. Nanotechnology approaches for ocular drug delivery. *Middle East Afr J Ophthalmol* 20: 26–37.

Xu, W., Jin, W., Li, Z. et al. 2015. Synthesis and characterization of nanoparticles based on negatively charged xanthan gum and lysozyme. *Food Res Int* 71: 83–90.

Yihong, Q., Yisheng, C., Geoff, G.Z., Zhang, L.Y., and Rao, V.M. 2017. *Developing Solid Oral Dosage Forms: Pharmaceutical Theory and Practice*. London: Academic Press, Elsevier.

Zerkoune, L., Angelova, A., and Lesieur, S. 2014. Nano-assemblies of modified cyclodextrins and their complexes with guest molecules: Incorporation in nanostructured membranes and amphiphile nanoarchitectonics design. *Nanomaterials* 4: 741–65.

Zhang, M., Xu, C., Liu, D., Han, M.K., Wang, L., and Merlin, D. 2017. Oral delivery of nanoparticles loaded with ginger active compound, 6-shogaol, attenuates ulcerative colitis and promotes wound healing in a murine model of ulcerative colitis. *J Crohns Colitis*. (Epub: ahead of print.)

16 Passive and Active Tumor Targeting of Polysaccharide Nanocarriers for Cancer Therapy

Miltu Kumar Ghosh and Falguni Patra

CONTENTS

16.1 INTRODUCTION

Cancer is now one of the foremost causes of morbidity and death. The unsatisfactory rate of cure with the currently available therapies substantiate the need for drastic improvement in their effectiveness. The complex nature of cancer necessitates the application of a combination of treatment strategies developed on the basis of a thorough understanding of its pathophysiology. Major chemotherapeutic agents for cancer treatments are limited by their specificity as they rapidly kill all proliferating cells as well as normal rapidly dividing cells (bone marrow, lymphatic system, red blood cell, and hair follicles, etc.) (Thibodeau and Voutsadakis 2018). When coupled with nonselective drug delivery systems, it is often required to administer the drug in high doses to attain an effective concentration of the drug in the tumor cells, causing toxicity in normal cells and limiting usefulness (Thibodeau and Voutsadakis 2018). This imposes a limit on the maximum allowable dose for the drug. In order to overcome these limitations, there is a growing emphasis on new therapeutic approaches and formulations with targeted drug delivery capability such as cell-specific drug targeting. This can be achieved by binding drugs to individually designed carriers. In recent years, studies on nanoparticles have demonstrated their potential to be employed as such a drug carriers. These nanoparticles carrying drugs and show controlled release of the drug to specific cells (Amreddy et al. 2017). Apart from being able to reduce toxic effects and maintain therapeutic concentrations for long periods of time, nanoparticles have the advantages of being biodegradable and small enough in size to pass through small capillary vessels.

Tumor cells get their nutrition through passive diffusion and as they increase in mass the supply is maintained by growing new blood vessels. These vessels are highly tortuous with leaky vascular structures due to rapid vascularization and allow accumulation of nanosized drug carriers in tumors with low lymphatic drainage. Besides, tumor cells also show an enhanced permeability and retention (EPR) effect that allows passive drug targeting by accumulation of nanoparticles at the tumor site (Ngoune et al. 2016). As some tumors lack this EPR effect, the application of drug delivery systems that depend only on passive targeting mechanisms are specificity-limited (Yin et al. 2014). In order to overcome these limitations, one alternative approach is to include a targeting ligand or antibody attached to the drug carrier system to achieve targeted drug delivery exploiting their higher affinity to bind with tumor cell surface receptors or antigens respectively (Dinarvand et al. 2012). Nanoparticles for this purpose are prepared by methods such as covalent crosslinking, ionic crosslinking, polyelectrolyte complexation, and self-assembly of hydrophobically modified polysaccharide using natural as well as synthetic polymers, lipids, and inorganic materials as drug delivery vectors. This method of preferential accumulation of the drug in the tumor zone is termed active targeting (Byrne et al. 2008).

Polysaccharides are a naturally available (animal, plant, algal) diverse class of polymers formed via glycosidic linkages of monosaccharides (Shukla and Tiwari 2012). These polysaccharides can have a linear or branched architecture depending on the nature of the glycosidic linkage between the monosaccharide units. In addition to structural diversity, polysaccharides have a number of reactive groups, including hydroxyl, amino, and carboxylic acid groups, indicating the possibility for chemical modification (Liu et al. 2008). Moreover, polysaccharide molecular weight can vary between hundreds and thousands of Daltons, further increasing diversity (Saravanakumar et al. 2012). The diverse characteristics of polysaccharides including biocompatibility, solubility, potential for modification, and innate bioactivity further strengthen their potential for use in nano drug delivery systems. Here we will discuss the passive and active tumor targeting of different polysaccharides as nanocarriers for cancer therapy.

16.2   ADAPTATION OF THE TUMOR MICROENVIRONMENT

The detailed understanding of the tumor microenvironment allows for the development of strategies based on the several different conditions prevalent there, such as pH, vascular characteristics, states of hypoxia, and metabolic states. These morphological conditions can be exploited to design drug delivery systems targeted specifically to these regions. Angiogenesis is a very important characteristic that allows the tumors to thrive providing them an enriching supply of oxygen and nutrients. It is regulated by a systematic control of activators and inhibitors (Eftekhari et al. 2017). Immature tumor vasculature undergoes extensive remodeling resulting in irregular shaped and dilated blood vessels (Viallard and Larrivée 2017). In 1971, eminent scientist Judah Folkman suggested that tumor growth might be curtailed by prevention of the recruitment of new blood vessels (Sung et al. 2007). This very finding formed an important basis of active tumor targeting to endothelial cells by nanosystems (Danhier et al. 2010). During the initial stages of tumor growth, the cells primarily use diffusion to obtain nutrients limiting their size to approximately 2 mm^3 (Herman et al. 2011). Accordingly, the tumor cells must begin to recruit new blood vessels in a process called angiogenesis. The blood vessels then continue to proliferate rapidly producing a severely irregular and aberrant vasculature (Cook and Figg 2010), thus resulting into regions with high blood or poor blood supply. Tumor vessels can become excessively leaky due to deficient basement membranes and incomplete endothelial linings caused by the extremely compromised ability of endothelial cells to completely envelop the proliferating cells forming the vessel walls.

There are some additional factors present intracellularly at elevated levels, which pose a significant contribution to neo-angiogenesis, thus recruiting an extensive network of blood vessels that feed the tumor (Birbrair et al. 2014). Some of these factors comprise of the vascular endothelial growth factor, the basic fibroblast growth factor, bradykinin, and nitric oxide (Deger et al. 2016). More notably, the vascular endothelial growth factor (VEGF) increases the permeability of blood vessels by causing a significant increase in the quantity of fenestrations or rather minute openings between cells (Bates 2010) (Figure 16.1).

16.3 DRUG TARGETING

There are so many problems currently associated with systemic drug administration, such as even biodistribution of pharmaceuticals throughout the body, the lack of drug-specific affinity toward a pathological site, the necessity of a large total dose of a drug to achieve high local concentration, non-specific toxicity, and other adverse side effects due to high drug doses. Drug targeting, i.e., predominant drug accumulation in the target zone independently on the method and route of drug administration, may resolve many of these problems. There are so many methods of drug targeting like passive drug targeting, "physical" targeting, magnetic targeting, targeting using specific "vector" molecules and active targeting.

16.3.1 PASSIVE TARGETING

In passive targeting, macromolecules including nanoparticles, accumulate preferentially in the neoplastic tissues as a result of the enhanced permeability and retention (EPR) phenomenon, first described by Maeda and Matsumura (Bazak et al. 2014). The EPR is based on the nanometer size range of the nanoparticles and two fundamental characteristics of the neoplastic tissues, namely, the leaky vasculature and impaired lymphatic drainage (Figure 16.2A).

One of the studies showed paclitaxel-loaded chitosan nanoparticles achieved improved biodistribution compared to Taxol®, having a higher drug accumulation in the liver and spleen, and lower drug concentrations in the heart and kidney due to passive targeting (Liang et al., 2016).

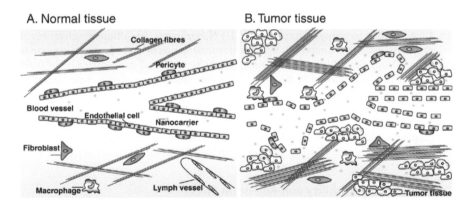

FIGURE 16.1 Differences between normal and tumor tissues that explain the passive targeting of nanocarriers by the enhanced permeability and retention effect. A. Normal tissues contain linear blood vessels maintained by pericytes. Collagen fibers, fibroblasts, and macrophages are in the extracellular matrix. Lymph vessels are present. B. Tumor tissues contain defective blood vessels with many sac-like formations and fenestrations. The extracellular matrix contains more collagen fibers, fibroblasts and macrophages than in normal tissue. Lymph vessels are lacking.(Reprinted from *J Control Release* 148, Danhier, F., Feron, O., and Préat, V. To exploit the tumor microenvironment: Passive and active tumor targeting of nanocarriers for anticancer drug delivery, 135–46, Copyright 2010, with permission from Elsevier.)

A. Passive targeting

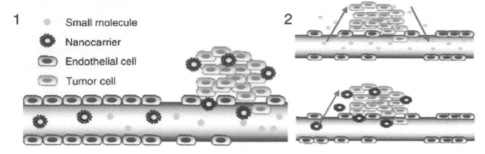

B. Active targeting

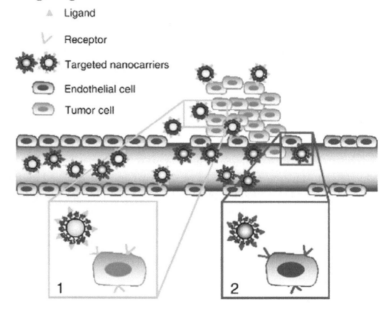

FIGURE 16.2 A. Passive targeting of nanocarriers. (1) Nanocarriers reach tumors selectively through the leaky vasculature surrounding the tumors. (2) Schematic representation of the influence of the size for retention in the tumor tissue. Drugs alone diffuse freely in and out the tumor blood vessels because of their small size and thus their effective concentrations in the tumor decrease rapidly. By contrast, drug-loaded nanocarriers cannot diffuse back into the blood stream because of their large size, resulting in progressive accumulation: the EPR effect. B. Active targeting strategies. Ligands grafted at the surface of nanocarriers bind to receptors (over)-expressed by (1) cancer cells or (2) angiogenic endothelial cells. (Reprint from *J Control Release* 148, Danhier, F., Feron, O., and Préat, V. To exploit the tumor microenvironment: Passive and active tumor targeting of nanocarriers for anticancer drug delivery, 135–46, Copyright 2010, with permission from Elsevier.)

16.3.1.1 Enhanced Permeability and Retention Effect

Drug delivery should be site specific to avoid any non-specific distribution. Currently, the principal schemes of drug targeting include the direct application of a drug into the affected zone, passive drug targeting which is an approach of spontaneous drug accumulation in the areas with leaky vasculature, or EPR effect (Dreaden et al. 2012). Hydrophobically modified glycol chitosan nanoparticles show an excellent tumor-homing efficacy along with prolonged blood circulation. This preferential accumulation at the tumor site due to the EPR effect results in improved therapeutic efficiency (Kim et al. 2008).

16.3.1.1.1 Effect of Size

Maeda et al. reported that 10–100 fold higher concentrations could be achieved in murine solid tumors due to the well-noted EPR effect when polymer-drug conjugates were administered intravenously as compared to free drug administration (Vicent and Duncan 2006). The permeability of compromised vasculature and retention can lead to the accumulation of even macromolecules thus increasing their tumor concentration by 70-fold (Bae and Park 2011). The foremost advantage in treating cancer with advanced, non-solution-based therapies is this very inherent leaky vasculature present in the pathologically compromised cancerous tissues. This leaky and defective vascular architecture created due to rapid vascularization which is a vital cog in enriching the ever-growing malignant tumors, coupled with poor lymphatic drainage allows the for famous EPR effect. Various important factors such as circulation time, targeting, and the capability to overcome barriers are heavily reliant on the shape, size, and the surface area of these particles. Passive targeting is a diffusion-mediated transport, which makes size a critically important factor. Conveniently the upper limit of nanoparticles to undergo diffusion is around 400 nm (Kamaly et al. 2012). The optimal size range of 40–200 nm will ensure longer circulation time, increased accumulation within the tumor mass, and lower renal clearance (Trédan et al. 2007).

16.3.1.1.2 Effect of Shape

The shape of the nanoparticles is another important factor in enhancing drug permeability and retention within the tumor cell. The effect of shape and geometry of contact of spherical and non-spherical microparticles during phagocytosis by alveolar macrophages was studied (Yhee et al. 2017). In the case of elliptical disk-shaped microparticles, it was found that when the macrophage initially made contact with these particles along the major axis, the particles were swiftly internalized in less than 6 minutes. However, when the primary contact was along the minor axis, the particles were not internalized for a very long time ranging up to 10 h. It is only because of their symmetry that these spherical particles were swiftly internalized (Yhee et al. 2017). Conventionally, it has been noted that a nanoparticle must be at least 10 nm in diameter to avoid clearance by first pass renal filtration (Greish 2010). Dreher et al. showed that the diameter of 100 nm nanoparticles has a greater proclivity to accumulate in the tumor tissue, passively. They showed that with dextran as a model macromolecule, the permeability and extent of penetration of a drug molecule is severely reduced, as the molecular weight is increased from 3.3 kDa to 2 MDa (Greish 2010). It was reported that spherical particles were taken up around 5 times more than rod-shaped particles, thus stressing the influence of the shape of the nanoparticles on the uptake mechanism (Greish 2010). The general gist of the discussion states that rigid, spherical particles, which are particularly 100–200 nm in size, have the greatest propensity for prolonged circulation because they are large enough to avoid any liver uptake, but at the same time, are optimal in size to avoid filtration in the spleen.

16.3.1.1.3 Effect of Surface

Internalization of nanoparticles into cells depends on the surface characteristics of nanoparticles. The surface can be modified by the polymer composition, thus governing an extra amount of hydrophobicity or hydrophilicity to these particles. Surface modification of these polymers by the addition of polyethylene glycol (PEG) has been known to protect the nanosystems from opsonization and subsequent clearance by the reticulo-endothelial system (RES) (Georgieva et al. 2011). Increasing the molecular weight of PEG chains will also increase the circulation time of these nanoparticles. Particularly for negatively charged nanoparticles, this PEG shield will confer more protection and thus prevent the immediate clearance of these particles. Passive targeting thus can be regulated by modifying the size, shape, or in some cases, the surface dimensions of these nanoparticles. However, one major drawback of passive targeting is that it may not be able to distinguish the healthy tissue from the diseased one just like a chemotherapeutic regimen (Mann et al. 2016).

16.3.2 Active Targeting

The most important challenge in active targeting is defining the most suitable targeting agent or agents to selectively and successfully transport nanoparticle systems to cancerous tissue thus avoiding any kind of toxicity in the process. These strategies then also rely on the targeting agents' or ligands' capability to bind to the tumor cell surface with an extremely strong affinity to trigger receptor endocytosis. With such kinds of interactions, the therapeutic agents will then be delivered into the tumor-specific regions (Figure 16.2B).

16.3.2.1 Ligand-Based Targeting

A number of targeting moieties have been used to functionalize the surface of nanoparticles including peptides (such as transferrin) and short amino acid polymers, as well as small molecules (such as folic acid). Such targeting moieties have a very high selectivity and avidity to their target receptors making them attractive tools for targeting cancer cells.

16.3.2.1.1 Transferrin-Based Targeting

Internalization of iron takes place through transferrin receptors. The upregulation of transferrin receptors on metastatic and drug-resistant malignant cells (which may reach up to 100 fold higher than that in normal cells), the extracellular status of transferrin in the body, and its internalization by cells make transferrin and transferrin mimicking agents suitable for delivery of cancer therapies (Daniels et al. 2012).

16.4 ACTIVE AND PASSIVE TARGETING OF POLYSACCHARIDE-BASED NANOCARRIER IN CANCER THERAPY

Biocompatibility, biodegradability, and stability are the basic characteristics of polymers used as biomaterial for the preparation of nanoparticles for targeted controlled release. Natural polymers, polysaccharides are safe and non-toxic. Several polymers are used in highly targeted controlled drug release. The polysaccharides can be used either in the preparation of nanoparticles, coating material, or to form polysaccharide drug conjugates (Barreto et al. 2011).

16.4.1 Polysaccharides

Polysaccharides are large carbohydrate molecules which are constituted by repeating monosaccharide units and linked by glycoside bonds. Polysaccharides have a large number of reactive groups on their molecular chain which contributes to varying chemical and biochemical composition. So, they have a higher diversity in their structure and properties. They can be homopolysaccharides or heteropolysaccharides depending on their monosaccharides units. If the polysaccharide containing monosaccharides are the same then they are called homopolysaccharides. When monosaccharide components are different then they are called heteropolysaccharides. Homopolysaccharides and heteropolysaccharides also have different positive charges and negative charges on their backbone (Swierczewskaa et al. 2016).

Whereas, exopolysaccharides are heterogeneous with a high molecular weight. They are composed of monosaccharides and non-carbohydrate functional groups. Most natural polysaccharides have several hydrophilic groups (carboxide, hydroxide, and amino groups) which help their stability in water and with the formation of non-covalent bonds with biological tissue and mucosal membranes resulting in bio adhesion and mucoadhesion. Hydrophilic nanoparticles also have the advantage of extended circulation in the blood which increases the probability of passively targeting nanoparticles into tumor tissue (Poli et al. 2011).

16.4.1.1 Chitosan

Chitosan (Figure 16.3) presents important characteristics such as low or no toxicity, biodegradability, biocompatibility, low immunogenicity, and antimicrobial properties. Lysozyme hydrolyzed chitosan. The degraded products of chitosan are also non-toxic, non-carcinogenic and non-immunogenic which is absorbed completely in the human body. A strong electrostatic interaction is present between chitosan and the negatively charged mucosal surface as well as macro molecules such as DNA and RNA. This strong electrostatic interaction can be helpful in the treatment of solid tumors (Morile et al. 2008). Chitosan also has a considerable entrapment efficiency of the drugs which is greatly dependent on its molecular weight. At low degree of decelylation ($\leq 40\%$) chitosan is soluble until a pH value of 9.0 while at a higher degree of decetylation ($\geq 85\%$) it is only soluble up to pH 6.5 (Zhang et al. 2010).

Considerable research has been directed toward developing efficient chitosan-based NP drug delivery systems. In comparison with the other biological polymers, positive charges target the chitosan carriers to the negatively charged cell membrane and have mucoadhesive properties to increase the uptake of nanoparticles, and prolong the retention time of chitosan in the targeted locations (Arya et al. 2011; Hosseinzadeh et al. 2012). Table 16.1 presents chitosan-based nanocarriers which are used as passive targeting agents for several anticancer hydrophobic drugs.

The design of chitosan-based nanoparticle systems to incorporate anticancer drugs, doxorubicin, and gemcitaline are already published (Arya et al. 2011; Hosseinzadeh et al. 2012). Chitosan-based nanoparticles have a great potential and are promising nanocarriers for anticancer drugs. Wilson et al. developed tacrine-loaded chitosan nanoparticles by spontaneous emulsification. The developed nanoparticles exhibited a good drug entrapment efficiency. In vitro release studies showed that after the initial burst, all the drug-loaded batches provided a continuous and slow release of the drug (Wilson et al. 2010). Hossenizadeh and colleagues developed chitosan nanoparticles by ionic gelation with tripoly phosphate in the presence of pluronic F-127 for the targeting of the anticancer drug gemcitabine and it performed with positive results. There are several researchers who have prepared chitosan nanoparticles by an ionic gelation process to get effective positive results (Hosseinzadeh et al. 2012). Table 16.2 shows several investigated chitosan derivative nanoparticle-conjugated ligands to target their specific receptors.

16.4.1.2 Dextran

Dextran (Figure 16.4) is a water-soluble polysaccharide. Glucose chains form complex branches with glucan chains of variable length which forms a dextran chemical structure. Dextran-based microspheres have been explored in vitro, in vivo, and most recently, in clinical trials of breast, colon, hepatic, and pancreatic tumors. Dextran microspheres can carry the vast majority of drugs and improve the solubility of insoluble antitumor drugs.

Mitomycin C (MMC) drugs, delivered with the help of dextran microsphere vehicles, are potent anticancer agents that function through bioreductive activation. However, it shows much acute and chronic toxicity and several limitations in clinical application. To overcome these problems, oxidized dextran microspheres loaded with MMC are used for targeted drug delivery to the hypoxic regions of solid tumors.

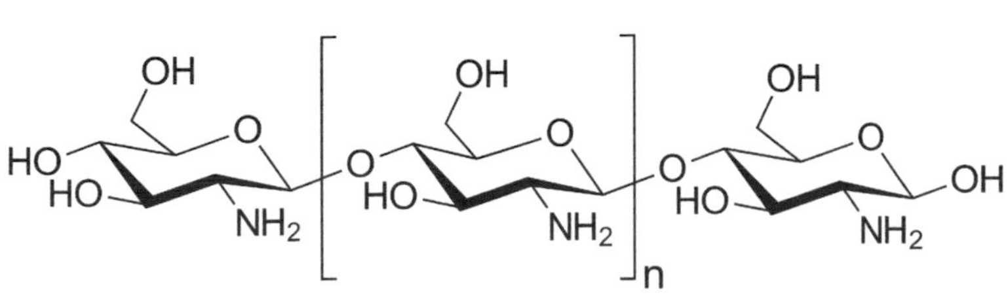

FIGURE 16.3 Chemical structure of chitosan.

TABLE 16.1

Chitosan-Based Nanocarriers Used as Passive Targeting Agents in Cancer Drug Delivery

Nanocarrier Component	Loaded Drug	Type of Cancer	Efficacy/ Mechanism	Evaluation	Reference
Chitosan nanocarrier	Gemcitabine	Lung, ovary	Oral adsorption	In vitro	Derakhshandeh et al. 2012
Chitosan/poly(ethylene glycol)	Gemcitabine	Lung	Reduce the burden of frequent dosing and higher toxicity	In vitro and in vivo	Garg et al. 2012
O-carboxymethyl chitosan	Curcumin	Various immune cells	Increase drug solubility	In vitro	Anitha et al. 2011
N-octyl-O-sulfate chitosan micelles	Paclitaxel (PTX)	Breast, epithelial ovarian,	Solubilization of hydrophobic drugs	In vitro	Zhang et al. 2008
Hydroxyapatitechitosan nanocomposite	Celecoxib	Colon	Sustained release patterns, desirable hemocompatibility, and enhanced cytotoxicity on cancer cells	In vitro and in vivo	Venkatesan et al. 2011
N-octyl-O-glycol chitosan, OGC	Paclitaxel (PTX)	Breast and ovarian	Enhanced long-term stability in aqueous solution, high drug-loading efficiency	In vitro	Huo et al. 2010

TABLE 16.2

Investigated Chitosan-Based Nanocarriers for Ligand–Receptor Active Targeting Delivery

Nanocarrier	Conjugated Ligand	Loaded Drug	Type of Cancer	Targeted Receptor/site	Evaluation	Reference
N-trimethyl Chitosan encapsulated	Galactose group	Lactosylnorcantharidin (Lac-NCTD)	Liver, Hepatic carcinoma	Asialoglycoprotein Receptor (ASGP-R)/ hepatocyte membrane	In vitro, in vivo	Guan et al. 2012
Chitosan nanoparticles conjugated 5 aminolaevulinic acid (5-ALA)	Folic acid	5-aminolaevulinic acid (5-ALA)	Colorectal cancer	Folate receptor	In vivo	Yang et al. 2010
Galactosylated chitosan–polycaprolactone (Gal-CH–PCL)	β-D-galactose and Nacetylgalactosamine	Curcumin	Liver, Hepatic carcinoma	Asialoglycoprotein/Hepatocyte membrane	In vitro	Zhou et al. 2013
Chitosan-coated liposomes (CCLs)	Folate	Fluorescein	Testicular, breast, and cervical	Folate receptor	In vitro	Yang et al. 2013

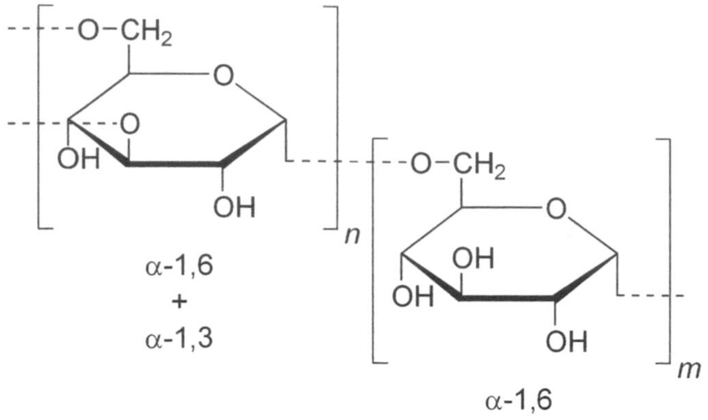

FIGURE 16.4 Chemical structure of dextran.

Dextran nanospheres exhibit biodegradability, biocompatibity, non-toxic, and non-immunogenic properties. These nanospheres are water soluble. When conjugated to antitumor drugs, dextran is rendered immunogenic and non-biodegradable which has hampered clinical trials several times. Dextran nanospheres have also shown side effects such as platelet dysfunction, anaphylaxis, and cerebral edema. Wasiak et al. (2016) found that different chemical moieties (e.g., drugs such as doxorubicin) can be attached to the dextran NPs via a pH-dependent bond that allows release of the drug with a lower pH.

Conjugated chitosan and dextran can self-organize into nanoparticles for incorporating drugs for tumor targeted delivery. Doxorubicin-loaded self-organized nanoparticles prepared by complexation with folic-acid-grafted chitosan showed folate receptor-targeted delivery in a tumor xenograft model (Lee et al. 2014).

Dextran-peptide conjugates of chemotherapeutic agents have been reported as a promising strategy for tumor-targeted delivery via the mediation of two widely known tumor-associated enzyme matrixes metalloproteinase II and matrix metalloproteinase IX. Optimization of linker property and charge of the backbone allowed for a high sensitivity of the conjugates toward the targeted enzymes along with satisfactory stability of the new conjugates in serum (Chau et al. 2004). Conjugates of dextran with a recombinant apoprotein of the antitumor antibiotic lidamycin integrated with enediyne showed highly a potent antitumor efficacy with selective accumulation and retention at the tumor site in epidermoid carcinoma and lung carcinoma tumor xenograft mice models (Li et al. 2014).

16.4.1.3   Pullulan

Pullulan (Figure 16.5) is a exo-polysaccharide consisting of both α-(1→4) and α-(1→6) linkages naturally available from the fungus *Aureobasidium pullulans*. It is a biodegradable, non-toxic, non-mutagenic, and non-carcinogenic polymer soluble in aqueous and several organic solvents. It can be derivatized into pullulan-drug conjugates that can be used for targeted drug delivery as well as targeted gene delivery for the treatment of various diseases in the liver, lungs, brain, and spleen (Jung et al. 2004). Scomparin et al. studied pullulan polymers with a main focus on tumor cell therapy. The group synthesized two pullulan derivatives i) conjugated pullulan with doxorubicin and ii) conjugated pullulan with doxorubicin and folic acid. To get proper functionality pullulan was activated by an oxidation and reduction conjugate with cysteamine. Both pullulan derivatives contained a similar doxorubicin concentration i.e., ~6% (w/w), with the second having 4.3% (w/w) folic acid. In the treatment of folate receptor-overexpressing human cervical carcinoma KB tumor-bearing mice, the folated-pullulan conjugate strongly inhibited tumor growth (Scomparin et al. 2015).

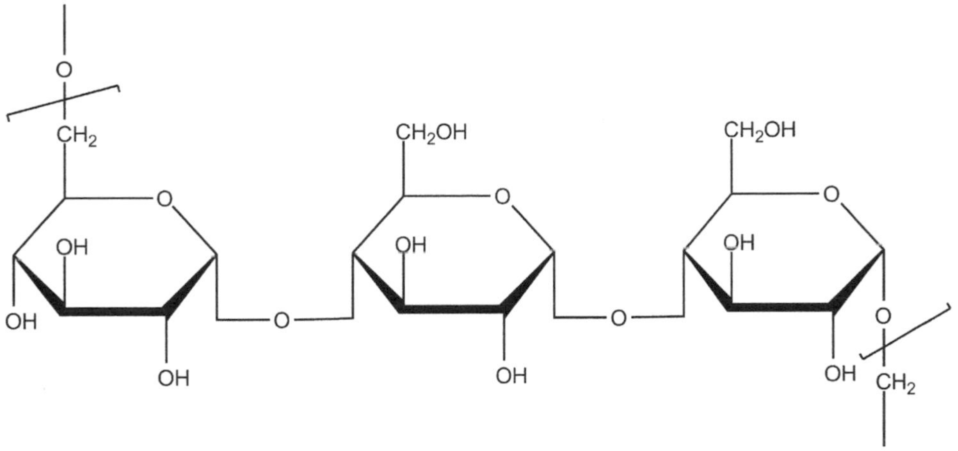

FIGURE 16.5 Chemical structure of pullulan.

Pullulan-stabilized gold nanoparticles have been used in the delivery of the anticancer drug 5-flurouracil (5-Fu) targeting the folate receptor. In vitro cytotoxicity tests were conducted in free 5-Fu and 5-Fu gold nanoparticles against HepG2 cells with over-expressed folate receptors (Zwicke et al. 2012). Biodistribution studies in male Wistar rats showed no excessive toxicity in untargeted healthy cells with the 5-Fu gold nanoparticles-folic acid bioconjugates and this result has set the groundwork for a novel approach in active liver cancer targeting (Qin et al.2012).

In another study Sang et al. (2015) investigated to see if folic-acid-conjugated pullulan/poly(DL-lactide-co-glycolide) graft copolymer nanoparticles could target the folate receptor of tumor cells (Lee et al. 2015). As the folate receptor is significantly upregulated on many human tumors such as ovarian carcinomas, osteosarcomas, and non-Hodgkin's lymphomas, such nanoparticles are a promising candidate for active targeting of anticancer agents (Kim and Oh, 2010).

16.4.1.4 Hyaluronic Acid

Hyaluronic acid (HA) (Figure 16.6) is widely used in anticancer drug delivery, since it is biocompatible, biodegradable, non-toxic, and non-immunogenic; moreover, HA receptors are over-expressed on many tumor cells including breast, ovarian, colon, lung, and stomach cancer (Coley 2008). Exploiting this ligand-receptor interaction, the use of HA is now a rapidly-growing platform for targeting CD44-overexpressing cells, to improve anticancer therapies (Liu et al. 2011). Liu et al. have shown that conjugation of HA to silica nanoparticles in colon cancer therapy could result in an enhanced uptake of 5-FU through CD44-mediated endocytosis uptake and could result in significant antitumor efficacy (Liu et al. 2015).

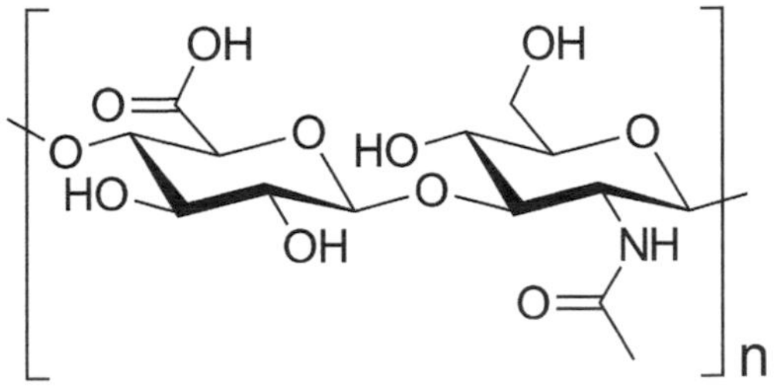

FIGURE 16.6 Chemical structure of hyaluronic acid.

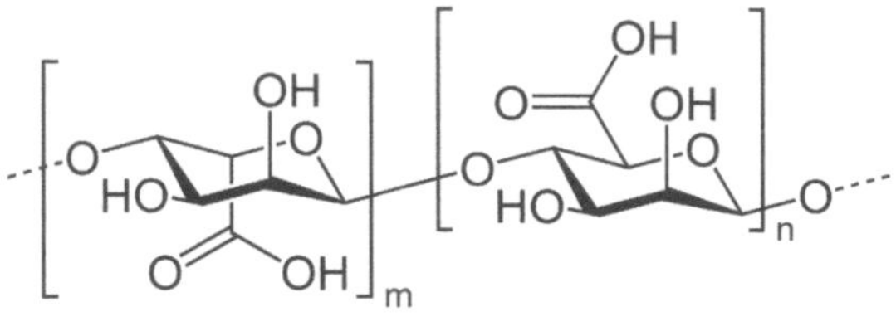

FIGURE 16.7 Chemical structure of alginate.

16.4.1.5 Alginate

Alginate (Figure 16.7) is a commercially available hydrophilic anionic polysaccharide copolymer of linear α-L-guluronate and β-D-mannuronate residues linked by (1–4) glycosidic linkage. Due to its many favorable properties like biodegradability, biocompatibility, non-toxicity, ease of gelation, and mucoadhesion, it has been widely used in drug delivery systems (Lertsutthiwong and Rojsitthisak 2011).

Active targeting can be achieved by conjugating a suitable targeting ligand to the alginate nanoparticles, thereby allowing preferential accumulation in the tumor site and tumor bearing organ. Glycyrrhetinic acid has a higher accumulation in the liver because of the abundant receptors for it on hepatocyte membranes. Glycyrrhetinic acid-modified alginate prepared by covalent attachment can be used to make nanoparticles with potential for targeted drug delivery to the liver. Doxorubicin-loaded glycyrrhetinic acid-modified alginate nanoparticles showed lower cardiac distribution compared to liver tumors as well as a higher tumor growth inhibition rate when administered to a Kunming mice model of liver cancer (Zhang et al. 2012).

Chitosan and alginate are polyelectrolyte polymers of opposite charges. Chitosan-alginate polyionic complex is formed through ionic gelation due to the ionic interactions between the amine group of chitosan and the carboxylic group of alginate. Several researchers have investigated the delivery potential of the chitosan-alginate bi-polymer nanoparticles and chitosan-coated

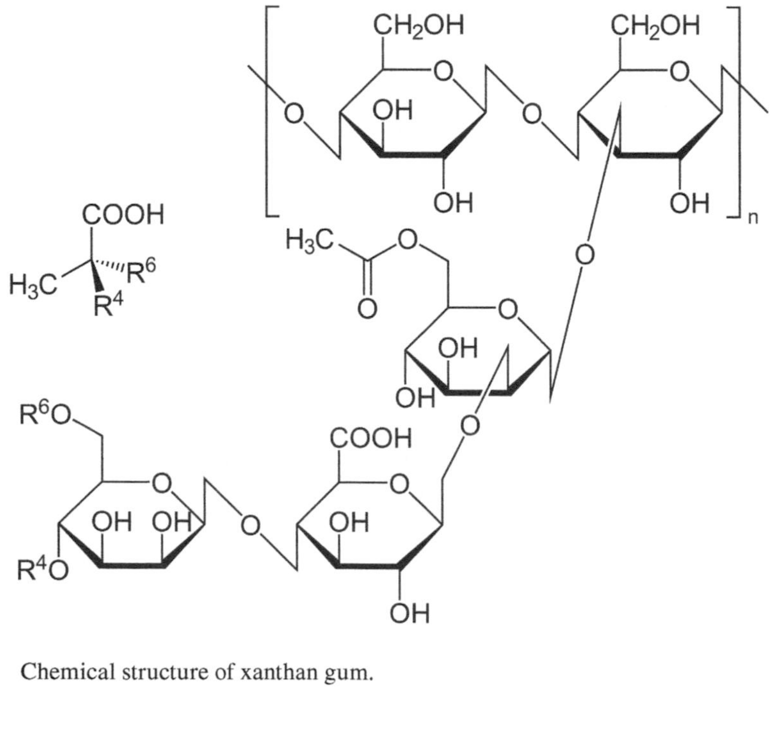

FIGURE 16.8 Chemical structure of xanthan gum.

alginate nanoparticles for delivery of drugs. Coating paclitaxel-loaded alginate nanoparticles with folate-chitosan by a double emulsion crosslinking electrostatic attraction method showed improved stability and cellular uptake of nanoparticles on HepG2 cells demonstrating its potential in anticancer drug targeted delivery systems (Wang et al. 2016).

16.4.1.6 Xanthan Gum

Xanthan gum (Figure 16.8) is an exopolysaccharide naturally available from the bacteria Xanthomonas campestris. It is a water-soluble polymer that is stable over a wide range of temperatures and acidic and alkaline conditions, as well as being resistant to enzymatic degradation (Becker et al. 1998). Xanthan gum has been used as a reduction agent in the synthesis of gold nanoparticles. These nanoparticles have a high drug loading, stability and are capable of targeted drug release (Pooja et al. 2014).

16.5 CONCLUSION

Current chemotherapy agents are associated with challenges such as non-selective distribution, cytotoxicity, short circulation half-life, and unwanted side effects to normal tissues. To overcome these drawbacks, nanosized carriers have been investigated to improve their permeability, retention effect, and delivery properties via passive and active mechanisms. Targeted delivery of drugs is critical in improving therapeutic efficacy and minimizing side effects. Many approaches are currently available to deliver the drugs to the specific site of action. Polysaccharides show variability and versatility, due to their complex structure, which is difficult to reproduce with synthetic polymers. Thus, native polysaccharides and their derivatives are emerging as one of the most used biomaterials in the field of nanomedicine, especially being chosen by a lot of researchers as carriers in the preparation of nanoparticulate drug delivery systems.

REFERENCES

Amreddy, N., Babu, A., Muralidharan, R., Panneerselvam, J., Srivastava, A., and Ahmed, R. et al. 2017. Recent advances in nanoparticle-based cancer drug and gene delivery. *Adv Cancer Res* 137: 115–70.

Anitha, A., Maya, S., Deepa, N., Chennazhi, K., Nair, S., Tamura, H. et al. 2011. Efficient water soluble O-carboxymethyl chitosan nanocarrier for the delivery of curcumin to cancer cells. *Carbohydr Polym* 83 (2): 452–61.

Arya, G., Vandana, M., Acharya, S., and Sahoo, S.K. 2011. Enhanced antiproliferative activity of Herceptin (HER2)-conjugated gemcitabine-loaded chitosan nanoparticle in pancreatic cancer therapy. *Nanomedicine* 7 (6):859–70.

Bae, Y.H. and Park, K. 2011. Targeted drug delivery to tumors: Myths, reality and possibility. *J Control Release* 153 (3): 198.

Barreto, J.A., O'Malley, W., Kubeil, M., Graham, B., Stephan, H., and Spiccia, L. 2011. Nanomaterials: Applications in cancer imaging and therapy. *Adv Mater* 23 (12).

Bates, D.O. 2010. Vascular endothelial growth factors and vascular permeability. *Cardiovasc Res* 87 (2): 262–71.

Bazak, R., Houri, M., El Achy, S., Hussein, W., and Refaat, T. 2014. Passive targeting of nanoparticles to cancer: A comprehensive review of the literature. *Mol Clin Oncol* 2 (6): 904–08.

Becker A., Katzen F., Puhler A. and Ielpi L. 1998. Xanthan gum biosynthesis and application: A biochemical/ genetic perspective. *Appl Microbiol Biotechnol* 50: 145–52.

Birbrair, A., Zhang, T., Wang, Z.M., Messi, M.L., Olson, J.D., Mintz, A. et al. 2014. Type-2 pericytes participate in normal and tumoral angiogenesis. *Am J Physiol Cell Physiol* 307 (1):C25–38.

Byrne, J.D., Betancourt, T., and Brannon-Peppas, L. 2008. Active targeting schemes for nanoparticle systems in cancer therapeutics. *Adv Drug Del Rev* 60 (15): 1615–26.

Chau, Y., Tan, F.E., and Langer, R. 2004. Synthesis and characterization of dextran– peptide– methotrexate conjugates for tumor targeting via mediation by matrix metalloproteinase II and matrix metalloproteinase IX. *Bioconjug Chem*15(4): 931–41.

Coley, H.M. 2008. Mechanisms and strategies to overcome chemotherapy resistance in metastatic breast cancer. *Cancer Treat Rev* 34 (4): 378–90.

Cook, K.M. and Figg, W.D. 2010. Angiogenesis inhibitors: Current strategies and future prospects. *CA Cancer J Clin* 60 (4): 222–43.

Danhier, F., Feron, O., and Préat, V. 2010. To exploit the tumor microenvironment: Passive and active tumor targeting of nanocarriers for anti-cancer drug delivery. *J Control Release* 148 (2): 135–46.

Daniels, T.R., Bernabeu, E., Rodríguez, J.A., Patel, S., Kozman, M., and Chiappetta, D.A. et al. 2012. The transferrin receptor and the targeted delivery of therapeutic agents against cancer. *Biochim Biophys Acta (BBA)-General Subjects* 1820 (3): 291–317.

Deger, A., Deger, H., and Taser, F. 2016. The role of neoangiogenesis and vascular endothelial growth factor in the development of carpal tunnel syndrome in patients with diabetes. *Niger J Clin Pract* 19 (2): 189–95.

Derakhshandeh, K. and Fathi, S. 2012. Role of chitosan nanoparticles in the oral absorption of Gemcitabine. *Int J Pharm* 437 (1–2): 172–7.

Dinarvand, R., Cesar de Morais, P., and D'Emanuele, A. 2012. Nanoparticles for targeted delivery of active agents against tumor cells. *J Drug Deliv* 2012.

Dreaden, E.C., Austin, L.A., Mackey, M.A., and El-Sayed, M.A. 2012. Size matters: Gold nanoparticles in targeted cancer drug delivery. *Ther Deliv* 3 (4): 457–78.

Eftekhari, R., Esmaeili, R., Mirzaei, R., Bidad, K., de Lima, S., Ajami, M. et al. 2017. Study of the tumor microenvironment during breast cancer progression. *Cancer Cell Int* 17 (1): 123.

Garg, N.K., Dwivedi, P., Campbell, C., and Tyagi, R.K. 2012. Site specific/targeted delivery of gemcitabine through anisamide anchored chitosan/poly ethylene glycol nanoparticles: An improved understanding of lung cancer therapeutic intervention. *Eur J Pharm Sci* 47 (5): 1006–14.

Georgieva, J.V., Kalicharan, D., Couraud, P.O., Romero, I.A., Weksler, B., Hoekstra, D. et al. 2011. Surface characteristics of nanoparticles determine their intracellular fate in and processing by human blood–brain barrier endothelial cells in vitro. *Mol Ther* 19 (2): 318–25.

Greish, K. 2010. Enhanced permeability and retention (epr) effect for anticancer nanomedicine drug targeting. In: Grobmyer, S.R., and Moudgil, B.M. (Eds.), *Cancer Nanotechnology, Methods in Molecular Biology* 624:25–37. New York: Humana Press.

Guan, M., Zhou, Y., Zhu, Q.L., Liu, Y., Bei, Y.Y., and Zhang, X.N. et al. 2012. N-trimethyl chitosan nanoparticle-encapsulated lactosyl-norcantharidin for liver cancer therapy with high targeting efficacy. *Nanomed Nanotechnol Biol Med* 8 (7): 1172–81.

Herman, A.B., Savage, V.M., and West, G.B. 2011. A quantitative theory of solid tumor growth, metabolic rate and vascularization. *PLoS One* 6 (9):e22973.

Hosseinzadeh, H., Atyabi, F., Dinarvand, R., and Ostad, S. N. 2012. Chitosan–pluronic nanoparticles as oral delivery of anticancer gemcitabine: preparation and in vitro study. *Int J Nanomedicine* 7, 1851–63.

Huo, M., Zhang, Y., Zhou, J., Zou, A., Yu, D., Wu, Y. et al. 2010. Synthesis and characterization of low-toxic amphiphilic chitosan derivatives and their application as micelle carrier for antitumor drug. *Int J Pharm* 394 (1–2): 162–73.

Jung, S.W., Jeong, Y.L., Kim, Y.H., and Kim, S.H. 2004. Self-assembled polymeric nanoparticles of poly (ethylene glycol) grafted pullulan acetate as a novel drug carrier. *Arch Pharm Res* 27 (5): 562.

Kamaly, N., Xiao, Z., Valencia, P.M., Radovic-Moreno, A.F., and Farokhzad, O.C. 2012. Targeted polymeric therapeutic nanoparticles: Design, development and clinical translation. *Chem Soc Rev* 41 (7): 2971–3010.

Kim, I.S. and Oh, I.J. 2010. Preparation and characterization of stearic acid-pullulan nanoparticles. *Arch Pharm Res* 33 (5): 761–7.

Kim, J.H., Kim, Y.S., Park, K., Lee, S., Nam, H.Y., Min, K.H. et al. 2008. Antitumor efficacy of cisplatin-loaded glycol chitosan nanoparticles in tumor-bearing mice. *J Control Release* 127 (1): 41–9.

Lee, K.D., Choi, S.H., Kim, D.H., Lee, H.Y., and Choi, K.C. 2014. Self-organized nanoparticles based on chitosan-folic acid and dextran succinate-doxorubicin conjugates for drug targeting. *Arch Pharm Res* 37 (12): 1546–53.

Lee, S. J., Shim, Y.H., Oh, J.S., Jeong, Y.I., Park, I.K., and Lee, H. C. 2015. Folic-acid-conjugated pullulan/poly(DL-lactide-co-glycolide) graft copolymer nanoparticles for folate-receptor-mediated drug delivery. *Nanoscale Res Lett* 10:43.

Lertsutthiwong, P. and Rojsitthisak, P. 2011. Chitosan-alginate nanocapsules for encapsulation of turmeric oil. *Die Pharmazie* 66(12): 911–15.

Li, B., Liu, X.J., Li, L., Zhang, S.H., Li, Y., Li, D.D. et al. 2014. A tumor-targeting dextran–apoprotein conjugate integrated with enediyne chromophore shows highly potent antitumor efficacy. *Polymer Chemistry* 5(19): 5680–8.

Liang, N., Sun, S., Hong, J., Tian, J., Fang, L., and Cui, F. 2016. In vivo pharmacokinetics, biodistribution and antitumor effect of paclitaxel-loaded micelles based on α-tocopherol succinate-modified chitosan. *Drug Deliv* 23 (8): 2651–60.

Liu, C., Kelnar, K., Liu, B., Chen, X., Calhoun-Davis, T., Li, H. et al. 2011. The microRNA miR-34a inhibits prostate cancer stem cells and metastasis by directly repressing CD44. *Nat Med* 17 (2): 211.

Liu, K., Wang, Z.Q., Wang, S.J., Liu, P., Qin, Y.H. Ma, Y. et al. 2015. Hyaluronic acid-tagged silica nanoparticles in colon cancer therapy: Therapeutic efficacy evaluation. *Int J Nanomed* 10: 6445–54.

Liu, Z., Jiao, Y., Wang, Y., Zhou, C., and Zhang, Z. 2008. Polysaccharides-based nanoparticles as drug delivery systems. *Adv Drug Del Rev* 60 (15): 1650–62.

Mann, S.K., Czuba, E., Selby, L.I., Such, G.K., and Johnston, A.P. 2016. Quantifying nanoparticle internalization using a high throughput internalization assay. *Pharm Res* 33 (10): 2421–32.

Ngoune, R., Peters, A., Von Elverfeldt, D., Winkler, K., and Pütz, G. 2016. Accumulating nanoparticles by EPR: A route of no return. *J Control Release* 238: 58–70.

Poli, A., Di Donato, P., Abbamondi, G.R., and Nicolaus, B. 2011. Synthesis, production, and biotechnological applications of exopolysaccharides and polyhydroxyalkanoates by archaea. *Archaea* 2011: 693253.

Pooja, D., Panyaram, S., Kulhari, H., Rachamalla, S.S., and Sistla, R. 2014. Xanthan gum stabilized gold nanoparticles: Characterization, biocompatibility, stability and cytotoxicity. *Carbohydr Polym* 110: 1–9.

Qin, J.M., Yin, P.H., Li, Q., Sa, Z.Q., Sheng, X., Yang, L. et al. 2012. Anti-tumor effects of brucine immuno-nanoparticles on hepatocellular carcinoma. *Int J Nanomed* 7: 369.

Saravanakumar, G., Jo, D.G., and H Park, J. 2012. Polysaccharide-based nanoparticles: A versatile platform for drug delivery and biomedical imaging. *Curr Med Chem* 19 (19): 3212–29.

Scomparin, A., Salmaso, S., Eldar-Boock, A., Ben-Shushan, D., Ferber, S., Tiram, G. et al. 2015. A comparative study of folate receptor-targeted doxorubicin delivery systems: Dosing regimens and therapeutic index. *J Control Release* 208: 106–20.

Shukla, R.K. and Tiwari, A. 2012. Carbohydrate polymers: Applications and recent advances in delivering drugs to the colon. *Carbohydr Polym* 88 (2): 399–416.

Sung, S.Y., Hsieh, C.L., Wu, D., Chung, L.W., and Johnstone, P.A. 2007. Tumor microenvironment promotes cancer progression, metastasis, and therapeutic resistance. *Curr Probl Cancer* 31 (2): 36–100.

Swierczewska, M., Han, H., Kim, K., Park, J., and Lee, S. 2016. Polysaccharide-based nanoparticles for theranostic nanomedicine. *Adv Drug Del Rev* 99: 70–84.

Thibodeau, S. and Voutsadakis, I.A. 2018. FOLFIRINOX chemotherapy in metastatic pancreatic cancer: A systematic review and meta-analysis of retrospective and phase II studies. *J Clin Med* 7 (1): 7.

Trédan, O., Galmarini, C.M., Patel, K., and Tannock, I.F. 2007. Drug resistance and the solid tumor microenvironment. *J Natl Cancer Inst* 99 (19): 1441–54.

Venkatesan, P., Puvvada, N., Dash, R., Kumar, B.P., Sarkar, D., Azab, B. et al. 2011. The potential of celecoxib-loaded hydroxyapatite-chitosan nanocomposite for the treatment of colon cancer. *Biomaterials* 32 (15): 3794–806.

Viallard, C. and Larrivée, B. 2017. Tumor angiogenesis and vascular normalization: Alternative therapeutic targets. *Angiogenesis* 20 (4): 409–26.

Vicent, M.J. and Duncan, R. 2006. Polymer conjugates: Nanosized medicines for treating cancer. *Trends Biotechnol* 24 (1): 39–47.

Wang, F., Yang, S., Yuan, J., Gao, Q., and Huang, C. 2016. Effective method of chitosan-coated alginate nanoparticles for target drug delivery applications. *J Biomater Appl* 31(1): 3–12.

Wasiak, I., Kulikowska, A., Janczewska, M., Michalak, M., Cymerman, I.A., and Nagalski, A. et al. 2016. Dextran nanoparticle synthesis and properties. *PLoS One* 11 (1): e0146237.

Wilson, B., Samanta, M.K., Santhi, K., Kumar, K.S., Ramasamy, M., and Suresh, B. 2010. Chitosan nanoparticles as a new delivery system for the anti-Alzheimer drug tacrine. *Nanomed Nanotechnol Biol Med* 6 (1): 144–152.

Yang, K.K., Kong, M., Wei, Y.N., Liu, Y., Cheng, X.J., Li, J. et al. 2013. Folate-modified–chitosan-coated liposomes for tumor-targeted drug delivery. *J Mater Sci* 48 (4): 1717–28.

Yang, S.J., Lin, F.H., Tsai, K.C., Wei, M.F., Tsai, H.M., Wong, J.M. et al. 2010. Folic acid-conjugated chitosan nanoparticles enhanced protoporphyrin IX accumulation in colorectal cancer cells. *Bioconjug Chem* 21 (4): 679–89.

Yhee, J.Y., Jeon, S., Yoon, H.Y., Shim, M.K., Ko, H., Min, J. et al. 2017. Effects of tumor microenvironments on targeted delivery of glycol chitosan nanoparticles. *J Control Release* 267: 223–31.

Yin, H., Liao, L., and Fang, J. 2014. Enhanced permeability and retention (EPR) effect based tumor targeting: The concept, application and prospect. *JSM Clin Oncol Res* 2 (1): 1010.

Zhang, C., Qu, G., Sun, Y., Yang, T., Yao, Z., Shen, W. et al. 2008. Biological evaluation of N-octyl-O-sulfate chitosan as a new nano-carrier of intravenous drugs. *Eur J Pharm Sci* 33 (4–5): 415–23.

Zhang, C., Wang, W., Liu, T., Wu, Y., Guo, H., Wang, P. et al. 2012. Doxorubicin-loaded glycyrrhetinic acid-modified alginate nanoparticles for liver tumor chemotherapy. *Biomaterials* 33 (7): 2187–96.

Zhang, H., Ma, Y., and Sun, X.L. 2010. Recent developments in carbohydrate-decorated targeted drug/gene delivery. *Med Res Rev* 30 (2): 270–89.

Zhou, N., Zan, X., Wang, Z., Wu, H., Yin, D., Liao, C. et al. 2013. Galactosylated chitosan–polycaprolactone nanoparticles for hepatocyte-targeted delivery of curcumin. *Carbohydr Polym* 94 (1): 420–9.

Zwicke, G.L., Ali Mansoori, G., and Jeffery, C.J. 2012. Utilizing the folate receptor for active targeting of cancer nanotherapeutics. *Nano Rev* 3 (1): 18496.

17 Polysaccharide-Based Nanocarriers Loaded with Drugs for the Management of Obesity

Sandipan Dasgupta, Souvik Roy,
Tania Chakraborty, and Nilanjan Sarkar

CONTENTS

17.1   INTRODUCTION

Obesity is a disorder comprising of excess body fat which is associated with an increase in health problems. A person with a body mass index (BMI) of over 30 kg/m^2, is measured as obese, where BMI is obtained by dividing a person's weight by the square of the person's height. In 2016, more than 1.9 billion adults, 18 years and older, were overweight, of these over 650 million were obese. This means 39% of adults aged 18 years and over were overweight in 2016, and 13% of these were obese. In highly populated countries obesity correlates to higher morbidity compared to underweight individuals. Forty-one million kids below the age of 5 were overweight or obese and more than 340 million children and adolescents aged 5–19 were overweight or obese in 2016. One of major causes of obesity is imbalance between calories taken in and calories used. Globally, there has been: (i) an increased uptake of energy-dense foods loaded with fat (Lau et al. 2007); (ii) few cases may be due to genetics, medical reasons, or psychiatric illness (Bleich et al. 2008) and (iii) an decrease in physical inactivity due to sedentary nature of various forms of work, varying modes of transportation, and increasing development of current society (James 2008). Changes in dietary and physical activity patterns are often a consequence of environmental and societal changes associated with the evolution and absence of steady arrangements in sectors such as health, agriculture, transport, urban planning, environment, food processing, distribution, marketing, and education.

There are numerous possible pathophysiological components engaged with in the development and maintenance of obesity (Flier 2004). This field of research has remained almost unexplored until the discovery of the leptin gene in 1994 by J.M. Friedman's laboratory (Zhang et al. 1994). While leptin and ghrelin are produced peripherally, they control appetite through their actions on the central nervous system. Specifically, the appetite-related hormones act on the hypothalamus, a region of the brain central to the regulation of food intake and energy expenditure. Several circuits within the hypothalamus contribute to its activity in integrating appetite, from which the melanocortin pathway is the most elaborately studied (Flier 2004). The circuit generates within the "arcuate nucleus" area of the hypothalamus, that has outputs to the lateral hypothalamus (LH) and ventromedial hypothalamus (VMH), the brain's feeding and satiety centers, respectively (Boulpaep and Walter 2003). The primary treatment for obesity includes dieting and physical exercise (Lau et al. 2006). The most efficient way to treat obesity is bariatric surgery (Colquitt et al. 2014) other than that five medications are designated for long-term use orlistat, lorcaserin, liraglutide, phentermine-topiramate, and naltrexone-bupropion.

The main function of orlistat is preventing the assimilation of fats from the diet by acting as a lipase inhibitor, thus reducing the intake of calories. Lorcaserin diminishes appetite by triggering a type of serotonin receptor known as the 5-HT2C receptor in the hypothalamus of the brain, which is associated with control of appetite (Shukla et al. 2015). Liraglutide is used as a long-acting glucagon-like peptide-1 receptor agonist and binds to the same receptors as the endogenous metabolic hormone GLP-1 to stimulate insulin secretion. Phentermine-topiramate is a combination medication used for weight loss. Phentermine and topiramate moderately promote weight loss by improving weight-related comorbidities such as improved blood sugar, cholesterol, and decreased blood pressure. Bupropion/naltrexone is another combination drug used for weight loss in individuals who are either obese or overweight associated with weight-related illnesses (Plodkowski et al. 2009). Current and potential anti-obesity drugs may operate through one or more of the following mechanisms: appetite suppressants, increase the body's metabolism, or interference with the body's ability to absorb specific nutrients in food.

In the past years, many drug delivery systems have been planned and have materialized based on medical requirements (Peppas 2013). The principles of drug delivery systems are to enhance the in vivo behavior of drugs via passive and active targeting. The uses of many drugs are restricted by low efficacy, non-site specificity, toxicity, rapid clearance, and random distribution. Various drug delivery systems provide methods to overcome all the above-mentioned shortcomings. Nanoparticles are thoroughly investigated in this aspect because of their ability to target ailing tissues and their potential to remain in circulation for longer periods in the human body (Zhang Nan, 2013). Nanoparticles are chemically stable structures that can be designed through different chemical and biological routes that are environment friendly and cost effective (Khan NT, 2017). Nanoparticles are so designed that they can easily diffuse inside cells by interacting with specific cellular components, permitting their selective targeting and accumulation in specific locations. They can accumulate in the fluid environment of the cell for weeks without being degraded, thus making them very suitable candidates for drug delivery systems. A few examples of different types of nanoparticle drug delivery systems are polymerosomes, nanocapsules, silica nanoparticles, quantum dot, amphiphilic nanoparticles, dendrimers, graphene, carbon nanotubes, metal-core nanoparticles, oligopeptides, and supramolecular polymers. Polymers and particularly polysaccharides are being thoroughly studied and engaged with in the production of nanocarriers able to deliver different drugs, owing to their promising physical and biological properties. This technology is considered to be the future for clinical and biomedical applications and in the treatment of numerous diseases. Nanocarriers are now being analyzed for their functions in drug delivery and their exceptional characteristics validate their potential use in chemotherapy and diabetes. Furthermore, nanocarriers could also be used in various other diseases where a targeted drug delivery is to be achieved. Currently, NPs to target the browning of fatty tissue were designed by Dr. Robert Langer at MIT and Dr. Omid Farokhzad at Brigham and Women's Hospital, respectively. It was observed by the team that mice treated with nanoparticles had smaller fat cells, more blood vessels, and increased levels of brown fat markers. These findings indicate that the targeted nanoparticles reduced weight gain by browning of the adipose tissue. This study can lead the way for a novel and improved method for targeted drug delivery of anti-obesity medication (Peppas 2013).

17.2 CONVENTIONAL METHODS FOR THE MANAGEMENT OF OBESITY

Obesity in individuals can be managed by lifestyle changes, medications, or surgery but dieting and physical exercise still remain the main form of treatment in obesity. Weight loss may be achieved by diet programs but temporarily retaining weight loss is very difficult and should therefore include exercise and low calorie as part of one's lifestyle. Overweight and obese individuals ideally should be managed by a multidisciplinary team which includes a physician, nutritionist, exercise therapist, and in certain situations psychiatrist/psychologists or other specialists.

17.2.1 SURGERY

The most efficient way to treat obesity is bariatric surgery (Colquitt et al. 2014). Surgery can induce long-term weight loss and is associated with decreased mortality. It is only opted for in severely obese individuals who have not attained weight loss through dietary modification and pharmacological treatment. The two most common principles involved in weight loss surgery are reducing the bulk of the stomach (e.g. by adjustable gastric banding and vertical banded gastroplasty), that induces an early sense of satiation, and by shortening the length of the intestine that comes into contact with food to reduce absorption (by gastric bypass surgery or endoscopic duodenal-jejunal bypass surgery) (Sullivan 2015; Muñoz et al. 2015). However, such surgeries are not free of complications and the patient may develop bowel obstruction, dumping syndrome, causing diarrhoea, nausea, or vomiting. But surgery is associated with long-term weight loss and is capable of decreasing overall mortality. Bariatric surgery also causes a dip in the risk of diabetes mellitus, cardiovascular disease, and cancer (Sjöström et al, 2007). Weight loss occurs during the first few months following surgery and is sustained in the long term. Studies have revealed that gastric bypass techniques are found to produce 30% more weight loss as compared to banding procedures one year following surgery (Tice et al. 2008). Liposuction is a cosmetic surgery that removes fat from the human body but it does not appear to affect obesity-related problems. Some studies have shown benefits while others have not (Klein et al. 2004).

17.2.2   ANTI-OBESITY MEDICATIONS

Various anti-obesity drugs are approved by the FDA for utilization in long-term use and marketed formulations of all these molecules are available for the treatment of obesity.

17.2.2.1   Orlistat

Orlistat is used frequently to treat obesity and is marketed as Xenical® by Roche in most countries. It is the saturated derivative of lipstatin, a potent natural inhibitor of pancreatic lipases, but orlistat was chosen over lipstatin as an anti-obesity drug because of its relative simplicity and stability (Pommier et al. 1995). Its function is to prevent the absorption of fat from the human diet by acting as a lipase inhibitor, thus reducing the intake of calories. It is generally used in conjunction with a reduced-calorie diet under the supervision of a healthcare provider (Shukla et al. 2015). Orlistat works by breaking down triglycerides in the intestine via inhibition of gastric and pancreatic lipases. When lipases are inhibited, triglycerides present in the diet cannot be hydrolyzed into absorbable free fatty acids and are excreted unchanged. Orlistat primarily effects the local lipase inhibition within the GI tract after an oral dose and is eliminated through the feces. The side effects of the drug include steatorrhea (oily, loose stools with excessive flatus due to unabsorbed fats reaching the large intestine), fecal incontinence, and frequent or urgent bowel movements.

17.2.2.2   Lorcaserin

Lorcaserin is sold under the trade name Belviq® and Lorqess®, developed by Arena Pharmaceuticals, and is presently being used to treat and shrink obesity. It reduces appetite by triggering a serotonin receptor (5-HT_{2C}) in part of the hypothalamus in the brain, which is known to control appetite (Thomsen et al. 2008). Lorcaserin is a specific 5-HT_{2C} receptor agonist, (Thomsen et al. 2008) and studies demonstrated reasonable selectivity for 5-HT_{2C} over other related targets (Smith et al. 2005. 5-HT_{2C} receptors can be found only in the choroid plexus, cortex, hippocampus, cerebellum, amygdala, thalamus, and hypothalamus of the human brain. Stimulation of 5-HT_{2C} receptors in the hypothalamus activates proopiomelanocortin (POMC) production and thus promotes weight loss through satiety (Spreitzer 2010). The most common side effects of Lorcaserin include headache, upper respiratory tract infection, nasopharyngitis, sinusitis, and nausea. Depression, anxiety, and suicidal ideation were uncommon and cardiac valvulopathy was reported in some subjects consuming the drug in phase 2 trials.

17.2.2.3   Sibutramine

Sibutramine was manufactured under the brand name Meridia® among others and acts as an appetite suppressant, but it has been withdrawn. Until 2010, it was promoted and used as an additional treatment for obesity with proper diet and exercise. Studies reveal increased cardiovascular events and strokes with the use of sibutramine and thus it has been removed from market in several countries. Sibutramine acts as a monoamine reuptake inhibitor (MRI) and decreases the reuptake of norepinephrine, serotonin, and dopamine, thus increasing their levels in synaptic clefts and helps achieving satiety. Side effects include: dry mouth, paradoxically increased appetite, nausea, strange taste in the mouth, upset stomach, constipation, trouble sleeping, dizziness, drowsiness, menstrual cramps/pain, headache, flushing, or joint/muscle pain. Occasionally occurring side effects that require serious and immediate medical attention are cardiac arrhythmias, paresthesia, and mental/mood changes (e.g., excitement, restlessness, confusion, depression, rare thoughts of suicide).

17.2.2.4   Rimonabant

Rimonabant is an anorectic anti-obesity drug that was approved in 2006 but due to serious psychiatric effects had to be withdrawn in 2008. Rimonabant acts as an inverse agonist for the cannabinoid receptor CB1 and was the first drug to be approved in this class.

17.2.2.5   Exenatide/Liraglutide

Exenatide is an analogue of the hormone GLP-1, which is secreted in the intestines whenever food is detected. GLP-1 defers gastric emptying time to promote a feeling of satiety. Exenatide is currently used to treat diabetes mellitus type 2 and some patients have reported that they lost a significant amount of weight while taking it. Disadvantages of using exenatide include patient compliance as it must be injected subcutaneously twice daily, and in some patients it causes severe nausea. The use of exenatide is recommended only for patients with type 2 diabetes mellitus. Symlin, is another drug available for treating diabetes and is also being tested for obesity treatment in non-diabetics (Sauer et al. 2015). Liraglutide or saxenda is another GLP-1 analogue.

17.2.2.6   Phentermine/Topiramate

Phentermine and topiramate, is a combination therapy used for the treatment of obesity. Phentermine amine which acts as an appetite suppressant and stimulant is a sympathomimetic amine and topiramate works as an anti-convulsant which includes weight loss as one of the side effects. The precise mechanism of action is unknown for the combination. The most common side effects include paraesthesia (tingling in fingers/toes), dizziness, dysgeusia (altered taste), insomnia, constipation, and dry mouth. Phentermine/topiramate extended release is contraindicated in hyperthyroidism, pregnancy, glaucoma, and in patients with hypersensitivity or idiosyncrasy to sympathomimetic amines. Phentermine/topiramate extended release can elevate the heart rate at rest.

17.2.2.7   Bupropion/Naltrexone

Bupropion/naltrexone is another combination drug used for weight loss in overweight or obese individuals. Both drugs are effective in weight loss individually, and their combination also produces some synergistic effects on weight loss. Bupropion is a reuptake inhibitor of norepinephrine and a nicotinic acetylcholine receptor antagonist and it works by activating proopiomelanocortin (POMC) neurons in the hypothalamus as a result there is a loss of appetite and increased energy output. The POMC is controlled by endogenous opioids via opioid-mediated negative feedback. Naltrexone is a pure opioid antagonist and assists bupropion's activation of the POMC (Greenway et al. 2008). This combination can affect mood and increase suicidal tendencies in individuals.

17.3   NANOPARTICLES IN DRUG DELIVERY

Nanotechnology is the controlling of matter in the 1–100 nm dimension range. This technology has been used in medicine to develop nanoparticles, so that novel therapeutic and diagnostic modalities can be obtained. Nanoparticles have special physicochemical properties, such as ultra-small size, large surface area to mass ratio, and high reactivity, which are dissimilar to the bulk materials of the same composition. These properties can be utilized to overcome the shortcomings in the present therapeutic agents. The drug could be dissolved, entrapped, encapsulated, or attached to a nanoparticle matrix. Nanoparticles, nanospheres, or nanocapsules are obtained on the basis of their methods of preparation. Recently, biodegradable polymeric nanoparticles, coated with hydrophilic polymers like as poly(ethylene glycol) (PEG), have been utilized as potential drug delivery devices due to their ability to circulate for a prolonged period time, target particular organs, carry DNA in gene therapy, and deliver proteins, peptides, and genes (Komma Reddy et al. 2005). Currently nanoparticles are being used to treat a variety of cancers and are being investigated in diseases like leukemia, diabetes, and sexually transmitted diseases (Maysinger et al. 2010). The most important points to remember while designing a delivery system with nanoparticles is to control particle size, optimize surface properties, and modulate the release of pharmacologically active agents to achieve a site-specific action of the drug at the ideal rate and dose.

17.3.1 THE ADVANTAGES OF USING NANOPARTICLES AS A DRUG DELIVERY SYSTEM

1. Passive and active drug targeting can be achieved by modification of particle size and surface characteristics of nanoparticles.
2. An increase in the therapeutic efficacy and reduction of side effects of a drug can be achieved using NPs as they can control and modify the drug release while transportation and also at site of localization thus leading to alteration of organ distribution and subsequent clearance of the drug.
3. Variation of the matrix constituents can modulate the particle degradation and release characteristics of NPs. NPs have relatively high drug loading capacity and hence drugs are incorporated with ease into the system, without any unwanted chemical reaction. This is an essential factor in maintaining the activity of the drug.
4. Magnetic guidance or targeting ligands to the surface of particles can allow us to achieve site specific targeting of the therapeutic molecules.
5. Administration of such NPs can be achieved either by oral, nasal, parenteral or intra-ocular etc.

Regardless of these advantages, NPs have a few confinements. Particle size aggregation is often encountered due to their small size and large SA, thus making their physical management difficult in liquid and dry forms. This issue must be overcome before nanoparticles can be utilized clinically or made industrially accessible.

17.3.2 THE VARIOUS TYPES OF NANOPARTICLES USED IN DRUG DELIVERY

There are the various types of nanocarriers used to deliver drugs to the target organs and tissues mentioned in Figure 17.1.

17.3.2.1 Liposomes

Liposomes contain a hydrophilic and a hydrophobic part in its structure and are thus amphiphilic in nature. These structures can form themselves spontaneously into closed spherical shell-type structures at a predetermined concentration (critical micelle concentration). This vesicular structure form composed of phospholipids, such as phosphatidylcholine, phosphatidylserine, or phosphatidyl ethanolamines are called as liposomes. The most popular method of production of liposomes is the solubilization of the phospholipids in an organic solvent, with agitation followed by evaporation with a rotary evaporator (Düzgünes and Gregoriadis 2005). The film is then rehydrated with an aqueous solution to acquire vesicles. Multilamellar (MLV) or unilamellar vesicles (ULV) can be obtained depending on the entry of the formulation through extrusion equipment and the colloidal association of amphipathic lipids (Severino et al. 2012). Liposomes can be used for the loading of

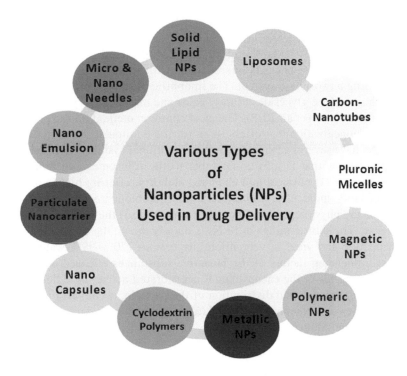

FIGURE 17.1 Different types of nanocarriers.

both hydrophilic and lipophilic active pharmaceutical ingredients (APIs). The hydrophilic moieties are trapped in the inner core of the liposomes, whereas the lipophilic ones are positioned within the acyl chains of the fatty acids that are linked to the glycerol component of the phospholipids. The use of liposomes provide various benefits, for instance, the capacity to incorporate both hydrophilic and lipophilic APIs by virtue of their biocompatibility, biodegradability, and non-immunogenic nature. Their greatest limitation is the small residual time in blood following injection, because they are exclusively removed from the circulatory system by monocytes and macrophages present in the liver, lungs, spleen, and bone marrow creating a prompt localization of these cells in the reticulo-endothelial system (Barenholz et al. 2001). Moreover, the excessive cost of the raw materials is not appealing from a business prospective.

17.3.2.2 Solid Lipid Nanoparticle

Solid lipid nanoparticles (SLNs) have been produced as a contrasting option to encapsulate drugs as compared to the traditional systems for example emulsions, liposomes, and polymeric nanoparticles. The benefits of using SLNs is their physicochemical stability, that provides better protection of drugs, including thermolability and susceptibility to chemical or physical degradation, such as proteins. Besides, SLNs offer sustained release and transport of drugs to preferred sites and targeted tissues, hence making it more therapeutically effective (Souto et al. 2013). The most important feature of these systems is the utilization of physiological solid lipids that can fuse numerous lipophilic drugs inside its lipid layers or potentially between the chains of unsaturated fats or even in already initiated flaws in the physical structure after the solidification of lipids. This lipids could be glycerides, ceramides, waxes, or fatty acids (Souto et al. 2013; Souto et al. 2011). By combining various lipids and fatty acids, the release patterns of these drugs can be made to suit specific needs. Moreover, SLN dispersions are cost effective, free of organic solvents, and are made up of raw materials which have been labeled as safe by the FDA. The most important feature of SLN dispersions is the capability to dissolve the drug in molecular form through the lipid matrix, which provides greater protection of the molecule and offers a sustained release profile with high API loading. Furthermore, owing to the nanometer size, the ratio of surface to area can be increased for the purpose of therapeutic targeting of tissues and also increasing its effectiveness (Mueller et al. 2000; Muller et al. 2002). These lipid systems resemble emulsions; but the oil phase is interchanged with solid lipids, and surfactants act as a stabilizer, constituting a two-phase system. The lipophilic drug is mostly spread in the lipid layers between the chains of the glycerides of fatty acids and also in the crystal imperfections after the lipids recrystallize (Souto et al. 2013). The most common method for the production of SLNs is high-pressure homogenization that offers room for the manipulation of the SLNs to produce various sizes. SLNs have several advantages over conventional systems based on route of administration and applications that is also comparable to the liposomes and nanoemulsions. The chief advantages include (1) physical and chemical stability, offering higher protection against the degradation of labile molecules, (2) biotolerability and biodegradability accompanying low toxicity because of the physiological lipid composition, and (3) the lipid matrix responsible for a controlled release. The shortcomings of SLNs is mainly due to the expulsion of the drug after polymorphic transition and yield in very dilute dispersions (70%–99% water) (Wissing et al. 2004). The most influencing factors of the bioactive substances released by SLNs are: (1) the physicochemical properties of the encapsulated/incorporated active ingredient, (2) its dispersal in the lipid matrix, (3) the size and distribution of the particle, (4) the arrangement of the lipid matrix, (5) the varieties of surfactants used, and (6) the procedure and parameters utilized in the fabrication (Mehnert and Mader 2001).

17.3.2.3 Polymeric Nanoparticles

Polymeric nanoparticles act as transporter within the submicron size (lower than 1 µm) and are made up of natural or synthetic polymers (Souto et al. 2012). Polymeric nanoparticles can entrap, disperse, and dissolve within the matrix or absorb APIs onto the surface of NPs thus making them a standout amongst the most utilized systems nowadays. Polymeric nanoparticles are made up of biodegradable or non-biodegradable polymers. Biodegradable polymers have a few advantages over non-biodegradable, as biodegradable polymers are not needed to be surgically removed after the end of their activity (Sionkowska et al. 2011). Some examples of synthetic polymers that are non-biodegradable in nature are polystyrene and polyacrylamide, while those of biodegradable nature include polyalkylcyanoacrylates and aliphatic polyesters. Natural polymers as rules of thumb are biocompatible and biodegradable; but, they are less predictable in their composition and can sometimes be mildly immunogenic. Examples are chitin, chitosan, alginate, hyaluronic acid, pullulan, gliadin, collagen, keratin, silk, and elastin. The decision of which material to use must agree with the physicochemical characteristics, such as viscosity, hygroscopicity, biocompatibility, and ability to release the solvent completely of the different materials utilized during the encapsulation process. The advantage of using these particles is the opportunity to chemically modify the structure of the polymer as well as the synthesis of copolymers. This alteration helps to decrease the toxicity of the polymers and can project the particles to specific points (Kumari et al. 2010). Additionally, the improved polymer stability and durability may extend their storage at room temperature and lengthen the shelf life of the APIs.

17.3.2.4 Microneedles and Nanoneedles

Microneedles and nanoneedles (MNs) are devices that cross easily through the SC painlessly. These least invasive devices are micron-scale needles gathered on one side of a supporting base or patches (Tuan-Mahmood et al. 2013). The treatments that utilize this innovation provide transcutaneous delivery, supporting a dependable and promising drug delivery system for high and low molecular wt molecules. They are useful for the delivery of hydrophilic APIs, and skin irritations are negligible when compared to absorption promoters of general transdermal formulations (Donnelly et al. 2009). The chief resources used to manufacture MNs are silicon, metals, polymers, glass, and ceramics. The "dissolving MNs" are formed using biodegradable polymers. They are more affordable than silicon ones and are safer in nature, as they are biocompatible and completely dissolved in the skin. Polymer MNs are easily produced and show excellent hydrophilic molecule release (Hong et al. 2014). Once the polymer is dissolved, the release of the molecule is very efficient from the API-loaded polymeric matrix of these systems. The advantages of these types of drug delivery systems include (i) delivery of macromolecules, (ii) safe and easy application (iii) can be used for potent drugs, (iv) biocompatibility and ability to hold a large amount of drug. Even though there are many advantages of such delivery systems it also presents us with some limitations such as (i) flow resistance, (ii) specialized and expensive techniques, (iii) poor mechanical strength.

17.3.2.5 Nanoemulsion

Nanoemulsions are a biphasic dosage form consisting of an aqueous continuous phase in which nanoranged size oil droplets are enclosed with surfactant molecules (Acosta 2009; McClements et al. 2009; McClements et al. 2007).

17.3.2.6 Particulate Nanocarriers

Particulate nanocarriers such as nanocapsules, polymeric nanoparticles, solid lipid nanoparticles, inorganic nanoparticles, polymeric conjugates, carbon nanotubes, and dendrimers have been extensively studied.

17.3.2.7 Nanocapsules

Nanocapsules consist of a liquid core generally an oil surrounded by surfactants or polymers. Generally, lipids like vegetable oils and triglycerides with medium- and long-chain fatty acids are commonly used for the lipid cores. The drugs are confined to the lipid core, which serves as a reservoir to allow a high drug loading for hydrophobic drugs and a slow release profile. Thus, nanocapsules are pharmaceutically attractive for water-insoluble drugs.

17.3.2.8 Dendrimers

Dendrimers are one type of multibranched polymer which consists of a central core, branches of repeating units, and an outer layer of multivalent functional groups. These functional groups can electrostatically interact with charged polar molecules, whereas the hydrophobic inner cavities can encapsulate uncharged, non-polar molecules through a number of interactions.

This complex structure consists of different functional groups which can allow for controlled delivery of the drug. This structure can be modified to control the release of drug in a certain pH or when encountered by specific enzymes; targeting molecules, such as the RGD peptide or mAbs are also used.

17.3.2.9 Cyclodextrin Polymers

Cyclodextrin polymers with a transferrin targeting moiety delivery system is frequently used in the treatment of MDR cancer (Davis and Brewster 2009). Cyclodextrin polycation is a one of the components of this system used for nucleic acid condensation and the other component is a transferrin linked PEG adamantane to stabilize the particle and to target the cell surface receptors (Davis and Brewster 2009).

17.3.2.10 Metallic and Magnetic Nanoparticles

Gold nanoparticles (Au-NPs) are extensively used for biomedical imaging and biosensing. Likewise, anti-HER2 was attached to nanoparticle surfaces to improve the cellular internalization of gelatin/albumin and gold nanoparticles (Van Vlerken and Amiji 2006).

Due to the photo-physical property of gold nanoparticle they can conjugate with other materials easily through ionic and co-valent bonds. They are considered as non-toxic and the therapeutic constituents can be released in a controlled manner. Various drugs with small particles like DNA, RNA can also be delivered by attaching to the gold particles. The anticancer agents can be formulated as Au-NPs by physical adsorption, ionic bonding, and/or covalent bonding (Chen 2007; Podsiadlo 2008).

17.3.2.11 Super Paramagnetic Nanoparticles

Iron oxide (Fe_3O_4) nanoparticles are a newer approach to treating the cancer. The drug can be delivered into targeted sites by local hyperthermia or by applying oscillation strategies. Magnetic fields can also be used to guide the drug to the intended target area within the body.

17.3.2.12 Carbon-Based Nanoparticles/Carbon Nanotubes

Carbon nanotubes having needle-like structures can penetrate through the tumor cell very easily and can deliver drug molecules into the intended site. Because of their special structure they have a large surface area which leads to high entrapment of drug molecules and large number of attachment sites. These carbon nanotubes also have electrical and thermal conductivity, which may prove to be useful in future cancer therapy applications such as thermal ablations.

Recently carbon nanotubes have been used to integrate various anti-neoplastic agents such as doxorubicin and paclitaxel, nucleic acids including anti-sense oligonucleotides, and SiRNAs (Fabbro 2012).

17.3.2.13 Pluronic Micelles

Micelles are the most basic colloidal drug delivery systems and are formed spontaneously in nature. In the body, colloidal micellar species comprising endogenous surfactants and lipid digestion products (i.e., bile salt mixtures) facilitate the absorption of highly insoluble fatty acids and fat soluble vitamins. Micelles have a particle size normally within a 5–100 nm range, and are thermodynamically stable and form spontaneously by the association of amphiphilic molecules, such as surfactants, under defined concentrations and temperatures.

17.4 POLYSACCHARIDES AS DRUG DELIVERY SYSTEMS

Polysaccharides include a varied class of polymeric materials of natural (animal, plant, algal) origin formed via glycosidic linkages of monosaccharides (Shukla and Tiwari 2012). Depending on the nature of the monosaccharide unit, polysaccharides either have a linear or a branched style. Other than having astructural diversity, polysaccharides have hydroxyl, amino, and carboxylic acid groups, indicating the opportunities for alteration through chemical modifications (Liu et al. 2008). Moreover, the molecular weight of polysaccharide varies between hundreds to thousands of Daltons adding more diversity to such molecules (Saravanakumar et al. 2012).

17.4.1 Advantages of Polysaccharide-Based Drug Delivery Systems

The various advantages of using such molecules as drug delivery systems are discussed below.

17.4.1.1 Biodegradability and Biocompatibility

Polysaccharides have very low toxicity levels in contrast to the many different kind of synthetic polymers used nowadays (Dang and Leong 2006). Dextrans are biopolymers that are composed of glucose α-1,6 linkages, with possible branching from α-1,2, α-1,3, to α-1,4 linkages, that exhibit low toxicity and high biocompatibility. Thus, dextran forms the basis of biocompatible hydrogels for controlled release deliveries (Coviello et al. 2007). Dextrans have exhibited extensive biocompatibility when they are formulated into microspheres, as suggested by absence of an inflammatory response following subcutaneous injection in animals (Cadee et al. 2001). Most polysaccharides are subjected to enzymatic degradation due to their natural presence in the body. Polysaccharides are broken to their monomer or oligomer units by enzyme catalysis and are further used for storage, structural support, and cell signaling applications (Jain et al. 2007). Glycosidases can catalyze the hydrolysis of many different glycosidic linkages (Jain et al. 2007). Hyaluronidase, for example, degrades the polysaccharide hyaluronic acid (HA) by cleaving β-1,4 linkages between D-glucuronic acid and D-N-acetyl glucosamine (Jain et al. 2007). Some polysaccharides are particularly susceptible to degradation by lysosomal enzymes, including glycosidases, esterases, and proteases, following endocytosis (Mehvar 2003). Thus, enzymatic degradation for polysaccharide-based carrier systems provides a mechanism of release for drugs in such systems (Mehvar 2003).

17.4.1.2 Solubility

The functional groups associated with polysaccharide backbones, namely hydroxyl and amine groups, yield high solubility in aqueous solutions. This solubility however, can be adjusted by monomer modification. Chitosan, made up of β-1,4 linked N-acetyl-D-glucosamine and D-glucosamine, is prepared by deacetylation of chitin molecules. Varying the degree of deacetylation the solubility of chitosan in acidic conditions can be altered. An increased number of protonated free amino groups is associated with higher degrees of deacetylation consequently, enhances solubility (Morris et al. 2010). Similarly, glucomannan, a polysaccharide formed via O-acetylation of β-1,4 linkage of D-mannose and D-glucose, can modulate the formation of intermolecular hydrogen bonds with water, thus altering solubility (Alonso et al. 2009).

17.4.1.3 Ease of Modification

Polysaccharides are easily subjected to modification. Polysaccharides, such as amylose, amylopectin, glycogen, and cellulose, offer a large number of free reactive hydroxyl groups that is easily modifiable (Jian et al. 2012). Polysaccharides possessing both hydroxyl and carboxylic acid groups are easily modified. For example, alginate, a polysaccharide composed of β-D-mannuronic acid and α-L-guluronic acid with 1,4 linkages, can be modified to produce a variety of different physiological behaviors. The hydroxyl group upon oxidation can increase biodegradability, while sulfonation causes a heparin-like polysaccharide that increases blood compatibility (Kumar et al. 2004). The alteration of chitosan has also been studied and it was noted that quaternization of the primary amines with various alkyl groups can be used to increase solubility and vary bioactivity of chitosan (Mourya and Inamdar 2009).

17.4.1.4 Bioactivity

Many polysaccharides show a variety of native bioactivity, like anti-microbial, anti-inflammatory and mucoadhesive properties. Mucoadhesion is the interaction of a material with a mucosal layer, such as the nasal pathway or airway and gastrointestinal (GI) tract. Chitosan, a positively charged polysaccharide can bind with the negatively charged mucosal layers via charge interactions (Bernkop and Dunnhaupt 2012). Thus, the use of chitosan for oral drug delivery has been extensively studied. For negatively charged polysaccharides like hyaluronic acid, hydrogen bonding provides a way for mucoadhesion (Reddy et al. 2011). Chitosan exerts an anti-microbial nature owing to a strong interaction of the protonated amines with the negatively charged bacterial cell wall (Dai et al. 2011). A well-known polysaccharide for reducing inflammation is heparin, composed of repeating disaccharides of β-Dglucopyranosiduronic acid or α-L-idopyranosiduronic acid linked to N-acetyl or N-sulfo-D-glucosamine, having a strong negative charge that can interact with a variety of proteins. Thus, the activity is believed to be due to binding with some immune-related complement proteins (Young et al. 2008). Heparin can also bind to the lysine-rich region of anti-thrombin thus assisting the catalysis blood clotting inhibitory proteins (Olson et al. 1981). There are various kinds of polysaccharides have been used in drug delivery system, some of them are mentioned below as they are used frequently in Table 17.1.

TABLE 17.1

List of Polysaccharide Frequently Used as Drug Delivery Systems

Name	Structure Composition	Properties	Advantages
Alginate	Anionic copolymer based on chemical structure with a backbone of (1→4) linked β-D-mannuronic acid (M units) and α-L-guluronic acid	1. molecular weight can be varied, based on the enzymatic control during the course its production and on the degree of depolymerization caused during its extraction. 2. the structure can be stabilized in a rigid gel form because it has a high content of guluronic acid that can form crosslinks. 3. contain many free hydroxyl and carboxyl groups along the backbone of the compound that are highly reactive which can modify the properties of the polymer like solubility, hydrophobicity, physicochemical, and biological characteristics.	1. a characteristic polymer well-suited with a wide assortment of substances, which does not require various and complex drug encapsulation process. 2. since it is mucoadhesive and biodegradable and, subsequently, it can be utilized in the preparation of controlled drug delivery frameworks accomplishing an upgraded and superior bioavailability. 3. it is abundant in nature, low in price and produces very low toxicity. 4. it has likewise been widely considered in nanomedicine, as a drug delivery device on the grounds that the rate of drug release can be adjusted by differing the drug polymer interaction in addition to chemical immobilization of the drug in the polymer backbone utilizing the responsive carboxylate groups.
Chitosan	A linear polysaccharide composed of units of glucosamine and N-acetylglucosamine linked by (1→4) β-glycosidic bonds	1. linear polyamine composed of reactive amino and hydroxyl groups. 2. it can chelate with many transitional metals. 3. it is capable of bonding with mammalian and microbial cells antagonistically. 4. assists the development of osteoblast that is used for bone formation. 5. also acts as a homeostatic, fungistatic, spermicidal, antitumor, CNS depressant, and immunoadjuvant	1. its polyelectrolyte nature is used for the absorption of heavy metal ions. 2. can be used as biomaterials in wound healing or as prosthetic materials as it is easily biodegrade in the system by enzymes. 3. chitosan can be useful in delivery systems intended to lengthen the residual time of the drugs at the site of absorption because of its bioadhesive properties. 4. chitosan has a polycationic character, reactive functionalities and is easily degraded by enzymes to produce non-toxic degradation products making it a suitable matrix for controlled release nanoparticles.

(Continued)

TABLE 17.1 (CONTINUED)
List of Polysaccharide Frequently Used as Drug Delivery Systems

Name	Structure Composition	Properties	Advantages
Hyaluronic acid	This polysaccharide Structure is composed of iterating disaccharide units of D-glucuronic acid and N-acetyl D-glucosamine joined by β (1–3) and β (1–4) glycosidic bonds	1. this polysaccharide has shown positive effects in several cellular mechanisms like angiogenesis and regulation of inflammation. In general, this polymer is biodegradable, bioactive, non-immunogenic, non-cytotoxic and negatively charged.	1. this polysaccharide has been used for surface modification of various biomaterials used in prosthetic cartilage, vascular graft, guided nerve regeneration and drug delivery. 2. it is a very efficient drug delivery carrier because of its polyanionic characteristics. This allows for minimal non-specific interaction between the polymer and serum components. 3. liver tissues with Hyaluronic acid receptors can be targeted very specifically with this polymer.
Dextran	The structure contains a large number of α(1→6) glycosidic linkages in its main chain, and an adjustable amount of α-(1→2), α-(1→3) and α-(1→4) linkages in the branched chain	1. this is a neutral, water soluble, biocompatible and biodegradable. 2. the features of this polymer can be varied depending upon the molecular mass, type and degree of branching. The type and degree of branching depends on the bacterial synthesis or post synthesis reactions of the polymer.	1. it can be used as plasma volume expander, adjuvant, emulsifier, carrier, stabilizer and thickening agent. 2. it can be used as carriers of nanoparticular systems and also to cover these systems. 3. this polymer comes very handy in the formulation of nanoparticles of drugs due to its superior availability, biocompatibility and biodegradability.
Pullulan	This polysaccharide is composed of glycosidic linkages between α-(1→6) D-glucopyranose and α-(1→4) D-glucopyranose units in a 1:2 ratio	1. the backbone of this polymer behaves as a random expanded flexible coil in aqueous solution, suggesting that this flexibility may be due to the α-(1→6) linkage. 2. new physico–chemical properties, like increasing its solubility in organic solvents or introducing reactive groups can be imparted to this by chemically derivatizing it.	1. the polymer can be used in drug and gene delivery, tissue engineering and wound healing because it is hemocompatible, non-immunogenic, non-carcinogenic in nature. 2. chemical derivatization of the polymer backbone leads to a polymeric system capable of forming hydrogels and nanogels. 3. hydrophobic molecules can modify the backbone of the polymer to obtain hydrophobized molecules of pullulan which can self-assemble in water solutions to obtain nanostructures acting as drug carriers.

(Continued)

TABLE 17.1 (CONTINUED)
List of Polysaccharide Frequently Used as Drug Delivery Systems

Name	Structure Composition	Properties	Advantages
Guar gum	The backbone of this polymer contains linear chains of $(1\rightarrow4)$-β-D-mannopyranosyl units with α-D-galactopyranosyl units attached by $(1\rightarrow6)$ linkages creating short side-branches	1. can hydrate in cold water to form a viscous solution containing nine hydroxyl groups that are capable of forming hydrogen bonds with other molecules, it can still maintain a neutral charge owing to the absence of dissociable functional groups. 2. viscosity of the polymer is reduced in the presence of strong acids and alkalis due to the hydrolysis of the hydroxyl groups. 3. It is sparsely soluble in most hydrocarbon solvents.	1. it is commonly used as a thickening agent due to its ability to produce highly viscous aqueous solutions. 2. it is susceptibility to microbial degradation in the large intestine and has a drug release retarding property making it a suitable candidate for colon targeted drug delivery. 3. a crosslinked product obtained via a spacer arm between the polymer chains produces an insoluble compound with a wide range of pH and good mechanical stability that can be used in cell culture, tissue engineering and as drug carriers. 4. guar gum can stabilize nanosuspensions during their synthesis process.
Pectin	This polymer contains a heterogeneous chemical structure founded on large amounts of poly (D-galacturonic acid) bonded via α-$(1\rightarrow4)$ glycosidic linkage	1. pectin is degraded by pectinases, which are secreted by the bacterial inhabitants of the human colon, but it remains intact in the stomach and small intestine. 2. the gelling activity of pectin is determined by the type and concentration of pectin, modification of hydroxyl groups, pH, temperature and the presence of cations.	1. calcium pectinate, which is sparsely soluble in water and are stable at low pH, can act as a drug carrier for colon-specific delivery in different formulations 2. pectin, containing amide groups and crosslinked with calcium has decreased biodegradability and can tolerate pH variations and fluctuations in calcium, can also be used for colonic delivery. 3. the degree of swelling and change mechanical properties like stability of the drug and controlling the drug release can be modified by combining pectin with another polymer.

17.4.2 Nanoparticle Preparation from Polysaccharides

17.4.2.1 Covalent Crosslinking

The polymeric chains in crosslinked NPs are interconnected by crosslinkers, leading to the formation of a 3D network (Berger et al. 2004). Factors that determines the properties of a crosslinked NP are drug release and mechanical strength, and crosslinking density that is determined by the molar ratio between the crosslinker and the polymer. The nature of the crosslinking agents determines the kinds of crosslinked NPs, namely covalently crosslinked NPs and ionically crosslinked NPs. In a covalently crosslinked NP a permanent network structure is obtained since irreversible chemical links are formed unless biodegradable or stimuli-responsive crosslinkers are employed. In ionically crosslinked NPs reversible ionic crosslinking can be obtained since no harsh preparation or toxic crosslinkers are used these NPs are generally considered biocompatible (Berger et al. 2004).

17.4.2.2 Polyelectrolyte Structures

Polyelectrolyte complexes (PEC) are formed by direct electrostatic interactions of oppositely charged polyelectrolytes in solution. PEC offers another biocompatible option for drug delivery since it makes used of non-toxic covalent crosslinkers.

17.4.2.3 Layer-By-Layer Assembly

Layer-by-layer (LbL) assembly of polyelectrolyte NPs is a new form of polyelectrolyte-based nano-sized delivery system. This technique is based on electrostatic interactions and employs alternate adsorption of oppositely charged polyelectrolytes (Ai et al. 2003).

17.4.2.4 Self-Assembly

When hydrophobic moieties are attached onto a hydrophilic polysaccharide it leads to the formation amphiphilic copolymer. In aqueous media the amphiphilic copolymers self-assemble into NPs comprising of a hydrophobic inner core and hydrophilic shell. The hydrophilic shell functions as the stabilizing interface between the hydrophobic core and the external aqueous phase (Allen et al 1999). This self-assembly process is governed by hydrophobic interactions to reduce interfacial free energy (Liu et al. 2008; Park et al. 2010).

17.4.2.5 Polysaccharide-Drug Conjugates

The polymer-drug conjugates modify the biodistribution and circulation time of free drugs, which, post conjugation are capable of being selectively delivered and accumulating at the tumor site due to the enhanced permeability and retention effect.

17.4.3 Polysaccharide-Based Nanocarriers As Drug Delivery Systems

Nanocarriers have been extensively studied and their application in the treatment of complex diseases has changed the face of the pharma industry. Approval of abraxane (ABI-007) and analbumin-taxol nanoparticles by The Food and Drug Administration for the treatment of cancer has opened several avenues for the development of nanoparticulate drug delivery aiming toward concentrating more drug inside the target tissue and less in healthy ones (Perez 2005). The attraction of these nanoparticles for use in medical purposes is centered on their unique features, such as large surface to mass ratio, quantum properties, and ability to absorb and carry other compounds.

Nanoparticle drug carriers have the following advantages (Jung et al. 2000):

1. They can pass through small capillaries due to their tiny volume and can avoid clearance by phagocytes so that they can remain for a longer time in the blood stream;
2. They can easily infiltrate cells and tissue gap to reach their target organs;

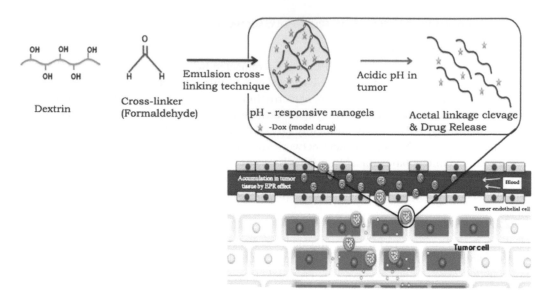

FIGURE 17.2 Schematic concept of the preparation of dextrin nanogels and their pH-responsive drug release. (Reprinted from *Carbohydr Polym* 126, Manchun, S., Dass, C.R., Cheewatanakornkool, K., and Sriamornsak, P. Enhanced antitumor effect of pH-responsive dextrin nanogels delivering doxorubicin on colorectal cancer, 222–30, Copyright 2015, With permission from Elsevier.)

3. They can exhibit controlled-release properties depending on biodegradability, pH, ion and/ or temperature sensibility of materials;
4. They can improve the efficacy of drugs and reduce toxicity and other side effects; etc.

Polysaccharide-based nanoparticles are receiving significant attention as they are considered one of the most favorable nanoparticular delivery systems because of their innate unique potentials. Nanocarriers like micelles and polymeric nanoparticles have given us an exclusive method of obtaining desired pharmaceutical and pharmacokinetic properties for various drugs. A variety of methods can be applied to prepare polymeric nanoparticles depending on the nature of the polymer and the drug to be encapsulated (Bawarski et al. 2008). Some of the methods may not be applicable to biopharmaceuticals owing to the use of heat, vigorous excitation, sonication, or organic solvents. Nanoparticles can also be formed by electrostatic interactions preventing the use of aggressive conditions, thus reducing the chances of degradation of the drugs during the development of such particles (Kumari et al. 2010). A variety of natural and synthetic polymers are available to form nanoparticles (Hillaireau and Couvreur 2009). Some natural polymers used for oral delivery of nanoparticles are chitosan, dextran, gelatin, alginate, and agar (Prego et al. 2006). The synthetic polymers used for oral drug delivery are poly(lactide) acid (PLA), poly(glycolide) acid (PGA), poly(lactide- co-glycolide) PLGA, poly(cyanoacrylates) (PCA), polyethylenimine (PEI), or polycaprolactone (PCL) (Jong et al. 2008).

Conventional therapies can be improved by encapsulating drugs into nanocarriers which confer prolonged circulation time and enhanced accumulation in targeted tissues via enhanced permeability and retention. Preparation of pH-responsive nanocarriers is a promising strategy because pH-responsiveness is independent of cellular chemical substances and does not require the exact location of drug delivery for triggering release compared to other stimuli-responsive systems mentioned in Figure 17.2 (Zhang et al. 2017).

17.5 DRUG DELIVERY CHALLENGES

Various biological barriers are found in every level from body to organism and tissue to cells up to a sub-cellular or molecular level. Due to these reasons successful drug delivery has become challenging. The main problem with anti-obesity drug delivery is the localization of the drug molecule into the intended site. Maximal drug response of a compound can only be possible if the compound will concentrate on the target site otherwise it can damage the other healthy cells resulting in toxicity and adverse drug reactions. So, the main aim to treat adipose cells is a targeted drug delivery system. Although this appears to be a simple goal achieving this result can be an expensive and time consuming process, without guaranteed success.

17.5.1 Strategies in General For Overcoming Obesity Treatment Using Nanotechnology

The research community is of the opinion that targeted nanomedical approaches could facilitate the development of more effective management strategies for the treatment of metabolic diseases like obesity and diabetes. The research is now focused on screening other drug candidates to test their therapeutics on higher animals.

17.6 NANOPARTICLES AND POLYSACCHARIDE-BASED NANOCARRIERS AS A TARGETED DELIVERY SYSTEM FOR ANTI-OBESITY DRUGS

Continuous research in the field of drug delivery techniques has provided solutions to address the limited efficacy and high toxicity of many drugs. Nanosized drug carriers are accepted because their size allows for selective accumulation at the targeted site. Polysaccharides being non-toxic and biodegradable natural polymers, can serve as the basis for these nanosized carriers. Polysialic acid (PSA) is a highly hydrophilic polysaccharide that may decrease uptake by the reticuloendothelial system and prolong the duration of action of the drug.

A study has shown that angiogenesis, i.e. promoting the growth of new blood vessels, can help convert adipose tissue and lead to weight loss in mice. Natural resources like chitosan (CTS), water-soluble chitosan (WSC), microparticles (MPs), and nanoparticles (NPs) reduces weight and retains safety standards in high-fat diet animal models and thus has shown that it is very significant for weight management in humans (Zhang et al. 2012).

Both in vitro and in vivo studies with nanoparticle (nanoceria) have tried to interfere with the adipogenic pathway by reducing the mRNA transcription of genes involved in adipogenesis (formation of adipocyte), and by turning down the triglyceride accumulation in 3T3-L1 pre-adipocytes. Nanoceria in Wistar rats did not have the standard toxic effects, but effectively worked on trimming the weight increase and also bringing down the plasma levels of insulin, leptin, glucose, and triglycerides (Rocca et al. 2015). Human adipose tissue is highly vascularized and possesses anti-angiogenic properties. A pro-apoptotic peptide ligand bound with a significant nanoparticle/nanocarrier which, when administered to obese adipose tissue, causes depletion of endothelial cells increasing cell apoptosis (Hossen et al. 2013).

Nanoparticles have proven to be effective in the treatment of particular locations of the body through a targeted delivery system. They work efficiently enhancing half-life of drug molecules, by regulating particle size, altering surface character, enhancing permeation, flexibility, etc., and thereby modifying the release of therapeutically active agents in order to deliver target-specific activity at a controlled rate (Shi et al. 2010).

Nano drug molecules bind to proteins found in the lining of the blood vessels that surround adipose tissue or bind to receptors on the outer surface of the adipose tissue and burn it. Studies have revealed that promoting angiogenesis, can aid transformation of adipose tissue thereby leading to weight loss in mice. However, drugs that promote angiogenesis can exhibit detrimental effect on the rest of the body and further investigation is required to target fat cells with minimal side effects (Rocca et al. 2014). A study in a diet-induced mouse model showed that a programmed death of endothelial cells by anti-angiogenic drugs (TNP-470) removes vascular tissues and effectively reduces weight in animals (Rupnick et al. 2002).

In obesity, expansion of adipose tissue and its transformation depends on the active growth of new blood vessels; hence, angiogenesis presents a prospective target for the treatment of obesity associated morbidity. Yuan Xue (2016) formulated two peptide-functionalized nanoparticle (NP) platforms in order to deliver either a peroxisome proliferator-activated receptor gamma (PPAR gamma) activator rosiglitazone or prostaglandin E2 analog (16,16-dimethyl PGE2) to adipose tissue vasculature. These NPs were engineered through the self-assembly of a biodegradable triblock polymer made up of end-to-end linkages between poly(lactic-coglycolic acid)-b-poly(ethylene glycol) (PLGA-b-PEG) and an endothelial-targeted peptide. In this design, released rosiglitazone promotes the transformation of white adipose tissue (WAT) into brown-like adipose tissue. In addition it also augments angiogenesis, which in turn facilitates the housing of targeted NPs into adipose angiogenic vessels, thereby amplifying their delivery (see Figure 17.3).

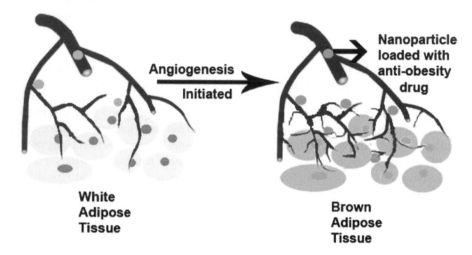

FIGURE 17.3   Nanoparticles in angiogenesis for the treatment of obesity.

In a study, the effect of chitosan (CTS) and water-soluble chitosan (WSC) microparticles (MPs) and nanoparticles (NPs) were evaluated in rats with high-fat diet-induced obesity. CTS and WSC MPs and NPs exhibited significant reduction in the final amounts of epididymal and perirenal white adipose tissue. Decrease in liver weight was observed in the CTS-MP group compared to rats fed with high-fat diet. The WSC-MP and CTS-MP groups showed a maximal reduction in serum total cholesterol and low-density lipoprotein cholesterol amongst the other treatment groups where the reduction was also significant. Significant reduction in triacylglycerol levels were observed in the WSC-NP group compared to the high-fat group. These results imply that CTS and WSC MPs and NPs have superior effects than commercially available CTS and WSC, and may be used as potential anti-obesity agents (Zhang et al. 2012).

In the year 2017, Chunhui Jiang and his team undertook a new approach to convert white adipocytes into beige adipocytes (browning) (Jiang et al. 2017). They established an alternative approach to stimulate browning using nanoparticles (NPs) consisting of FDA-approved poly(lactide-co-glycolide) that allows for sustained local release of a notch inhibitor (dibenzazepine, DBZ). These DBZ-loaded NPs facilitate rapid cellular internalization and obstruct notch signaling in adipocytes.

In another work, orlistat-loaded nanoparticles were prepared to overcome the drawbacks of the raw drug. The study design was intended to formulate orlistat in an alternative way compared to the existing practice and examine its efficacy in the inhibition of gastrointestinal lipases. The benefit of the selected technical procedures is nanosized orlistat with increased in vitro dissolution rate in contrast to raw drug, physical mixture, and marketed products. Moreover, nanosuspension exhibited appreciably higher in vitro lipase inhibition in comparison to the aforesaid products (Dolenc et al. 2010).

Liang and team in 2016 investigated the targeting of adipose tissue macrophages in obesity with polysaccharide nanocarriers. They found that polysaccharide-based biocompatible glucose polymers can effectively concentrate on adipose macrophages in obese mice wherein it was observed that following regional peritoneal administration, larger dextran conjugates efficiently distributed to visceral adipose tissue and selectively associated with macrophages. This observation presents strong evidence that critical factors leading to obesity comorbidities can be inhibited effectively by nanomaterial-based delivery strategies and provide us with a unique transport mechanism for drug delivery to visceral tissues (Liang et al. 2016).

It can be promising in future to control obesity by using nanotechnology for targeted vascular therapy as an anti-angiogenic agent given in Figure 17.3. Based on the passive drug delivery approach numerous nanotechnology formulations have been approved by the FDA in the US.

17.7 CONCLUSION

Nanotechnology-based drug delivery into obese adipose tissue will enhance opportunity in the pharmaceutical industry. The extensive study of targeted drug therapy will provide new breaks in the pharmacotherapy of weight management. Nanotherapy can be a door to new anti-obesity formulations with systematic and advanced administration. It can revolutionize clinical trials and understanding of vascular targeted drug delivery for obesity control.

A cumulative approach for treatment of obesity using strategies with polysaccharide-based nanocarriers loaded with anti-obesity drugs is most important for its success. Due to some important characteristic polysaccharides are a good choice for drug delivery systems. Polysaccharides are easily subjected to modification. Polysaccharides, such as amylose, amylopectin, glycogen, and cellulose, offer a large number of free reactive hydroxyl groups that are easily modifiable.

The functional groups associated with polysaccharide backbones, namely hydroxyl and amine groups, yield high solubility in aqueous solutions. Also polysaccharides have very low toxicity levels in contrast to the many different kind of synthetic polymers used nowadays.

It is highly important to look for new targets. Knowing the recently developed targets help to study the origin of obesity to treat the complications. Due to their size, nanomaterials and nanocarriers are similar to cellular organelles such as mitochondria, lipoproteins and also surface receptors, siRNA, micro RNA, genes, and unknown proteins. Thus, nanocarriers can easily interfere with different biomolecules. The flexibility of platforms or carrier developed with the help of nanotechnology has paved a fortunate and rapid invasion of these molecules into the adipose tissue.

REFERENCES

Acosta, E. 2009. Bioavailability of nanoparticles in nutrient and nutraceutical delivery. *Curr Opin Colloid Interface Sci* 14(1):3–15.

Ai, H., Jones, S.A., and Lvov, Y.M. 2003. Biomedical applications of electrostatic layer-by-layer nano-assembly of polymers, enzymes, and nanoparticles. *Cell Biochem Biophys* 39: 23–43.

Allen, C., Maysinger, D., and Eisenberg, A. 1999. Nano-engineering block copolymer aggregates for drug delivery. *Colloids Surf B* 16: 3–27.

Alonso-Sande, M., Teijeiro-Osorio, D., Remuñán-López, C., and Alonso, M.J. 2009. Glucomannan, a promising polysaccharide for biopharmaceutical purposes. *Eur J Pharm Biopharm* 72: 453–62.

Barenholz, Y. 2001. Liposome application: Problems and prospects. *Curr Opin Colloid Interface Sci* 6: 66–77.

Bawarski, W.E., Chidlowsky, E., Bharali, D.J., and Mousa, S.A. 2008. Emerging nanopharmaceuticals. *Nanomedicine: Nanotechnology, Biology and Medicine* 4: 273–82.

Berger, J., Reist, M., Mayer, J.M., Felt, O., Peppas, N.A., and Gurny, R. 2004. Structure and interactions in covalently and ionically crosslinked chitosan hydrogels for biomedical applications. *Eur J Pharm Biopharm* 57: 19–34.

Bernkop-Schnurch, A. and Dunnhaupt, S. 2012. Chitosan based drug delivery systems. *Eur J Pharm Biopharm* 81 (3): 463–9.

Bleich, S., Cutler, D., Murray, C., and Adams, A. 2008. Why is the developed world obese? *Annu Rev Public Health (Research Support)* 29: 273–95.

Boulpaep, Emile L. and Boron, Walter F. 2003. *Medical Physiology: A Cellular and Molecular Approach.* Philadelphia: Saunders.

Brian, S., Charles, A., Gilson III., Jeffrey, S., and Jeffrey, S., US patent 7704993 Benzazepine derivatives and methods of prophylaxis or treatment of 5HT2c receptor associated diseases, published 2004-16-06, issued 2010-27-04.

Cadee, J.A., Brouwer, L.A., den Otter, W., Hennick, W.E., and van Luyn, M.J.A. 2001. A comparative bio-compatibility study of microspheres based on crosslinked dextran or poly(lactic-co-glycolic)acid after subcutaneous injection in rats. *J Biomed Mater Res B* 56: 600–9.

Colquitt, J.L., Pickett, K., Loveman, E., and Frampton, G.K. 2014. Surgery for weight loss in adults. *Cochrane Database Syst Rev* 8: CD003641.

Chen Y.H., Tsai C.Y., Huang P.Y. et al. 2017. Methotrexate conjugated to gold nanoparticles inhibits tumor growth in a syngeneic lung tumor model. *Mol Pharm* 4: 713–22.

Coviello, T., Matricardi, P., Marianecci, C., and Alhaique, F. 2007. Polysaccharide hydrogels for modified release formulations. *J Controlled Release* 119: 5–24.

Dai, T., Tanaka, M., Huang Y.Y., and Hamblin, M. 2011.Chitosan preparations for wounds and burns: Antimicrobial and wound healing effects. *Expert Rev Anti Infect Ther* 9: 857–79.

Davies A., Jordanides N.E., Giannoudis A., Lucas C.M., Hatziieremia S., Harris R.J., Jørgensen H.G., Holyoake T.L., Pirmohamed M., Clark R.E. et al. 2009. Nilotinibconcentration in cell lines and primary CD34_ chronic myeloid leukemia cells is not mediated by active uptake or efflux by major drug trans-porters. *Leukemia* 23: 1999–2006.

Dang, J.M. and Leong, K.W. 2006. Natural polymers for gene delivery and tissue engineering. *Adv Drug Deliv Rev* 58: 487–99.

Dolenc, A., Govedarica, B., Dreu, R., et al. 2010. Nanosized particles of orlistat with enhanced in vitro dis-solution rate and lipase inhibition. *Int. J. Pharm* 396: 149–55.

Donnelly, R.F., Morrow, D.I., Mccarron, P.A., David Woolfson, A., Morrissey, A., Juzenas, P. et al. 2009. Microneedle arrays permit enhanced intradermal delivery of a preformed photosensitizer. *Photochem. Photobiol* 85: 195–204.

Düzgünes, N. and Gregoriadis, G. 2005. Introduction: The origins of liposomes: Alec bangham at babraham. In: D. Nejat (Ed.), *Methods in Enzymology*. New York: Academic Press.

Fabbro C., Ali B.H., Da R.T. et al. 2012. Targeting carbon nanotubes against cancer. *Chem Commun (Camb)* 48: 3911–26.

Flier, J.S. 2004. Obesity wars: molecular progress confronts an expanding epidemic. *Cell* 116: 337–50.

Greenway, F., Whitehouse, M.J., Guttadauria, M. et al. 2009. Rational design of a combination medication for the treatment of obesity. *Obesity (Silver Spring)* 1: 30–9.

Hillaireau, H. and Couvreur, P. 2009. Nanocarriers' entry into the cell: Relevance to drug delivery. *Cell Mol Life Sci* 66: 2873–96.

Hong, X., Wu, Z., Chen, L., Wu, F., Wei, L., and Yuan, W. 2014. Hydrogel microneedle arrays for transdermal drug delivery. *Nano-Micro Lett* 6: 191–9.

Hossen, M.N., Kajimoto, K., Akita, H., Hyodo, M., and Harashima, H. 2012. Vascular-targeted nanotherapy for obesity: Unexpected passive targeting mechanism to obese fat for the enhancement of active drug delivery. *J Controlled Release* 163: 101–10.

Hossen, M.N., Kajimoto, K., Akita, H., Hyodo, M., Ishitsuka, T., and Harashima, H. 2013. Therapeutic assess-ment of cytochrome c for the prevention of obesity through the endothelial cell-targeted nanoparticulate system. *Mol Ther* 21: 533–41.

Jain, A. Gupta, Y. and Jain, S.K. 2007. Perspectives of biodegradable natural polysaccharides for site specific drug delivery to the colon. *J Pharm Pharmaceut Sci* 10: 86–128.

James, W.P.T. 2008. The fundamental drivers of the obesity epidemic. *Obesity Rev* 9: 6–13.

Jian, F., Zhang, Y., Wang, J., Ba, K., Mao, R.Y., Lai, W.L. et al. 2012. Toxicity of biodegradable nanoscale preparations. *Curr Drug Metabol* 13: 440–6.

Jiang, C., Cano-Vega, M.A., Yue, F., et al. 2017. Loaded nanoparticles induce local browning of white adipose tissue to counteract obesity. *Mol Ther* 25(7):1718–29.

Jong, W.H.D. and Paul, J.A.B. 2008. Drug delivery and nanoparticles: Applications and hazards. *Int J Nanomedicine* 3 (2): 133–49.

Jung, T. Kamm, W. Breitenbach, A. Kaiserling, E. Xiao, J.X., and Kissel, T. 2000. Biodegradable nanopar-ticles for oral delivery of peptides: is there a role for polymers to affect mucosal uptake? *Eur J Pharm Biopharm* 50: 147–60.

Khan, N.T. 2017. Nanoparticles mediated drug delivery. *J Pharmacogenomics Pharmacoproteomics* 8: 172.

Klein, S., Fontan, L., Young, V.L. et al. 2004. Absence of an effect of liposuction on insulin action and risk factors for coronary heart disease. *N Engl J Med* 350 (25): 2549–57.

Kommareddy, S., Tiwari, S.B., and Amiji, M.M. 2005. Long-circulating polymeric nanovectors for tumor-selective gene delivery. *Technol Cancer Res Treat* 4: 615–25.

Kumar, M.N., Muzzarelli, R.A., Muzzarelli, C., Sashiwa, H., and Domb, A.J. 2004. Chitosan chemistry and pharmaceutical perspectives. *Chem Rev* 104: 6017–84.

Kumari, A., Yadav, S.K. and Yadav, S.C. 2010. Biodegradable polymeric nanoparticles based drug delivery systems. *Colloids Surf B Biointerfaces* 75: 1–18.

Lau, C.W.D., Douketis, D.J., Morrison, M.K., Hramiak, M.I., Sharma, M.A., and Ehud, Ur. 2007. 2006 Canadian clinical practice guidelines on the management and prevention of obesity in adults and children summary. *CMAJ* 176 (8): S1–13.

Liang, Ma., Tzu-Wen, L., Matthew, A.W., Iwona, T.D., Lawrence, W.D., Erik, R.N., Kelly, S.S., and Andrew, M.S. 2016. Efficient targeting of adipose tissue macrophages in obesity with polysaccharide nanocarriers. *ACS Nano* 10 (7): 6952–62.

Liu, Z., Jiao, Y., Wang, Y., Zhou, C., and Zhang, Z. 2008. Polysaccharides-based nanoparticles as drug delivery systems. *Adv Drug Delivery Rev* 60: 1650–62.

Liu, Z.H., Jiao, Y.P., Wang, Y.F., Zhou, C.R., and Zhang, Z.Y. 2008. Polysaccharides-based nanoparticles as drug delivery systems. *Adv Drug Deliv Rev* 60: 1650–62.

Maysinger, D., Kujawa, P., and Lovrić, J. 2010. Nanoparticles in medicine. In: A.V. Narlikar and Y.Y. Fu (Eds.), *Oxford Handbook of Nanoscience and Technology: Volume 3: Applications*. New York: Oxford University Press.

McClements, D.J., Decker, E.A., Park, Y., et al. 2009. Structural design principles for delivery of bioactive components in nutraceuticals and functional foods. *Crit Rev Food Sci Nutr* 49(6):577–606.

McClements D.J., Decker E.A., Weiss J et al. 2007. Emulsion-based delivery systems for lipophilic bioactive components. *J Food Sci* 72 (8): R109–24.

Mehnert, W. and Mader, K. 2001. Solid lipid nanoparticles: Production, characterization and applications. *Adv Drug Deliv Rev* 47: 165–96.

Mehvar, R. 2003. Recent trends in the use of polysaccharides for improved delivery of therapeutic agents: Pharmacokinetic and pharmacodynamic perspectives. *Curr Pharm Biotechnol* 4: 283–302.

Morris, G.A. 2010. Polysaccharide drug delivery systems based on pectin and chitosan. *Biotechnol Genet Eng Rev* 27: 257–83.

Mourya, V.K. and Inamdar, N.N. 2009. Trimethyl chitosan and its applications in drug delivery. *J Mater Sci Mater Med* 20: 1057–79.

Mueller, R.H., Maeder, K., and Gohla, S. 2000. Solid lipid nanoparticles (SLN) for controlled drug delivery—A review of the state of the art. *Eur J Pharm Biopharm* 50: 161–77.

Muller, R., Radtke, M., and Wissing, S. 2002. Nanostructured lipid matrices for improved microencapsulation of drugs. *Int J Pharm* 242: 121–8.

Muñoz, R. and Escalona, A. 2015. Chapter 51: Endoscopic duodenal-jejunal bypass sleeve treatment for obesity. In: S. Agrawal (Ed.), *Obesity, Bariatric and Metabolic Surgery: A Practical Guide*. Cham, Switzerland: Springer.

Olson, S.T., Srinivasan, K.R., Bjork, I., and Shore, J.D. 1981. Binding of high affinity heparin to antithrombin III. Stopped flow kinetic studies of the binding interaction. *J Biol Chem* 256: 11073–9.

Park, J.H., Saravanakumar, G., Kim, K., and Kwon, I.C. 2010. Targeted delivery of low molecular drugs using chitosan and its derivatives. *Adv Drug Delivery Rev* 62: 28–41.

Peppas, N.A. 2013. Historical perspective on advanced drug delivery: How engineering design and mathematical modeling helped the field mature. *Adv Drug Deliv Rev* 65: 5–9.

Perez, E. 2005. American pharmaceutical partners announces presentation of Abraxane survival data. In: 22nd annual Miami Breast Cancer Conference, Miami, FL.

Plodkowski, R.A., Nguyen, Q., Sundaram, U. et al. 2009. Bupropion and naltrexone: A review of their use individually and in combination for the treatment of obesity. *Expert Opin Pharmacother* 10 (6): 1069–81.

Podsiadlo P., Sinani V.A., Bahng J.H. et al. 2008. Gold nanoparticles enhance the anti-leukemia action of a 6-mercaptopurine chemotherapeutic agent. *Langmuir* 24: 568–74.

Pommier, A., Pons, M., and Kocienski, P. 1995. The first total synthesis of (-)-lipstatin. *J Org Chem* 60 (22): 7334–9.

Prego, C., Torres, D., Fernandez-Megia, E., Novoa-Carballal, R., Quinoa, E., and Alonso, M.J. 2006. Chitosan–PEG nanocapsules as new carriers for oral peptide delivery: Effect of chitosan pegylation degree. *J Controlled Release* 111 (3): 299–308.

Reddy, K., Mohan, G.K., Satla S., and Gaikwad S. 2011. Natural polysaccharides: Versatile excipients for controlled drug delivery systems. *J Pharm Sci* 6: 275–86.

Rocca, A., Mattoli, V., Mazzolai, B., and Ciofani, G. 2014. Cerium oxide nanoparticles inhibit adipogenesis in rat mesenchymal stem cells: Potential therapeutic implications. *Pharm Res* 31: 2952–62.

Rocca, A., Moscato, S., Ronca, F., Nitti, S., Mattoli, V., Giorgi, M. et al. 2015. Pilot in vivo investigation of cerium oxide nanoparticles as a novel anti-obesity pharmaceutical formulation. *Nanomed: Nanotechnol Biol Med* 11: 1725–34.

Rupnick, M.A., Panigrahy, D., Zhang, C.Y., Dallabrida, S.M., Lowell, B.B., Langer, R. et al. 2002. Adipose tissue mass can be regulated through the vasculature. *Proc Natl Acad Sci India* 99: 10730–5.

Saravanakumar, G. Jo, D.G., and Park, J.H. 2012. Polysaccharide based nanoparticles: A versatile platform for drug delivery and biomedical imaging. *Curr Med Chem* 19 (19): 3212–29.

Sauer, N., Reining, F., Schulze Zur Wiesch, C., Burkhardt, T., and Aberle, J. 2015. Off-label antiobesity treatment in patients without diabetes with GLP-1 agonists in clinical practice. *Horm Metab Res* 47 (8): 560–4.

Severino, P., Moraes, L.F., Zanchetta, B. et al. 2012. Elastic liposomes containing benzophenone-3 for sun protection factor enhancement. *Pharm Dev Technol* 17: 661–5.

Shi, J., Votruba, A.R., Farokhzad, O.C., and Langer, R. 2010. Nanotechnology in drug delivery and tissue engineering: From discovery to applications. *Nano Lett* 10: 3223–30.

Shukla, A.P., Kumar, R.B., and Aronne, L.J. 2015. Lorcaserin HCl for the treatment of obesity. *Expert Opin. Pharmacother* 16 (16): 2531–8.

Shukla, R.K. and Tiwari, A. 2012. Carbohydrate polymers: Applications and recent advances in delivering drugs to the colon. *Carbohydr Polym* 88: 399–416.

Sionkowska, A. 2011. Current research on the blends of natural and synthetic polymers as new biomaterials: Review. *Prog Polym Sci* 36: 1254–76.

Sjöström, L., Narbro, K., Sjöström, C.D. et al. 2007. Effects of bariatric surgery on mortality in Swedish obese subjects. *N Engl J Med* 357 (8): 741–52.

Smith, B. M., Smith, J. M., Tsai, J. H., et al. 2005. Discovery and SAR of new benzazepines as potent and selective 5-HT2C receptor agonists for the treatment of obesity. *Bioorg Med Chem Lett* 15 (5): 1467–70.

Souto, E.B., Fangueiro, J.F., and Muller, R.H. 2013. Solid lipid nanoparticles (SLNt). In: I.F. Uchegbu, A.G. Schatzlein, W.P. Cheng, and A. Lalatsa (Eds.), *Fundamentals of pharmaceutical nanoscience*. New York: Springer.

Souto, E.B., Severino, P., and Santana, M.H.A. 2012. Preparacao de nanopartículas polimericas a partir da polimerizacao de monomeros-parte I. *Polimeros* 22: 96–100.

Souto, E.B., Teeranachaideekul, V., Boonme, P. et al. 2011. Lipid-based nanocarriers for cutaneous administration of pharmaceutics. *Encyclopedia Nanosci Nanotechnol* 15: 479–91.

Spreitzer, H. 2010. Lorcaserin. *Austrian Pharmacist Newspaper.* 64 (19): 1083.

Sullivan, S. 2015. Endoscopic treatment of obesity. In: S.S. Jonnalagadda (Ed.), *Gastrointestinal Endoscopy: New Technologies and Changing Paradigms*, 61–82. New York: Springer.

Thomsen, W.J., Grottick, A.J., Menzaghi, F. et al. 2008. Lorcaserin, a novel selective human 5-Hydroxytryptamine2C agonist: In vitro and in vivo pharmacological characterization. *J Pharmacol Exp Ther* 325 (2): 577–87.

Tice, J.A., Karliner, L., Walsh, J. et al. 2008. Gastric banding or bypass? A systematic review comparing the two most popular bariatric procedures. *Am J Med* 121 (10): 885–93.

Tuan-Mahmood, T.M., Mccrudden, M.T., Torrisi, B.M. et al. 2013. Microneedles for intradermal and transdermal drug delivery. *Eur J Pharm Sci* 50: 623–37.

Van Vlerken, L.E. and Amiji, M.M. 2006. Multi-functional polymeric nanoparticles for tumour-targeted drug delivery. *Expert Opin Drug Deliv* 3 (2): 05–216.

Wissing, S., Kayser, O., and Muller, R. 2004. Solid lipid nanoparticles for parenteral drug delivery. *Adv Drug Deliv Rev* 56: 1257–72.

Young, E. 2008. The anti-inflammatory effects of heparin and related compounds. *Thromb Res* 122: 743–52.

Zhang, H.L., Zhong, X.B., Tao, Y., Wu, S.H., and Su, Z.Q. 2012. Effects of chitosan and water-soluble chitosan micro-and nanoparticles in obese rats fed a high-fat diet. *Int J Nanomed* 7: 4069.

Zhang, L., Pan, J., Dong, S. et al. 2017. The application of polysaccharide-based nanogels in peptides/proteins and anticancer drugs delivery. *J Drug Target* (8): 673–84.

Zhang, N. 2013. Polysaccharide-based nanocarriers for improved drug delivery. Dissertations - ALL. Paper 40.

Zhang, Y., Proenca, R., Maffei, M. et al. 1994. Positional cloning of the mouse obese gene and its human homologue. *Nature (Research Support)* 372 (6505): 425–32.

Index

T - #0172 - 111024 - C382 - 254/178/18 - PB - 9780367571016 - Gloss Lamination